Notes on ICU Nursing

Critical Care FAQ Files From the MICU

Second Edition

Mark Hammerschmidt, RN

Editor: Jayne Mulholland, RN, CEN, CCRN

Jayne: this book, and everything else, as always, is for you.

Edit Date 10/2007

<u>Please make sure to read the disclaimer at the beginning of this book!</u>

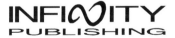
INFINITY PUBLISHING

ISBN 978-0-7414-1705-3

Published by:

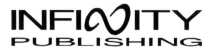

INFINITY PUBLISHING
1094 New DeHaven Street, Suite 100
West Conshohocken, PA 19428-2713
Info@buybooksontheweb.com
www.buybooksontheweb.com
Toll-free (877) BUY BOOK
Local Phone (610) 941-9999
Fax (610) 941-9959

Printed in the United States of America
Published July 2007

Please Read This Disclaimer!

This book is a little different: it is not meant to be an authoritative reference text. In fact, it's sort of the opposite – pretty much straight from the bedside, it's a collection of opinions, experiences and impressions that the author and the editor have gained as RNs, with about 40 years of ICU experience between them. Mark is a seriously burnt night nurse, working in the MICU of one of the big teaching hospitals in Massachusetts, and Jayne is now the boss of the cardiac labs at another one: cath, EP, stress, and so on. Currently our licensure is as diploma grads (Mark has a BA in something else, and Jayne is in diploma-to-MSN school. "Gradual School"). Someone asked us a while back: "What's your source material?", to which we answered: "Well, we made 'em up as we went along!"

For better or worse, the articles here were written from the standpoint of a preceptor: "from the shop floor." Both of us have put in our time "in the trenches", ankle-deep sometimes in the you-know-what, plus that other stuff, and those lumpy things that float around in it, too. (Jayne has to take off her white coat first.) We're not academics in any way.

The result is that these articles reflect our experiences and points of view, and not our professions' as a whole. **Please remember that everything you read in them has not been impartially peer-reviewed.** Our peers like them – does that count? We hope you find them useful too, but please: **always check with your local authorities and references!**

These articles were originally posted on our website at www.icufaqs.org – leave us a note there, or an email, send us error corrections when you find them (we'll happily give you credit if you like), and let us know what you think. Thanks!

Thanks to:

Jayne – you are the most patient of editors, best of friends, and still the world to me…

Ruth, Ben and Ray – you too.

Coworkers: over the years you have been really good about putting up with me as I have bugged you: about reading rough copies, filling in gaps, and providing endless encouragement. You are the best - you do it all, happy or complaining, sad, excited, bored, tired, frustrated, but always there, always holding the highest standard. Thank you all so much. A few names, purely at random… Fletch. Gloria. Jacqueline. Terry. Jessica. Oldest of sisters, best of friends. Younger sisters: the Katies. The Amandas. AnnMarie, Kerin. The Keris. Caitlyn. Adele, the boss. Lillian. Rabih – always a brother.

A really special thanks to Dr.Cristina Hendrix, DNS, FNP, Professor of Nursing at Duke University, who appeared one day out of the ether with an amazing invitation, and who has continued to do unexpected and astonishing things in support of this project.

To the email correspondents: I think that the responses you all have sent in have been the most affecting aspect of the whole project. We always worried - we still do - that we were way out in some weird area of left field, muttering to ourselves, writing things down, with somebody making sure we didn't hurt ourselves... instead, we seem to have struck something really responsive in our profession. We're not sure exactly what it is, but we hope to keep going. Thanks so much.

A word about images, copyrights, and our responsibilities: A note about the images in this book: there are quite a few of them! Some are from scans that we made ourselves, some are from websites, some from correspondents. In <u>every case</u> we have gone back and tried to locate the sources they came from, and requested permission for their use. Images with web addresses underneath are used by permission. Some of the websites have disappeared or gone down, but we were very careful in every case. If we have violated a copyright requirement despite our "due diligence", please let us know, and we'll fix the problem immediately. Our sincere thanks go to all our sources!

The First Question: What is a FAQ?

A FAQ (people pronounce it as "fak") is a list of Frequently Asked Questions on any given topic. The usual plan is to list the questions in some kind of meaningful order up front, and then the person who wants the answer to any particular question or group of questions just has to look in the document for the answer with the same number.

<u>Contents:</u>

A note on the images:

There are a lot of photos and diagrams in this book – many more than the first time around. Many of them were found from websites, many we made ourselves, strips we printed out, and so on. Of the images we got online, we have tried to contact the site owners in every single case for permission to use them. Some of the sites have disappeared since we found the images for the original articles. We feel that we have really been diligent about requesting permissions in every case. If by some error we've violated a copyright, please let us know immediately, and we'll fix the problem right away. Thanks!

A couple of comments on the second edition:

How time has flown! Four years since the first edition, and in something like six years since the website went up, the articles have all been substantially updated and revised – lots of new images… a lot of work, and an enormous reward of satisfaction. We've gotten emails from students, nurses, physicians, EMTs, paramedics, medical students, medical transcriptionists, social workers…

Some emails stand out in memory. This one came not long after Hurricane Katrina:

Hi, Mark!

I am a nurse educator at Medical Center of Louisiana (Charity Hospital) in New Orleans.

I have come across your icufaqs, and they are really neat. Our services are slowly returning, and we have many nurses who will be coming back and needing refreshers/instruction on many of the topics covered in your icufaqs. Our educational resources are EXTREMELY limited right now, and we were hoping we could reproduce and use these materials as information that our staff would find helpful.

Another request is that we would like to consider placing links to your site from our intranet.

Please let me know your thoughts. This would be so helpful. We have limited resources, as I am sure you are aware, and this would be an excellent support for our staff.

Thanks!
Ecoee Rooney, RN, MSN
Inservice Instructor
Education/Staff Development
Medical Center of Louisiana at New Orleans

We framed that one…

Starting Out: A New RN In the MICU

1- What kinds of patients come into the MICU?

2- How do families interact with the MICU staff?

3- Who are the nursing staff in the MICU?

    3-1- Who are the resource nurses?
    3-2- Who is the nurse manager of the MICU?
    3-3- Who is the Clinical Nurse Specialist?
    3-4- How are the assignments made?
    3-5- Who are the CCTs?
    3-6- Who are the OAs?
    3-7- Who are the USAs?

4- Who are the doctors in the MICU?

    4-1- How are the physican teams organized?

5- What does Respiratory Therapy do in the MICU?

6- Who are the other staff in the unit?

7- What are the routines that we use in the MICU?

    7-1- How do I manage my time during my shift?
    7-2- How do I use the flow sheet to organize my time?
    7-3- How should I give report?
    7-4: What is "routine prophylaxis"?

8- What do I need to know about the monitors?

    8-1- Should I believe everything the monitors tell me?
    8-2- What can the monitor do?
    8-3- How does the information get from the patient into the monitor?
    8-4- How should I react to the alarms?

9- What are the different pumps used for in the unit?

    9-1- What are microinfusion pumps?

10- What are all the lines going into these patients?

    10-1- How does the line connect the patient to the monitor?
    10-2- What are the inflated white bags for, that hang on the poles in the rooms?
    10-3- Why do they use that stiff tubing for the transducers?

To start with…

In thinking about how to organize this FAQ, it certainly seemed that there was a whole lot of material to cover – where would you start? Obviously from somewhere… a little later, we realized that a good way to put things together would be to describe them in the same way that we give shift report – in the same way that we try to cover all the bases when we do that, starting with age, gender, history, where admitted from, and then a system-by-system review of the patient, ending up hopefully with a coherent picture of the current situation. So we thought this might be a useful way to break up a description of the ICU: into manageable chunks that, while they could be described separately, should add up to a whole system for treating whatever comes in the door. Let us know what you think! Please remember that this material is in no way 'official' – it is meant to represent information as it would be passed from a preceptor to a new ICU nurse. As usual, mistakes – and there will be plenty of them – are ours. Please let us know when you find them, and we'll work the answers in and update the file. Thanks!

To start with – here's a scenario that we remember all too well. It was a little extreme, but it's a true story, and it helps illustrate a lot of what makes working in the ICU so different: (lots of the details have been changed to protect identities).

A patient comes in as a transfer from another hospital. He'd been brought down from somewhere in New Hampshire, where he'd been eating home-cured meats and apparently drinking home-made liquor. He'd gotten a stomach ache, so he took "a handful" of aspirin. When this didn't help, he apparently repeated the dose. Probably a bad idea - he developed an enormous lower GI bleed, became hypotensive, and by the time he finally got to us, he'd infarcted much of his bowel, knocked off his kidneys, gone into shock liver, and when I first saw him he was postop, having had a large segment of his bowel removed. He'd required so much fluid peri-operatively that the surgeons had been unable to close him – instead, his abdominal wound was open, covered with a clear, adherent OR drape, and he had normal saline infusing into the wound continuously from several IV pumps for irrigation. The wound was being drained by several salem sumps laid into and across the incision. He was in ARDS, so he was vented, sedated, and chemically paralyzed. He was extremely septic, hypotensive, and he was on at least two pressors. He was on TPN. To correct his renal failure he'd been started on CVVH (bedside dialysis). I'll put each part of the report that I might give in quotes, and I'll try putting the topic being discussed into some kind of dialogue: "Holy cow, this guy is in tough shape."

1- What kinds of patients come into the ICU?

"This is Chuck M. Chuck is a 38-year-old gentleman who came in yesterday from an outside hospital, where he ingested too much aspirin after apparently eating and drinking home-cured meat and whiskey…"

Patients come into the MICU from a variety of places: the floors, the ER, as transfers from other hospitals, as postops, as boarders from other services, and sometimes as "direct admits", bypassing the ER. The interesting thing about the MICU is that we literally see a bit of absolutely everything, unlike the specialty ICUs. If you work here long enough, you'll see patients that would normally be in every other ICU environment (except maybe fresh postop cardiothoracic patients – that ICU will bump more stable patients out to make room). We see cardiac patients, sometimes with intra-aortic balloon pumps; we see neuro patients, occasionally with monitored bolts in place, we've done adult ECMO a few times, and we even sometimes get general-surg postop cases when there is no room in the SICU , including the occasional fresh liver transplant.

2- How do families interact with the ICU?

"Chuck has a girlfriend here who's been in and out a few times – I'm not sure what the relationship is, and I'm not sure who could sign for consent on his procedures, so would you speak to her and figure that out? Then maybe we can help her find a place to stay nearby. We may need to do some teaching with her because she gets very upset when she's been in the room for a more than a few minutes…"

There's been a lot of discussion and planning over the years about the ways that we can involve patients' families in the MICU. At this point we have no fixed visiting hours, but access to the patients is strictly at the discretion of the nurses. The emphasis is on allowing access for families at any time of day, but our first responsibility is the direct care of the patient. The family may be advised to remain in the waiting areas until the patient can be visited. We try to keep the number of visitors to two at a time, to prevent crowding in the room. As well, usually we try to identify a family member who will be willing to act as family "spokesperson" – all questions and answers to be relayed to other family members through that person, so the nurses don't have to spend a lot of time explaining things to many sets of visitors. This goes for phone calls too – you can refer callers to the spokesperson.

3- Who are the nursing staff in the ICU?

"I took report from Susie. You know, I am so totally intimidated by her, because she's been here so long? I mean, she's really nice, but I don't know, I just feel so stupid around her..."

The MICU nurses have a wide range of experience, ranging anywhere from three months to upwards of twenty years. (You can tell who those are right away.) I've been working in this unit since 1986, and I realized around my last birthday that I've spent a third of my whole life working with some of these people. We have nurses with diplomas (I'm one of them), but most of us have finished BSNs. Some of us are, or have been CCRNs, and some of us have special areas of expertise – CVVH, or balloon pumping, or leadership, or skin care, or IV insertion – learn who these people are and make use of them!

3-1- Who are the resource nurses?

Shift-to-shift leadership is provided by the resource nurses, who carry no patients, for the very good reason that the whole ICU is their assignment.. They make out staff assignments, and arrange for admissions and discharges with the supervisors and the house officers. They are also there to be your "resource" for any situation or question you may have. Use this resource any time you think you need to. **Always** run any question you may have by your resource nurse. At the same time, try to be merciful, and remember that they are keeping a lot of balls in the air at once!

3-2- Who is the nurse manager of the MICU?

Our nurse manager is a master's prepared RN, with many years of experience in a variety of leadership settings. She had already been a head nurse in our hospital, some years back, before becoming a nursing supervisor.

An important point to remember about our nurse manager: like the rest of us, she is doing a job that requires keeping a very large number of balls in the air at the same time. Most of us senior nurses shake our heads in wonder sometimes, as we watch the nurse manager field staffing crises, unusual clinical situations, and that most difficult of managerial problems – staff politics. The boss has an extremely complex job, and unlike the rest of us, she is "on" 24/ 7. I have been impressed over the years with her consistent willingness to face tough problems and see them through.

Another point: the role of the nurse manager in the MICU is clinically "hands-off". The management model tries to shift most of the clinical management responsibility issues to the clinical nurse specialist. So it's been a while since the boss wore scrubs. You will find however that she is very up-to-date in her clinical knowledge, and that she works very hard to keep it that way.

3-3- Who is the clinical nurse specialist?

The role of the clinical nurse specialist basically centers around clinical staff support. This is the person to go to when you have a clinical question, a question about a medical issue, about a nursing issue, about procedures, equipment, policies – anything that has to do with immediate bedside care.

Our clinical nurse specialist joined us a year and a half ago. She has a very broad background of ICU experience, including many years in surgical intensive care, and previous experience as a CNS in another hospital. (You mean there are (gasp) – "other" hospitals?) A tradition of our institution is that other hospitals are always referred to in chart notes as "OSH"s – "outside hospitals": "Yeah, well, that MRI was done at the outside hospital, so, you know, they're goIng to have to do it again here to make the staff happy." Or: "I just do not understand what in the world they thought they were doing with this patient at that outside hospital. I mean, 30 centimeters of PEEP? For two days? And they were surprised when the patient started popping pneumos? What the heck…?"

For all the complaining that you'll hear us do, we are very proud of where we work. We would never allow ourselves to be treated anywhere else in the world. Not in our own ICU however – and it has come up! We go into the CCU… I guess I can put in an unusual anecdote here: a year or so ago, one of our really prominent staff physicians flew over to Europe to assess one of the most powerful people in the world. He brought the person back – very nice person – on a private jet. What ICU, of all the ICUs in the world, did this patient choose to be treated in? And you know, we took care of him meticulously, just like the street person in the next room! We are very good at what we do…

3-4- How are the assignments made?

Assignments are made with lots of considerations in mind: we try to give primary/associate nurses their own patients first, and we try to keep the same nurses assigned to the same patients every day if possible. This may vary if, for example, the patient goes on CVVH and their primary can't run it. We try to make really acute patients one-to-one, but since this closes a bed, we watch these situations closely to see if things have improved enough to allow for the patient to be doubled later on. Most assignments are doubles, and we try to work in all the issues: primary/associate relationships, acuity, distance between rooms, skills of the RNs available, etc. Very rarely a nurse will get a triple assignment – usually this means that one of the patients is about to be discharged to the floor. Once a year, maybe, a patient will be two-to-one: this actually happened recently, with a patient who required upwards of 200 (true story!) blood components during the course of a day before going to the OR.

3-5- Who are the CCTs?

We have a number of critical care techs in the unit. Generally these people tend to be made of solid gold. They are available to help you in a number of ways: baths/bed changes, blood draws from A-lines or peripheral sticks (including blood cultures), room setups for admissions, line setups for transduced lines, foley insertion, trach care, chest tube dressings, EKGs, "road trips", and general feats of strength. They check all emergency equipment: transport boxes, intubation boxes, pacer boxes, travel equipment, MRI kits, EKG machines, defibrillators, and Zolls. They can't do some things, and you should never ask them to: for example to touch, run or silence any of the infusion pumps. They are not allowed to touch IV's, but they can DC them, and they can DC unsutured A-lines. They are not allowed to tracheally suction patients. They are allowed to silence a room alarm only if an RN tells them to, and is present in the room.

3-6- Who are the OAs?

We also have a group of Operational Associates in the unit, headed up by an Operational Coordinator: these are the people who sit behind the front desk. They make the unit run; they get us what we need: equipment, paperwork, blood products; they transcribe our orders for us; they field our questions and problems of every description; they contact personnel all over the house for us; they speak to patients' families for us, and they follow up to make sure things were done right. Be merciful with the OAs – they also keep many balls in the air at once.

3-7- Who are the USAs?

USAs on the unit are the people who take care of the unit's physical environment. Some of them have been in their positions longer than any nurse in this unit. They have a tough, detail-oriented job. Notice sometimes how clean this unit is.

4- Who are the doctors in the ICU?

"The junior on tonight is Ralph – you remember him from last year? The red intern is Marcia, and the blue intern is Helmut, who I think is from Germany. The fellow was in talking to them about an hour ago, but they've been lining up another patient, so I don't know if they changed plans on this man or not. Howie is the visit, and I think he's actually here, so we can ask him what the latest plan is...I really hope they don't want another MRI."

4-1- How are the physician teams organized?

Ours is a teaching hospital, and so the doctors are organized into teams with a senior resident as the boss, junior residents under them, interns at the bottom, often with med students attached. We actually have two senior residents leading two teams in the unit at a time, changing every first of the month. The unit as a whole is supervised by a medical director and an assistant director, both pulmonary/intensivist attendings from the in-house group, who are also called 'visits'. These people take monthly turns leading rounds, so you'll hear people say "Who's the visit this month?". There are also pulmonary/critical-care fellows attached to the unit. They are available for questions that the team may have during the day, and they're pageable for problems at night. Fellows place PA lines for the team – sometimes they'll come in just for that purpose during the night, and they'll help figure out complicated management strategies.

The two resident teams in our unit are called 'red' and 'blue' – both teams are present in full force during the day, so the floor gets pretty crowded. At night, the teams alternate putting a junior in charge of the whole unit, along with an intern from each team who split the patients between them. There is a senior resident 'covering the house' available to support them if they need it, and there's a second, or 'backup' senior to help out as well. (As an ancient night nurse, you'll notice that I make lots of references to the night shift in these articles - this is because the night shift is where all the real nursing in the unit goes on. Hey – just telling it like it is! Day-shift nurses may say that their shift rules – don't listen.)

The consult services are still available at night – the anesthesia resident is available (and has to be called) for emergency intubations; sometimes we will call the renal fellow for questions about CVVH management at night, sometimes we talk to cardiology. The other night a urology resident was paged to deal with a foley problem involving hematuria – the point is, there's someone in the house available to deal with every kind of problem. These specialty services exist for a reason - you need to see that your patient gets proper care...

5- What does Respiratory Therapy do in the ICU?

"So, let's see, Chuck seems to be going into ARDS, and they were having a lot of trouble ventilating him, so we paralyzed him – Joanne is on for respiratory, and she's been giving a lot of good advice about the vent settings, so check in with her when you need to..."

Obviously, a large number of our patients have trouble breathing. There are all sorts of technologies and strategies available to help them, and it's important to remember that respiratory therapists are not people who "just make vent changes." These are the people with the specialty training to help the whole team make judgments about pulmonary management. If you think your patient is in trouble, the respiratory therapist is there to help you and the medical team figure out what to do. Use their expertise to help your patient.

Specific things you may find an RRT doing for your patient: setting up a vent, making recommendations about vent management, giving inhaled meds through the vent circuit (make sure that they know your patient has been ordered for these, and get them to sign off on the med sheets), setting up alternate vent systems like face-mask ventilation, mask CPAP or mask bi-pap, high-flow O2 setups, nitric oxide treatment systems, heliox treatment systems - and if you're lucky, you'll get to watch them running an ECMO system.

Here's your part in this: make sure that there are clear lines of communication from the team to respiratory and to nursing. Changes in vent settings, or in vent modes must be entered into the computers as orders. You can certainly get the team to write orders that give you some leeway – such as "Wean FiO2 to keep O2 saturation greater or equal to 95%" – absolutely okay. But don't let things happen without making sure that decisions are being made properly, and documented properly.

6- Who are the other staff in the ICU?

"I hate working days. I mean, I know some of the staff love days, but there are so many people around..."

Other specialty services are available in the ICU – pharmacy is available for questions 24/ 7. Social service is always available, and frequently help us with family and patient issues. Nutrition rounds on patients and makes recommendations for appropriate treatment. Physical therapy, chest PT, OT people all get involved.

It's complicated. But the part that I like is the fact that all of these systems, pointed like beams of light on your patient, are focused through the nurse at the bedside. You are the one who controls the flow of everything into and out of your patient.

Realize that you have entered a new world, which in complexity is right up there with "nuclear submarine", and take the time (it takes years) to learn how to apply all these tools of your trade. Be patient with yourself.

7- What are the routines of the ICU?

"Give me a second while I write these signs down from this paper towel - I get totally lost if I don't get it down on the flow sheet right away, because then I forget what happened and when. See, here is where he got acidotic, and then we started a bicarb drip, and see, when his pH got better, we were able to wean his pressors - a little, anyway…"

7-1- What are the routines of the ICU?

Time is carefully structured in the ICU – obviously we use routines to help us organize our activities, so that we can tell which ways the patients are going. A lot of this has to do with recording information: flow sheets, med sheets, intake and output totals, lab results…

These routines form another part of your set of tools: learn to use the numbers on the sheets as indicators of trends: "Wow - look at how his heart rate has gone up during the day. I mean, look, yesterday, all day, his heart rate was in the 80s, and since he spiked, it's been in the 100's, and now he's about three days in the hospital, and how long ago did they say was his last drink? You think he might be withdrawing? Or is his rate up because he's hot? Or both?" Or: "Wow - look, as his temp came down he came right off the Levo, and his heart rate is down, and his pO2 came up. So maybe his pneumonia and sepsis are getting better, and we can think about extubating him soon?" Or: "Look, his crit has been dropping over the past two days, and he's been TBB positive about 2 liters every day, so do you think he's actually losing blood somewhere, or is he just getting diluted?"

7-2- How do I use the flow sheet to organize my time?

The hourly vital sign check is only the baseline for recording patient info – with any change in condition, you need to start recording more frequently. The idea is that if the patient does something, and you have to make a change in treatment as a result, like changing a pressor rate, or a CZI drip, - then you have to clearly document what they did, what you did to respond, and how they responded to what you did. Sometimes you have to record vital signs every five minutes until a patient stabilizes. Sometimes you can't even get to the flow sheets because your hands are moving too quickly: hanging blood, maybe two or three units at once, changing fluid and pressor rates, suctioning, bagging – I've written signs on the sheets, on my scrubs – and then transcribed them a little later. (Better yet, get somebody to help you out.)

Other routines in the ICU are just baseline too – daily x-rays happen in the morning for example, but they can be ordered anytime necessary – did your patient suddenly become hypoxic? Rounds happen in the morning – but if a patient becomes critical in the middle of rounds, things may have to get flexible for a while. But the routines form the structure of all the number crunching that is so important to figuring out which ways the patients are going.

An important word about routines – nurses can often get compulsive in the ICU. (They say that somewhere in the world, there is a perfect job for every mild kind of craziness.) This is actually a very useful personality trait to have in the unit. Unless something critical is happening, I always enter a room at the beginning of a shift and follow my routine: look at the patient. Then the monitor. Then the vent. Then the drips.Then I zero the lines. Then I adjust the alarm limits. **(Always check your alarm limits!)** Then I check when the last set of labs went out – do they need rechecking now? Then meds. Then TBB. Always the same routine, like clockwork. This way, I don't have to ask myself later – did I zero the lines? Have my patient's alarms not been showing his heart rate of 24, while I was bathing my other patient, because I forgot to check the limits? I know that I have those bases covered, because I rely on the fact that I keep to a routine.

At the same time, sometimes routines have to go out the window. You may find yourself writing down signs every five minutes, or every two hours if a stable patient has been made a "floor-boarder", or you may be calling them out to another nurse recording during a code while you do compressions. Remember that the routines are a set of tools - make them work for you.

I always ask preceptees: what is your goal for this shift? Always keeping in mind: "What's wrong with this patient?" – this will be your guiding idea among the forest of all the new equipment, procedures, meds, labs, etc. Priority setting should help you figure out what you need to be doing, and in what order. As an example, a GI bleed – do you want to spend a lot of time doing a head-to-toe assessment at first, or do you want to make sure that the pressure is up, the heart rate is okay, the airway isn't threatened, and that you know when and what the last CBC was? You should be able to assess all that within about 20 seconds, standing in the doorway at the beginning of the shift. You can, and should learn to do your detailed assessment as you work your way through the first hour or two of the shift – what you observe will make more sense to you as you get a feel for which way the patient is going.

Take time to do the basics: get the vitals written down every hour. Get the meds in on time. Make sure the TBB gets done. Send the routine labs on time, and extras when needed. Document changes in the patient's condition on the flow sheet promptly, so that changes you make in treatment are clearly linked to what the patient is doing.

A few more words about the basic routines: TBB's (Total Body Balance – also called I and O totals), are calculated every six hours, and tallied up at midnight. Daily labs should be sent about 4-5am, although other labs obviously get sent whenever they need to. Orders are reviewed at rounds, but can be updated at any time. Remember to check the computer at least every hour or so to check – if the doctors have given you verbal orders, repeat them back to the doctor, and insist that they get written into the computer the way they were told to you. I keep a sheet in the front pocket of the flow book for to help me keep track – I can't hold too many things in my head anymore, and the more I write down, the better I can find the information when I need it.

Remember: verbals are really discouraged. Policy is: orders must be in the computer before they are acted on.

The last piece of routine that needs describing is the shift report. The goal is simple, but report needs to be more than just reading off the numbers – you need to communicate two basic things: what's wrong with this person, and what are we doing to fix it? For example, I might start report: "Uh, this is a 27 year old man who went down in a nightclub, and was intubated at the scene by the paramedics. They think he aspirated his stomach contents, and now he's on the vent with lousy blood gases. He had a tox screen that was positive for ETOH of 2300, benzos, and colace." (Creative!)

So there's the overall picture. Then go on to the detailed numbers: temp is this, heart rate is that, gave Tylenol and heart rate came down to this, temp came down to that, pressure has been so-and-so, weaned the Neo to this --- you get the idea. Try to see the forest and not all those trees – again, to do that, keep in your mind the idea: what is wrong with this patient, and how are we applying the tools of the unit to make her better? That will guide your report. Use a routine, (some people "start with neuro and work their way downwards" – brain, then lungs and heart, then GI, then kidneys) and try to do it the same way every time – cover the bases, system by system, the meds, the labs, the TBB, always thinking of the big picture. Airline pilots land a plane by going through a checklist, every flight, every time – so they never forget to put the wheels down. A routine method for report will help you the same way.

7-3- How should I give report?

Your report should always center around the single idea: "What's wrong with this patient?" People get so lost, "Well, she has a PA line, and she's vented, and she spiked, and we had to shock her, and she's on dobut, and…" – all correct! But what's the BASIC problem? Is she having a huge MI? And now has line sepsis? Start with the essence of the problem, and move outwards from that.

There's – finally! – been some serious discussion about making reports systematic, like the checklists that pilots use – every single time – before every takeoff, every landing. "Hey Chuck! The wheels down? Oh DAMMIT…"

Y'know? I happen to think this is a great idea. Start with name, age, allergies, quick history, then a quick – just a word: "pneumonia sepsis". Make sense? Then go on to all the systems and details and whatnot. "He got run over by a truck." Simple.

7-4: What is "routine prophylaxis"?

Every patient that gets stuck in a bed is probably going to develop problems alongside what's "officially" wrong with them – and certain routine treatments are usually applied to prevent them . For example, huge numbers of these people will develop DVT's and… what? – if they're not prevented? So: subcutaneous heparin, or fragmin, or lovenox for almost all of them. And air boots.

A lot of them will develop spontaneous gastric stress irritation. So - ranitidine. Protonix maybe.

Then it turns out that bunches of "ventilator-associated pneumonias" can be prevented by simply sitting intubated patients up at least 30 degrees at all times. Prevents reflux aspirations. Also oral chlorhexidine, twice a day.

Decubitus ulcer prevention: we turn the patients every couple of hours, and use fancy beds with mobile surfaces. Some of the younger nurses have never seen deep ulcers the size of their fist… or maybe both fists…

These routine practices prevent a LOT of problems. Make sure they're in place.

8- What do I need to know about the monitors?

"I know the patient is sick when every channel on the monitor has something on it."

8-1- Should I believe everything the monitor tells me?

The monitors are your second major bedside assessment tool – the first is your eyes. Always <u>look</u> at the patient first – the monitor may be crisis-alarming for VT, or asystole – but is the patient smiling, waving at you? The 02 sat may say 30% - is the patient pink, and eating dinner? Things like that. Remember that <u>the monitor has no brain</u>. (Sometimes it seems like the doctors…never mind.)

8-2- What can the monitor do?

The monitor has a screen that is divided into sections – each section looks at a different part of the patient. The monitor can see a number of different things: EKG (we usually have the monitor display lead II and V1 at the same time), pressures of different kinds, O2 saturation… the monitor can count respirations (not always very well), and can monitor the heart rate off an arterial line or a sat probe. It can be set to beep with heartbeats, or not to – it's a very useful tool. But use your eyes first.

8-3- How does information get from the patient into the monitor?

There are a lot of cables coming out of the monitor – the first, which fits in the green slot on the left side of the 'brick' is the EKG cable, which goes to five (or more) chest electrodes on the patient. The cables with red plugs go into the next three slots, and they are for monitoring pressures through transducers: arterial lines, CVPs, PA lines, etc. The brown slot is for a cardiac output cable, that you use with a PA line. The last slot on the right is black, and is where the noninvasive BP cuff plugs in. Below the row of cables is a blue socket, which is where the O2 sat probe goes.

The monitor has software built into it that is supposed to recognize arrhythmias – and there are different levels of alarms, from 'warning' to 'crisis', that tell you if your patient has done something to alert the software. Often the crisis alarm will go off, which is triggered if the monitor thinks it's seen asystole, VF, or a run of VT. Do <u>not</u> get into the habit of ignoring the alarms just because the first four ones were from "motion artifact": the patient shaking the wires, or scratching herself, because the next one may be real. (Actually, the law of hospital karma says that if you ever ignore an alarm, it probably <u>will</u> be real. This is the same kind of thing as looking around and saying "Jeez, it's quiet tonight" – almost a criminal act.)

8-4- How should I react to the alarms?

Alarm awareness is very important in the ICU. Try to remember that if you hear an alarm of any kind go off, <u>no matter whose patient it is</u>, you need to start thinking about what it means. Learn what the different alarm sounds are. Try to be aware that you may be tuning things out, especially if you are focusing really hard on your own patient. If you hear a 3M pump go off – is that the flush line for someone's pressors? If you hear a minipump – is that the pressor itself? Are the main arrhythmia alarms going off in the hallways?

You have to respond. You are not allowed to ignore any alarm, at any time. You can certainly ask the nurse assigned to the room if she needs help, and she can tell you that she'll get the pump in a minute, that it's her potassium dose finishing up. But don't let alarms go un-answered.

At the same time, remember that it does take time to learn what the noises mean and how to prioritize them in your head. But what you want to avoid is some situation like this (I make these up to sound particularly awful): alarms go off, and for whatever reason no one responds right away, the patient extubates himself, climbs out of the bed, pulls out his CVP, and is found bleeding from the site. It is a critical part of your ICU skills that you learn to respond to alarms appropriately, every shift, every time.

A couple more words about the monitors – learn to find your patient on the central monitor screen in the hallways. Learn to reset the alarms using the mouse at the central screen. Learn to change the paper in the printers, and respond to the low-level alarm that reminds you if they're empty. Lastly, biomedical engineering is always available if the monitors give you serious trouble.

9- What are the different pumps used for in the unit?

"Bill says that it's sort of a bad sign when there are more than six drips running…anyhow, Chuck is on nimbex at 6 for paralysis, and fentanyl at 600 mikes an hour, which is holding him pretty well. He's on levo at 35 and neo at 400 – they say to try to wean the levo first and the neo afterwards (but they told me the opposite on some patient I had last week). He's on TPN, and D5 with 3 amps of bicarb running at 250 an hour, and he's on an insulin drip at 4."

Many of the medicines we give in the ICU are dosed by micrograms per minute, or in units per hour, or in milligrams per minute - which means that they have to be given by pumps that deliver really precise rates of flow.

You're probably used to using the 3M pumps for things like heparin on the floors – here we use them for almost everything, because you really want to be sure that fluids are running at precise rates.

One common use for them is to run what we call 'flush lines' - these are lines that are usually running saline at some fixed rate, sometimes KVO, sometimes more, but always at a fixed rate.

To these we add other infusion meds – often we'll use the introducer for all our pressors for example, and a 3M pump will run the flush line that keeps everything flowing along. We also use these pumps to deliver precise volumes for IV boluses, or for slow timed meds like AmphoB that run over several hours – lots of uses. You can also program them to run bag mixes of pressors, because they have a 'dose-rate-calculation' function that you probably never bothered with on the floors.

9-1- What are microinfusion pumps?

The pumps you probably haven't seen before are our syringe pumps – also called 'microinfusion' or 'minipumps' – these are used for meds in syringe mixes that have to be titrated very tightly, sometimes in increments of 10 mikes per minute or less. They're very precise, but remember that if you change the flow rate on the flush line (they're usually plugged into a flush line), then your delivery isn't precise any more. Likewise, if you disconnect a med, remember that the flush line is still full of that med, starting from the port where you unplugged it. Last week we couldn't figure out why a patient's blood pressure was still low after we'd unplugged the labetolol for an hour – then we realized that the flush line was running at 10cc/hr, and the drug had been plugged in way up the line, so the patient continued to get the med, as the line was still full of drug. We took the line down, aspirated the line, and the patient's pressure began coming up within 10 minutes. Syringe pumps are useful – like any other device, you have to get used to them.

10- What are all the lines going into the patient?

"So okay, Chuck has a swan (www.icufaqs.org/PALinesApril04.doc), he has a left radial A-line, he has a femoral Quinton on the right for the CVVH. He came up with like 5 peripheral IVs (www.icufaqs.org/PeripheralIVs.doc) , but he's so swollen I couldn't get any blood return out of most of them, so I pulled them - there's one in his left antecub that I'm running the bicarb through because it wasn't compatible with anything, and it does have a good blood return. I mean, we're using every port on the guy, and I don't know where to run my insulin drip…"

You start hearing a lot about "lines" as soon as you set foot in the ICU – there are several kinds that you need to learn about, but they have things in common that it'll help you to understand.

10-1- How does the line connect the patient to the monitor?

The thing to remember is that some of the lines that we use in the unit monitor one pressure or another inside the patient, continuously. Let's take the example of an arterial line: an "A-line" is an ordinary 20-gauge IV catheter that is put into (usually) the patient's radial artery, in the wrist where you feel your pulse. (www.icufaqs.org/ArterialLines.doc) Now, you want to see that pressure up on your monitor screen – how does the information get there? The catheter is connected to a long piece of clear tubing which is rather stiff – which connects to a device called a transducer. The transducer is a pressure sensor – it 'feels' the pressure as it varies. Remember that with systole and diastole, the pressure in the arteries is going up and down. The transducer changes what it 'feels' into a varying electrical signal that goes to the monitor through a cable, where it's displayed as a varying line, over time, going from left to right on the screen. This catheter-line-transducer-cable-monitor-display setup is the same for every kind of invasive line that we use – which makes it easier to remember how they get set up.

10-2- What are those inflated white bags for, that hang on some of the poles around the ICU patients' bed?

Invasive lines often lead to pressurized areas of the patient's body – for example the arterial line above. If that catheter were attached to a regular IV gravity bag, the patient's blood pressure would drive blood right back up that line until the bag overfilled with blood – you get the idea. So the trick is to pressurize the line right back into the patient. The transducer looks at the pressure coming out of the patient, and at the same time lets a pressurized flow go back towards the patient at about 3cc/hr, to keep the line clear. You'll see these setups on arterial lines, monitored CVP lines, and PA lines. The exception is intracranial "bolts" – these use the transducer, but are never pressurized. (www.icufaqs.org/ICPMonitoring.doc)

10-3- Why do they use that stiff tubing for the transducers?

Here's the way I understand it: you want the pressure waves to get to the transducer clearly. Soft tubing absorbs the vibrations, so that by the time they get to the transducer they're all flattened out and meaningless. Stiff tubing reflects the waves back into the saline inside, so the waves get transmitted to the transducer without vanishing along the way.

10-4- What should I worry about when using these lines?

A word about pressurized lines – I've learned the hard way to check that the connections are tight. For whatever reason, these lines like to gently unscrew themselves, usually at a really unpleasant time – for example I always check the place where the art-line stopcock connects to the catheter tubing – they love to loosen themselves up. Likewise, check all the places where meds and infusions plug into flowing lines – a hub can come loose, and your pressor will infuse very nicely into the bed while your patients' pressure bottoms out, and you run around the room trying to figure out what's wrong. Be alert to wet spots in unexpected places.

More things to watch out for: **always make sure that you've set the alarm limits properly**. Make sure the lines are dated. Make sure that they're levelled correctly. Make sure the bags stay pumped up to pressure. Make sure that your waveforms look reasonable – you need to know if your PA line has slipped back into the RV, for example. Watch for bubbles in the stiff transducer tubing – they'll ruin your waveforms. Use air filters between the bag and the transducers for patients on balloon pumps (on the root line), and for patients who have a PFO (patent foramen ovale) – the idea being that you <u>really</u> don't want patients to risk a big air embolus into the arterial circulation. Nice big bubble, right to the brain...?

10-5- How should I organize the lines?

Neatness counts. This is not just the compulsive part of me talking, (well, it's <u>partly</u> the compulsive part of me talking) - suppose you follow some nurse into a room where a patient is on six infusion drips, and the lines are running every whichy-way all over the bed and the patient, crosswise, not labeled...suppose this patient gets into trouble – where are you going to push your meds? Or if she's agitated, where are you going to give her Ativan? Suppose she arrests – quick, which line do you use? Are you just going to guess? Is the person covering for you at lunch going to guess? Kind of nasty to see your bicarb line crystallize when you give calcium through it. Get into the habit of organizing the lines – take the time to check them thoroughly at the beginning of the shift, so you'll know things are tight, and straight. If my patient has more than three infusions going, I usually label the lines at the connector with the name of whatever is going through them, and sometimes I label the pumps too.

11- What kind of labs do we send on the ICU patients? (www.icufaqs.org/LabsUpdated.doc)

"The last crit I sent was at 6pm and that was 42, but I'm sure that won't last, because I'm emptying his Jackson-Pratts every hour or so. For blood! They want us to send CBCs every four hours, and coags every six. And the insulin drip means we send chems every two hours, and his last blood gas wasn't very good, so I guess you'll be sending a lot of labs tonight."

We send a lot of labs. Obviously the labs ought to have some clear relationship to what exactly is wrong with the patient - blood gases for respiratory patients, hematocrits and coags for bleeding patients, etc. When we admit a new patient from the EW, we usually send off the basic "one of everything": CBC, coags, what some people call a Chem 20, a blood gas if needed, cultures as needed. We also send a VRE stool swab, and a MRSA nasal swab off for screening with every admission. We send blood gases with most vent changes or with any change in the patient's condition, and the same idea should guide you in sending other labs as well – if you suspect a crit drop, send a CBC.

11-1- What do I do with the results?

The thing about labs is: follow up! If you treat a low K+ on a patient with ectopy, check it again to see the response. If you went up on the insulin drip, recheck the glucose in two hours (insulin drips require glucose checks every two hours anyway.) If you transfused them, send a CBC an hour later. Simple enough.

About blood gases: it takes a while to learn to interpret blood gases. Get someone to help you interpret them, because they can mean lots of things.

12- What is the procedure for admitting a patient to the ICU?

"I swear, it was such a mess getting him in here – you know how they are in the OR. I don't know how they get the lines wrapped around the patient's body like that. Anyway that took a while, and I've got some of the admission paperwork done, but would you work on the checklist for me? I'll keep him as a primary, but I'm a little nervous about running the CVVH alone…"

How an admission goes depends on how acute the patient is, and sometimes where the patient is coming from, but the priorities are usually the same. The first thing when the patient arrives is to quickly do a visual assessment. Has he tolerated the transfer well? Is he being bagged? Is he nice and pink, or dusky? Seizing, comatose, or smiling and waving? Bleeding? Always keep in your mind: what's the admitting diagnosis, what is wrong with this patient? Keep it simple: is he having a heart attack? Asthma attack? Brain attack? Killer tomato attack?

Follow the routine: hook her up to the monitors, slide her into the bed, start writing down vital signs, do an intake EKG, but… assess! Is the patient hypotensive? Does someone need to go get a pressor for you because the patient lost his blood pressure between the ER and the unit? Did you check the transport monitor to see if she was in a stable rhythm on arrival? Assessment comes before routine – remember that nothing replaces your eye as a monitoring device.

12-1- Admitting from the OR?

Admitting a patient from the OR is a little different - postop procedures follow their own routine. The essential point is that we do initial recovery of postops <u>with</u> the anesthesia person – they are responsible for supervision of post-anesthesia recovery.

Once the patient is in the MICU bed and monitored, and once the initial set of vitals have been taken, the nurse takes postop report from the anesthesiologist. You want to know exactly what was done. You want to know about total fluids in and out during the case, the EBL (estimated blood loss), blood products given, labs sent during the case. You want to know if the anesthesia or intraoperative paralysis was reversed, and when. When the last dose of pain medicine was given, and what it was, and how much. You want to make sure you know which surgical team to page if you have questions. Then you have to document vital signs at least every 15 minutes for the first hour. I usually send "one of everything" labs if they weren't sent during the case, get an EKG, ask if they want any postop x-rays – after all this, the regular ICU routine will usually do. Don't forget that they'll be in pain when they wake up!

12-2- What are "boarders"?

Sometimes we have patients in the MICU that belong to other services: usually surgery of one kind or another. We take patients from burns, thoracic, general surgery, neurosurg, neuro-med, and once in a while an OB/GYN person who may have developed problems. This is one of the neat things about working in this particular unit: here you will definitely get exposed to the widest possible range of patients and problems. We do it all.

13- What do I need to know about giving meds in the ICU? (<u>www.icufaqs.org/MedTips.doc</u>)

"He went into rapid a-fib at a rate of about 170 at about 2:30 this afternoon. He actually kept his pressure up with that rate, so we hung a loading dose of Amio, and started a drip at 1 – that's another port tied up. Is Amio compatible with anything? We can look in the computer…"

Giving meds in the ICU is definitely different from giving them on the floors – one of the biggest differences is the use of IV pushes. It's true what they teach you: once you push it in, it's gone, and you're not going to get it back. So think, and recheck labels before you push. And remember: in general, <u>push slowly</u>. Drugs pushed too rapidly can <u>kill</u>. Check the drug references for guidelines on how fast to push different meds.

Meds that we commonly push include diuretics: lasix, diuril, sometimes edecrine; cardiac meds: lopressor, digoxin, verapamil, sometimes adenosine (I hate adenosine – 10 seconds of pure terror); sedatives: ativan, valium, haldol; pain meds in small doses like morphine – there's a long list. Initial doses of some of these meds must be given by, or in the presence of a physician. **Be**

sure that you know what these meds are about before you push them. The simplest example – when you push lasix, the first thing I ask the new nurses is: why is the patient getting this med? Then: what's the patient's K$^+$? Then, what's her BUN and creatinine? - the higher they are, the harder it will be to diurese her. Or is the BUN high, but the creatinine normal – she may be dry to start with. Then: will she need K$^+$ replacement? And: is she having ectopy? (Why do I ask that one?) Last: did you empty the foley bag after the dose so you'll know what her output really was? I know it's a lot of questions, but these are exactly the kinds of things you need to think about, every time. After a while, you'll find that you've noticed most of those things already – you'll have put the picture together. It does get easier, but it takes a couple of years to get comfortable (don't get too comfortable!) – part of your job is to be patient with yourself.

13-1- What are pressors?

Another group of meds that you won't see much until you get into the ICU is pressors: actually there's a varied family of drugs that come under the name of "vasoactives" – drugs that make blood pressure go up or down. There's another FAQ about these, take a look over there for more on the subject. (www.icufaqs.org/PressorUpdate.doc)

13-2- What other drips do we use?

Other specialty drugs: unusual sedative drips like propofol, or continuous benzos like ativan; continuous opiates like fentanyl or morphine for pain; paralytics like nimbex (cisatracurium) or vecuronium; antiarrhythmics like amiodarone – these all have their own attributes that you need to learn about. An example: paralytic drips + stress-dose steroids = _serious_ badness in the form of myopathy: the patient may not be able to move for quite a while after the paralysis is shut off.

About sedation and paralysis: let's see how clear I can make this. Listen up, now: **sedation and paralysis are not the same!** If I _ever_ hear another nurse tell me that his patient was sedated with nimbex, I think I'm going to say, "Is that how you want us to sedate you when it's your turn?" Fortunately the teams usually get this one right, but for some reason a lot of the nursing staff get a little confused about this. If you don't know sedatives from paralytics, then you really do not belong in the ICU... okay? (www.icufaqs.org/finalsedationupdate.doc)

13-3- How do I make sure I'm giving all these meds correctly?

References: check yourself frequently, and always check if you're not sure. One thing you'll notice about experienced ICU nurses is that we're continually asking each other if this is right?, is that right?, looking things up, crosschecking... seriously, if you have a question, get a definitive answer before you proceed. Check with your peers, check with the doctors, check with pharmacy. Nobody is perfect, and two or three heads are always better than one.

14- What are some of the tests that ICU patients may have done in the unit?

"Then of course they wanted all sorts of weird films, and of course they had to be shot in the room. Then ultrasound was up looking at his gallbladder, - they were talking about putting in a percutaneous drain, and then the medical student told me they were thinking about a portable

CT scan – I just looked at him, and I guess he realized that I was about to snap like a twig, because he left the room in a hurry…"

Lots of tests get done in the unit: the commonest of course are x-rays and lab draws. Others you'll see: ultrasounds and echoes, portable CT scans (these are almost worse than the ones you travel for), trans-esophageal echoes, upper and lower endoscopies – you may be needed for help with these. You need to know what they're for, what they showed, and how to get the patient through them safely.

15- What tests are done on ICU patients that they might have to travel out of the unit for?

"So of course then the team wants to know if the patient can travel to CT scan, and I just was not comfortable with that. I'm really not sure that this man would survive a trip to the scanner!"

The commonest test that requires travel is to CT scan. The scanners are several floors below us, and you may have to pack up your pressor-and-vent-dependent patient, and roll him down the halls and down elevators to get there and back. This can be a truly terrifying experience for the newer nurse, because you are really it – if the patient decides to do something scary, you're on the spot.

15-1- How do I take a patient to CT scan?

Let's walk briefly through a trip to the scanner. The scanner tech calls and tells you that your patient was booked for an abdominal CT scan with gastrografin contrast about an hour ago, and what do you mean no one told you?, and what do you mean the patient hasn't had their gastrografin, and can you be there in five minutes?

Or at least it seems that way. And this is a patient whose pressure has been jumping all over the map, and every few minutes you've been running in and out of the room dialing her levo up or down. And her blood gases are awful. And she's agitated, and you know she's never going to lie still in the scanner, and maybe she doesn't speak English, and come to think of it, you're getting pretty agitated yourself.

Believe it or not, much of the decision about travelling for this test is absolutely your call, your judgment (but run the situation by the resource nurse too). It's true, this dilemma has to be referred upwards through the medical chain of command, with the point being clearly made about your reservations and fears. You can always, and legitimately insist that a house officer accompany you with the patient if you think the situation may become unstable. But you are going to be directly responsible for getting the patient through this ordeal safely – therefore, the trip must be a controlled experience. And you must be the one in control.

First off, I would have no problem asking that the test be rescheduled: the patient needs time to absorb the gastrografin, and you need to stabilize her blood pressure as much as you can. You need to make a coherent plan about travelling with respiratory – are the blood gases so bad, is the patient so acidotic, that you think the patient might arrest at any time now? Does this patient need to be ambu-bagged during transport? You need a sedation plan: does the patient need to be sedated for the test? Is the patient intubated? Does she need to be intubated, so she can be safely sedated, so she can be CT scanned? And it would be a good thing if somebody would please tell the nurse exactly why the patient is going for this test anyhow? You'd be amazed how the practicalities of something that seems simple can completely evade the minds of the doctors ordering these tests. Do they realize that this patient has been as agitated as a trout in the bottom of a canoe for the past six hours?

The point is that while you do have to do your best to get the scan done promptly, you must do it such that make you sure that your patient will be safe. Nothing else will do. Anything less would be negligence. And your legal responsibility is no less than any doctor's. So take your time, and do it the right way.

So, now we've rebooked the scan for an hour later. Gastrografin doses are going in every 20 minutes. You've arranged with respiratory to transport the patient (who _is_ intubated - that helps!), and the CCT has agreed to push the vent down to the scanner suite for you. You've pulled the team into the room, and after having actually seen the patient trying to leap out of the bed, they agree to let you run propofol for the length of time it takes to do the scan. (Did they think you were lying when you said the patient was agitated?) This lets the patient start to ventilate a little better, and their blood gas looks a little better, and the blood pressure stabilizes, and maybe this won't be so bad after all.

Get your travel gear together: travel monitor with batteries, code drug tackle box, portable defibrillator with battery – remember how to work it? Practice now and then – I mean, you know what I mean – don't actually defibrillate the bed, or your co-workers or anything, but make sure you know how it works. Make sure you have gel with you – it should be in your tackle box. Oxygen tank – check the meter to see how full it is. Ever see a patient arrive from somewhere on an empty tank? – well, don't be the first!

Turn off the tube feeds and aspirate your patient's stomach contents. An aspiration event from an even partly-full stomach because your patient had to lie flat… not good. Turn off the insulin drip for the trip. Try to travel with as few pumps and junk attached to your bed as possible – the fewer lines you have to travel with, the better. I usually disconnect and cap the cvp transducer, leave it behind.

Next – unplug your pumps and your bed, coil up the lines, hang them so they won't fall under your feet or the bed wheels. You can lie the transduced lines with their bags right in the bed next to the patient – the pressures will read reasonably well at that level when they're connected to the travel monitor.

Got everything? Unlock the bed wheels, and move off a couple of feet. Anything left connected to the wall? No? Off you go. Respiratory will bag the patient. Your position is at the bottom of the bed, watching or listening to the travel monitor as you go. What I do is to turn on the sat-probe beeper. This can be set not only to beep with each pulse, but also to beep in a higher or lower tone if the sat should rise or fall, so that you have some idea of what the patient is doing, even if you look away to steer around corners.

15-2- What do I do at the scanner?

At the scanner – again, this is your show, you're responsible. Take your time as you get the patient moved onto the scanner table. Watch that you have enough slack on your lines – if you don't, then stop the scan until you do. Don't be afraid to ask the radiology staff to help you move equipment around, and to stop the movement of the table to make sure that the lines will reach all the way in. Position the travel monitor so that you can see it through the control room windows throughout the entire scan (ask to borrow their binoculars – or am I the only one?). Watch that monitor – it alarms, but softly. If the patient needs a pressor change, tell the radiology people, and they'll stop the scan. Take the time you need to keep the patient safe. Write down vital signs during the scan to document how well the patient tolerated it.

Done? Right. Back to the unit, the same way, just backwards.

A word about the big scary thing– a code in the CT scanner. This is really not any kind of fun, and sometimes happens if a nurse is pushed into taking a patient down who may really be too sick to go. Which is no help when you're down there and it happens. Try to keep that possibility in mind when the team pushes really hard for a scan requiring travel, and make your concerns very clear. This is the situation in which you have a house officer come to the scanner with you.

If the patient does code – you know what to do, so do your best. Have the radiology techs call the code on the phone. Have them call the unit for help. Start compressions – watch the monitor. Get someone bagging the patient. Identify your line for pushing meds. Delegate as quickly as people arrive – get someone bagging, someone doing compressions. Your position as the RN who knows the patient best should probably be pushing meds, and speaking with the resident running the code. You may be surprised at how well things go. (Take ACLS.)

15-3- What other scans do patients travel for?

Other scans off the unit: MRI is the big one. This can be a scary, prolonged experience, especially with a pressor-dependent patient, since you have to run special long IV tubing into the scanner room because the metal IV pumps can't go in there. They do have a better monitor for blood pressure now – it will read an art-line now, instead of only using a noninvasive cuff. But pay special attention to your pump setup. Pre-prime the long tubing with pressor before you go down to the scanner. Then get the lines all set up, quickly move the patient into the magnet room, reconnect with the long lines, and watch the patient until their pressure is stable to your satisfaction. When things look right to you, the scan can go ahead. Important point about the MRI room – **the patient must come out of the room if bad things happen!** Remember that nothing ferrous can go into the MRI scanner room. There was a story that went around about someone forgetting this, at some hospital or other, and a code cart apparently got physically pulled up off the floor, flew through the air, and got yanked into the magnet. Bummer.

Lastly: angio. I hate angio, because it usually means someone is trying to bleed to death, and it's a race between you hanging blood, the doctors trying to find and plug the leak, and the patient exsanguinating. (Some nurses actually enjoy the adrenaline of this situation. Myself, I like a nice unstable cardiogenic shock patient on twelve drips and a balloon pump…) Sometimes you have to stay and hang blood at a frantic pace with the nurse in the suite, sometimes not. Do your best.

16- What do I need to know about IV access?

"So ask the team – I don't know exactly where we are going to put another line in this patient, but I need someplace to run antibiotics, and I don't want to interrupt anything. Oh, you know what, I think I can run some of these through the CVVH circuit, right? Let me ask Karen..."

They say that timing is everything in life – sometimes that's true, but in the ICU, access is everything. You just can't have enough IV access. Even a low-acuity ICU patient – say, a "soft" rule-out for an MI, should have two heplocks. Make it three. What if they rule in, have ectopy or chest pain, and the one IV you do have turns out to be no good? Do you want to futz around putting in another one, or do you want to be ready with a backup? Simple enough.

In the world of IV's, size matters. Bigger is better, and bigger is usually farther up the arms. If you think that a benign-looking patient can't suddenly turn into a frightening GI bleed, and need rapid infusions of blood and IV fluid – just ask an older nurse. And you can't run blood through a 22 gauge butterfly. Choose your access goals with an eye towards what's wrong, or what you think might be wrong, with the patient.

16-2- Central Lines:

I love central lines, because you can run anything through them: fluids, meds, blood products – you can transduce them and measure CVP's – they're wonderful. (www.icufaqs.org/CentralLines.doc)

I hate central lines - they can be deadly: an undressed central line site can suck air into the venous circulation, or provide entry for killer germs. Be very careful with these.

16-2-1- Where should they go?

The preferred site of central lines is somewhere in the neck or upper chest, going for either an internal jugular vein or a subclavian. The problem here of course is that the big finder needle that the docs use to insert these lines can easily drop a lung, especially if the patient is on a lot of PEEP, and the upper lobes of her lungs have been pushed up to the level of her ears. This doesn't mean they've done the insertion wrong – it simply happens sometimes. Or the line could make a wrong turn and go up into the neck towards the brain. So unless it's a code, you must get a chest film to make sure the line is in the proper place before you use it. (Do you want to be the nurse who became infamous for infusing pressors towards a patient's brain?) A quicker site for a central line is the femoral vein – this tends to be a dirtier insertion site, but if you're dealing with a hypotensive situation, and you don't want to have to wait for chest x-rays to start pressors – that's the place to go.

A trick of the trade: remember that all of the great veins, which is where you want your central lines to go, have arteries right next to them. It's always possible that a central line can go into one of these by accident. If you're not sure which vessel the line is in, hook it up to a transducer – even in a hypotensive patient, the venous number is always going to be lots lower than the arterial one.

16-3- Should I put in my own IV lines?

My own feeling has always been: the more you can do for your patient, the better. I think that all ICU nurses should be competent and comfortable with putting in their own peripheral lines – central lines of course are left to the docs. But I've been in codes before where the physicians are working like mad to get a femoral or chest line in some poor patient, while a nurse working on one of the arms quietly pops in an 18-gauge, stands up, and says, "I've got a good line here, folks."

16-4- What do ICU nurses give through IVs in the unit?

We give much the same kinds of things that patients get on the floors, except that we often give more, and more quickly – such as blood products in treating a GI bleed. We also give rapid infusions of IV fluids, and as discussed above, we give a lot of IV meds, some of which are pushes, and some of which are very precisely controlled drips. It can never be stressed enough: **be very aware of what is going through your lines**. This sounds almost stupid until you realize what would happen if you hung an antibiotic through a line with levophed in it…not a lesson you want to learn twice, much less once!

16-4-1- Crystalloid:

We use all sorts of clear IV fluids in the unit – I guess I show my old SICU background when I think of these as 'crystalloid', an old name for them. The main point to keep in mind about IV fluids: your goal is to keep careful track of how much the patient absorbs. Some units do this hourly – we do it every six hours, and we do totals at midnight. You may find that you have to keep running totals in your head – as in GI bleeds, when you need to know where the patient is, "net" – that is, total, positive or negative, at any given time.

16-4-2- Blood products:

We give lots of these, and you'll have to pass a transfusion test before you can hang blood. Transfusion reactions are quite dangerous, but we see even suspected ones only rarely. Scrupulous attention, every single time, to the rules of checking blood products before transfusion will keep you and your patient out of trouble. Even in the worst GI bleed situations, when you'll see two RNs checking blood for the one hanging the bags in the room, while members of the team are running about getting the patient intubated, placing lines - those two nurses will be very calmly standing there, carefully reading numbers off to each other, co-signing slips, numbering the bags, and passing them in for transfusion. Remember – there really is enough time in any situation to do things right. Seriously– next time a crisis comes up, take five or ten whole seconds, and just stand there, and collect your thoughts. Ten seconds is actually a long time. You could even take fifteen. (Of course, people will look at you and wonder…)

A couple of things to add about transfusion: you can run more than one blood product at once, which you may have to if you're chasing a big bleed, but you have to get an order written saying so.
You can save a lot of time by using multiple-use transfusion filters. Ours are orange – they plug into standard large-bore tubing (<u>not</u> transfusion tubing, use regular IV tubing), and you can run a

total of ten units through them – packed cells and/or FFP. Not platelets, I don't think. Put a sticker on the tubing numbered 1-10, and cross the numbers off as you go.

If you have a large-volume blood transfusion situation, you can get an ice chest up from the blood bank that holds all the available blood products that are closest to expiration – this will give you a larger number of units to have on hand – a good idea if GI thinks that your recently embolized variceal patient might very well "open up" overnight. (www.icufaqs.org/BloodUpdated.doc)

16-5- IV meds:

We make a lot of our own mixes in the med room – remember to use very careful technique doing this. Remember the 5% rule of mixing – if your additive will equal more than 5% of the total mix volume, then withdraw and discard as much from the bag as you will be adding in. Remember to check mix compatibilities – some meds like nipride must be mixed only in D5W, for example. Use the reference books in the med room, call pharmacy if you have questions, check the IV med policy books, check with your co-workers – you get the idea. Do it right. Take careful, detailed pride in your profession.

17- What are some of the common emergency situations that come up in the ICU?

"I was surprised that he was able to keep his pressure up when he went into the rapid AF. The team said that if it dropped we'd cardiovert him out of it, but he did fine, and the Amio load went in, and his rate is slower now." (www.icufaqs.org/BedsideEmergencies.doc)

17-1- Some basic thoughts about emergencies:

Before getting to specifics, let me make one quick point: take the time to figure out what your plan is. <u>There is always time to think</u>, even in a code. Take that time, and use it. There is no need to get really scared – help is always at hand. In fact, you'll notice that a well-run code is actually pretty quiet : no yelling, no pushing, just calm orders coming from the person running the situation, and steady application of the basics, which do not change: Airway, Breathing, Circulation.

Sometimes it helps to think your way ahead of time through a given situation: for example, suppose your patient stopped breathing. First – "Annie, Annie, are you all right?" (grin!) Next – call for help. Next? Got an oral airway handy? Got an ambu-bag? Hook it up, insert the airway – is the patient moving air with bagging? Now – is there a pulse? Is he responding? What if his name isn't Annie?

Now – suppose you saw VT on the monitor. You pelt over to the patient: is he smiling at you? Once, a very green ICU nurse ran over to where he saw VT on a monitor, and forgetting to first assess the patient for responsiveness, well… he thumped the patient precordially. The sleeping patient did not appreciate this: "What the hell did you do that for!?". Which of course didn't help either, after the nurse found out that the "VT" was actually monitor artifact, generated by water in the patient's corrugated O2 mask tubing… Or it really is VT, and the patient really is unresponsive? Think the scenario through – should you thump her? Probably. (What does ACLS say about this nowadays?) Call for help. Get an airway – know where it is? It really does get easier after the first few times.

17-2- Cardiac/Hemodynamic situations:

"He did drop his pressure when Gloria was with him downstairs yesterday in the scanner, and they tapped his belly – she is amazing, she whipped him back up here, and she called ahead and got the OA to order up some blood products – he's got a standing order to stay ahead something like 8 units of red cells - and got them up and running with the team within ten minutes…"

17-2-1- Hypotension:

This is one of the commonest situations you'll see. The question to ask yourself – and the team – is simple: why is the patient doing this? The answer may not be so simple, but usually has something to do with the three basic parts of a blood pressure: pump, volume, or arterial squeeze. There's more about this subject in the FAQs on pressors/vasoactives, and PA-lines, to help you learn to sort these issues out. Meantime, think: does your patient need fluid?, or pressors?, or is their pressure low for some cardiac reason having to do with rhythm, or low EF? As you gain experience, you'll learn to figure things out quickly.

The commonest moves you'll be ordered to make in a hypotensive situation: give a fluid bolus, usually NS, usually 250cc, sometimes repeated. Run the bolus right in, either wide open on gravity, or set a pump at 999, which will give the bolus in 15 minutes. Make sure the IV site will tolerate the rate. If you use a pump bag to infuse crystalloid rapidly, **make sure you pre-spike the bag, and get all the air out** – you don't want that going into the patient when the bag is empty.

Used to be, we could use only one pressor peripherally: dopamine (using what we call the 'peripheral mix' of 200mg/250cc) can run up to 300mcg/minute through a peripheral line, although in a code, you do whatever you have to do. Nowadays we can also use pheynlephrine at a concentration of 10mg in 250, up to about 300 mcg/minute.

Remember that drugs like levophed and neosynephrine work by causing vasoconstriction – if you run them through a peripheral vein, and the med gets extravasated into the tissue, the patient could lose an arm, or at least end up with a really nasty wound – I've seen them skin-grafted in the past.

17-2-2- Arrhythmias:

"I think the levo didn't help the whole situation with the a-fib, so maybe we could change him over to neosynephrine instead."

We don't see as many lethal arryhthmias as we used to, for the simple reason that most MI patients get clot-busted nowadays. It was always the big "rule-ins" that generated most of our big scary arrhythmias. You will see them though, and ACLS is a very useful experience to have gone through when it happens, but it's just one of those things – you have to go through it a few times. You should be absolutely clear on the basics of defibrillation. The essentials don't change:

assess for unresponsiveness, call for help, get what you need. Some people do maintain a pressure with arrhythmias, some don't, so be ready with a defibrillator. (www.icufaqs.org/ArrhythmiaReview.doc) (www.Defibrillation.doc)

17-2-3- Not-quite-so-scary arrhythmias:

You need to be familiar with these. We see just about every weird rhythm eventually, but the most common ones nowadays are the ones that go with sepsis and pulmonary disease: a-fib, rapid and not-so-rapid; a-flutter, occasionally SVTs. Try to be familiar ahead of time with the use of adenosine, metoprolol and verapamil, and know the procedures for shocking a patient out of a-fib. Anesthesia is supposed to be present during elective cardioversions, because the patient might go into something really unpleasant, like VF. Push the sync button! Remember too that sometimes septic patients go into these rhythms because they want to go fast – that's their reflex to try to maintain blood pressure. Think carefully about whether or not you should be blocking a reflex tachycardia.

17-2-4- "Flashing":

A sort of cardiac/respiratory 'double whammy' that we see sometimes in the unit is the infamous 'flash' of CHF. This is usually due to an episode of ischemia, or fluid overload, or both. If you're very good, and very quick and lucky, you may be able to actually head this one off with aggressive treatment: remember LMNOP, for lasix, morphine, nitrates, oxygen, and position. That is, diurese him, give him morphine for pain, nitrates for ischemia, oxygen for ischemia/shortness of breath, and sit him way up in a high Fowler's position. A pillow under each arm is helpful. Watch the blood pressure! Get EKGs with the onset of pain/ angina/ chest pressure/ whatever, and get another one afterwards. The goal is to see that the ischemic changes on the EKG go away with treatment. I personally think that ICU nurses ought to be able to read EKGs on a basic level to see if there are bad things happening. This is actually not very hard – a FAQ on this topic was put together recently, so take a look! (www.icufaqs.org/ReadingEKGs.doc)

17-2-5-Codes:

"Oh s-word."

I hate codes. Jayne likes them. Each to their own, I guess. I'd rather do my best to head one off, than pump some poor person's chest. Again – the basics apply: take the time to think through your plan.

You can call a code whenever you need to. There's a code button in the room, or you can get on the intercom, or you can lean out into the hall and shout – briefly. Your job is simple: get help, and start the ABC. Simple as that. Get the airway open – oral airway, jaw lift, ambu. Get the board under the patient, get the EKG machine hooked up, start CPR. Your position should probably be "pusher" – as the nurse assigned to the patient, you know where to push meds. Make sure someone is recording the meds for you as you give them. Responders to a code will be what seems like everyone including Santa Claus: anesthesia, the medical seniors, the rest of the team, medical students, respiratory, pharmacy, nursing supervisors, operational associates – I think even security responds to a code, to escort family members out of the room if necessary.

The code 'boss' is the medical senior resident - make sure that orders are coming from one source only, since this is not the time to have contradictory orders flying from various places.

Nurses from our unit also respond to floor codes. In practice this is usually the resource nurse, but it may be another senior staff person. I usually try to get in to the bedside and help to get things flowing smoothly, although the nursing supervisor may be doing this already. Once the situation is stabilized, your role as a "first-responder" is done – check with the supervisors to see where the patient will be headed, then come back to the unit.

17-3- Respiratory situations:

"His sat dropped after he got here – I think the vec wore off postop, and he began to get asynchronous with the vent, and his pH went to 7.06 with a PC02 in the 80s, so we had to paralyze him…"

Respiratory distress: this is another common ICU scenario. The goal here is actually to be planning ahead – you want to try not to let the beginnings of respiratory distress get away from you. If you can. For example, if you think your patient is going into CHF, you want to be all over it: treating it, assessing them for response to treatment, documenting sats and blood gases and lung sounds …the secret is: have a plan. If you think your patient may need intubation during your shift, tell the team so, tell the resource nurse, tell respiratory, and tell your co-workers. Impending intubation is something the medical teams may not want to hear about, because it indicates that the patient got worse under their care – not what some aspiring residents want to tell the attendings in the morning. But you have no less of a responsibility than they do.

Common situations in the MICU involving the respiratory system: pneumonia, CHF (or both!); ARDS, sometimes BOOP – this one is unusual, but we see it enough to remember it. The letters stand for Bronchiolitis Obliterans with Organizing Pneumonia. Discovered, I believe, by the famous Dr. Betty, of the same name, at the Warner Brothers School of Medicine and Animation. BOOP is a tissue pathology diagnosis that they make by doing an open-lung biopsy. There's two kinds of this actually, the kind with pneumonia, and the kind without – you want to have the kind with, because in cases where it looks like pneumonia provoked the disease, then those people do better. People with just plain BO do worse. Now and then we see people with pulmonary hypertension, or pulmonary fibrosis – we work with a drug called flolan on the first group, which takes some careful watching and learning – the second group is sometimes being worked up pre-transplant.

Again, guiding your plan in staying ahead of the patient's condition is remembering: "What is wrong with this patient?". I mean, it seems obvious. But you can get so lost in sat probes, and blood gases, and arterial lines, and vents and nebs and this and that, and all the trees, that you totally lose sight of the forest. Basic ideas: does the patient need diuresis? Suctioning? Nebs? All three? Intubation? Sometimes you can't avoid intubation: do you want to wait until the last minute, or do you want to do it electively? Use your team-mates to help you make your plan with the doctors.

There's lots more information on the specifics of what we do in the unit as regards respiratory matters in the FAQs on "Vents and ABGs" (www.icufaqs.org/ventFAQ.doc) , and "Intubation". (www.icufaqs.org/IntubationFAQ.doc)

17-4- ID Issues:

"I sent cultures from all the lines as they went in, and there's no urine to send, but I guess we could straight-cath him to see what he's got. Chris cathed him yesterday and said he got "bladder dust"…"

For some reason I always lump ID issues in with the respiratory system. Probably a bad habit, but so many of our infections have to do with pneumonia… remember that an infection can hide in lots of places, and you as the person at the bedside are probably in the best position to help figure out where it is. Be prepared to do a lot of culture-draws in the MICU. Check with the team if your patient spikes a fever – she may have been 'cultured up' that day completely, or the team may want a whole new set.

17-5- Renal Failure:

"The renal fellow said he really couldn't call it one way or the other if Chuck's kidneys are going to come back or not, so I guess he's going to be on CVVH for the duration. How long do we keep people on CVVH anyhow?" (www.icufaqs.org/CVVH.doc)

We see a lot of renal failure in the MICU. It can be chronic, or acute, or "acute-on-chronic", and we think a lot about how to avoid making things worse. As a primary nurse, you definitely want to keep your patients' BUN and creatinine in mind. One thing to remember is that the kidneys are very sensitive to blood pressure – they hate to be underperfused, even for a short time, and will sometimes turn right around and bite you by going into ATN. This can take a long time to come out of – weeks sometimes, sometimes less, and now that more and more of the nurses are competent with CVVH, we do more and more of it. CVVH looks like the octopus from hell, but it really does sort itself out after you work with it for a while – all of us look at it in terror at first.

17-5-1- Urology problems.

Under renal failure comes urology, I guess. We don't see many patients with urological surgeries, but we do see the occasional nephrostomy tube. More importantly, be careful about foleys and where they actually are, as opposed to where they are supposed to be.
(www.icufaqs.org/FoleyCatheters.doc)

Tips: do not inflate the foley balloon on a male until, 1: the catheter has been advanced all the way to the Y, where the balloon port comes off, and 2: until you see urine in the tubing. Use similar precautions for women. Even if the catheter has advanced smoothly, you may have to stand there for a minute before urine starts flowing - or you may see it right away. Do not force the foley in under any circumstances. Call the team. If you aren't satisfied, speak to the resource nurse, and think about getting urology to come and look. Inflating a Foley balloon anywhere but all the way into the bladder can be a disaster, and can mean possible surgery later on. Another obvious maneuver that gets overlooked – is the foley plugged? A sharp nurse saved her patient from CVVH recently by changing a foley and discovering that the patient's kidneys were working after all…

A word about Murphy drips: gravity drip only. No pumps, no way. If the drainage lumen of your patient's three-way foley plugs with a clot, you do not want that drip pushing fluid through the other lumen, into the bladder…

17-6- GI problems:

"I don't think we're going to be able to use his gut for a long time. I mean, with that kind of surgery plus all the fentanyl he's on, he probably won't have a single bowel sound for the next week or so anyway, so it's a good thing they started the TPN right away."

17-6-1- GI Bleeds:

Nothing comes to mind under the GI category quicker than GI bleeds, which as you probably know come in two main varieties: upper bleeds, which are as I understand it above the pylorus, and lower ones. We see plenty of both, and we get to know the endoscopy fellows pretty well: they come in and scope the patients, then sclerose or band bleeding esophageal varices at the bedside. Basic principles: access is everything – they'll order "two large bore IVs at all times", but you probably want to get the team to put in central access as soon as possible, because these patients can really move fast. A clue to trouble coming: watch the heart rate. Even before a patient drops BP from a GI bleed, her heart rate will rise. Even an increase of 10 bpm from baseline gets me all nervous. Send labs as you think you need to: the orders are usually for a CBC, and maybe coags after every set of transfusions, or for any clinical change. Send labs even if you suspect a clinical change, and you'll be way ahead of the game. A second main principle with upper GI bleeds: think carefully – should this patient be intubated for airway protection? My feeling is, better safe than sorry, but hey, I'm old – do you think I worry too much?

Other GI bleed scenarios: we see the occasional Blakemore tube- a soft NG tube with inflatable balloons that GI will insert, and use to tamponade bleeding sites in the esophagus or upper stomach. This is held in place with a cord-and-pulley traction setup that attaches to the foot of the bed – it's a good idea to know where it is ahead of time: it hangs on the wall in the equipment room.

Now and again we'll send a GI patient to angiography, where they try to plug a GI bleed from inside the vasculature: they use fluoro and dye studies to locate the bleeding source, and inject sterile gelfoam (is that what they still use?), and plug the bleeding vessel from the inside. Or even more fun: sometimes we'll take the patient to angio for an emergent TIPS procedure. This involves threading a line down the jugular vein into the liver, and using a trocar (think of a small harpoon) to poke an opening to connect up parts of the hepatic vessel structure – this opening allows blood to bypass part of the stiff, cirrhotic liver, and lets the portal circulation pressure fall, therefore shrinking esophageal varices. It's exactly the same as a porto-caval shunt, as I understand it, except different.

17-6-2- Liver Failure:

We deal with a lot of liver failure patients. Some of them are pre-transplant, some of them are treatable, some not. Often they're transfusion dependent – be very aware of their heme lab values. We give a lot of lactulose – we follow ammonias daily. Be careful with blood draws – we see lots of people with hepatitis.

17-7- Neurological situations:

"His neuro status: about the only thing I can assess is his pupils - they're equally responsive at 2mm bilaterally. And his heart rate goes up sometimes when you talk near him – actually it went way up when his girlfriend was talking to him, so maybe he's not really sedated enough under the paralysis. I have the BIS on him, but I'm not sure if it's reading right."

Every patient is at risk for neuro/ mental-status changes while in the MICU. We don't get a lot of the really acute neuro patients in the MICU, but it happens once in a while. You want to be very alert for changes in the patient's neuro exam: any change in the size of either pupil compared to the other, or change in mentation, or strength of an extremity, calls for an immediate check-in with the team. We do some continuous seizure monitoring with EEG machines, that are left hooked up to the patient for a given period of time. We used to turn them on periodically so that the neuro people could look over the strips in the morning, but nowadays they use a computerized EEG that apparently stores the information for them. You should know what a therapeutic dilantin level is, what valproate is, and you should know what benzos are usually used for acute seizure activity.

BIS monitors are the latest and the greatest in the sedation monitoring line.

17-7-1- What should I worry about?

The biggest thing we worry about in many of these patients is increasing intracranial pressure. The thing to remember is that the very first sign of this is decreased mentation – it's very clear – the patient suddenly becomes hard to arouse. Any patient in the midst of a neuro event who does this probably needs an immediate head CT, and maybe mannitol, depending. The famous triad (Cushing's triad?) of dropping heart rate and respirations, along with widening pulse pressure (systolic heading up, diastolic down) is, as I understand it a late sign of increasing ICP – you do not want to let this develop. The goal of mannitol treatment is to shrink the brain: doesn't sound very nice, but it's better than having it try to escape down through the foramen magnum. Treatment with mannitol is titrated to the osmolality ("Hey, what's this guy's osm?") level – remember: high is dry, and the goal is usually something like "greater than 310", normal being something like 280-295.

Neuro patients often have tight blood pressure goals – too high and they might bleed, or rebleed; too low and they might not perfuse. The neuro team will tell you what range they want – you may find yourself titrating nipride or labetolol to bring a pressure down. Or the other way: recently we've seen pressors used to hypertensively perfuse ischemic brain tissue. Remember to run nipride alone, without even a flush line. (I sometimes flag the ports on the IV tubing that has nipride running through it, so that no one will accidentally plug in an antibiotic).

17-7-2- Bolts.

If you do have a patient with a bolt – lucky you! Use the chance to learn all about them, because we see them very rarely. I always ask the nurses in the neuro ICU to come down and inspect the setup to make sure everything is right. (www.icufaqs.org/ICPMonitoring.doc)

I mean, neuro is not my strong point, and I'm not sure I'd know a bolt unless they screwed one into my head, but the essentials of the exam will always serve you well: if a patient has equal strengths and pupils and is telling jokes one hour, and is totally out of it the next hour with one pupil blown… you get the idea. Check with the team even if you think that there might be, say, a slight change in mentation – catching things early is always better!

17-7-3- A zebra. (A nursing student hears hoofbeats out the window. Does he think of a horse?)

A last neuro scenario that we see once a blue moon, but which you need to know about is the infamous "neuroleptic malignant syndrome", or "NMS", which is a rare side effect of antipsychotic meds like haldol and zyprexa. This is when your patient has developed a really high fever – we recently saw a patient hit 107 – in response to one of these meds. They become very rigid, and I think their CPK bumps impressively. NMS and its cousin "malignant hyperthermia" (which shows up sometimes in response to gas anesthesia) are both treated with a drug called dantrolene. Pretty orange color. Works very well. Just something to put in the back of your mind.

17-8- Psychiatric situations:

"It sounds like he may be sort of a tough character – I mean, eating home-cured meat and drinking moonshine – was that really true? And that whole story about taking so much aspirin – it's hard to imagine he didn't know that would hurt him. So maybe we should have a plan when we wake him up…"

We have a lot of patients who have psychiatric problems, and you'll see lots of patients being treated with antidepressants, or antipsychotic meds like haldol. Be aware that haldol can prolong the QT interval to the point where the patient can have dangerous arrhythmias (torsades de pointes?). Something to watch for.

17-8-1- Overdoses.

Our mainstay psych situation is OD. We see these regularly, and there are a couple of things to keep in mind. First is toxicity: what did he take, and is it trying to kill him? Some meds are dialyzable, lots are not – we give a lot of charcoal, we clean up a lot of stool. (A lot of stool.) Timing seems to be most of the battle in this one - how much did he take, how long has he had to absorb it? These patients must be placed in leather restraints – ordered by the acute psych service – and these can only be removed when the patient is "cleared" by psychiatry – not otherwise. Leathers come up with the patient from the EW, but they're supplied by security and have to be returned there.

A word about restraints in general: your goal is to keep your patient safe. If your patient is lined up, or intubated, or just a bit confused, you do have the authority to restrain him, although you have to notify the doctors immediately, and they have to enter an order. The order specifies how much restraint can be used, for how long, and why. Make sure you understand the restraint documentation policies, and fulfill them. Every time.

Speaking of overdoses, this is a good time to bring up the topic of weaning - we often run patients on sedative drips for long periods of time, and if someone has been on morphine or fentanyl for more than a couple of weeks, they may have habituated enough to require careful weaning. Even then, they may have withdrawal symptoms. The basic guideline that we've used in the past has been: wean 25% of the drip every day. This does not mean weaning in four days – it means weaning 25% of what's running every day. So a patient on 1000mcg of fentanyl/hour will go to 750mcg on the first day of the wean, then 562mcg the second day, then 420 the third, 315 the fourth – always subtracting 25% of what's up.

For the tachycardia and hypertension that come with withdrawal, we've sometimes used clonidine, either po or as a patch, which apparently blocks a lot of the adrenergic release. Works pretty well. Useful thing to know.

18 - How do I deal with my own stress in the ICU?

The first thing for a new person to realize is that coming to the ICU is like being a new grad all over again. Everyone goes through this: feeling scared, feeling stupid, feeling isolated. (Too many of us still feel that way…)

You have to remember that this is one of the very hardest, and most complex jobs ever invented – as mentioned earlier, right up there with "nuclear submarine." People will point this out to you, but it may not sink in until you find yourself crying in the bathroom for the third time in a week – can you seriously think of a harder or more stressful job? It involves being in "crisis mode" almost every day – how many people do you know out in the regular world who have ever seen someone who may be bleeding to death? If they see something like that once in a lifetime, it may be a story they tell forever. But you'll see things like that every week, maybe every day. Be patient with yourself. Senior staff RN Jane says: "It takes a year just to learn which way to turn the stopcocks!"

18-1- Being scared.

Specifically, as for being scared – read my lips: we all get scared. Sometimes the older staff is more scared than you are, because we know more about what might be coming! If you're in a scary situation, there is only one way out: don't let yourself get isolated. If you don't have your preceptor around any more, then talk to the resource nurse when you have problems. She should know about them anyhow. If the resource nurse isn't around, go after your team-mates. Be a squeaky wheel if you have to, because the patient won't benefit if you don't speak up when you think she needs something done.

18-2- Feeling stupid.

As for feeling stupid: look, here we are surrounded by university-level academic doctors. How could we not feel stupid?

But remember this: residents spend one month out of each year in the unit, over a three-year residency – something like that. You, on the other hand, are in the unit year-round. Which means that after one year, you have four times the ICU experience that a resident gets all told. Your opinion counts. Don't forget that.

Another thing to remember (this should be printed backwards on our foreheads so we can read it in the mirror): "**There is no such thing as a stupid question.**" Watch the senior staff – after 15 years, we still check with each other constantly to make sure we've got things right.

18-3- What do I do if I make a mistake?

"I hung his Vanco at 4, but I got distracted because he started bleeding from his Jackson-Pratts, so I forgot to hang the other half of the dose – I guess I should've put it on a pump instead. I told the doctors, and they said it was fine, because with his renal failure that dose is going to go round and round inside him for a long time. But I felt terrible, and I know I'm going to worry about this all night."

The only thing you can do if you find you've made an error is to let the team know right away. There is just no other way to handle it. Reporting the error quickly will help fix things the fastest.

But the worst part for many nurses is feeling so bad about it afterward. Well, think of this: what kind of nurse would you be if you didn't feel so bad about it afterward? Remember your mistakes, and learn from them. Better yet, learn from other people's mistakes, and avoid making your own. But we are all of us only human. You have to learn to forgive yourself eventually, or the job will eat you alive. Ice cream seems to help. Heath Bar Crunch, or maybe Waffle Cone…

My own way to avoid mistakes is to be extremely systematic and compulsive, because I find that doing things by routine helps me remember every single thing: I check my med sheets every hour. I check the computer for new orders every hour. (Good thing I'm not like this at home. Do I check with my spouse for new orders every hour? Not telling…)

18-4- What do I do if I find someone else's mistake?

"Wow, look. Susie didn't write down the vent settings, and he's on too much O2. I guess she is human!"

Tell the team right away, and check with the resource nurse about followup. Make out an incident report. Tell the nurse you followed, but be gentle about it. We are here to catch each other when we slip on the ice, not to hurt each other. We are all we have – we need to take better care of each other.

18-5- What do I do if I think the doctors are telling me to do the wrong thing?

This is always a very difficult situation, and sometimes it happens. ICU nurses tend to sum up overall situations very quickly: "Will somebody please tell me why they insist on coding this patient with liver mets!?" And you could make a good case: that the nurses are so close to the patients that we understand their suffering in ways the doctors don't. But you'd be surprised – I know I've been surprised – to see more than a few of these patients that the nurses were sure would never, ever get better… actually leave the unit.

It's easy for us to fault physicians for standing back – but maybe it's that distance that lets them see what we don't see, up so close.

On the other hand, sometimes there's a real difference in making a judgment call. The situation I always think of is a team waiting too long to intubate a patient, who's increasingly in respiratory distress. Clearly, if the p02 keeps going down, and the Fi02 keeps going up, then where those two lines meet on the graph is going to be a plastic tube. But the residents are sometimes concerned that intubating a patient means that they haven't managed them correctly, which is hardly ever true.

The only way to work on a situation like this is to be gentle and persistent. Be a genuinely friendly, insistent pain in the butt. Enlist the resource nurse, enlist respiratory, and work on the team steadily, but as nicely as you can. In a pre-intubation setting I would bring the team in to look at the patient with each blood gas, or every time I had to blind suction him, and try to let the evidence convince them. That way there's no big adversarial fight, and no one can say that you were unreasonable. Which helps!

18-6- What if I think the doctors aren't listening to me?

Try not to get mad – getting into a fight will really make your effort at persuasion tougher. On the other hand, what kind of caring nurse would you be if you didn't get mad? And you can be as mad as you want to be, but if you dump it all over the team they probably not only won't listen, but they certainly won't listen. Steady application of cheerful pressure is really the only way. "Uh, Hildegard? I really do just have to tell you, and I know I've been after you all night, but I'm really afraid that if we wait too long to intubate Mr. Fink-Nottle, that we might have a code situation on our hands – I mean, look at how his gases have gotten worse in the past few hours…" If Hildegard is smart enough to become a doctor, she should be smart enough to listen to you.

18-7- How should I go up the chain of command if the doctors don't seem to listen to me?

Gently. Talk to the resource nurse and see if she'll go to bat for you. If you and the resource nurse agree that there's a real problem, you can tell the team that you'd like to run the situation past the house senior – this often helps resolve these situations. (Once again, I'm describing this as if everyone only worked on the night shift…) If the pulmonary fellows are around, you can drag them into the discussion. Even the attendings (sometimes especially the attendings) are usually ready to listen to the concerns of the nurse at the bedside. The trick is - and this of course is the really hard part - to stay calm and friendly, even if you think they're acting dismissively towards you, and just steadily make your case. Document that you did so. Tell them that you did.

18-8- How should I involve the resource nurse?

Let her know early on if you think a situation is developing that might need intervention from higher up the chain, and keep her posted about developments. If you think something is happening that may endanger your patient, let her know right away. "Listen, Mary - I'm really afraid for my patient. His pressure stinks, and I think he needs central access right away…"

18-9- What do I do if I think that my patient's treatment is unethical?

A lot of people have trouble with this issue, and that's because it's genuine. We provide a lot of what often looks like futile care, especially at the ICU nurse's distance of six inches or less. It can be terribly frustrating.

Try to broaden your perspective of observation. Maybe it looks futile in retrospect, maybe it looks that way while we're doing it. I'm not going to say I don't agree – of course I agree. But the fact is that the way our society is structured just now – the legal environment, our technical abilities, the incentive of the teaching hospital to teach – there are all sorts of forces at work that combine to put your patient in her bed, there in front of you.

Here's my feeling: I can't change those social forces. I can't change the legal environment that makes families likely to sue, or not. I can't change the attitudes of a family who want "everything done" for a patient with an obviously (to me) terminal illness. And no matter how bad I feel for a patient that I may agree is being made to endure a long painful course in the unit, it is not my place to speak for them, or to pre-empt what they might have wanted. It's their life, isn't it?

So what I am faced with is: a patient in a bed. What to do? Take care of them! A quote I read somewhere: "What then must we do? We must care for those that God places before us." I mean, it may as well be me, because what I <u>can</u> do, the difference that I <u>can</u> make is that I can advocate for that patient with all my skill and experience, so that their distress is minimized, and their outcome – whatever it is, whatever <u>they</u> have decided, is the best it can be. And it's only the nurse at the bedside who does that. Who else is up in the middle of the night to hold the hand of some dying person, maybe no family, just the two of you, and maybe the Great Nursing Supervisor…?

But it is a tough proposition. Tough on us, I mean. This is not a job to take lightly, taking care of people on the edge of life and death. It has the deepest effects on you as a person. The suffering, or even what you perceive as the suffering of the patients, can threaten to eat you up.

It can be dealt with, even if it seems overwhelming. Even if it <u>is</u> overwhelming. (Ask me how I know.) Each of us has to find her own way. My spouse has the same job that I do, and we vent to each other, and that helps a lot. I have two dogs, who help a lot too. But here's one thought you might hold in mind: every day, when you walk out of that ICU, don't you look down at your feet, walking there under you, and say to yourself: "how priceless"? Aren't you glad that you can just breathe in and out on your own? Drink coffee? For me, that's the gift I get, every day, working in the unit. The gift that only nurses get. "Chop wood, carry water – how amazing!". Well, it is, isn't it?

19- A word about levity:

Dear reader: it may seem to the un-initiated that there is some inappropriate humor in this article. I think that any nurse with any experience of ICU nursing in particular, or nursing in general, will tell you that if you can't keep your sense of humor – especially black humor – in a setting like an ICU, you are definitely sunk. Humor of this kind does not mean that anyone involved is less than serious – on the contrary, it is an effective way of dealing with what is ultimately serious:

the great matter of life and death. As well, there are inevitably descriptions of frustration with nearly all aspects of this job – personnel, tasks, attitudes and institutions all come in for criticism. This is also a kind of healthy emotional venting, and it needs to take place nearly all the time. Please do not get the impression that the opinions expressed in this way mean that ICU nurses are cynical, or dysfunctionally angry. Actually, the reverse is true, or they wouldn't be there. So forgive us if we seem a little burnt around the edges. Thanks!

Arrhythmia Review

Hi all – here's another one – this one took a while, but it was a lot of fun to hunt around for strips and images. As usual, please remember that this file is not meant to be a final medical reference of any kind, but is meant to represent knowledge passed on by a preceptor to a new orientee. Please let me know when you find mistakes, which I'm sure you will!

What is an arrythmia?

The nodes: SA and AV.

The normal complex:

1-1: What is a P-wave? What is the P-R interval?
1-2: What if there's no P-wave?
1-3: What is the QRS complex?
1-4: What if there's no QRS complex?
1-5: What is the T-wave? What is the QT interval?
1-6: What if there's no T-wave?
1-7: What is the isoelectric line?

2- Why do people have arrhythmias?
3- What is the difference between a bad arrhythmia and a not-so-bad arrhythmia?
4- What is "ectopy"?
5- What does "supraventricular" mean?
6- What are the supraventricular arrhythmias that I'm likely to see in the MICU, which ones do I need to worry about, and how are they treated?

6-1: Sinus arrhythmia
6-2: Sinus bradycardia
6-3: Sinus tachycardia
6-4: Paroxysmal Atrial Tachycardia (PAT)
6-5: PAC's
6-6: Atrial bigeminy
6-7: A-flutter
6-8: A-fib
6-9: Wandering Atrial Pacemaker & Multifocal Atrial Tachycardia (MAT)

Continuing southwards...

6-10: Nodal beats
6-11: Junctional "escape" beats
6-12: Escape capture bigeminy
6-13: Junctional rhythms
6-14: Accelerated junctional rhythms

6-15: What if the atria and the ventricles aren't talking to each other? How can I tell?

6-15-1: What is A-V dissociation?
6-15-2: What does "marching out" mean?

Even Further On South... how this FAQ is organized.

What ventricular arrhythmias am I likely to see in the MICU, when should I worry about them, and how are they treated?

7-1: PVCs
7-1-1: What are couplets? Triplets?

7-2: Ventricular bigeminy? Trigeminy, quadrigeminy?
7-3: What is a "run"? What is a "salvo"? What is "Non-sustained ventricular tachycardia"?
7-4: VT
7-5: VF
7-6: What is the difference between "narrow complex" and "wide complex" tachycardia?
7-7: What do I do if I see VT on the monitor?
7-8: What if the patient is still awake?
7-9: What if the patient rolls up her eyes and becomes unresponsive?
7-10: What is a precordial thump? Does it work?
7-11: What if I see VF on the monitor?
7-12: Torsades des Pointes
7-13: AIVR
7-14: Asystole

Things we left out the first time:

8-1: SVT – Supraventricular Tachycardia
8-2: WPW – Wolff-Parkinson-White

9- Quiz Questions

What is an arrhythmia?

By the time they get to the MICU, most people have a good basic idea of what arrhythmias are all about, but enough new people are coming in that we thought it might be helpful to put together a quick review.

The idea that helped me the most in actually understanding what arrhythmias do to people was correlating, or maybe I should say learning to visualize in my head, what the heart was actually doing during one arrhythmia or the other. Each part of the normal cardiac cycle has a specific mechanical event associated with it, and if you can get a mental image in your head of what is, or isn't happening, then the effects of the arrhythmias become much clearer.

The Nodes:

Take a look at the diagram that follows.

Remember these? These are the "intrinsic pacemakers". Not too hard – there's only two of them. First is the sino-atrial node – which lives in the right atrium, in something called the coronary sinus, which I have no idea what exactly is, exactly. Jayne knows – she works in the EP lab… anyhow, there it is in the picture, in yellow up at the top. This is the one that generates P-waves. P-waves travel from the SA to the AV, or atrioventricular node, which lives at the place where the atria and the ventricles join. As the signal travels through the RA, both atria contract.

This is the key thing: **as the signal goes through its part of the heart, that same part of the heart responds mechanically, with movement**.

Well – it's <u>supposed</u> to! (grin! – what if it doesn't? What's that called? What would you do?)

That movement, of one set of chambers or the other – atria or ventricles - is what you want to try to visualize mentally as you think your way through arrythmias. So: **P-wave – atrial contraction**.

Next comes the AV node, which is also called the "junction", and sometimes confusingly called "the node" – even though its sibling up above is also called a node. (I have no idea where this second name came from – anybody know?) The signal that came from the SA node gets to the junction, and is passed along to travel through the ventricles, producing the QRS complex on the EKG. In response to this part of the signal, the ventricles contract. So this time: **QRS – ventricular contraction**.

Let's take a second to look at how **lead II** works:

Negative electrode goes here

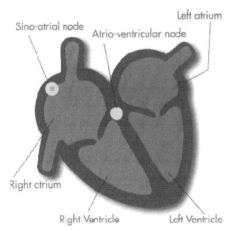

Positive electrode here www.arrhythmia.org/ general/whatis/

43

The point here is that the normal pathway that the signal takes is going <u>from</u> the negative electrode, <u>towards</u> the positive one. See that? Going towards the positive electrode, the signal makes an <u>upward</u> blip on the cardiac monitor.

This is actually really important, and I'll probably make this point too many times, but <u>the direction in which the signal is moving tells you where the beat is coming from</u>. If it makes an upward blip on a lead II, then it has to be moving in the normal direction, towards the positive electrode. So it must be coming from somewhere in the normal pathway: either the SA or the AV node. If the signal goes downwards – meaning, the signal is going the other way, backwards towards the negative electrode – where's it coming from?

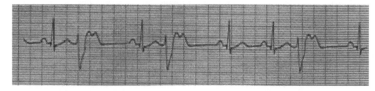

Like these guys. They go downwards, mostly, right? So – they're going the wrong way. Hm. So that means they must be coming from where?

Well… they're PVC's, right?

Premature… aha! - <u>ventricular</u> contractions! They're going backwards because they're <u>coming from the other end of the heart</u>, down in the ventricles, and heading backwards towards the negative electrode in lead II… so the signal goes <u>downwards</u>… bing! Lightbulb go on? Which way are the normal ones headed?

See why Lead II is used as the standard monitoring lead? It reflects the normal conduction path.

A word about depolarization - my son wanted to explain this, because he's figured out what it means. "Depolarization is when you take one of those white bears, and take it away from the arctic – it gets depolarized!" - just so everybody's clear on that one…

The Normal Complex:

Now let's take a quick look at the normal cardiac cycle on the EKG:

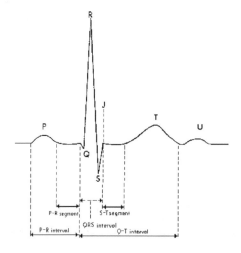

www.bilgi.umedia.org.tr/ yayin/tejm/ekg.htm

This is a pretty good diagram – looks like lead II from a 12-lead EKG. Let's say it again: Lead II is used as the basic reference lead for looking at cardiac rhythms, because it reflects the normal path of the signal moving through the heart. In lead II, the positive electrode is near the apex of the heart - the bottom of the cone formed by the ventricles, pointing southeast; (that's "down and towards the right" for you non-map people – ow! Violent daughter. Who exactly do you think paid for drivers' ed, anyhow?) The negative electrode is up on the right chest near the clavicle, northwest. Now imagine a line drawn connecting the two electrodes. Got that? The normal signal follows that path, moving through the chambers, always towards that positive electrode, making an upward blip on the ekg trace as it does. See those upward blips?

Now – everybody knows where the electrodes go, right?

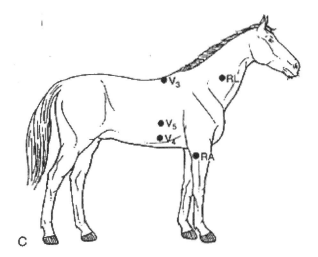

(What do you mean, "Nice picture of your first girlfriend!"?)

1-1: What is a p-wave? What is the PR interval?

So. In lead II, as the signal goes through the small muscle mass of the atria, it generates a small upward wave – you guessed it, the P-wave. Atrial depolarization ends, sort of obviously, at the AV node – at the beginning of the QRS. Actually we ignore the Q-part of the complex in measuring the PR interval. A normal PR interval is supposed to be equal to, or less than .20 seconds (5 little boxes, or one big box on the EKG paper.)

1-2: What if there's no P-wave?

No p-wave means that the SA node hasn't generated a signal. No signal, <u>no atrial</u> <u>motion</u>. Can you live without atrial motion? – probably, although you lose your atrial kick – which they say accounts for something like 25% of your total cardiac output.

1-3: What is the QRS complex?

As the contraction signal gets passed along through the large muscle mass of the ventricles, it generates a large waveform. The QRS is not supposed to be longer than .12 seconds – three little boxes. Longer means the signal is taking longer than it should to get through – maybe there's a bundle branch block?

1-4: What if there's no QRS complex?

No QRS complex means that no signal has gone through the ventricles. No signal, <u>no ventricular motion</u>. Can you live without ventricular motion?

1-5: What is the T-wave? What is the QT interval?

Now that both sets of chambers have contracted, the electrical system resets itself – producing the T-wave. The significant thing we worry about as regards an otherwise normal T-wave is the length of the waveform: from the beginning of the QRS to the end of the T-wave, called the QT interval. A "corrected" QT interval that lasts too long can mean that bad things may be developing – usually one kind of drug toxicity or another – which may show up as nasty tachyarrhythmias like VT. Haldol is infamous for this.

1-6: What if there's no T-wave?

Well – if there's no QRS, there won't be a T-wave. Otherwise, the ventricles are definitely going to have to reset themselves – producing a T-wave of one kind or another. It's very important to remember that T-waves, or more correctly the ST segment of the complex, can change if the patient goes through an MI, or is having an ischemic, or anginal episode. If the T-waves on your patient look different at the end of your shift – get suspicious. There's lots more on ST segments and what they're trying to tell you in the FAQ on "Reading 12-lead EKGs".

1-7: What is the isoelectric line?

Let's look at a normal sinus rhythm strip.

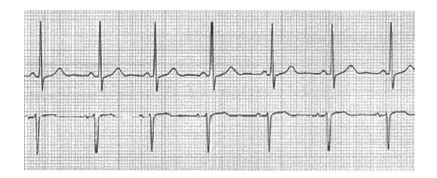

Do you see the area where the line is flat between the beats? After the T-waves, and before the next p-waves? That's the "isoelectric line". When ST segments go up, as in an MI, or down, as in ischemia, what you're hoping is that they will come back to their original positions with treatment, and that position is: where they started out, on the isoelectric line.

2- Why do people have arrhythmias?

Lots of reasons, but if you think about things that are going to make a heart unhappy, then those are the things that will produce arrhythmias acutely: cardiac ischemia, hypoxia, MI, changes in electrolytes…obviously in a situation like this you are going to be treating the underlying problem – either with anti-ischemic treatments in situations like anginal CHF (remember "LMNOP"- Lasix, Morphine, Nitrates, Oxygen and Position); or clot-busting an acute MI – and hopefully this will minimize or even reverse the conditions that are producing the arrhythmias in the first place.

Chronic changes that produce arrhythmias have to do with processes that make cardiac chambers do things over long periods of time that they don't want to do, usually producing an abnormal change in their size. Anything that makes a chamber "stretch" chronically will produce chronic arrhythmias – the classic example is cor pulmonale ("lung-heart" – meaning, heart problems caused by the lungs.) The lungs, remember, are supposed to be nice and soft, and the relatively thin-walled right ventricle doesn't have any trouble sending blood through them. Any process that makes the lungs stiffen up - whether acute or chronic - will increase the pressure needed to send blood through them. Now the RV has to work harder, and since it's not built too powerfully to start with, if it's made to work harder over time, it's going to grow – like your biceps do during weight training (mine never did…).

This chamber growth is actually not a happy thing, because the heart wants to stay small – it works better that way, small and tight – and the bigger it gets, the more stretched and boggy it gets, and this stretching and bogginess characteristically produces arrythmias. I was taught that a stretched-out RV and RA produces atrial fibrillation – the classic arrhythmia of smokers and COPDers. And liver patients. Make sense?

We had another neat example of chronic chamber stretch recently: patient came in with a primary liver tumor that had been treated for a while. He was in a-flutter, probably because the impaired perfusion through the liver had kept his right sided pressures high for a long time. (His CVP was 20, and he was not wet – wasn't making much urine.) Right-sided stretch.

Likewise, anything that makes the left side of the heart grow and stretch will produce arrhythmias – usually the more unpleasant ventricular ones. These will be your CHF patients with low EF – they will often have a certain amount of ventricular ectopy at baseline, and you'll hear people say "Is Mr. Yakowitz allowed to have triplets, or should we wake up the team to look at him?", and someone will answer, "Oh yeah, he has them all the time whenever his K gets below 4, and we're not supposed to call the team unless he starts having long runs."

3- What is the difference between a bad arrhythmia and a not-so-bad arrhythmia?

The key concept: is the patient able to make a blood pressure? I mean, clearly there are lots of other things to consider – for example, a patient may go into VT and maintain a blood pressure nicely, talking to you, maybe complaining of chest pain – would you shock that patient? You would need to know that in VT, a patient may sometimes maintain a pressure for a while, and then lose it abruptly – does this happen with other arrhythmias? It takes time, study and experience to learn your way around these situations – <u>don't</u> feel bad if you find that it takes you quite a while. It takes years to get comfortable in the ICU. I'm still waiting…

Let's try the visualization thing to see if it helps to analyze the threat that is produced by one arrhythmia or the other. Here's an example – you've probably seen people with this.

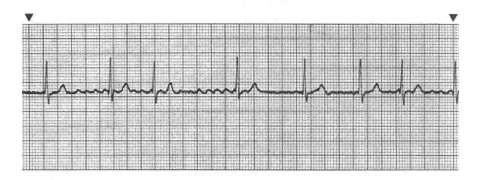

Right – here we are in A-fib. Are there P-waves? Hmm – maybe? What are those fluttery looking waves along the isoelectric line? Not really p's. So - no P-waves means: no kind of normal atrial contraction. Are there QRS's? Definitely. So there are <u>ventricular</u> contractions – and how many in a minute? This looks like a six-second strip - count the QRS's and multiply by 10 to get the ventricular contractions in one minute. Everybody get 70? (Don't count that last QRS at the end – it's beyond the 6-second measurement).

Should this patient be able to maintain a nice blood pressure with a rate of 70? Probably – the ventricles need time to fill up, and at this rate they're probably filling very nicely. A lot depends on the strength of the ventricle – the "ejection fraction". There's all sorts of good stuff about EF, and filling pressures and the like in the PA-line FAQ.

Now the mental part. (My wife laughs at this point.) In my mind, when I see a-fib, I think of the atria, uh… fibrillating. Remember the "bag of worms", which is how they describe what a fibrillating ventricle looks like? Same thing, but up on top. The ventricles, I can see, should be pumping properly, because there is a normally upright QRS – this means that the path of conduction is travelling in the right direction through the ventricular muscle mass, just the way it normally should – so they're at least conducting okay.

> The important points in this situation:

> - I recognize this as A-fib, which is a fairly "stable" arrhythmia – it may be cheating in a FAQ for new RNs to say that the old guy already recognizes the rhythm, but we learn by example, right?

> - The ventricular rate is not too fast. This is a very important concept in grasping the significance of arrhythmias: speed matters - usually we're talking about ventricular speed here. Ventricles beating at a rate of 200 bpm have no time to physically fill up with blood – therefore they don't have much blood in them to pump out – therefore cardiac output and blood pressure fall, and other bad things like death may ensue. Too slow a rate may have the same result – sure, the ventricles have all the time they

need to fill, but at such a slow rate, the cardiac output is still too low to maintain a blood pressure. What's the ventricular rate in the strip above – 70, we said? Sounds good to me. If the ventricular rate is kept around this range, the patient will probably do fine.

- A helpful basic concept: the ventricles do most of the pumping in generating a blood pressure. The rule is, no matter what else is happening, if the ventricular rate is somewhere near the normal range of sinus rhythm – say 60 to 100 bpm, then the resulting blood pressure will probably be all right. Probably. (grin!)

4- What is "ectopy"?

"Ectopic" means: "something occurring where it isn't supposed to". Pregnancy anywhere in the body but the uterus is "ectopic pregnancy". Seizures result from ectopic electrical activity in the brain. If the signal that starts a heartbeat originates from someplace other than it's supposed to, it's also called ectopic.

Two points to make here: first, you'll remember learning years ago that cardiac tissue has the property of "automaticity" – which means it is able, all of it in one way or another, of acting as a pacemaker, not connected in any way to the normal, built-in pacemaker/conduction system.

Second, the heart responds to the fastest signal it receives. This means, for example, that if the AV node should wake up and start feeling frisky and quick, it could capture and pace the heart if it were generating a rate faster than the SA node. (CCU nurses in the audience – what arrhythmia would this be?)

The result is that electrical pacemakers can pop up just about anywhere – in the atria or in the ventricles, and if they produce a beat sooner than the current pacemaker (I'm talking about built-in, natural pacemakers here) does, that ectopic beat will capture the heart. For example, a single PAC. Or a single PVC. The idea is that these signals are premature, arriving sooner, at a faster rate than whatever else is normally pacing the heart. As a result, they capture.

Or, if it's a sequence of rapid signals, it will capture the heart for as long as that sequence lasts – any examples from the audience? VT for sure. SVT also for sure – rapid Afib as well. (Pardon me – supposed to say: "A-fib with RVR" – rapid ventricular response...) The normal, slower rhythm will not recapture the heart until the faster rhythm is controlled – and if the rapid rhythm doesn't allow the ventricles enough time to fill, there you have your lethal arrythmia situation. More on these later.

5- What is "supraventricular"?

You'd think that this meant "atrial" in reference to arrythmias, but I believe we're supposed to add AV-nodal (sometimes called "junctional", or just "nodal") rhythms to this group.

6- What are the supraventricular arrhythmias that I'm likely to see in the MICU, which ones do I need to worry about, and how are they treated?

Let's begin by looking at normal sinus rhythm – the normal supraventricular rhythm:

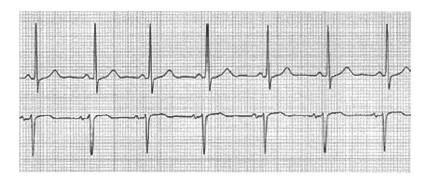

Look familiar? Normal intervals, rate in the 70's – nice! Everybody see the p-waves – the little ones in front of the big ones? Then the QRS's, which are the big ones. Then the t-waves, coming after the QRS's...

Here are some of the common supraventricular arrythmias – some aren't really so common, but you should have a basic grip on them anyhow.

6-1: Sinus arrhythmia

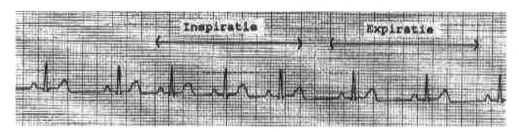

This is not one to worry about, as far as I know. Sinus arrhythmia is when the normal sinus rate speeds up and slows down slightly, varying with respiration. In 26-odd years I've never seen any physician show the slightest concern about this one. (French website...)

6-2: Sinus Bradycardia

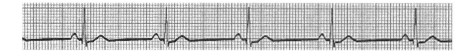

Here's a nice sinus bradycardia, rate in the 50's. Everyone remember what the intrinsic rate is for the SA node: 60 to 100bpm, right? Is this rhythm coming from the SA node? Sure – see the p-waves? But it's slow, isn't it? – "bradycardia", of sinus origin. Sinus bradycardia is sometimes a good thing – it means your patient has finally fallen asleep, or that her metoprolol is finally starting to work. A <u>really</u> slow bradycardia is not such a good thing – clearly, you don't make much of a blood pressure with a rate of 20.

Scenarios causing sinus bradycardia:

- Inferior MIs – "IMI"s – are classically famous for producing brady episodes, where the patient's rate drops to the twenties, and you run into the room and give a milligram of atropine, and start looking around for the external pacing pads. If I'm getting a patient with an acute IMI, I put a vial of atropine in the room just for good voodoo. Mojo. Whatever.

- Sedation: being sedate will drop most people's heart rates.

- Ischemia: definitely. If you think about it, you'll remember that there are three main coronary arteries – these perfuse the SA and AV nodes, and if the nodes become unhappy, then arrhythmias certainly result. As with an IMI, in the case of ischemia in inferior territory, the RCA is usually the problem… there's lots more on the coronary arteries, where they go, and how they show up electrocardiographically in "Reading 12-lead EKGs".

6-3: Sinus Tachycardia

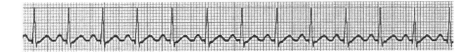

Sinus tachycardia – pretty easy. P-waves? Yes. So the rhythm is coming from the sinus node. What's the rate – somewhere near 130? So, faster than the normal range of 60-100. Tachycardia. Let's do the mental thing just quickly: P-waves mean that the atria are contracting, QRS's mean that the ventricles are too, and in the right order, atria first, ventricles second. Which is of course better than if they're doing it backwards – or even simultaneously, which does happen sometimes.

Reasons for sinus tachycardia:

- Agitation, pain or distress – pretty easy.

- Fever – also pretty easy.

- Dehydration – anything that decreases the circulating volume for any reason will produce a rise in heart rate, as the body tries to keep blood pressure up. Dehydration would mean a relative loss of water in the circulation, but certainly blood loss will do the same thing. There's lots more on how blood pressures work in "Pressors and Vasoactives", and "PA – Lines".

- There can certainly be combinations – it wouldn't be unusual at all to see all three of these conditions at once in a septic patient. Remember – sinus tachycardia is usually something the body is doing on purpose, for a reason, such as trying to maintain a blood pressure. Don't be too anxious to start giving drugs like beta-blockers in tachycardic situations until you have some idea of why the patient is doing what they're doing. (The exception would be during an acute MI. Hearts get tachycardic during MIs, usually because their owners are in pain, or terrified, or both. Bad.)

6-4: Paroxysmal Atrial Tachycardia (PAT)

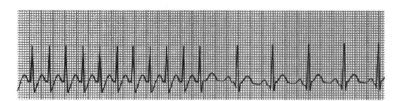

PAT is a very rapid supraventricular rhythm that comes from the atria – usually it runs at a very rapid rate, about 250-300bpm. You sometimes see young people have short bursts of this rhythm, which in my experience doesn't last more than a couple of seconds. How much caffeine did they drink today? This strip shows the PAT breaking spontaneously to NSR. It may set your alarms off – unless it persists, most physicians don't get too involved with this. Document it. If it persists – as what you would then probably call SVT - things could get ugly, in the sense that the blood pressure might suffer – what drugs would you think about having on hand for this? Might need a machine, too.

6-5: PAC's: (Premature Atrial Contractions)

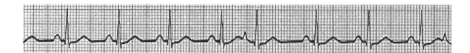

Here are some nice premature atrial contractions. That is, we assume that the heart is contracting in response to these signals. Anyhow, if you look at the early beat – 5th complex, right? – you'll see that it has a different P-wave shape (the impressive word for shape is "morphology"), meaning that it comes from someplace other than the normal sinus node. (My son loves to find little words that mean the same as big ones. "Yo Ralphie! Your face has a weird morphology!") Ectopic. The other thing you'll notice is that it comes too soon – it's premature. Coming sooner than the normal SA node impulse, the PAC captures the heart, just for that one beat – then that ectopic source (an ectopic pacemaker is often called a "focus") shuts off again, and the regular sinus rhythm comes back. To speak impressively, remember to say that the different p-wave "has a different morphology, arising from an ectopic focus". Wooo….

PACs don't get physicians worried, as a rule. The thing to worry about is: if they start getting too frequent, it may mean that a-fib is coming.

6-6: Atrial bigeminy – this means that every other beat is a PAC. Again – afib may be coming.

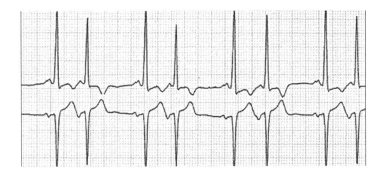

6-7: Atrial Flutter

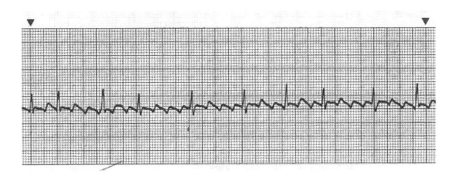

Right – here we are in atrial flutter. Pretty! Remember: a normal, upward QRS means that the conduction from the AV node on down is in a normal direction – assuming this is a lead II. That means that conduction through the ventricles is happening the way it's supposed to.

So what are the atria doing here? Who said "fluttering"? (I seem to be visualizing an audience here.) You in the back, very good. How did you guess? You get to buy lunch. Right – the atria, if you looked at them, would be contracting at about what rate – you guys know how to count boxes to determine rates, right? We'll get to that later – in a-flutter, the atria contract at a rate around 300 bpm. Are all the signals from the atria being conducted to the ventricles? No? Good thing! Would the ventricles have time to fill if every atrial signal made the ventricles contract – at a rate of 300 bpm? Nope! What's the ventricular rate? Six-second strip, count the QRS complexes, multiply by 10 – about 100 – close enough to a normal sinus rate to tell us that the patient is probably going to generate a decent pressure with this rhythm.

What's the ratio of atrial to ventricular contractions here? 300 atrial bpm, 100 ventricular bpm – I would call this "3-to-one a-flutter", and I would document the rhythm carefully strip-wise, but seeing this rhythm wouldn't make me very nervous. A-flutter is usually transient – people don't stay in it too long, because they're usually on the way towards developing a-fib.

Another point worth mentioning – the ventricles are responding to roughly one out of three signals here, right? This is called the "ventricular response rate". Duh. But obviously, it matters a lot, because if the response rate gets too high, then the chambers don't fill, and the pressure drops, and etc. What if the ratio were 2-to-1? What would the ventricular response rate be? Around 150 – not too too fast, but pretty darn fast, faster than I'd like to see my patient go, especially some older MICU patient who gets ischemic very easily – what in this case would be called "rate-related ischemia". I would definitely wake up the team for an episode of 2:1 flutter, for that very reason – in the old days physicians would compress one of the carotids to try to provoke the "carotid body response" – namely, bradycardia, specifically by slowing AV node conduction – partly a diagnostic, and partly a therapeutic maneuver. (We used to call this "doing the neck thing", as in "Are they gonna do the neck thing?") You would look for the ratio to change – fewer QRS's.

I got lucky hunting around – here's a really neat strip of someone "doing the neck thing", otherwise known as "carotid sinus massage".

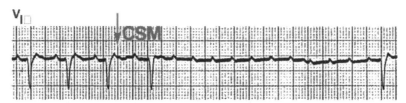

**Atrial flutter with 2:1 block responding to corotid
sinus massage (CSM)**

Nowadays they don't do the neck thing much any more, since people with carotid disease don't usually enjoy it too well – threatens the brain, and all – although some physicians will do it if they don't hear any carotid bruits on exam. Instead you may see maneuvers with verapamil, sometimes metoprolol, sometimes adenosine – I've seen all of them work, but my experience leans toward verapamil in this situation. I hate adenosine – ten seconds of total terror…

6-8: Atrial fibrillation –

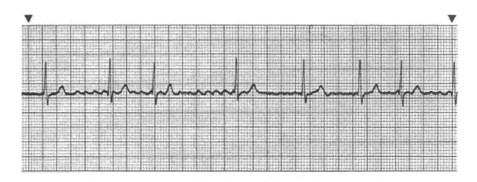

Okay, here's the nice picture of a-fib that we looked at earlier. A-fib is a pretty similar scenario to a-flutter – the atria are doing the worm dance, and only the occasional signal gets conducted through the AV node to the ventricles, which is a good thing! Remember, you want the ventricular rate to be something like what the normal sinus rate would be – 60's to about 100. Let's do the mental thing – what are the atria doing? Is there a nice stable p-wave? No. Can you visualize the motion of the atria? Bzzzzz – fibrillating, and not contracting in any organized way. Signals are not coming from organized sources, or "foci", but from all over the atrial tissue, simultaneously. Some signals are getting through the AV node and being delivered to the ventricles – again, they speak of "ventricular response rate" – you'll hear people describe an episode of "rapid afib with RVR" – rapid ventricular response – which may require a quick cardioversion back into sinus rhythm to restore a failing pressure. Or the patient might need IV blocking agents of one kind or another – betas, calciums, digoxin maybe (takes a day to work), to bring the RVR down to a rate that produces a better pressure.

Once brought under control rate-wise, afib in and of itself is a stable arrhythmia, but it does have a couple of significant bad things that go with it:

First, fibrillating atria don't empty themselves very well. The result is that clots can form in them, and if the a-fib suddenly converts back to sinus rhythm, those clots will get shot out into the circulation – arterial or venous, or both – off to the lungs if on the right side, producing a PE, or if on the left, then off to all sorts of interesting places down the arterial tree, such as brain, or foot, or mesenteric artery (producing bowel infarct), or elsewhere. "Paroxysmal a-fib" as a result is seen, rightly, as very dangerous. What could you do to prevent this from happening – not the a-fib, I mean, but the clots? Audience? Right – anticoagulation. Acutely, with heparin, long-term with coumadin. What if the patient was HIT positive?

Continuing southwards…

Working our way south from the SA node, the next source of arrythmias is the AV node, otherwise called the "junction" – or just "the node", as in producing "nodal rhythms".

6-9: Wandering Atrial Pacemaker & Multifocal Atrial Tachycardia

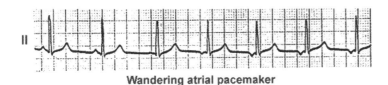

Wandering atrial pacemaker

Here's a rhythm you see once in a while – see how the p-waves have a number of different morphologies? (79 cents for the word, please.) The idea here is that the atrial focus shifts from the SA node to the atrial tissue, in various places, each of which generates it's own signal, which goes on to capture. If the rate is less than 100, they call it WAP – if it's over 100, the name changes to Multifocal Atrial Tachycardia.

6-10: Premature nodal beats

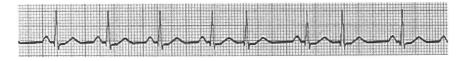

Everybody see something strange in beats 5 and 7? Are they early? Sure. Are they PACs? There's no p-wave, is there? But look – the direction of the QRS is normal – this means the signal is moving in the normal direction through the ventricles.

These are premature nodal, or junctional beats. No p-wave means they're not coming from the atria. What's happening here is that sometimes the junction, for reasons of its own – will accelerate somewhat and send out premature beats, which very nicely depolarize the ventricles in the normal southward direction. My experience is that these are considered benign – that doesn't mean that they are benign, but I've never seen anything done acutely about them.

6-11: Junctional "escape" beats

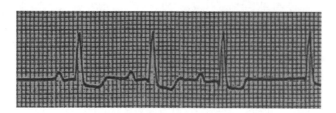

Here's the opposite of premature nodal activity. Here's a nodal beat – no p-wave, and normal QRS conduction, just like in a sinus beat. But is it early? No – actually it's a little late. This is a rescue situation, not unlike demand pacing. The SA node, for some reason, probably ischemia, is slowing – and the AV node, like a demand pacemaker, senses the time difference, and jumps in with a beat to replace the one from the SA that never came. They call this an "escape beat" – I think of it more as a "rescue beat". The AV node loyally sits there passing along beats from above, all it's life, and then one day, the SA node gets hit by some bad cheeseburger byproduct, and the AV node wakes up and starts delivering a rhythm on it's own. If you're lucky. If not – you know how to work the external pacemaker, right?

As you work your way through all these rhythms, try to get a sense of which beats are coming early, which are coming late, and why. The early, or premature beats are the ectopic ones, coming from someplace that they're not supposed to. The late beats, at least these nodal ones, aren't ectopic really, because they do come from an "intrinsic pacemaker", right? – the AV node. I think of the premature beats as "abnormal" more than I do the nodal ones, except that the nodal beats wouldn't be appearing if the SA node weren't in trouble…

6-12: Escape capture bigeminy

This is a complicated name for the rhythm in which sinus beats alternate with nodal escape beats. This is probably happening for an unhappy reason, like MI or ischemia affecting the SA node – the AV node is having to rescue the rhythm with every other beat – I'd worry if I saw this one, because heart block might be coming. Any disease process that affects the rhythm that much has probably done some real damage to the SA node. There's lots more (why do I keep hearing this phrase?) about heart blocks and pacemakers in the FAQ files with those titles.

6-13: Junctional rhythms

medlib.med.utah.edu/kw/ecg/mml/ecg_junctional.html

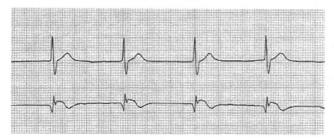

Everybody see what's different about this one – what's going on here? Let's be systematic about it: are there p-waves? I don't see any. But do the QRS's look normal? Yup, normal. So what have we got - let's visualize this please – you in the back, you all visualizing this? Are the atria doing anything? Not that I can tell, they aren't. Ventricles? Yes they are. And since the QRS's appear normal, this means that the rhythm has to be coming from the junction, and going southwards. Everybody see that? What about the rate? About 40. Perfect! Junctional! Dude!

6-14: Accelerated junctional rhythms

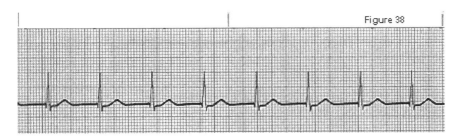

Figure 38

This ought to be pretty much the last of the supraventricular rhythms that we're going to look at. I'm sure there are more, but these cover pretty much the ones you run into in the MICU setting. As usual, please let me know what I've left out!

This is a junctional rhythm too, but obviously it's faster - 80's - than the normal 40-60 rate that you'd expect. Anybody know why this happens? – I have no idea. It's generally considered benign – one thing that does matter however is that the patient loses whatever atrial kick they had – this can be as much as 25% of the total cardiac output. Like a-fib…

6-15: What if the atria and the ventricles aren't talking to each other? How can I tell?

6-15-1: What is AV dissociation?

I'll explain this as I understand it (which is what everybody does, right?) – this can happen in a couple of different ways, for a couple of different reasons. Here's the first one:

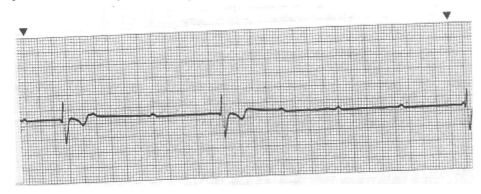

You all know complete heart block when you see it? Look at all those p-waves floating around, lonely, on an empty isoelectric sea with no QRS's to talk to. Here's how to tell if your patient's atria and ventricles aren't communicating: it has to do with the relative rates. What's the atrial rate here? Let's count boxes going to the right from the p-wave just above the "?" in the first line of this paragraph: 300-150-100-70 – somewhere in the sixties. How about the ventricular rate? Yow! – wicked slow, as we say up here in Mass. – somewhere around 20. And irregular, at that.

The SA and AV nodes aren't communicating very often, if at all, and the AV node isn't doing much, although it seems to be trying.

Is there:

- "a": any kind of visible relationship between the p's and the qrs's that you can see?

- Or "b": are the p's just sort of appearing in amongst the QRS's at random? I'd say "b". And is there any kind of predictable ratio between the p's and the qrs's? Such as 2:1, or even 8:1, or some varying number? Not really. Take a look at the "Heart Block" FAQ for more on this subject.

Oh, yeah – just by the way – why is this happening? What would you do in this situation?

Here's the second scenario:

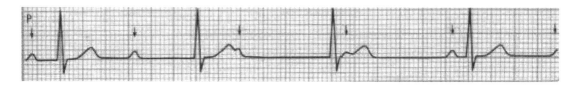

The folks who recorded this strip have helpfully put little arrows showing that the p-waves are actually popping up all over the place. Even though the last complex looks normal, that's actually just a lucky hit – the atria are doing their thing, and the ventricles are doing theirs, but they're not on speaking terms. Ready for another question? Where are the QRS's originating?

This is almost the same thing as complete heart block – actually, it probably is complete heart block, but difference is in the ventricular rate. Complete heart block usually describes the first situation, in which the junction isn't generating much of a rate at all.

This second strip describes the situation that people call "A-V dissociation" – it involves the same kind of non-communication, and probably for the same reasons: ischemia or MI, but produces a different effect. This person is a bit luckier than the one above. Clearly! This time the AV node is still able to work in "escape", or "rescue" mode. But the signal isn't going across the little bridge there, from the a's to the v's.

Now – just because this one looks a bit better doesn't mean that things are ok! Something has hit the signal transmission system, hard!, (what kind of MI would it probably be?), and you'd better know who's on in the cath lab… remember, the AV node is not a reliable pacemaker – it can poop out at unpredictable times, and there you are, up the cardiac creek without an escape rhythm to paddle with.

But do you see how the clue to dissociation is that the rates are different? – that's the clue that the nodes aren't communicating. Usually the atria are inhibited in a junctional tachycardia – sometimes a signal coming from the AV node will actually depolarize the atria backwards – upwards! This can show up in a couple of ways: the p-wave may be abnormally short, maybe upside down, maybe on top of the QRS. All in all – something isn't right, because the signal transmission isn't happening the right way. Watch these folks carefully.

6-15-2: What does "marching out" mean?

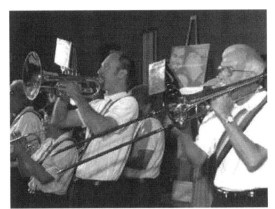

This is actually simple – it means that impulses, or signals, no matter where they're coming from, are coming regularly: either p-waves, or QRS's. This is where calipers come in handy. Take another look at the first strip of complete heart block above. Now take your calipers, and point one end at one of those sad little p-waves floating around all alone, and put the other end on the p-wave nearest to it. Now, holding the calipers with the points in that position, see if the p-waves coming before and then after those two are coming in regular rhythm, which on EKG paper means: "the same distance apart". They do on this strip, right? They march out. The caliper points always touch two p-waves, no matter which one you use to start with. So now you know that at least one pacemaker is trying to work properly. Which one is it? How about the AV node? Do the QRS's march out? Can you even tell? How about in the second strip?

Even Further On South...

Everybody's starting to realize how this file is organized, right? The first part is about arrhythmias coming from the upper part of the heart, and we're moving downwards in sequence. Just making sure everyone was awake…

7- What ventricular arrhythmias am I likely to see in the MICU, when should I worry about them, and how are they treated?

7-1: <u>PVCs</u> - Premature Ventricular Contractions

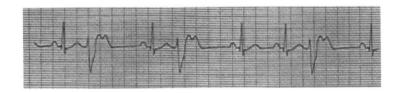

These are pretty easy to recognize. A couple of points to make:

<u>Premature</u> ventricular contractions – they're early, as in the strip above- which is to say they come sooner, or faster, than the sinus beat would. Since they're faster, they capture.

<u>Ventricular</u>: They're ectopic, coming from a focus somewhere in, uh… the ventricles!

Why do they look so strange? Let's put this one to the audience. Why do PVCs look the way they do? The clue is: which way is the signal travelling?

Why are they happening? Context is everything. If your patient has been in perfect sinus rhythm, and suddenly develops PVCs, your task is to figure out if something has changed. Or the other way – have the PVCs suddenly gone away? Then again, some people have chronic ventricular ectopy – they may even have short bursts of VT – these will usually be patients with stretched, boggy hearts: people who have had a couple of MIs, people with cardiomyopathy, CHF patients – you get the idea. We say: "Oh, he's allowed to have short runs, he has lots of ectopy all the time. What's his last Mag?"

Things that cause PVCs: by now this should be clear enough – anything that interferes with the delivery of blood; things that make the heart unhappy: ischemia, MI, hypoxia, electrolyte problems.

PVCs may or may not make a blood pressure. You can observe this really well if your patient has an a-line – just look at the arterial waveform following the PVC – is the wave lower than one following a sinus beat? Probably. If your patient has a run of PVCs – are they all lower than the sinus pressure? Did your patient lose pressure completely with the run? You'll see nurses respond to a VT alarm by going over to the central monitor, looking at the printer strip, and saying "Wow, he doesn't perfuse those beats very well! Sure looks like VT to me - the team has been having a hard time figuring out exactly what the rhythm is. Whatever it is, he doesn't like it very much."

This is an essential point of "surviving" the arrythmias that you will run into in the MICU. Your patient may make a fast rhythm of one kind or another, the cardiologists may have a great time debating whether it's "type-2-accelerated-idioventricular-rhythm", or "rapid-a-fib-with re-entrant-something", or "nonsustained-supraventricular-tachycardia with pre-excitation syndrome of the Lown-Ganong" something else… – your immediate problem is what? All together now: Is the patient making a blood pressure? If she is, this does not mean (obviously) that you can now go downstairs for lunch! Get the patient seen by the team, don't leave the room - the rhythm may deteriorate into something you will recognize – as bad!

7-1-1: What are couplets? Triplets?

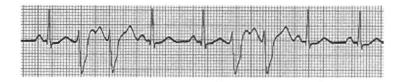

Couplets are easy – two PVCs in a row. Again, context is everything. Has your patient had couplets before? Or never before? Is she doing something clinically – having chest pain, getting hypoxic, sweating, getting restless? Is her K+ low, or magnesium? Is she acidotic?

Or is this an improvement? Has she been having long runs of VT, which are now going away because you started lidocaine?

Are you sure that's actually your patient? (Not a stupid question when you're using remote central monitoring.)

So, couplets: easy to recognize, but don't forget to try to figure out what they're telling you.

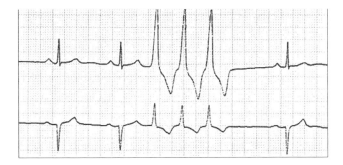

Triplets: same as couplets, except three PVCs in a row.

7-2: What is bigeminy? Trigeminy, quadrigeminy?

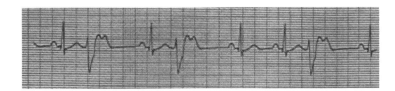

Bigeminy means that every other beat is ectopic. Trigeminy means the same, for every third beat. Quadrigeminy for every fourth. This strip goes from bi- to tri-. Once again – put this into context: is this acute or chronic? Does his ectopy go away if his K, or his Mag is low? How would you treat the low K? Would you take KCl on an empty stomach? What do BUN and creatinine have to do with giving K replacement?

7-3: What is a "run"? What is a "salvo"? (Ahoy!) What is "non-sustained VT?"

These are all pretty much interchangeable terms for a series of PVCs that's "longer than a triplet". Some runs are short – maybe 6 beats long, some are lots longer, but the main idea is that the run stops by itself, and the rhythm goes back to whatever (hopefully stable) it was before. You'll hear the alarm go off, and the board will say "VT alarm" – your job is to check things out: go to the patient's room, then go over to the printer and look at the strip printout.

Round up the usual suspects: are the runs coming when the patient is doing something else that might indicate trouble? Angina, diaphoresis, changes in electrolytes, hypoxia, fluid overload, evolving an MI? What is this run of VT trying to tell you? Or is the patient "allowed to have runs of VT"? Maybe he shouldn't!

A lot of the VT alarms are artifact caused by people moving, or scratching. Water in corrugated O2 tubing can collect in the bend where the tube hangs down, and vibrate as the air is pushed through – I've seen this produce artifact that looks just like VT. Chest PT will do it.

What you have to do though, is to darn well go down to that printer and check the alarm printout <u>every single time</u>. No exceptions. You might think: "Well, Mr. Gerbilowitz has had artifact 32 times already this shift", but you'd hate to be wrong… Often artifact problems can be fixed by changing chest electrodes – I usually take them all off, and replace the whole set. Another useful trick is to move the electrodes inwards on the chest towards the borders of the heart – people who have lost cardiac muscle mass often have very small ekg complexes, and you can see them much better this way.

7-4: VT

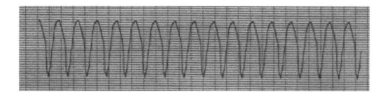

<u>www.mediscan.co.uk</u>

Now things are starting to get a little scary. Now is when you need to remember your ACLS class, and/or your defib class. Take a look at the faq on "Defibrillation".

Same phenomenon as a triplet, except "sustained". VT is really one of the scariest things that comes up in the MICU, along with it's nasty cousin VF. This might be a good place to talk about lethal emergencies.

> - <u>Rule one</u>: do your best to keep from getting panicky. Always remember that the MICU is a group process. You are never, ever alone. Senior staff nurses are always around.

> - Subrule to rule number one: the only way to get over being afraid of these situations is to spend a lot of time in the unit doing them. Everyone has trouble with this at first.

> - <u>Rule two</u>: remember the basics, and keep it simple.

Let's take a minute at this point, and walk through a scenario briefly. The VT alarm goes off – you turn your head to look at the central monitor, and there it is – the real thing. You immediately go into VT yourself, but because you are probably about a third of your patient's age, you still make a blood pressure, so you can still stay upright. You bolt for the patient's room.

First move is? Call for help as you run.

Second move? Always the same – let us stress this: **look at the patient.** Is she smiling at you? Comatose? Seizing? This is what the CPR course means by "establishing unresponsiveness". You need to know that some patients can make an adequate blood pressure with VT, maybe for a short time, maybe for quite a while. They may be awake, may be having chest pain, may not be feeling anything at all. You do **not** want to start running a code on a patient who is awake! This is what ACLS is all about – learning what to do in different situations.

Let's take the unresponsive scenario. Very important, you must say the following words very loudly: "Annie, Annie, are you all right?". This usually works in class, anyhow. She never says much though – unresponsive. You've run down the hall, called for help, you arrive in the room, you determine that the patient is not responsive. Is the rhythm still VT? Old guy that I am, I would thump this patient – I've done it enough through the years to know that it works sometimes. This has become a debatable move nowadays, and it's been a while since I took ACLS – can anybody clear this up from the group?

I remember one episode: I was standing by the bed in the patient's room, and the crisis alarm went off – I heard it coming from her bedside monitor, about a foot above my head as well as from the hallway. I looked up – VT! Low, or no blood pressure on her A-line trace. I looked down – her eyes had closed, she was shivering – maybe seizing? I thumped her – this all happened in about the space of seven seconds. She broke immediately into sinus rhythm. The team came bolting into the room at the call of the nurses at the station, who'd seen the rhythm on the central monitor – and came to a screeching halt, burning rubber. They looked at the monitor, looked at the patient, looked at me, standing there with my fist in the air. I looked at the monitor, looked at the patient, looked at them. Yikes!

Where were we? – oh yes. Keep it simple. Remember that stuff in Basic Life Support CPR about A, B and C – Airway, Breathing, and Circulation? Same deal applies. Lethal arrhythmia?- sure, you want to shock them, but remember to get the backboard under them, start compressions, establish an airway – here, let's scenario-ize this one too.

Alarm goes off. Mr. Hamsterowitz is in VT – not artifact this time. You run down the hall from the central monitor, you're calling for help, you try not to plow into the other nurse coming from the opposite direction. There's Mr. Hamsterowitz – not looking too good. Bedside monitor clearly shows VT. No BP – well, maybe a little BP on the A-line trace. Not enough to perfuse his head, clearly, since he is really not responsive. First move? I'd thump him. I understand that this has to do nowadays with "witnessed" vs. "unwitnessed" events – as far as I'm concerned, in the MICU they're all witnessed, so I'd thump him. Do not let thumping or anything else get in the way of defib maneuvers, however.

Second move – did he break from VT with the thump? No? Get him lying down, get the board under him – one poor nurse I know, in her first code, swung the backboard over the bed and clocked the nurse on the other side, right upside the head. Start compressions. Is the airway open? No? Is he in VT because he aspirated a piece of steak? Did you have to push his dinner tray out of the way when you got into the room? How are you going to clear his airway in this position?

Or: airway's open? Got an oral airway in place? Good motion of the chest with the ambu-bag? Holding his chin the right way? Remember how to hold his chin?

Here's an important point that I try to emphasize: take your time. Doesn't sound right, does it? But look, you're in a very controlled environment. You have all the personnel and equipment around you that you need. You have what – 3 to 6 minutes before the patient sustains anoxic brain damage, and that's if you're not doing <u>anything</u>! So you really do have all the time you need. Take a deep breath, and take a few seconds, and just think of the ABCs – then get on with the fancy stuff.

Okay, here comes the defibrillator. What's the rule nowadays? – it's been a while since I did ACLS. For VT, I learned that the maneuver to make was to do a synchonized cardioversion. Let me lean over and ask my wife, who is an ACLS instructor. Okay – here's the word. For pulseless

VT – shock the patient as if they were in ventricular fibrillation; that's to say, unsynchronized DC countershock, starting with 200 joules. Didn't work? 300 joules. Still didn't work? 360 joules. For VT with a pulse, if they're unresponsive but very hypotensive, she says you can try doing a synchonized cardioversion at 200 joules, but it may not be worth it. Make sure they're not awake! Don't forget the paddle gel! (Update comment – recently we changed to the new biphasic defibrillators, and the joule numbers are different. Assignment to the class – somebody look these up and send them in.There's more on defibrillators, how they work, and what joules and things are in the Defibrillation FAQ. We'll have to update that one too.)

One more point. There really is no reason to yell and scream and shout in a code. A well-run code is quiet. There may indeed be lots of activity, but the basics, the basics, the basics are being done – A, B, and C are established, IV access is established, drugs are coming in, equipment is being used – you have a great deal to contribute by staying calm, and communicating your sense of calm to the others. You'd be amazed how much this can help. Don't yell. Speak clearly. Make sure someone is in command – it may have to be you at first! Give the process time – I always say that the first, oh, 125 codes are the toughest…(grin!)

7-5: VF – Ventricular Fibrillation

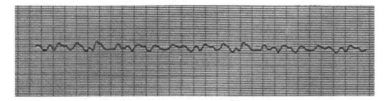

Here's another big scary one. For this one you want to shock them as soon as possible, no cardioversion, no synchronization, no nothing but electricity, 200 joules, as quickly as possible, followed if necessary by 300, then 360 joules. Keep the paddles on the patient's chest between shocks. Establish ABC, get ACLS going.

7-6: What is the difference between "narrow complex" and "wide complex" tachycardia?

We're speaking honestly here? Well honestly, I think there's a reason why the Great Nursing Supervisor invented cardiologists. Narrow or wide complex, my concern is: are they making a blood pressure? If they are – call for help and monitor closely. If they're not, call for help and start a code. This is not to say that narrow versus wide doesn't exist, or matter – they do, and it does, and you will see this kind of thing. But the practical principle for you as the person at the bedside is always the same – is the patient perfusing with this rhythm? Get all the help you need. I guess I should say that my own interpretation is that wider complexes tend to be coming from lower down, and therefore are probably VTs – and that narrower complexes are probably coming from higher up, and may be things like SVTs – supraventricular tachycardias. Compare the VF strip to the PAT strip, and you'll clearly see the difference.

7-7: What do I do if I see VT on the monitor?

Pretty much as described above. Try to remember which patients are DNR… make sure you get the strip from the printer. If the run breaks on it's own, count the beats in the run, and document it that way: "Patient had two episodes of wide-complex tachycardia (ha!), one 22 beats, the other 30 beats. Potassium and magnesium repleted, am levels pending., O2 sat > 95%, strips taped to flow sheet."

7-8: What if the patient is still awake?

Don't shock her! Don't thump her either. Call for help, get the team to the bedside, monitor her closely because she may lose her pressure at any time – at which point you <u>can</u> thump, or shock her. Patients in this situation are <u>very tenuous</u> - watch them very carefully. Usually the goal here is "chemical cardioversion" – up until very recently all these maneuvers were made with lidocaine boluses and drips, followed sometimes by procainamide, but just recently I understand that amiodarone has come into the situation. Here's my wife, also a MICU old-timer, speaking from the couch on this subject: "People still use lidocaine in this situation because that's what they always did, so they just keep doing it, but it's of indeterminate value." (Can you tell that she's in grad school?) "There have been no studies that show that lidocaine is really effective – it's all anecdotal. There's been one really good study out of Seattle called the ARREST study, that showed significant improvement in this kind of situation when people were treated with amiodarone." Whoa! You go, my girl!

Update: yup – amiodarone. Either 150 or 300mg IV followed by an appropriate drip…

7-9: What if the patient rolls up her eyes and becomes unresponsive?

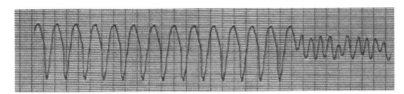

This is why you were watching them…

7-10: What is a precordial thump? Does it work?

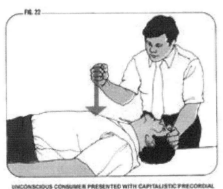

UNCONSCIOUS CONSUMER PRESENTED WITH CAPITALISTIC PRECORDIAL CHEST THUMP IN ORDER TO STIMULATE ECONOMIC ACTIVITY.

Jayne says that they don't teach this maneuver any more in ACLS, but that most experienced folks use it. The thump is a carefully delivered punch in the chest – (my parents always taught me not to hit people, so this is hard for me). The idea is to strike downwards with your fist onto the middle of the sternum, right around where you'd do compressions, from a height of about 18 inches, full force, hitting with the fleshy part of your fist instead of the knuckles. I've seen this work myself, as I've mentioned above, and I'd always want people to know how useful it can be. You'll hear the old nurses stand up when they see VT, and yell down the hall: "Hit him!"
http://www.medgadget.com/archives/img/thump.jpg

7-11: What if I see VF on the monitor?

Make sure you look at the patient before you code him! Here's a relevant story from awhile ago – during the last Ice Age, seems to me. I was working with a new nurse on one of the floors. She had a patient on a monitor, portable job outside in the corridor, and the nurse's task was to read the monitor every hour, and document the rhythm. A really frightened shout from the nurse down the hall – I bolt down there – the patient's wires had come loose, she'd seen something scary on the monitor… next night, same nurse, same patient, another shout from down the hall – the patient was in unresponsive VF. Full code. No go. Holy cow – that was literally twenty years ago, the last time I did mouth-to-mouth…something you don't forget.

7-12 What is Torsades des Pointes?

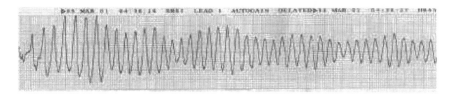

http://www.ekgreading.com/AVB_torsades.jpg

This is a weird one, and a bit rare, but you should know about it. Torsades is an unusual kind of VT. In "normal" VT (ha!), you could think of the electrical signal going through the heart, back and forth, through the tissue, zipping along, but always along one axis, one direction of travel. In Torsades (they also call it "polymorphic VT" – actually, whichever one you call it, they'll call it the other one…), the axis actually rotates as the arrhythmia goes along – it swings, rotating around the heart, as though around a pin stuck in the middle of the heart. There's a lot of scholarly debate about what to do for this arrhythmia – my experience is by the time we've done shocking them in the regular ACLS way, there's not much point in arguing. The question then becomes: why did they get it? My understanding is that certain meds are usually the problem – they cause the QT interval to get longer and longer, which in turn tends to set off this unpleasant problem. I've seen Haldol do this, and I've seen patients sedated with Haldol get taken off it, as their QT interval has been seen to get longer. Does this happen in quinidine loading? Procainamide loading? I forget – anybody know? I need to look this one up again…

Update – magnesium turns out to be just the thing for Torsades.

7-13: What is AIVR?

Here's how I understand it: the ventricles can generate their own escape rate, just as the AV node can, called the "idioventricular rhythm" – it's very slow, around 20-40bpm, and it looks like this:

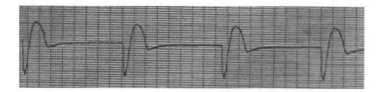

See any p-waves? No p-waves. Wide and bizarre? (What do you mean, "Your mom was wide and bizarre!"?) Pretty bizarre, anyhow – this and the rate tells you where the rhythm is coming from – low down in the ventricles. Very slow – not really fast enough to do what, group?: (all together now) "Generate a blood pressure!!" Right. Thank you.

The "A" in AIVR stands for "Accelerated". Meaning exactly that – the strip shows an idioventricular rhythm: no p's, coming from the ventricles (remember how to tell if it's coming from the ventricles in lead II?) – but an AIVR will be faster than the "normal" idioventricular rate of 20-40 bpm. Maybe 60, or faster even. Will this rhythm perfuse? Maybe... hhe ventricles will pump, if sort of slowly. Will this patient have, or not have, the benefit of atrial kick?

The mechanism here is like the escape, or "rescue" mechanism in the accelerated junctional rhythm. The AV node speeds up, for reasons of it's own which I certainly don't know about, (but which the cardiologists don't seem worried about), and so can the ventricular pacemakers speed up – and, they capture – assuming they're running faster than whatever the underlying rhythm is. Let's say you've aggressively beta-blocked your patient down to, say, a sinus rate of 50. That's somewhere around the intrinsic junctional rate, correct? A frisky nodal, or even ventricular pacemaker might wake up and capture at a similar rate... "A" - IVR. As long as it's fast enough, it will provide a cardiac output the same way that (slow) ventricular pacing would.

People don't get upset much about regular AIVR - the feeling seems to be: so the ventricle woke up and captured, so the patient is a little too beta-blocked, big deal – hold the next lopressor dose, I'm going to bed. There's a rare second kind of AIVR, just in case you really wanted to know – irregular AIVR. This one is dangerous – I seem to recall being told that it's functionally the same as complete heart block. I don't think I've ever seen it, unless while watching that sad "rhythm of death" you see on the monitor just before your patient passes away...

7-14: Asystole

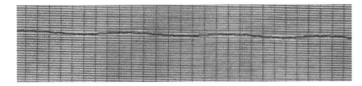

Oh dear…

8: Things we left out the first time:

8-1: SVT: Supraventricular Tachycardia

SVT is nasty, it's fast, it's kind of the same as VT except different... let's think about this one for a second. If ventricular tachycardia comes from the ventricles, and is therefore wide and bizarre (Hey! Don't talk about my aunt like that!)... and SVT is supra-ventricular, coming from someplace above the AV junction...then what's it going to look like?

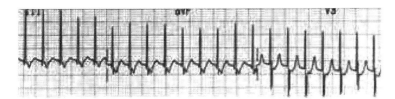

Is it going to be wide? Nope, probably not, because it isn't coming the place where the wide beats come from…

This is where the whole discussion about narrow-versus-wide complex tachycardias raises its head. Which is this one?

What to do? SVT is not the most common arrhythmia, but you need to be ready – as with all of them, your worry is: is my patient making a pressure with this rhythm? And will it get worse?

Well – of course it's never really that simple…it turns out that there's about twelve kinds of SVTs…if you really want the workup, you'll have to call Jayne and make an appointment in her EP lab!

As a practical matter, I've seen regular SVTs-with-a-pressure treated with adenosine: 6mg IV, then 12mg; and SVTs-with-a-horrible-BP treated with synchronized cardioversion.

8-2: WPW – Wolff-Parkinson-White Syndrome

(Do they call it "Dubya P. Dubya" in Texas?)

Nothing very new about this one, and it's kind of rare, but it's cool, and pretty interesting to an old CCU geek like me.

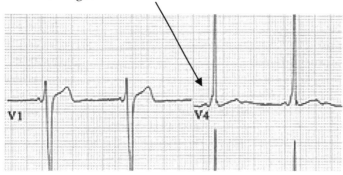

WPW stands for "Wolff-Parkinson-White" syndrome. See what the arrow is pointing at? At the beginning of the R-wave, after that really short PR interval, there's a short diagonal segment – called the "delta wave" - leading up into the normal part of the R-wave at an angle. Hard to see. "Subtle" is the word they use. Not to worry! – after about a decade of reading EKGs you'll have no problem at all. Maybe two. Yeesh!

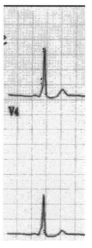

http://www.medlib.med.utah.edu/kw/ecg/mml/ecg_12lead018z.html

Here's some more – see the delta waves?

The significance is actually serious: people with WPW have an extra conduction tract built into their hearts by accident, called the "accessory pathway", which goes around the AV node, connecting the atria and ventricles directly. The accessory tract lets conduction signals go back around and around into the normal pathway instead of having them sent along towards the ventricles, producing a very rapid paroxysmal SVT. Treating the SVT: valsava maneuvers, putting the face in ice water (hmm – not sure how I feel about that one…), or verapamil, or adenosine. (Giving adenosine always makes me feel like I've gone into an SVT… and no matter

68

how much of a valsava I do, it doesn't seem to fix the patient. Maybe I should start putting my face in ice water...)

Here's a quote from the "Virtual Naval Hospital": "Patients with WPW should not be treated with maintenance dose verapamil or digoxin, regardless of the response of their PSVT to acute administration. Symptomatic patients with WPW should be treated with cardioversion or IV procainamide, and referred to a cardiologist for electrophysiologic evaluation."

http://medlib.med.utah.edu/kw/ecg/mml/ecg_12lead018z.html .

Quiz Questions

As usual, our sense of humor invades everything here at ICU faqs central... these quiz questions are not designed to be comprehensive, complete, or authoritative. They are meant to help you think a little, maybe smile a little... let us know if you have questions to add...

1- **An arrhythmia is defined as:**

    a- an alteration in the normal rhythm of the lungs
    b- any rhythm that comes from someplace that it shouldn't, like Queens instead of Brooklyn
    c- any rhythm that begins with the letter "a"
    d- any cardiac rhythm apart from normal sinus rhythm

2- **People develop arrhythmias because:**

    a- their electrolytes are out of whack
    b- they're having myocardial ischemia
    c- they're confused
    d- one or another of their cardiac chambers has become stretched
    e- all except c, except maybe sometimes

3- **The bedside difference between a bad arrhythmia and a not-so-bad arrhythmia is:**

    a- a bad arrhythmia will kill a person, and the other kind won't
    b- bad rhythms don't make a viable blood pressure, and the other kinds do
    c- bad rhythms usually come from lower down in the heart, rather than higher up (although not always)
    d- there are no "bad arrhythmias", and we shouldn't be so judgmental!

4- **Ectopy is:**

    a- spelled "ectopy"
    b- spelled "ectopi"
    c- something that shows up where it shouldn't be, like Dad at a rave club: "Mom! It's me! Dad's being ectopic again!"
    d- animals that live in the ocean, with tentacles, that squirt ink
    e- a and c

5- Supraventricular means:

    e-   much better than ventricular
    f-   coming from anywhere except the ventricles
    g-   coming from anywhere above the AV node
    h-   that my ventricles are better than somebody else's

6- Sinus arrhythmia is:

    a.   the one that shows up when you get a head cold
    b.   a really dangerous arrhythmia
    c.   the one that young people often get, in which the heart rate varies a bit with their breathing, and which is considered benign
    d.   there's no such thing as sinus arrhythmia

7- Sinus bradycardia:

    a.   should always be treated with atropine
    b.   should never be treated with atropine
    c.   should be observed, and considered in the context of what's going on with the patient
    d.   might be treated with atropine if it causes dangerously low perfusion pressure
    e.   might be the result of a pressor bolus
    f.   c, d and e

8- Sinus tachycardia:

    a.   should always be treated with atropine
    b.   should never be treated with atropine
    c.   should be observed, and considered in the context of what's going on with the patient
    d.   might be treated with atropine if it causes dangerously low blood pressure

9- PACs:

    a.   are also known as APCs
    b.   are also known as PVCs
    c.   are also known as FLBs
    d.   were what they called girls in the British army during World War II

True or False:

10- Atrial bigeminy is a horrible, terrible, terrifying, lethal arrhythmia that needs immediate cardioversion, defibrillation, and external pacing.

11- Atrial flutter is a horrible, terrible, terrifying, lethal arrhythmia that needs immediate cardioversion, defibrillation, and external pacing.

12- Atrial fibrillation is a horrible, terrible, terrifying, lethal arrhythmia that needs immediate cardioversion, defibrillation, and external pacing.

13- Nodal beats:

    a. come from the SA node, which is also known as "the junction", or "the node"
    b. come from the AV node, which is also known as "the junction", or "the node"
    c. are like sick sinus beats, coming when the patient has a cold in the node
    d. may represent ischemia of the AV nodal territory
    e. b and d

14- "Escape" beats are:

    a. ectopic beats that come from the brain
    b. ectopic beats that come from anywhere besides the heart
    c. ectopic beats from anywhere in the conduction system, but usually the AV node, which take over the job of generating a rhythm, and therefore chamber contraction, if the normal SA – node beats don't show up on time
    d. dramatic drumming soundtracks used in adventure movies

15- AV dissociation is:

    a. the club that the nerds belonged to in high school, who ran the film projectors at assembly
    b. what's happening when the atria don't talk to the ventricles, and each set of chambers beats independently, probably as the result of ischemia or infarct
    c. when they remove the letters between A and V in the alphabet
    d. an alteration in cardiac output, potential
    e. an alteration in cardiac output, actual
    f. b, probably d, and usually e

16- Marching out means:

    a. being a band geek on St. Patrick's day
    b. being a band geek on Stonewall day
    c. the interval between p's remains the same, the interval between QRS's remains the same, even if the p's and QRS's aren't connecting to each other
    d. the intervals between the p's and the QRS's remains the same

17- PVC's are:

    a. large off-road vehicles used by the National Cardiac Forest Service
    b. early beats coming from the ventricles
    c. a sign of ischemia, sometimes
    d. a sign of electrolyte disturbances, sometimes
    e. b,c and d

18- Couplets are:

   a. lethal, and need to be treated immediately with lidocaine, amiodarone, potassium, and kayexelate
   b. twin babies with cardiac problems
   c. a form of poetry, usually romantic
   d. two PVCs in a row, something to be monitored in the patient's clinical context

19- Triplets are:

   a. even more lethal than couplets, and need to be treated immediately with potassium, magnesium, lidocaine, amiodarone, atovaquone, and ECMO
   b. three babies, but with no cardiac problems
   c. not usually poetic
   d. three PVCs in a row, a little more worrisome – this could signal a long run of VT coming

More True or False:

20- Patients in VT should be immediately defibrillated.

21- Patients in VF should be immediately defibrillated.

22- Patients in Torsades des Pointes should be immediately defibrillated.

23- Patients in asystole should be immediately defibrillated.

24- There is no such thing as Wolff-Parkinson-White syndrome, and if there is, all patients with it should be immediately defibrillated.

Strips: no answers are given (grin!) – got to figure these out on your own!

   25- This is: http://tooldoc.wncc.edu/mi/mi8.JPG

25-

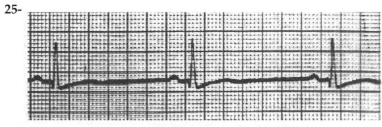

   a. supraventricular tachycardia, with aberrancy, Type 1
   b. supraventricular bradycardia, Lown-Ganong variant Type 3a
   c. an irritable focus flipping the bird
   d. sinus bradycardia

26- This is:

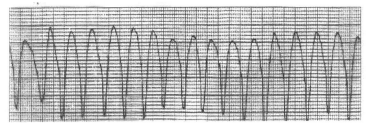

    a.   sinus bradycardia
    b.   ventricular bradycardia
    c.   ventricular brady-bunchia
    d.   wide-complex tachycardia, probably VT
    e.   I don't know what this is
    f.   all of the above
    g.   none of the above

27- This is:

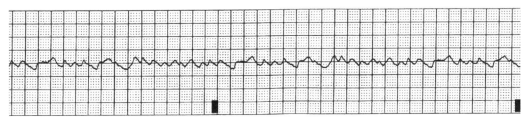

    a-   sinus something
    b-   ventricular something
    c-   the wires are off…
    d-   call a code!

28- This is:

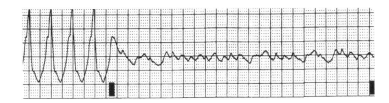

    a.   one real ugly thing turning into another real ugly thing…
    b.   VT turning into VF
    c.   who forgot to hit the bleedin' sync button on the cardioverter!
    d.   probably the result of the R – on – T thingy
    e.   all of the above

29- This is:

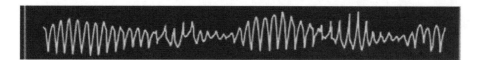

http://www.realcor.com.br/arquivo_digital/img/Torsades.jpg

    a- a totally fake arrhythmia
    b- torsades de pointes
    c- the march of the toreadors
    d- what happened to my rhythm when I ran with the bulls in Pamplona

30- This is:

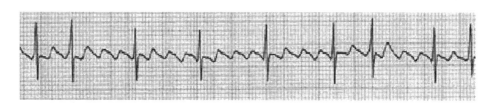

http://medicine.gotohamed.com/EKGs_files/Lectur14.jpg

    a- atrial trigeminy
    b- trigeminal neuralgia
    c- bigeminal atrialism
    d- atrial flutter with variable conduction

31- This is:

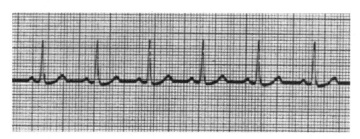

http://www.ce5.com/wpeD.gif

    a- normal sinus rhythm

Arterial Lines

1- What is an a-line?
2- What are the parts of an a-line?
3- Does it matter if the flush setup is made with saline or heparin?
4- What are a-lines used for?
5- What do I have to think about before the a-line goes in?
6- What is an Allen test?
7- Where can a-lines go besides the radial artery?
8- Who inserts a-lines?
9- How is it done?
10- What kinds of problems can happen during a-line placement?
11- How do I use an a-line to monitor blood pressure?
12- How should I set the alarm limits?
13- How do I draw blood samples from a-lines?
14- What order do I draw the tubes?
15- How often does the transducer setup have to be changed?
16- What kind of dressing goes on an a-line site?
17- What is the armboard for?
18- Does the patient's arm have to be restrained?
19- What if my a-line has a good tracing on the screen, but I can't draw blood from it?
20- What does "dampened" mean?
21- What if I lose the trace completely?
22- How often should I check the pulse at the a-line site?
23- How do I know if the patient's hand is at risk?
24- What do I do if the line disconnects at the hub/stopcock/transducer?
25- What do I do if the patient pulls out her a-line?
26- How do I know when it's safe to take out my patient's a-line?
27- How do I remove the line?

I thought it might be interesting to get away from big scary things like balloon pumps, PA-lines and defibrillation, and to try focusing on something that we use routinely, and try to look at it in detail. I read once that pilots will sit and argue about the right way to do anything – taxiing, turning, whatever – that they never stop trying to refine their skills at both the big things and the little ones. Close attention to little things really helps in the MICU, and looking closely at a tool like an a-line might be useful in showing how details matter…as usual, please remember that this is preceptor material, and not meant to be official in any way. When you find mistakes, let us know and we'll fix them. Thanks!

1- What is an A-line?

A-line stands for Arterial line. Our teams use the same 20-gauge straight IV catheters that they use for peripheral lines, and insert them into – usually – the radial artery in one wrist or the other.

2- What are the parts of an a-line?

We start with a bag of heparinized saline: 2units of heparin per cc. The bag is connected to a standard transducer setup: soft tubing from the bag to the transducer, and stiff tubing from the transducer to the patient (some of us old guys call this "Cobe tubing", named after the manufacturer of the tubing we used back in the last Ice Age. Anybody else remember Norton domes?) The stiff tubing goes from the transducer to a stopcock – the stopcock is connected to a short length of softer tubing that we call a "T-piece" (I have no idea why we call it a t-piece – doesn't look like a 't'.) The t-piece screws onto the stopcock at one end, and the other end plugs into the open end of the arterial catheter.

The bag of flush is pumped up to 300mm of pressure with a white pump bag – the transducer controls the forward flow of flush into the artery, keeping it open, at a rate of (I think) 3cc per hour. If the line weren't pressurized this way, the arterial pressure would make the patient's blood climb right back up the line.

3- Does it matter if the flush setup is made with plain saline or heparinized saline?

Actually I think that it doesn't matter in terms of keeping the vessel open – but it does matter if your patient is heparin-sensitive. We've been seeing more patients turning up positive for the heparin-induced-thrombocytopenia thing – lately when I'm making my own flushes for a new patient that I know nothing about, I use saline. If your patient's platelet count drops for no apparent reason, you can go ahead and change them to saline line flushes – apparently even a tiny bit of heparin can cause this problem, which seems to go away after the heparin does.

4- What are a-lines used for?

Two things mainly: blood pressure monitoring, and for patients who need frequent blood draws. Any patient on more than a small amount of any vasoactive drip really needs to have an a-line for proper BP management – if they're sick enough to be put in the unit and need pressors, then they're sick enough for an a-line. Non-invasive automatic blood pressure cuffs are useful, but if a person is labile – push for an a-line.

Certain situations absolutely require an a-line for BP monitoring: any use of any dose of nipride, for example. This is a truly powerful drug – it works very quickly, and your patient can rapidly get into all sorts of trouble unless you're monitoring BP continuously.

I've heard lately that there's a trend towards using fewer a-lines – it seems silly (and painful) to have your patient get stuck what seems like twelve times in a shift for labs and ABGs. Remember that it's always been our unit's policy for nurses to send ABGs after every vent change, or for any clinical change that the patient makes.

Update – this has changed a little: ABGs probably don't seem to be necessary for vent changes that are only going to affect oxygenation: changes in FiO2 or PEEP, since the O2 sat will keep you pretty well informed about where your patient's oxygenation is at. Changing something that is going to affect ventilation or pH is a different matter though – these probably still merit a blood gas.

5- What do I have to think about before the a-line goes in?

First – unless the patient is unresponsive, or has no proxy at hand – the team should get informed consent for this procedure. You need to remember that you're putting something in one of the two vessels that supply the hand with blood. Is the patient hypotensive – are you going to need a doppler to find the pulse in the first place? Is the patient anticoagulated? Which hand does the patient use to write with? – get the team to use the other one. Is the patient very agitated, and likely to pull the line out – does she need some sedation?

Oh yes – have a transducer setup ready to hook up to the new line. House officers do <u>not</u> always think of this, especially if they're just learning the procedure – they're trying to do it right and not hurt the patient. Hook the setup to the monitor with a cable, and zero the transducer so that you'll be able to see the waveform when the line goes in.

6- What is an Allen test?

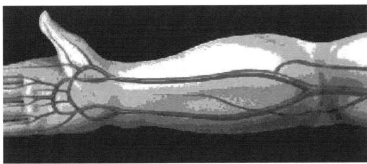

Two main arteries. Which is the radial, and which is the ulnar? The idea here is to figure out if the ulnar artery will supply the hand with enough blood, if the radial artery is blocked with an a-line. Here's the way I was taught: ask the patient to make a fist and hold it. Use your two thumbs to compress both the radial and ulnar arteries of the wrist, and have the patient open the hand. Now release the ulnar artery - the hand should quickly become nice and pink. Allen testing should be done before any a-line insertion, and maybe even before any blood gas sampling.
http://www.medicaexpress.com/cardiologia/car_02_01_37/car_02_01_37.htm

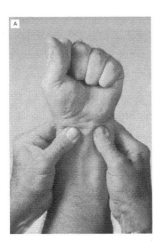

Uh, doc?…I think that was: release the <u>ulnar</u> artery, to see if the hand will perfuse…but see how well that hand pinked up? (He's probably checking both…)

http://www.sadekeen.8m.com/images/the_allen_test.jpg

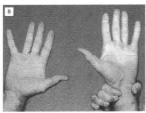

7- Where can a-lines go besides the radial artery?

I've seen ulnar a-lines, brachials, axillaries, and the occasional one placed in the dorsalis pedis – the foot.

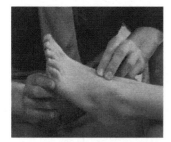

There are actually two pulses in the foot that you need to know about – this is one of them.

http://www.latrobe.edu.au/podiatry/vascular/pulses.html

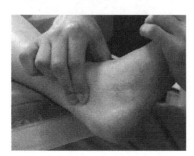

Which one is this?

What would you do if you couldn't find them?

Lots of patients come back from the cath lab with femoral artery sheaths in place. You <u>always</u> want to transduce any line that goes into an artery – what if it came disconnected? What could happen? Why would you want to know?

http://www.latrobe.edu.au/podiatry/vascular/pulses.html

8- Who inserts a-lines?

House officers put these in, sometimes medical students under direct supervision. A-lines are tricky – sometimes you may have to ask the junior to help out an intern who's tried a few times…

Now and again the team is just not able to place the line – the patient is very hypotensive, maybe he's vasculopathic and just doesn't perfuse too well anywhere; or maybe he's very "clamped down" – which means that the arterial bed is very tight, as in cardiogenic shock.

In tough situations, the thing to do is to have the team get in touch with the anesthesia resident on call – these people can usually put an a-line in a marble statue while they're asleep. They are also the folks who will use other sites than the radial artery – foot, axilla, etc.

9- How is it done?

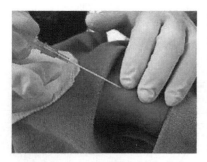

For the radial artery, the most common insertion, the arm is restrained, palm up, with an armboard to hold the wrist dorsiflexed. A straight number 20 IV catheter is inserted puncture-wise over the radial pulse, on something like a 30 degree angle from the skin. If nice bright red blood comes up into the catheter, the stylet is removed, and the catheter is pulled back a little until the blood really starts flowing – this means that the tip of the catheter is at the puncture site in the artery. Now a short guide wire is fed through the catheter, and because it's stiff, it will slide into and along the lumen of the artery. The catheter is slid down the wire, following it's path into the vessel, and the wire is removed. At this point the physician will put her sterile, gloved thumb over the end of the catheter to stop the blood flow. You want to pass the end of the transducer line with the t-piece to the physician, who will insert it into the catheter hub. Encourage her to place it firmly – it's very unpleasant if these two parts separate. Now take look up at the monitor. Good waveform? The catheter gets sutured in, and we apply a standard dressing.

http://www.ispub.com/xml/journals/ijh/vol3n1/aline-fig4.jpg

10- What kinds of problems can happen during a-line placement?

Think about what might happen to any part of the body if its perfusion were disturbed: the patient could develop a hematoma of one size or another – this could even produce a compartment syndrome in the arm if not watched carefully. Make sure that you always keep an eye on the stick site – check the pulse routinely, check the distal capillary refill and feel the warmth of the hand overall a couple of times during the shift. Any time your patient is stuck for an arterial specimen – hold and compress the site for a while afterwards. This reliably prevents hematoma formation, and will save your patient a lot of grief. (Was he anticoagulated?)

A-lines can sometimes be hard to place. Inexperienced team members will often go through a number of catheters, sometimes hitting the artery a couple of times. Arteries don't like this very much, and, (just like the doctors), sometimes they'll go into spasm, tightening up – the pulse becomes harder to find. Encourage the team to try the other arm if this happens, or to wait a while to see if the spasm goes away.

Another problem that "goes with the territory" when a-lines are going into hypotensive patients is the fact that they are, uh…hypotensive. It's going to be hard to find the pulse. Try turning up the patients' pressor drip – often very helpful.

11- How do I use an a-line to monitor blood pressure?

A transducer is a device that reads the fluctuations in pressure – it doesn't matter if it's arterial, or central venous, or PA – the transducer reads the changing pressure, and changes it into an electrical signal that goes up and down as the pressure does. The transducer connects to the bedside monitor with a cable, and the wave shows up on the screen, going from left to right, the way EKG traces do.

A couple of things to remember:

-      The transducer has to sit in a "transducer holder" – this is the white plastic thing that screws onto the rolling pole that holds the whole setup.

-      The transducer has to be levelled correctly. Use the spirit level in the room to make sure that it's at the fourth intercostal space, at the mid-axillary line.

-      Make sure there's no air in the line before you hook it up to the patient – use the flusher to clear bubbles out of the tubing.

-    Zero the line properly, and choose a screen scale that lets you see the waveform clearly.   This can be really important in situations like balloon pumping.

Let's take a second to look at a (hopefully) typical arterial waveform:

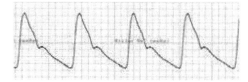

http://www.datascope.com/ca/images/millar_waveform3.jpg

The highest point is the systolic pressure, the lowest is the diastolic. Everybody see the little notch on the diastolic downslope? – there's one in each beat. A little after the beginning of diastole – the start of the downward wave – the aortic valve flips closed, generating a little back-pressure bump: called the "dicrotic notch". You'll need to remember that when the time comes for balloon pumping.

12- How should I set the alarm limits?

Set them meaningfully. Make sure that the limits will tell you if your patient gets into trouble. I always recheck all the alarm limits at the beginning of my shift. For example: the heart rate limits that are built into the monitor default at 50 and 150 – do you really want your patient's heart rate to go to 150 before the monitor will tell you?

13- How do I draw blood samples from a-lines?

Senior staff nurse Jane says: "It takes a year just to learn which way to turn the stopcocks!" This is really true: some stopcocks point to where they're open, and some point to where they're closed – it just takes some time to learn which is which. Drawing samples isn't hard – we use a vacutainer, draw a red discard tube of 5cc, and then plug the specimen tubes into the vacutainer the same way you would if you were doing a peripheral vein stick. The trick is remembering which way to turn the stopcock, and avoiding a mess. Don't forget to clear the stopcock, recap, and then flush the line. Keep things nice and sterile.

14- What order do I draw the tubes?

The trick here is remembering not to contaminate one tube with what might be left from the one before. The main one to watch for is the blue PT/PTT tube – if it gets contaminated by heparin from the line or the previous tube, you'll get results that have nothing to do with the patient. Draw the blue-top specimen right after the red discard tube.

15- How often does the transducer setup have to be changed?

The routine now is 96 hours – make sure that you label the line setup when you hang it. Obviously, change the line setup if it is contaminated in any way.

16- What kind of dressing goes on an a-line site?

Our routine is: scrub the site with a sterile 4x4 soaked in betadine, then paint about an inch away from the site – all around it – with benzoin. Cut a sterile piece of 4x4 to go on the site, and cover with a small clear tegaderm dressing. Try to resist the temptation to reinforce the site dressing with tape – this can make it really hard to get the dressing off without almost losing the line.

17- What is the armboard for?

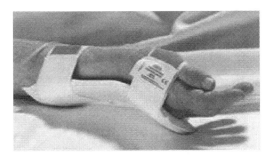

The armboard and roll holds the wrist in a (gently) dorsiflexed position, which keeps the catheter from kinking if the patient bends his wrist.

http://www.dalemed.com/images/armboard.jpg

18- Does the patient's arm have to be restrained?

It ought to be, if there is any chance that she might lose the line by moving around. If the patient is very sedate or chemically paralyzed, you'd probably be safe without a restraint. Be careful judging this: patients can lose blood rapidly from a disconnected a-line hub.

19- What if the a-line has a good tracing on the screen, but I can't draw blood from it?

This probably means that the artery being monitored has "clamped down", or gone into spasm. You need to think about things that might make this happen: is the patient very cold? Are his extremities poorly perfused? Is he on a "shipload" of pressors, making his arterial bed tighten up – is he "dry" as well? Sometimes arteries become unhappy with catheters in them, and you just have to convince the team that the patient needs a new one placed in another site.

20- What does "dampened" mean?

To me, dampening is what happens when the catheter can't see the patient's blood flow clearly – he's bent his wrist, kinked the catheter – sometimes the top of the catheter pushes up against the vessel wall. The waveform flattens out on the screen – doesn't look much like an a-line trace any more. The trick is to learn the difference between a dampened waveform and a hypotensive one! If straightening out the patient's wrist doesn't help, sometimes you can take the dressing down and back the catheter out just a bit – this often works well. (I think there's a more technical definiton of dampening – does anybody know? What's "ringing"?)

21- What if I lose the trace completely?

This could be a couple of things, and you need to do a little troubleshooting. The first thing to think about is: is the arterial catheter still in place? Yes? Try drawing with a 3cc syringe from the stopcock – if it draws normally, then you've got a hardware problem. Cables come loose? Once in a great while a transducer setup will fail – try a new setup. Did the screen scale get accidentally set to, say, 40, instead of 150 or 200mm of pressure?- you'll only see a flat line.

If the line doesn't draw – is there a clot in the hub? Try taking the site dressing down – is the catheter kinked going into the patient? Sometimes art-lines just fail – the artery spasms and won't open up – time for a new site.

22- How often should I check the pulse at the a-line site?

Strictly speaking, every hour. In practice, if your patient has tolerated having the line in place for some time, this can be loosened up a little, but try to remember that a-lines are a lot more invasive than IV's. A vasculopathic patient whose extremities may be poorly perfused is always at risk, even if his arteries don't have catheters in them.

23- How do I know if the patient's hand is at risk?

Usually this will be pretty obvious: the pulse will diminish, or go away altogether. The hand may look dusky, or be cold, or lose some sensation – remember to assess for coloring, sensation, motion, and capillary refill. If you think that the a-line is threatening the patient's hand, let the team know right away, and be ready to set up for another insertion somewhere else if the line is still necessary.

24- What do I do if the line disconnects at the hub/stopcock/transducer?

This is what alarms are for – the monitor should flash "line disconnect". You really want to get down to the room right away – the patient is definitely at risk for losing some blood in this situation.

If the catheter hub has come apart from the t-piece, the thing to do is to screw a syringe onto it, keeping it sealed and clean while you attach a clean t-piece (they're in sterile packages) to the stopcock. Get someone to hold the artery proximal to the catheter (north along the wrist, above the insertion site) while you remove the syringe and replace it with the new t-piece end. (Flush the line clear first!)

If the t-piece comes loose from the stopcock, try to see if the parts are still sterile – usually in this situation they haven't been tightened enough. Just screw the parts together to make a tight seal and flush the line.

If the stiff transducer tubing comes loose at the transducer itself, blood will back up quickly along the line. If the loose end is hanging, turn the site stopcock off to the patient to stop the blood flow, and put together a new transducer setup right away. Always make sure that your setups are screwed together tightly!

25- What do I do if the patient pulls out her a-line?

Compress the site with a sterile 4x4 for several minutes, longer if the patient is anticoagulated. Assess the perfusion of the hand. Try to see if the patient has ripped out her sutures or not…make sure you put the patient on the non-invasive cuff at meaningful intervals while you talk to the team about replacing the line.

26- How do I know when it's safe to take out my patient's a-line?

This is usually pretty obvious – the patient is hemodynamically stable, needs only one or two blood draws in a day, no more need for ABGs – you know all that stuff.

27- How do I remove the line?

You'll want to disconnect the cable from the monitor before you do this, which will automatically turn off the alarms. What I do is clamp the t-piece, which has a little line clamp on it like the ones on the lumens of a triple-port cvp line – that leaves a minimum of hardware connected to the patient while you work on removing the catheter. Take out the sutures in the usual way with a fresh sterile kit. Have a 4x4 ready, pull the catheter, and manually compress the site for at least 3 to 5 minutes. Make sure the patient's hand is still perfused. Check for hematoma or bleeding, put a compression dressing on the site (not too tight!), which you can then take off after about an hour. Recheck the site hourly for a few hours afterwards – a hematoma could still form, and since there isn't a whole lot of room in a wrist, you'd definitely want to know!

Quiz Questions

True or False:

1- Any patient, on any dose of any pressor, should have an arterial line.
2- Any patient on any dose of nipride should have an arterial line.
3- Allen tests are for sissies.
4- It's perfectly safe for a patient to have an arterial line.
5- Arterial line site dressings don't have to be sterile.
6- A-line blood pressures are more accurate than cuff blood pressures.
7- Radial a-line pressures are more accurate than ulnar ones. Pedal ones. Femoral ones.
8- Restraining an a-lined arm is for sissies.
9- The author of these questions is pretty darned flip!

Bedside Emergencies

Somebody asked me the other day why we were expected to take ACLS to work staff in the unit. She meant: we nurses weren't going to be intubating anybody anytime soon, or putting in central lines, or running codes, or anything like that. I could see her point, I guess.

But I think her point is missing something. Last time around for my continuing ed I did a course on "nursing and the law", which I thought might not be very interesting. Wrong. It turns out that when you look at the legal definitions of what it is that nurses are supposed to do in the course of their nursely duties, they vary. The duties. Nurses do all sorts of things, depending on where they are, what their supervision is, etc. And are held responsible. In other words, the judge may say to me one day:

"Nurse Markie – you've been an ICU since the last Ice Age, isn't that right?"

"Uh, yes ma'am, your honor. Sir."

"And so didn't you know that you're not supposed to shock asystole (even though they always do it on TV), or give epinephrine in the tube feeds, as has been verified by the expert witnesses during this proceeding? Aren't those pieces of nursely ICU knowledge that you are held responsible for knowing when you are a staff nurse in the ICU?"

"Uh, yes sir, I did know those things, and it is my responsiblility to know them. Ma'am. I am supposed to know the procedures for defibrillation, and for giving meds."

"So then why did you allow those things to happen, nurse Markie, in the light of your knowledge and experience?"

"Uh… because the doctors were running the code?"

"You mean those same doctors who, over three years of residency, spend a total of three months in the MICU environment? Compared to your years of experience, spent working in the ICU since the time of the Crusades? You allowed them to tell you what to do, even though your experience told you that it might be wrong?"

Not that you should refuse orders … but are you responsible for knowing better if you're told by a doctor to do the wrong thing? Legally responsible? Especially if you have a lot of relevant experience?

The apparent answer is yes, documented over and over again by legal case after case. You are responsible. And especially since, in the course of one year, you collect roughly four times the ICU experience that a doc does in her entire residency. So you'd better know your stuff. But play closely with the team, and get orders written!

Disclaimer:

That said, the usual disclaimer applies to this article: the opinions and experiences described here are in no way to be taken as "official" – they are meant to represent the kind of information that a preceptor might pass along to a new ICU nurse, and are not particularly objective, although they do represent a lot of experience (about 45 years!) between the author and Mrs. Author. Please let us know when you find errors (and you will), and we'll fix them right away. Thanks.

At the beginning, it seems as though there is an endless stream of emergent situations that crop up in the unit, sometimes clearly in response to some prior event, sometimes all by themselves, and they can be genuinely terrifying. (An experienced ICU nurse may be a lot more nervous than a newbie simply because she knows what to be afraid of…) A key rule of the ICU: <u>any</u> patient is capable of doing <u>anything</u>, at <u>any</u> time. And might! Patients admitted with a lower-leg cellulitis may suddenly open up an impressive GI bleed, without anticoagulation, without NSAIDS, without any precipitant that anyone can think of. Patients can go into lethal arrhythmias without warning – which is why we get a steady stream of admissions from the airport. (Why is it always the airport?) This doesn't mean that anyone has made an error, or done anything wrong – some things just happen.

It's good to be ready.

Neuro:

1: What if my patient becomes unresponsive?
2: Has a change in mental status?
3: What if I have a change in mental status?
4: Climbs out of bed?
5: Climbs out of bed naked and runs around the unit?
6: What is APS?
7: What if my patient starts refusing treatment in an emergency?
8: What if my patient seizes?
9: Repeatedly?
10: Does repeated seizure activity really injure the brain?
11: What is a blown pupil?
12: What if they're both blown?
13: What if my pupils are blown?
14: Acute CVA?
15: Sudden rising ICP?

Sedation/Paralysis

16: What if my patient is undersedated?
17: Oversedated?
18: When should I use Narcan? Mazecon?
19: How do I know if my patient is withdrawing from something?
20: What if paralysis won't take effect?
21: Won't wear off?

CV (Pump, Volume and Squeeze)

Pump

22: What if my patient suddenly becomes bradycardic?
23: When do I give atropine?
24: Tachycardic?
25: Sudden VT? Narrow complex? Wide complex?
26: VF?
27: Rapid AF? What is RVR?
28: Asystole?
29: How do I work the Zoll?
30: How do I work a temporary pacing box?
31: What if my patient's K is 1.9?
32: 6.9?
33: What if my patient is having an acute episode of ischemia, or an MI?

Volume

34: What if my patient is dry? How do I know?

35: What if he's wet?
36: When should my patient get a central line?
37: Where should it go?
38: Should I give IV fluid?
39: Should I give blood?
40: What if my postop patient drops her pressure?
41: What if her abdomen/ arm/ neck/ leg is swelling?
42: What if he pulls out his arterial line?
43: Central line?
44: PA line?
45: Balloon pump?
46: What if he pulls out his only IV access and drops his pressure immediately?
47: Needs sedation immediately?
48: Has a rapidly enlarging hematoma at the line site?
49: Has trouble after a paracentesis?
50: Thoracentesis?

Arterial Squeeze

51: What if my patient suddenly drops her BP?
52: Has a sudden rise in BP?
53: Is becoming septic?
54: What if I turn her in the bed and her pressure drops?
55: How do I pick a pressor?
56: What if I turn up the pressor and nothing happens?

57: What if my patient gets a pressor bolus?
58: What if my waveforms and numbers just don't make sense at all?

CAD

59: What if my patient is having ischemia?
60: What if my patient has chest pain that won't go away?
61: What if my patient is having an MI?
62: What is cardiogenic shock?

<u>Respiratory</u>

Non-intubated:

63: What if my patient becomes short of breath?
64: What if she has COPD?
65: Is acutely hypoxic?
66: What if I gave her too much oxygen?
67: Is acutely hypercarbic?
68: When should I get a blood gas?
69: Suddenly starts wheezing?
70: What if my patient is "flashing"?
71: What is "guppy breathing"?
72: What if my patient stops breathing?
73: Obstructs her airway?
74: Has sleep apnea?
75: Plugs?
76: What does a pneumothorax look like?
77: Should we needle the chest or not?

Intubated:

78: What if my patient codes during intubation?
79: Bites the ET tube?
80: Extubates herself?
81: Extubates herself and runs down the hall extubating everyone else?
82: What if I can't get the ET tube cuff to seal?
83: How do I know if she needs to be reintubated?

<u>GI</u>

84: What if my patient pulls his NG tube?
85: Pulls his NG tube just far out enough to aspirate tube feeds?

86: Vomits?
87: Vomits tube feeds?
88: Vomits and aspirates?
89: Vomits "coffee grounds"?
90: Bright red blood?
91: What if he starts passing melanotic stool, or BRBPR?
92: What if my patient starts having severe abdominal pain?
93: What if he's pregnant?
94: What does appendicitis look like?
95: What does a bowel infarct look like?
96: What if my patient has lost bowel sounds, has a K of 6.7 and a pH of 7.10?

GU

99: What if my patient stops making urine?
100: Makes too much urine?
101: Pulls his foley out?
102: Twice?
103: Develops hematuria?
104: With clots?
105: Without clots?
106: What if his BUN and creatinine are doubling every day?

Neuro:

1: What if my patient becomes unresponsive?

Even though there may not be one apparent, things happen to patients for a reason. It's usually a matter of figuring out the context – this can be hard for a newbie who's still trying to figure out which way to turn the stopcock on an a-line. The thing to try to focus on however is pretty simple - keep in mind the basic question: "What's wrong with my patient?" This sounds stupid but actually isn't, since the poor newbie is still struggling to remember how to read the CVP – and it's definitely a fact that equipment of any kind has a genuine hatred for new staff. I remember flushing a toilet once in a patient bathroom during my first week at a job, and watching horrified as the plumbing came apart, off the wall, in front of my eyes, convinced I'd somehow flushed it wrong…

The goal for the new ICU nurse (for any ICU nurse) is to try to figure out what the patient is doing – but when your patient does something unexpected, there is just no substitute for experience. So go get some: go get the resource nurse, and go get the team. This points up the most basic principle of ICU nursing: it is a group process. Tattoo that backwards on your forehead so you can read it in the mirror. Several heads are always better than one. Don't get isolated in your room.

Anyhow. Patients can become unresponsive for lots of reasons – your clues will probably lie in the reasons why they were admitted in the first place. There's a neat maneuver that they do in the ER when a patient comes in unresponsive: they give a quick cocktail of meds that might reverse whatever is causing the problem: an amp of D50 for low sugar, an amp of narcan to reverse opiate OD, a dose of thiamine for (is it the Wernicke's alcoholic thing?) – there might be some others. What's a "banana bag"?

Unless the situation is really emergent (brand new seizures in a patient with a broken foot), you usually have some sort of diagnostic context to help you puzzle things out – is there an underlying neuro problem? Is their blood sugar too low? Blood pressure low? - have they flipped into some unpleasant cardiac rhythm? Rather than trying to think of every possible cause, my point is that you will almost always have something to go on.

2: Has a change in mental status?

This is so common in the unit (and I'm not just talking about the patients), and can have so many causes. All sorts of meds will do this for example, and often you'll discover that the Ativan you've been giving at bedtime makes Mr.Yakowitz confused, every time, but that he does fine with benadryl to help him sleep. Or the other way around. What's the patient's ammonia? Is his calcium really high? Is he "sundowning", or "sun-upping"? Is it "ICU psychosis"? Lots of things to think about – try to think about reasons having to do with his admitting diagnosis.

3: What if I have a change in mental status?

Otherwise known as "Alteration in Reality, Potential vs. Actual". I've been a night nurse for 20 years – I know about this one. Lots of reasons for your own mentation to change: not enough sleep, not enough caffeine, too much caffeine, low blood sugar…one time I had to do the "dad thing" to a young woman who insisted, as she was sliding down towards the floor, that she was just fine, she needed to go turn her patient right now… I had to speak to her firmly, stuck her in a chair, and someone got her some orange juice. How is it that some people "forget to eat"? Not to be antifeminist or anything, but this really is totally a chick thing. Guys never "forget to eat" – forget to eat? I carry power bars in my bag to eat standing, a bite at a time along with some Gatorade if I can't get out to the back room. What good are you to your patient if you've fainted on the floor?

The point is: this really is one of the hardest jobs there is. Not kidding. Nurses have such an ingrained sense of how little they matter that they have trouble perceiving their own value, much less the real impact of the anxieties and burdens that come with working in the ICU. Take care of yourself – you really took on the big one when you came to the MICU. You're in the majors now.

One more thought: is there another profession that sees death so often? In this job we may spend 25 years treating patients who are trying to die…give yourself credit, and wear the invisible golden badge (the one only your co-workers can see) with pride.

4: Climbs out of bed?

Happens all the time. Your responsibilities are simple: keep your patients safe. If your patient is competent, oriented, can get up and wants to, then you should help her. (If she's still intubated that might be a problem.) Keep the bed in low position. Know the hospital's restraint policies. Read more on this topic in "The House of God", by Samuel Shem. Kind of a dirty book, but hilarious. Not very accurate on nurses, though.

5: Climbs out of bed naked, and runs around the unit?

Well, this one does actually happen once in a while. He's still your patient though, isn't he? Call security, call the team, try to keep him safe until you can get him back into the bed. Something that came up recently in the "Med Tips" article might be useful to keep in mind – a patient who's pulled out all his IV lines can still be given safe sedation by nebulizing a dose of, say, 5 mg of morphine through a neb mask. Surprising but true – a year or so ago we had a similar situation, and the attending pulled that idea out like a rabbit out of a hat. Worked really well.

6: What is the APS?

This stands for our hospital's Acute Psych Service – this is an in-house resident psychiatry service available for emergency consults 24/7. Good to know.

7: What if my patient starts refusing treatment in an emergency?

Obviously this depends on the situation. An elderly patient with a terminal illness may be completely rational (and I believe in the right) if she decides to refuse being intubated for the fourteenth time.

A patient we had some months ago demonstrated a different scenario: a man in his fifties, I think with some degree of COPD at baseline, but with a clearly treatable pneumonia that was pushing him over the edge towards the snorkel. He began to refuse everything – nebs, meds, and began climbing out of the bed to go home. This is the kind of situation that legally requires a stat assessment of competency – we called the APS.

8: What if my patient seizes?

For the first time ever? For the third time in an hour? Intubated? Not? The basics are clear – get help, get the team, treat acutely with things like benzos (we usually use Ativan for acute seizures), try to keep the patient's airway clear and prevent aspiration. If he's intubated, try to get a bite block in place – we've seen patients bite through the pilot line, deflating the ETT cuff. Also, biting the tube closed is not usually a healthy thing – I've seen agitated patients arrest doing this once or twice over the years. The jaws are very strong. Put seizure padding on the bed rails, and check their dilantin level. Or valproate, or whatever.

9: Repeatedly?

Hopefully you've got the neuro service on hand (or their assessment and treatment plan). Is this a sudden change, increasing in frequency? Time for more benzos, more dilantin? Phenobarb? Time for neuro to come back and have another look? Time for another (don't say it!) CT scan? Ack!

10: Does repeated seizure activity really injure the brain?

I ran this one past Jayne, and her opinion is that it's the hypoxia that goes along with repeated seizures (if the patient isn't intubated) that causes the damage. We got a patient in last week who'd been in "status epilepticus" for 90 minutes without being intubated – she woke up and wanted to know what all the fuss was about. (How did she breathe that whole time?)

11: What is a "blown pupil"?

This refers to a pupil that's suddenly gone big, independently of the other one. This usually something acutely bad is happening on one side (the opposite side?) of the head. Jayne: is this because rising ICP compresses the area that holds one of the optic nerves? Pretty clear that I'm no neuro nurse.

12: What if they're both blown?

Make sure it's not just dark in the room. Has the patient's level of consciousness has changed? Everybody knows about "fixed and dilated" pupils – this is a true BBIT (big bad ICU thing), indicating a prolonged hypoxic injury to the brain.

A couple of exceptions: sometimes a patient will have a dilated eye exam done by opthalmology, and they may not remember to tell you that your patient's pupils are going to be sort of massively enlarged for a while. The other thing is that a patient who is post-code may have dilated pupils from atropine, rather than hypoxia – these should go back to normal after several hours.

13: What if my pupils are blown?

Don't forget to bring sunglasses after your eye exam. Otherwise, is the room candle-lit? You know what to do.

14: Acute CVA?

The single enlarged pupil may be your major clue if you have a patient who is otherwise sedated or chemically paralyzed. The critical piece of the puzzle is: is this an embolic or a hemorrhagic event? Quick trip to the CT scanner.

We had a really nice example of "brain attack" treatment a few weeks ago. Gentleman about 80 years old came into the ER, suddenly unable to move his left side, unable to speak, previously completely functional. Apparently the window for assessment and treatment is really short for this kind of event – two hours? – Jayne says it's three hours for an embolic stroke, as against the 4-6 hours that an MI patient has to get into the ER for lytic treatment. Anyhow, I guess the window was still open, and the man flew right through it, got his lysis, and by the time he was finishing up the dose, back in CT scan, he was able to speak and move freely. By the time he got to us, and when I was doing my resourcely nurse duties running around checking things out, he looked up at me.

"How are you doing, sir?" says I.

"I'm just fine, sir." says he, "How are you?" (Yeah, they call me "sir" now. Getting grey around the edges. Okay, more than just the edges.)

I guess I looked a little funny with this enormous goofy grin on my weary old-gome-nurse face, as I stood there in the doorway – he looked as if he was a little worried about me. "Saves" like that are so incredibly gratifying – we rescued this guy from being paralyzed and speechless, hopefully for the rest of his life. So cool.

15: Sudden rising ICP?

What year is it?

Not too long ago, a patient couldn't tell me who the President was, but he looked pretty much with it, so I asked: "Well then, who's Monica Lewinsky?" That got an enormous grin – I think he was pretty well oriented.

Everybody remembers the triad (is it "Cushing's" triad?) of symptoms: falling heart rate, depressed respiratory rate, and widening pulse pressure: systolic heads north, diastolic heads south. The "critical element" however, as they say, is much easier than that: mentation goes first. A patient who was previously arousable and oriented will abruptly become too "sleepy" to respond to questions. Intra-cranial bolts are nice I'm sure, and once or twice a year we get them, but the first real clue to rising ICP is the patient's decreased level of consciousness. (Whenever we get a bolt I always ask the neuro ICU nurses to come down and tell me if it's working right. Anything that I only see once a year makes me nervous.)

These changes can be really abrupt - here's a story by way of example: years ago, I think with Flo during the Crimean War, I was working in a medical CCU and, being the owner of the only open ICU bed in the hospital, I was sent the gift of a fresh post-op craniotomy patient for recovery. As my grandpa would say: "This, I know from nothing!" But, a nurse is a nurse is a nurse, right? Anyhow, I got explicit instructions on postop assessment from the neurosurgeons, and I just documented the crap out of that entire situation – the patient's answers to questions, strengths of extremities, pupil exams, tongue stuck out at midline (didn't Mark Green get into trouble with his tongue that way?), severity of postop pain – I'm sure there were others which now, 700 years later I don't remember. Anyhow, I sent the patient to the floor after the prescribed number of hours postop with a sheaf of documentation, after a surgical postop check to clear the transfer.

I got a call about 20 minutes later – had the patient been unconscious when he left the CCU? No way, I told them – check the assessment sheets. Between the unit and the floor, the patient had become suddenly unresponsive. Zapped to CT scan – she'd re-bled. Unbelievable. Be very careful!

Sedation /Paralysis:

16: What if my patient is undersedated?

This is a complex subject, and there's more than you probably ever wanted to know about it in the "Sedation and Paralysis" FAQ. Apparently the studies consistently show that nurses always think that their patients are undersedated, and doctors always think the opposite (what else is new?) The essential point: keep the patient safe, and as free of pain and distress as possible. Make sure that you communicate carefully with the team, and document your assessments.

17: Oversedated?
They do have to wake up sometime. Use your judgment, keep the patient safe. Jayne points out that new practice guidelines from the Society for Critical Care Medicine say that sedated patients need to be awakened every two hours to make sure that everything is working, neuro-wise. This seems kind of impractical to me, but I guess they know what they're talking about. I always try to document my sedated/paralyzed patients' neuro status carefully: a chemically paralyzed patient will still have pupillary reflexes, right? So if one pupil suddenly gets big – well, what you have there is sort of your basic clue.

18: When should I use Narcan/naloxone? Romazecon/Flumazenil?

Narcan is the drug that pushes opiates off of their little cell receptor sites, so it's used for opiate overdose situations, and sometimes for patients who aren't able to tolerate their prescribed pain meds too well. Romazicon is the same thing except different – it works on benzo receptors. You have to be careful with flumazenil – it can provoke seizures in chronic-benzo-using patients. Be careful with narcan too – a patient can become frighteningly agitated after a dose of narcan. I usually put soft restraints on the patient ahead of time. And maybe pad the ceiling.

19: How do I know if my patient is withdrawing from something?

Usually the picture is pretty clear: agitation, tachycardia, hypertension - and you'll have some idea of what to expect if your patient is admitted as an OD of one kind or another. If your patient is admitted intubated, maybe after being found down, maybe with an big aspiration pneumonia, maybe brewing ARDS, sedated with propofol, and two days along they start to become tachy, hypertensive…if the ER was doing it's job, they'll have sent a tox screen on admission, so you'll have that to work with. And the timetable does vary for withdrawal, but the thing I try to think about is DT's – usually the symptoms will start between 48 and 72 hours after the person's last drink.

20: What if paralysis won't take effect?

Some patients just don't paralyze. I'm sure there are very good, and horribly complex physiological reasons why they don't paralyze, but all I care about is whether or not my patient is ventilating, so would you all stop the intellectual discussion and give me a suggestion as to how we should control this guy before he codes? This is similar to the situation where the anesthesia resident stands there teaching the intern the fine points of intubation while the patient's sat is falling (which is being watched mainly by the nurse while this intellectual discourse goes on). And falling. While we remind them. Again.

Surgical intern says to me once, not very happy: "No one ever listens to me!" I suggested: "Try being a nurse." She didn't like that answer...

Where were we? Before starting paralysis, if possible, it's good to document a baseline "twitch", or train-of-four response, using a peripheral nerve stimulator, if only to document that they do or don't respond to it. This gets a bit into the voodoo realm sometimes – some patients just don't seem to paralyze, or twitch, or both. Twitch response may have to do with peripheral edema over the nerve that you're trying to stimulate – but remember that your first goal is not the twitch number – it's the patient's condition. You can twitch them every whichy-way, but the point is to get the patient into some sort of safer condition than the one they were in before you started. There's lots more about this topic in the "Sedation and Paralysis" FAQ.

21: Won't wear off?

Progress has definitely been made on this one, and without going into too much detail, suffice to say that titrating to the train of four has given us a way to keep from giving too much paralytic drug. In the old days, a patient was either "paralyzed" or "not-paralyzed" – and apparently they sometimes soaked up too much med over the time they spent on the drug. Titrating to one-out-of-four on the TOF let's us minimize the dose, so they won't have to cook off large amounts of drug after their lungs get better.

The other thing: paralytics and steroids seem not to mix. Certainly "pulse dose" steroids of something like a gram (!) of methylprednisolone seem to make the effects of paralysis linger on and on – and "stress" doses of 60mg may do the same. Something about "steroid myopathy" – as we say in Boston: "Alls I know is, don't give 'em togedda!"

CV: (Pump, Volume and Squeeze)

Pump

22: What if my patient suddenly becomes bradycardic?

Scary one. Two main possibilities for this: first, has the patient acutely obstructed her airway? Acute hypoxia produces bradycardia. Has she plugged her ET tube? With her thumb? Tootsie Roll? Anybody suctioned her lately?

A word about suctioning goes here. Somewhere along the line the word got out that using saline lavage while suctioning is not the right thing to do. This is simply wrong. As I read somewhere (on a different subject): "All the studies demonstrating this point are wrong, and should be burned." Just last week we had a vented patient whose respiratory rate had been rising all evening – it was currently in the 60's. I was the resource RN, and probably the senior nurse to the next by about 13 years. Actually, it might've been 20. (And that's another whole story too, isn't it?) After some discussion I went into the room with the respiratory therapist – we lavaged and suctioned her ET tube with ten cc's of saline a couple of times and produced a large, dryish plug. Her respiratory rate went to the 20's, her heart rate dropped forty points, her sat went up – use that saline!

Jayne: "You are just totally wrong on this one. I have a whole bunch of studies at work that show that what you're doing is opening up a sterile, closed system, and introducing something foreign into the system. Sending the saline down the tube will break up the mucus that's trapping the bacteria, and then if you ambu them, you're just pushing the bacteria down further into their lungs, and making them sicker!"

Myself: "Phooey. And we use the inline suction thing anyway. But I'm putting in your opinion, all right?"

J: "Yeah, well, I'm right, and you're wrong."

She has a tough job. We've been together for 25 years this August. I used to sit behind her in nursing school…

Sleep apnea people are at sometimes at risk for bradycardic events because they're obstructing – which of course is their problem, right? They obstruct every four minutes, wake up with a snort, and go back to sleep for another 90 seconds, all night long. Suppose they have COPD as well, and someone gets nervous and applies too much oxygen when the patient comes in with a flare – total setup for respiratory suppression, right? These patients easily become C02 "narced" (pronounced "narked"), which is to say "suffers an episode of hypercarbic narcosis" – or even better! – has an "alteration in gas exchange secondary to Pickwickian body habitus and history of toxic tobacco exposure resulting in chronic obstructive breathing pattern resulting in an alteration of the human spirit, potential versus actual…" – right. Sorry Aunt Nanda…(!)

Anyhow – that patient may get narced, stop breathing, obstruct his airway, and brady down. So be alert, and think ahead: what are you going to want to have on hand? Atropine? Sure, but maybe not if the reason for the bradycardia is a closed airway, which you then open with a jaw lift, or an oral airway, or both.

The heart rate ought to pick up once oxygen starts getting into the blood again. If you've given atropine, the heart rate may go up to a zillion – now you have a whole new set of problems. So: keep atropine nearby, sure, but take 30 seconds if you can to see if opening the airway and restoring some oxygen delivery fixes the problem. If not, and the BP is dropping significantly, then go push that atropine!

What else are you going to have on hand if you think this might happen? Oral airway? Ambu-bag, all hooked up? Suction at the bedside working? Plus (big plus here) – did you set your alarm limits nice and tight when you started your shift? If I have a patient who's unstable for any reason at all, I set my limits less than ten points above and below where the patient is at for heart rate and MAP – hey, if I waste printer paper on a bunch of artifact alarms, what does it matter? You can loosen the limits later if you think it's safe.

The other main reason for bradycardia of course is that some unpleasant cardiac thing is happening, usually in the form of some kind of inferior ischemia or MI. These folks will often show you what they're doing by vomiting, or having hiccups along with, or instead of - their chest pain. (Why?) You may know what's wrong just by looking.

Let's take a minute to look at a couple of the main bradycardic possibilites. Suppose you see this:

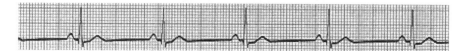

Everybody recognize sinus bradycardia? What's the rate – about 55? Does this patient need atropine? No? Remember that atropine is only for symptomatic bradycardia, meaning, "with a low blood pressure". Maybe he's getting lopressor loaded today. But what if the same patient's heart rate had been at about 100 for the whole day before this? And he was vomiting when he did this? And broken out in a sweat, with chest pain and a dropping O2 sat? Blood pressure dropping in this setting might mean some sort of acute inferior-territory problem – it all depends on the context. If this had been the patient's rate all day, with a good BP – probably no problem.

How about this one?:

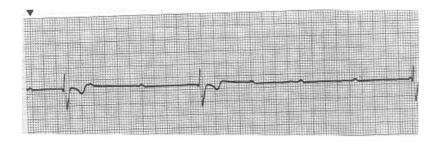

Yikes! Everybody recognize third degree heart block? Everybody know how to use the external pacemaker? Atropine may not help much here…
Here's another:

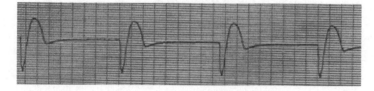

Ack! Even worse! "Idioventricular" rhythm, otherwise known as "physiology of death". Probably the next-to-last rhythm the poor guy will ever have.

And another:

That's real bradycardia! (Are the leads on the patient?)

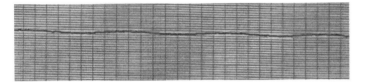

23: When do I give atropine? Do I need an order?

The policy is "Give atropine for symptomatic bradycardia." - lots of people get totally wound up, ready to give atropine when the patient is still making a pressure – and it's hard not to want to just charge ahead and do it. But try to wait just a little and see what happens. If the patient loses pressure, you are absolutely authorized to go ahead and give the atropine. (Make sure their airway is open. Yours too.)

24: Tachycardic?

This is usually going to be some kind of arrythmia. Sinus tachycardia happens, for sure, but usually it creeps up over the period of some hours at least, and is usually pointing to something happening: the patient is spiking a temp, or getting dry, or agitated, or some combination of the three. Sudden supra-ventricular tachycardia is often something like a burst of rapid PAT, which will likely stop as suddenly as it started, or rapid a-fib, which won't. The essential point here is: "Is the patient making a pressure or not?" If they are, then you have time to try different things – if they aren't, you don't. Take a look at the articles on "Arrhythmia Review" and "Defibrillation" for ideas on how to identify rapid arrhythmias, and how to go about treating them: some rhythms get defibrillated, and some don't, and it's a good idea to be ready to tell which is which. We'll do some basic review here.

25: Sudden VT? Narrow complex? Wide complex?

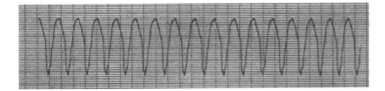

Ok, ready? VT? SVT? Narrow, or wide complex? That's all good stuff to know, but go back to the essential point: are they making a pressure? Yes? Sometimes you'll see a patient maintain a pressure in VT, and there are algorithms for that, but remember not to defibrillate someone who's awake! Stop making a pressure? Think it's VT? Pretty darn sure it's VT – nice wide complex? Patient's "out of it"? Try a precordial thump. This is something you see the old nurses do: they'll see VT on the central station monitor, and a newbie nurse assigned to the room may be standing there (no offense now, okay?), like a "deer in the headlights", and the old RNs will stand up in a group and yell "Hit him!" as they scramble for the defibrillator, cart, ekg machine, docs, etc. I've precordially thumped several patients back into sinus rhythm in my day – all I can say is that I think it's still useful, even though I think it's not part of the protocols any more.

This is the kind of situation where ACLS comes in handy – if you have the kind of mind that memorizes easily, then you'll have absolutely no trouble remembering what to do when everyone is yelling at everyone else in the middle of a code situation. I don't memorize well at all, but what I can do is to learn from experience – for some reason memories come up in my mind literally from years before, and I'll say "Hey, I've seen this, I know what to do."

ACLS is a wonderful thing, and it's way cool to be ACLS certified, but the basics of BLS still cover most of what you want to do in a code situation: A,B, and C. Let's do these individually for a minute:

A: Is the airway open? No amount of dramatic maneuvering with defibrillators, wires, or external pacemakers is going to make the least bit of difference unless the patient's airway is open. Some months ago we had a patient who brady'ed down with a low O2 sat, and people were in there doing all sorts of stuff, but having the chance to stand back a little, you could clearly see that the patient's airway wasn't open. We did a jaw thrust and things got better very quickly.

B: Breathing. Once the airway is open, get your ambu bag and mask and get some gas exchange going. Make sure the bag has good 02 flow. An oral airway will usually do a good job of keeping the airway open under the mask. Suction, suction, suction.

C: Circulation. You know this part. "Hut hut hoo!" (Wait – isn't that something else?)

Now's time to think about cardioversion and defibrillation. Take a look at the FAQ on the subject for lots of info and some nice pictures.

26: VF?

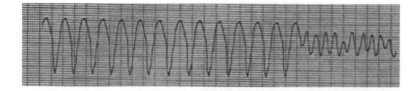

So - what happened here? Just when you were hoping that things couldn't get worse, they did. This is the thing about VT – even if your patient is making a pressure initially, they may lose it –

sometimes because they've gone into VF. This situation calls for immediate defibrillation – but try to get the airway open, too…

27: Rapid AF? What is RVR?

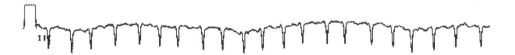

RVR stands for Rapid Ventricular Response – the ventricles are responding to so many atrial signals that they haven't got time to fill properly, so the blood pressure may drop impressively. That situation usually calls for <u>synchronized</u> cardioversion right away.

28: Asystole?

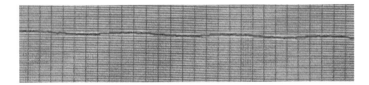

Ugly. We saw this one before – everybody remember the first thing to do? Are you going to call a code if the patient is eating dinner in this rhythm? Unresponsive? You or them? Okay – <u>now</u> call a code, get the Zoll, start BLS, bag the patient…what do you mean, you can't do all of that at once?

29: How do I work the Zoll?

External and internal pacing devices both work the same way – you pick a rate that you'd like to pace the patient at, then turn up the milliamperage output until you capture the patient. Obviously it's the delivery system that's different: in this case the electricity is being delivered through pads on the patient's chest and back. External pacing is tricky, and it makes a lot of sense to spend time looking over the box, the pads, the sensing and output cables – the whole setup, before you have to use it. Take a look at the FAQ article on "Pacemakers" for more on this topic.

30: How do I work a temporary pacing box?

This is the controller for an internal wire, as opposed to the external box we were talking about above. Same basic idea – the patient is not making enough intrinsic signals to generate a heart rate fast enough to make a decent blood pressure; something like ischemia, or an acute infarct involving the SA or AV nodes is disrupting the process. A wire is placed – almost always in the cath lab, although at really rare intervals you may see one "floated in" at the bedside – and is connected to a generator box. Same idea: set the "rate" control at some rate that you think will make a blood pressure, then increase the milliamp output until the heart is captured 100%.

Once the box is set you'll probably have to worry more about the wire being dislodged than working the box itself, although you need to have the basics in mind.

There is a third knob besides "rate" and "milliamps" on an internal controller, labeled "sensitivity" (doesn't always work on males). If the patient's heart rate does come up, you probably want to let it capture, because intrinsic rhythms are usually the best ones – setting the sensitivity lets the box sense the patient's intrinsic rate. Or not. In emergent situations with the patient's rate at 22, (or zero!), you usually want to set the box to just pace – not sense. In that situation, the knob is set to "least sensitive", or "asynchronous".

31: What if my patient's K is 1.9?

Well, how the heck did that happen? These things don't come out of the blue, y'know! This is sometimes the patient who got overdiuresed – too much lasix? I guess! This sort of underlines my fear about some of these drugs that we give patients to take home: here's a patient with heart trouble, probably CHF, probably prone to some arrhythmias anyhow, who gets sent home with a diuretic that makes him "dump" potassium. And, sure, he gets a scrip for potassium too – but what if he doesn't like the taste of it? Ack!

This person is going to need replacement treatment right away. Our rules are: no more than 20 meq of potassium through a central IV per hour, max. You can give a dose orally at the same time – but make sure the patient's creatinine is okay! (Why?) And make sure the patient stays on a monitor until you know he's not going to keel over in VT!

It really is amazing how, in some patients, replacing electrolytes can make arrythmias go away. Some people are very predictable this way: "Oh, did he have a run of ten beats? Yeah, he has one every night – did he get his Mag dose yet?"

32: 6.9?

Then again, there can be too much of a good thing! Is this result for real? Could it be a hemolyzed spec? (Quiz question for later – what does hemolysis have to do with it? Clue: draw specimens <u>gently</u> from arterial lines.)

If it is real, then the danger is severe – the patient may go into an arrhythmia just as she would if her K were low, or maybe brady down to about nothing. Couple of maneuvers to make here: first we might give a dose of regular insulin – 10 units IV push, followed by an amp of D50. (Jayne says to give the D50 first – makes sense to me. In the blood sugar world, sort of too high is much better than way too low.) The insulin will push the potassium from the plasma into the red cells circulating in the blood, so the plasma level will drop. That same insulin dose will of course drop the patient's blood sugar too, so that's why they get the D50. The problem is that the potassium will leak back out after a short while, so this only buys you some time. Giving calcium chloride is supposed to help protect the myocardium from irritability in this situation. I'd be pretty irritable myself.

The second maneuver works better, but takes longer: kayexelate. This stuff is an "exchange resin", which sits in the gut (it has to get into the intestinal tract to work), and swaps ions – one reference I looked at said that one gram of kayexelate will bind one meq of potassium – good to know. This stuff works pretty well, but of course you need to be thinking about what the problem is (isn't that just always the way?) – is the patient in acute renal failure? Everything always depends on the context.

You noticed that little key phrase up there "it has to get into the intestinal tract to work"? Apparently kayexelate doesn't work if it just sits in the stomach, and if your patient has some sort of ileus, then you can give doses through an NG tube all day, but they'll just bounce off the pylorus and come back up the next time you check an aspirate. We see a lot of opiate ileus's – the only thing to do in this situation is to give the med as a retention enema through a rectal tube.

Important things to remember about rectal tubes. First – they don't work very well. You can't give a large volume through one and expect the patient to retain it – what we do is to mix the kayexelate with some normal saline to make it dilute - it's very thick - and then give small amounts every half hour or so through the tube, maybe 100cc at a time. Clamp and unclamp things as necessary to let the dose dwell, then drain, then repeat. Works pretty well. Better than trying to give 500cc, having it leak everywhere, and then having to tell the team that it couldn't be done. This trick works with lactulose too. Don't forget to let the balloon down every four hours.

33: What if my patient is having an acute episode of ischemia, or an MI?

Why don't you ask an easy question, huh? Lots of stuff to think about in this situation, and you know, there's a reason why God created cardiologists…

Some basic thoughts:

Is the primary process MI or ischemia?

- If an MI, should the patient get "clot-busted"? (Are they liable to start bleeding from someplace if they do? Have they recently had surgery? Maybe lysis isn't such a good idea.)

- Should she get an aspirin?

- Should she go to the cath lab? If the goal is to reopen a plugged coronary artery – probably. Is the patient 26 years old? 126 years old?

- Is the patient having specific symptoms that need to be treated right away? The symptoms can vary a great deal, depending on where the MI is territory-wise. Inferior MI people may vomit and go bradycardic (atropine!), while anterior or lateral MI people may become horribly short of breath ("flashing" - although that can happen with an ischemic episode or an MI, and it's important to figure out which is which.) Lots of other arrhythmic possibilities exist too.

Either way, ischemic event or MI, some basic maneuvers usually apply:

- Morphine. (This is all, as always, with MD orders, right?) Make sure the patient has a blood pressure before (and after!) you give it.

- Nitrates – sublingual nitroglycerine is usually the first thing to try here, but if the patient is having an MI, this may actually not be what they need. Watch their blood pressure!

- Oxygen. This is the problem, right? - some part of the cardiac musculature isn't getting 02 – so apply some. Try to remember if the patient has COPD or not. (Why?)

- Is the patient short of breath? Sit her up, way up in a high Fowler's position with pillows supporting her arms. Watch her blood pressure. Does she need diuresis?

- Get lots of EKG's – in fact, leave her hooked up. If the pain comes and goes, try to get EKG's with the pain and afterwards, to see if things are changing. Take a look at the FAQ on infarct localization for help on interpreting these guys. It's not as hard as you think…really!

Volume

34: What if my patient is dry? How do I know?

Arguments can actually break out at the bedside on this one, and not for trivial reasons either. It can be really hard to sort out what a patient is doing if they show up short of breath, looking bad, getting worse, with a diffusely horrible chest x-ray that looks like "wetness". We've seen patients come in who were actually developing something unusual like ARDS after some precipitant like a car crash, or maybe BOOP (discovered by the eminent pulmonologist Betty, back in the 40's, at the Warner Bros. Med School. Didn't she do something else as well?) Or Wegener's, or whatever…

Anyway: is he making urine? Sodium up? BUN up? What's the BUN/ creatinine ratio? Here's a normal one: BUN/ creatinine of 10 / 0.7 .

Now look at this one: 60 / 0 .7 - look different? Clearly a higher ratio than the one before. Which one means "dry"?

Let's take a second to remember what the numbers actually mean. The BUN tells you how much nitrogen waste is floating around in the blood, while the creatinine tells you if the kidneys are actually working or not. If the creatinine is high, the kidneys are in real trouble – maybe "taking a hit". Then the BUN will go up because the kidneys can't get rid of it.

If however the creatinine is normal, then the kidneys are working properly. So if the BUN is high, it means that the patient is dry – their BUN is high because the patient has lost water. Dry. Less water means that everything floating around in the blood becomes more concentrated – red cells, electrolytes, BUN – see? So the hematocrit will go up, the sodium will go up, the BUN will go up…see? Right.

Here's a scenario: Mr.Yakowitz comes into the ER. He's 64 years old, and he's been feeling rotten for about ten days. Hasn't had much to eat or drink in that time. Getting a little short of breath. Chest x-ray is clear, EKG is normal (he's not having chest pain.)

He used to smoke for many years, but he "quit last week". He does wear two liters of 02 at home for COPD. Not making much urine. (Jayne the CNS : "Wouldn't he have RV strain pattern because of the COPD?" – Yeah, okay, smartypants!)

Quick look at the labs: Sodium is 147. Hematocrit is 52. (What reason does this guy have to walk around with a high hematocrit besides being dry?) BUN is 64, creatinine is 0.8. What do you think?

Yup, dry - real dry. I wonder if he's making any urine – these people can get so dry that they can get pushed into renal failure. (Is he pre-renal? Post-renal? Intra-renal? Renal-renal?) This is a classic situation: a COPD patient who gets pushed over the edge by a URI or community-acquired pneumonia. They come in "dry as a dog-biscuit", and their x-ray is clear because their infiltrates won't "flower" until they're hydrated. Then they may get into more trouble handling secretions….

35: What if he's wet?

Opposite problem. Of course there's wet, and there's wet, depending. "Wet" usually means that the patient is fluid overloaded to the point of hypoxia – pushed into a little CHF. If you give enough fluid, almost any patient can get into trouble (also depending) – but it gets a little complex if you have a patient whose blood pressure is low. Volume resuscitation in sepsis can add up to a lot of liters in a very short time – keep careful track! Respiratory "wetness" will usually show up as increasing hypoxia, shortness of breath, bilateral rales to one level or another – you know that stuff.

Another aspect: the patient may look "wet" because she's having myocardial ischemia. Someone with left-sided CAD who has an ischemic episode may develop a sudden problem with her mitral valve. (That's the one on the left side.) Remember the chordae tendonae? – the stretchy things that support the valve leaflets? Ischemia can make them suddenly go all floppy, and then the valve doesn't valve – blood starts leaking backwards with every contraction, back towards the lungs, which get congested, and leaky, and then the little alveoli start filling with water that transudes from the capillaries because of the backup pressure…and it can happen <u>really</u> fast. "Uh-oh. I think he's flashing".

So for sure this ischemic person is "wet" – but should you remove fluid? Probably, but you need to treat the underlying problem, which is the ischemia. So you do the little memory thing: LMNOP.

L: Lasix – most of the time they'll give some. But again, volume overload may not be the real problem.

M: Morphine for the pain, also helps lower BP ("afterload reduction") – which in English means "dilating the arterial system so that the heart doesn't have to work so hard to pump blood into it".

N: Nitrates. You know this stuff – sublinguals, nitropaste, IV nitroglycerine. If you can "fix" the ischemic situation, the valve may start valving again, and you may save your patient an intubation.

O: Oxygen is what the myocardium wants, right?

P: Positioning helps – sit her up straight with pillows under the arms.

36: When should my patient get a central line?

Not too hard to tell – any time your patient needs a pressor, for example. Some patients have terrible veins, and they come in with complex problems, and they start needing all kinds of good stuff like fluids, antibiotics, blood, drips of all description – access is everything in these situations.

37: Where should it go?

Depends. In a real emergency like a code, the team will go for a femoral site – you won't need an x-ray to confirm the position. (Although you can tease the team and ask if they want a KUB.) Not the cleanest insertion prep, but once the patient is stabilized you can go after a line in the neck or the subclavians.

A thing to remember: is your patient on a lot of forward pressure from a ventilator? A lot of PEEP maybe, or a lot of pressure suport combined with PEEP? The patients' lung apices will be pushed up almost to his ears – be careful with subclavians! Everybody know how to set up for a chest tube?

38: Should I give IV fluid?

Depends! Pump, volume, or squeeze? If the patient is "just dry", then the hematocrit will probably be up – most hypotensive situations are usually treated with a bolus or two of normal saline given over a few minutes. For a really rapid fluid bolus you can put the saline in one of the pressure bags that we use for pressurizing arterial and central lines. Remember two things – giving fluid this way through a peripheral vein may blow your only access. Second – (very important, this) - **purge the air from the saline bag before you infuse!** Otherwise the patient will get the air as a bolus. Bad.

39: Should I give blood?

Depends! Do they need it? How would you know?

40: What if my postop patient drops her pressure?

Always scary. The first move is probably to give some volume – it's important to know if your patient got a lot of IV fluid during the case in the OR (and if she made urine during the case). Big postop belly cases will "sequester" (there's a word!) lots of fluid in and around the very vascular tissues everywhere in the abdomen, so they'll act like fluid sponges for at least a day or two. These patients can scare the life out of MICU personnel who don't recognize what's happening.

Another thing that can happen is that the patient simply warms back up. If Mr. Shmulewitz comes back from the OR after a long procedure with his chest or abdomen physically open for several hours, he's going to be very cold indeed when he gets back. Cold makes blood vessels do what now? Constrict, very good. With what effect on the blood pressure? Raises it, correct. Also very good. So as the patient warms up, the vessels will, what?… dilate – excellent. (And after they dilate at about two in the morning, you barium, right?)

And when they dilate, their pressure will do what?

Okay – let's get very ICU here. Ready? Mr. Shmulewitz goes to the OR after it's been found that he's infarcted much of his bowel. He just had to smoke and take birth control pills at the same time, didn't he? Dummy. He's down there for three hours, comes back with a PA line, and the anesthesiologist gives you report. Since the patient has a history of CHF, they tried to run him dry during the case – in other words, they didn't give him a lot of IV fluids, and they used a little neosynephrine to keep his pressure up. He made about 150cc of urine during the case. Blood loss was 500cc, and he got two packed cells intra-op.
Right. You unsnarl the lines, hook everything up, blood pressure is pretty good, say 126 systolic with a MAP of 67. Let's hook up the PA line – core temperature reads 94 degrees.

Let's shoot some numbers: CO /CI /SVR /SV are, respectively: 2.8/ 1.8 /2050 /25 . CVP is 12, PCW is 17.

Vent settings are 60% FiO2, IMV at a rate of 12, tidal volume of 700, PEEP of 15.

Interpretation please? Everyone remember how to interpret cardiac-output/ SVR/ SV numbers?

Something seems to be wrong. Cardiac output is low, but no, he's not cardiogenic. He's tight, that's for sure. Let's check an EKG – no changes. So what's going on? Anybody? Anyone notice the stroke volume? Doesn't look right? Right – that's they key here. Remember the three parts of a blood pressure: pump, volume and squeeze? Which one isn't in good shape here? He's certainly not having any trouble squeezing; look at that SVR. The cardiac output is iffy – is there a pump problem? Only indirectly. If this were cardiogenic shock, which the pattern does look like, it's true, would he be able to empty his LV? No. Not well, anyway. So his wedge pressure would be up, down, or sideways? Up – correct. But this wedge isn't very high. How about the stroke volume? That would be down in cardiogenic shock, but down to 25? That doesn't look right.

In fact, it's very low – the usual SV range is something like 70 –110 cc. Mr. Shmulewitz is dry – they ran him dry during the case, remember? But his abdomen was also open for three hours, right? You think you have insensible loss on a hot day? – just try hanging around for three hours, even in a cold OR, with your abdomen open to the breeze! Enormous fluid loss there. Plus almost all the water component he's got in his whole body is flying to his belly now. No wonder he needs neosynephrine!

So, okay, now we know what's going on. Great – let's give him some IV fluid. But this is the MICU, remember? And the resident is very aware of the history of CHF – once she's persuaded that this isn't cardiogenic shock, she takes her courage in both hands and gives you an order for D5 1/2NS at 75cc an hour for One Liter Only! Maybe you should call the surgeon back.

Now Mr. Y. begins to warm up. Covered up with nice blankets, nice warming circuit running on the vent (still intubated postop) – what happens? He dilates. Are you ready to barium? Not yet! Pressure drops some more. Let's shoot numbers again, in the same order. This time: 2.2 / 1.5 /2400/ 18. CVP is 10, PCW is 16. Ack! Even tighter! Bet he's losing his peripheral pulses at this point, fingers are blue…what to do? (That SV is awful low…)

Anybody catch the ringer in this situation? (Meaning, I threw in something that really does happen, but makes the situation less obvious than it might usually be.) Stroke volume is really low – he's obviously dry. But the CVP and wedge pressures are fine – is he really all that dry?

The ringer is the PEEP. (Strictly speaking, this situation really is too hard for beginners. But this is the kind of thing that you're going to see, and it can't be bad to throw in an example of something complex. Come back and look at it again a year from now.)

PEEP does what exactly? It sets an expiratory pressure limit, which is to say, the patient can exhale, but only to a point. The vent will maintain "x" amount of forward pressure through the ET tube at the end of expiration. Forward pressure. Into the chest.

Increasing PEEP pressure means that the intra-thoracic pressure increases, and that means that any pressure that you read coming out of that patient's chest is going to be artificially raised. It's going to read higher than it really is. Your CVP and wedge pressure numbers are lying to you. (But mom!!)

The way I was taught it, back when the ICU was in the basement of the Great Pyramid: for every 5cm of PEEP <u>after the first five</u>, take away three from the wedge pressure. And presumably, the CVP as well.

So the situation here – this patient is on how much? - fifteen of PEEP? Okay, so we ignore the first five, right? That leaves ten, or two fives, okay? And for each of those, we take three away from the central pressures, okay? So a CVP of 10, and there's two fives of PEEP left over, so that makes actually two threes, so that's six, so we, uh…what was the question?

It's really pretty easy. 15 of PEEP. Take away the first five. That leaves ten, or two fives. For each of those fives, take away three from the wedge and CVP. Two fives – two threes. Got it? Three fives, three threes. See? So the CVP which says 10 actually isn't 10, it's actually 4. See? And the wedge which said 16 is actually 10. See?

The point is: if there's a lot of PEEP, then you have to suspect your central line numbers – they're probably too high. The patient may very well be "wicked dry" (Boston speak). Is he peeing?

The best thing might be to call the surgeon.

Okay – here's Dr. Yakowitz. (The patient's niece?) Orders: normal saline 500cc IV bolus times two over 10 minutes each. (Use the pressure bag trick. **Vent the air first!**) Then run D5 lactated Ringer's (why do surgeons always use Ringer's?) at 300/hour, and give 250cc of 5% albumin every 4 hours until she comes back for morning rounds. Transfuse for a crit less than 30.

So – the patient gets a rapid bolus of a liter of NS, and a bolus of 5% albumin too, or a bag or two of hetastarch (which I understand they make from Jello…kidding!) – and his pressure starts to rise. Wow – look how far we weaned the neo in an hour – let's look at the numbers. Well - first off, the CVP is now 16, and the wedge is 22! Let's talk to Dave from respiratory – yeah, his P02 is 246 – think we can wean the PEEP down?…what do you mean the medical team wants to diurese the patient – we just got hydration orders from the surgeon! (Gnashing of teeth, rending of clothes.)

Let's shoot the numbers: 3.2/ 2.6/ 1700/ 46. Wow! Look at this: CO is 3.8, up from 2.2, index is 2.6, up from 1.5, SVR is down from 2400 to 1700, and the stroke volume is 46, up from 18. And who was the one that wanted to start dobutamine, huh?

So what Mr. Y has done here is to open up, as we filled him up. Make sense? His arteries could afford to loosen, because they were fuller. See that? Isn't that so cool? He's still on the dry side though, isn't he – see, his stroke volume is still low, and he's going to be hiding God-only-knows how much fluid in and around his abdominal wound for the next couple of days, so you need to straighten out your fluid management orders right away.

No – it isn't always that complicated. But wasn't that <u>fun</u>? (Total geek, your preceptor.)

41: What if her abdomen/ arm/ neck/ leg is swelling?

Well, of course, that's the other thing. Postop bleeding happens sometimes – rarely, but it happens. Follow the hematocrit, follow the coags, tell the team, and what I do in belly situations is to measure the abdominal girth every couple of hours with a measuring tape, just as I would for any part of the body that was swelling. Time for an abd CT? Retroperitoneal bleeding, maybe? Last week we had a patient whose neck was swelling after a central line insertion – I've seen it happen after (traumatic) intubation as well, but for different reasons, right? Bleeding vs. subcutaneous air. Either way, that patient is at risk for airway closure – should the patient be tubed? Do you know where your trach kit is? (And the surgeon?)

Non-human example: we took our newly adopted greyhound to get spayed, and brought her home with a lump next to her incision which grew steadily, hour by hour. Went back to the vet, who reassured us repeatedly that this was a seroma, a collection of serous fluid. Seroma my butt. That poor dog wound up with hematomas extending down all four legs, and that was after she spent the night at another vet's hospital with a pressure binder on. The vet had missed a bleeder.

42: What if he pulls out his arterial line?

Oh, well, that's no big deal, right? They can just pop in another one, right? What if the patient is anticoagulated? This can be the source of significant blood loss. Grab the site, compress it, and think about sending a hematocrit. Hold pressure for about 10 minutes, apply a pressure dressing (not too tight!), tell the team, and come back to take the dressing off a few minutes later to see if everything is okay with the hand/ arm/ foot.

43: Central line?

Oh – I don't like this one. Very dangerous, because things could go either way, right? They could bleed outwards, or they could suck air inwards – or they could bleed into their tissues. And what if that's the only access they have? And they're getting their pressors/ sedation/ TPN/ paralysis and antibiotics through it? Nuh-uh: bad.

44: PA line?

Same kind of thing, except that if the line only gets pulled back to the RV – well, somebody tell me, what's the dangerous thing about that? And what if one of the proximal ports is hanging outside of the skin? With the levophed running through it?

Related question – what do you do if your PA line is stuck in wedge?

45: Balloon pump?

Don't let this happen. Make sure that the team knows if your balloon patient is getting confused (they often do), and keep her safe. Sometimes that may even involve intubation, so that the patient can be sedated safely with something like propofol.

46: What if he pulls out his only IV access and drops his pressure immediately?

Lost your pressor access? Well – do what you can. Get the team in the room – you're going to need quick central access, and for that you want a femoral line so that you don't have to futz around with x-rays and stuff. Or if there's any delay at all, you can try putting in a (hopefully) large-bore peripheral line and running some fluid along with some neosynephrine in a peripheral mix: 10mg in 250cc. We're only supposed to run that for as long as it takes to get a central line in; pressors and peripheral blood vessels really don't go together well. In a code? Do what you have to do, but go to a central line as soon as possible.

47: Needs sedation immediately?

Feeling nervous? Oh, the _patient_...I think we looked at this question somewhere else, maybe in "Med Tips". Here's a story I heard: a patient, young guy, maybe an OD? He'd been intubated and lined for apnea and hypotension, and I think also maybe had an aspiration pneumonia, so I think it wouldn't have been safe for him to extubate right away. Anyhow, the guy woke up, extubated himself (you know how to work the restraints, right?), yanked his IV's, and was halfway out of the bed by the time the nurses got down the hall. Looking a little blue, too, he was, and no IV's left. That was when they did the nebulized morphine trick. Worked like a charm.

48: Has a rapidly enlarging hematoma at the line site?

At the site where his line pulled out? Or where the new one went in? Not a good sign either way. Is he on heparin? Get the team – if it's really growing quickly, think it might be arterial? Once in a while a central line will wind up in the nearby artery, and if your patient is very hypoxic you may not be able to tell by the color of the blood in the line – likewise if she's hypotensive, it won't come out under pressure the way it normally might. Try hooking it up to a transducer and have a look at the pressure – even if the patient is hypotensive, the pressure will be lots higher in an artery than it will be in a vein.

For the hematoma itself nothing works like pressure at the site. Sandbags seem to have gone out of favor in recent years, and anyway a rapid bleed might need manual pressure, followed by one of those clamps that they use in the cath lab. Once the team takes a look you might want to ask if vascular surgery should take a look at the site; sometimes a patient will need a vessel surgically repaired. Check the distal perfusion – good pulses below? Know how to run a pulse-volume recorder?

49: Has trouble after a paracentesis?

Most of the problems that come after paracentesis have to do with blood pressure dropping after the procedure. The liver is going to start re-effusing ascites (out of the circulation, into the abdomen) as soon as you remove what was there, and it may happen at a pretty rapid rate. Usually the thing to keep in mind is that the patient may need volume replacement: we give one unit of 25% albumin IV for every liter of ascites removed. The albumin tends to stay in the circulation better than IV fluid would, so this works pretty well. Watch out for bloody drainage.

50: Thoracentesis?

This has generally gotten much safer since they got better at ultrasound-guided drainage. Even with really good x-rays, it was just never easy to know where the needle was going, exactly. Obviously the big problem to watch for is pneumothorax – everybody know what a patient with a pneumo looks like? Short of breath – sure. Get a chest film – you're going to get one anyhow to see how well the lungs are re-expanded, right? Know how to page surgery? Know how to needle the chest? Should you? Keep a pleurevac handy.

Arterial Squeeze

51: What if my patient suddenly drops her BP?

How long have you got for an answer? We talked about arrhythmic problems before – of the three parts of the blood pressure, that was "pump". Next would be "volume", and we talked about blood products and IV fluids some. This time it's the third part we're interested in: "arterial squeeze". Some people call this "tone". Not at all hard to grasp – think of the system of arteries as elastic tubes, which is what they are, that can dilate and constrict, which they do. If you have a fixed amount of volume being pumped around in the system of tubes, and the tubes all suddenly dilate, what happens to the pressure? Drops, right? So if you assume that the pump is working okay, and the volume is okay, then what do you do if the squeeze starts to unsqueeze? Anybody remember what an alpha receptor is?

53: Has a sudden rise in BP?

So why are you complaining? Lots of reasons for this – is the patient agitated? Can you tell if your patient is agitated, if he's chemically paralyzed? Not sedate enough maybe? We had a patient a while back who was intubated and who had some kind of expressive neuro deficit, and she really couldn't communicate. She was hypertensive and tachycardic for about two days until someone figured out that she hadn't stooled for a few days…after all sorts of maneuvers with IV meds and drips and this and that, what fixed the problem was a manual disimpaction.

What I worry about more is an inadvertent pressor bolus. There are several ways that this can happen, none of them good for the patient. **You need to try to keep your pressor delivery very constant**. If you're using a background IV flush with the pressors infusing along with it, try connecting the pressor using a manifold (triple stopcock) at the end of the flush line, closest to the patient. If you make a change in the pressor rate and the drip is connected to the flush line two feet away from the patient, she may not "see" the change for a long time if the flush is running at 10cc per hour. For that reason it's usually a good idea to run the flush at a faster rate while you're initially getting the pressors going – the patient will respond more rapidly to changes in the drip.

What you really don't want to do is to bolus the patient with pressor. If your patients' BP drops, yes, turning up the flush rate briefly will get some pressor into the patient. Did his blood pressure just go from 70 to 270 systolic as a result? 320? Not good. But look what else happened – you've neatly washed the flush line clear of pressor, and now the patient may bottom out again before the med gets back down the line. Also not good. Smooth delivery is the only way.

53: Is becoming septic?

Same problem, right? Dilated arterial bed – bacteremia, endotoxins, (and more lately as the theories say: problems in the clotting cascade? Think Xigris?)

The three rules of sepsis:

1: Fill the tank (fill up the dilated system with volume).

110

2: Squeeze the tank (that'll be your alpha pressor; probably neosynephrine).

3: Kill the bugs.

You're really going to want both central and arterial lines for this patient. It is not good practice to run pressors without an a-line, and for rapid volume administration nothing but a central line will do. We have large bore introducers – they really work well. (They run "like stink".) Useful for GI bleeds too.

54: What if I turn her in the bed and her pressure drops?

Jayne: Turn her back!
This happens sometimes, in my experience usually with septic patients who are in the really sickest phase of their disease course. The way it was explained to me once was that the patient is probably compressing her septic "focus" – her infectious "pocket", hidden away somewhere, and injecting purulent material into her circulation, causing an acute pressure drop. "Septic showering", they call it. Not a very good sign. Need another abd CT? Maybe IR can find a pocket to drain.

Then there are the patients who get turned in bed and arrest – it seems like the really acute, hypoxic patients who are on all kinds of PEEP, maybe 100% oxygen, maybe on pressors, acidotic, but early on – in the acute phase of whatever it is that they're doing – do this once in a while. Usually a brady arrest, it seems to me. Not a very good sign, but I can remember some patients who got better after doing things like this. I have no real clue why it happens.

55: How do I pick a pressor?

Obviously it varies with the hypotension's cause. Is your patient septic, arterially dilated? They're going to need fluid first, and then something to agonize the alpha receptors, which live in the arteries, right? Neosynephine/ phenylephrine is pure alpha, so it's a good choice for that.

What if they're cardiogenic? Well, which receptors live in the heart – the betas? Which pressor has a "b" in it's name? Dobutamine? Good choice! Except – do you really want to flog this hurtin' heart with something that is going to make it work even harder? I didn't think you did. This patient needs an intra-aortic balloon pump – before they came along, almost 100% of cardiogenic shock patients died.

There's definitely more than you ever wanted to know about this subject in the articles on "Pressors and Vasoactives", and "IABP Review". Don't say I didn't warn you.

56: What if I turn up the pressor and nothing happens?

Always scary. You have to work very hard at being patient. Make sure the flush line is running fast enough that the higher pressor dose is actually getting to the patient. Make sure the pressor is plugged in really close to the patient. <u>Don't</u> give a pressor bolus if it's at all possible – it will only create a whole new set of problems. Don't be afraid to turn the drip rate up on the med itself, but be ready to dial down quickly to avoid overshooting. I usually start cutting back as soon as I see any rise in the patient's blood pressure at all.

57: What if my patient gets a pressor bolus?

Now look - what did I just tell you?

This really isn't a good thing to happen, but it's very clear when it does: usually the blood pressure goes frighteningly high, maybe close to 300 systolic. That pressure surge usually causes a reflex bradycardia, which is the little carotid bodies saying "Slow down!" – exactly the reverse of the usual septic situation, wherein they say "Speed up!" The carotid bodies sit in the aortic arch, looking down into the LV – if the volume reaching them out of the LV suddenly pops up, they send out the message to slow down, and vice versa. That's how the reflex tachycardia occurs in sepsis. The bradycardia that comes with a pressor bolus should not need treatment – the heart rate will come back up as the pressure comes back down.

58: What if my waveforms and numbers just don't make any sense at all?

They're confusing enough when they working properly, aren't they? Sometimes you have to sort things out equipment-wise, especially coming back from a road trip to CT or MRI ; where they seem to have this ability to wrap all the lines and cables around the patient's body in coils – how do they do that? Cables sometimes get plugged into the wrong transducers during a transport, sometimes things get confusing. Start from scratch, and try to sort things out from the monitor to the patient cable by cable, re-zero and re-level everything.

Still not making sense? Here's a common scenario: often the first wedge pressure that gets read is the one that they do during the line placement, while the patient is still in a little bit of Trendelenburg, where they've been maybe for the past hour and a half, maybe getting agitated…yet everyone is surprised when you measure the number again after the patient has had a chance to recover. The fact is that all pressures usually rise and fall together – if your patient is agitated, with a BP of 190/ 110, then the wedge and the CVP will both be elevated too: "Well, yeah, but 32 was his "agitated" wedge. Now that he's sitting back up and gotten his pm ativan, his wedge is 18. Do you still want me to give the lasix?"

CAD

59: What if my patient is having ischemia?

You know this stuff from earlier on – do all that good anti-ischemia stuff.

60: What if my patient has chest pain that won't go away?

Not a good thing. This is often what buys the patient a ticket to the cath lab. The first thing to do is to make sure that it's actually a cardiac process going on – if it's not clear, try doing a Mylanta test. Try to figure out if the pain is actually coming from the chest tube that they put in the patient yesterday… if it turns out to be an ischemic event, do all those nice anti-anginal things that you did before. See if anything specific makes a difference in the patient's pain at all, and let the team know what it is. Make sure the patient is very well oxygenated. Watch for ectopy. Send cardiac enzymes. Do EKGs. If the patient does get a cath, plan for the possibility of a balloon pump.

61: What if my patient is having an MI?

What, you mean you left your copy of Braunwald at home? I mean, it only weighs 80 pounds! But we should be able to sum it all up in a couple of minutes…as always, it all depends on the context and the severity of the event. Send enzymes. Think about possible, sometimes even predictable problems: one example might be bradycardias and large fluid requirements in an IMI / RV infarct. Be ready for acute "flashing" of CHF in left-system infarcts. (Why?) Be ready for arrhythmias. Does the patient need lysis? Need an aspirin? You too?

62: What is cardiogenic shock?

Shock is the word used to describe the state that the body gets into when it's not perfusing the peripheral tissues very well, and each of the three components of a blood pressure has it's own version of shock to go with it – this time the name sort of gives it away. Almost by definition a cardiogenic patient is going to be in the middle of a big left-sided MI, diminishing the pumping ability of the LV. Poor pump, poor output, poor pressure, poor perfusion, acidosis, etc. Some patients with a poor EF will always have cardiogenic-looking numbers if you put a PA line in them…and make sure they're not just dry! There's altogether too much material on cardiogenic shock in the Balloon Pump Refresher…

Respiratory

Non- Intubated:

63: What if my patient becomes short of breath?

This is almost never going to happen out of context with the underlying problem – does the patient have heart disease – did she flash? Did she aspirate? Does she have her air boots on? (Why am I asking?) Did she plug? Anaphylax? See Vin Diesel on the TV? (My daughter explains these things to me.)

You won't go wrong by calling for help – get the team, get respiratory, get the resource nurse. Does the patient need to be suctioned? The good thing is that - as always - you don't have to work the problem by yourself. Let me restate this central principle yet again: get help. Ask questions. Work with the team, of which you are a part.

Not actually to be filed under the "short of breath" category, but a nice story anyhow, is the time that I was working on a floor, I think it was during the Pleistocene era (I try to remember which dinosaurs were around then besides myself), and a woman gave me a frantic wave from down the hall. Her roommate, a nice enough lady who never stopped talking, ever, under any circumstances including sleep, had done the classic aspiration thing of a piece of her dinner – just like they teach you in CPR. Obviously before the days of central sat monitoring. She was a very interesting color. I slid into the bed behind her – she was sitting up – did the Heimlich, and out it popped. So that works, anyhow. Or it did then. Good to know.

64: What if she has COPD?

These patients carry around their own set of problems. Oftentimes they'll come in with something that's pushed them over the edge – they're usually sitting there with their feet hanging over the edge anyway. Maybe a URI, maybe pneumonia, maybe a COPD flare. Remember that these folks won't tolerate much oxygen. Nebs, steroids, antibiotics maybe, and remember too that any sedation you give them may be just what they need to stop breathing…

65: Is acutely hypoxic?

Is he wet? Did he plug? Throw a PE? Come disconnected from the vent? Try to think of the possibilities, and try to fit things in with the diagnostic picture: "Oh, he needs to be diuresed again." Or: "Oh, he's just put his chewing gum over his trach again – you can always tell." You'll never go wrong by calling for help, and getting an EKG, a blood gas, and maybe asking for a stat chest x-ray.

66: What if I gave her too much oxygen?

Ah, big deal. So she has COPD and stopped breathing, so what? I mean really, this preoccupation with trivial details…

67: Is acutely hypercarbic?

CO_2 narcosis is definitely for real. A COPD patient will become unresponsive if they "retain" CO_2 when they get too much oxygen. Everybody understands how that works, right? No?

In five minutes or less: When you hold your breath, and your brain begins to scream "Breathe, dopey!", it's the chemoreceptors (also in the brain?) that are doing the yelling, because why? Because your pCO_2 is rising, up into the 50's maybe. So, you breathe.

Now – if you're dealing with a COPD patient, he probably walks around with a pCO_2 in the 50's all the time. "50?", he says, "Ha! It is to laugh! I don't worry about no stinkin' CO2! I got plenty of CO2! How about that, huh? What you got? You talkin' ta me?" Taxi driver, is he? Personality might be giving you a clue here…

Of course with a pC02 of 70 he might not be breathing much anyhow, because he'll be narcotized – patients with COPD will still do this – and will become unarousable, barely breathing. Time for a tube? Narcan? Romazicon? Sometimes you can head off intubation with something like a bipap mask – they work, but I hate them. The patients often hate them. And all they need to do is vomit into them…can you imagine? The word is that it takes 20cm of forward pressure from a mask device to start pushing air into the esophagus, inflating the stomach…I wouldn't be so sure about that.

Anyway. In the case of COPDers, walking around as they do with a chronically high pC02, the chemoreceptor thing is deactivated – doesn't work any more, exactly because of that continually high C02, as though they had become saturated, which maybe they are. So these people use a backup system (apparently it was the Great Biomedical Engineer up above who invented redundant systems – I mean was that smart or what?) – they get a stimulus to breathe when they become hypoxic, rather than hypercarbic. You'd think hypoxia would be the primary drive, but it ain't.

"So okay, they breathe when they're hypoxic, big deal." Well, the problem is, see, that if you then give them all the oxygen that they seem to want, why, then they may have no drive to breathe at all, 'cause they aren't hypoxic any more. Which is what they were depending on. And they may stop. Right in front of you. Because you put 100% on them. Bummer.

Actually it seems to be a progressive thing – they'll breathe less and less as they get a higher and higher FiO2. This is called "retaining", because they retain CO2 in response to getting oxygen - they exchange less gas, breathing more and more shallowly. You can actually document the rise with a series of blood gases, and it can be very abrupt: "Look, on 40% his pCO2 was 62, but on 60% it was 104!" "I guess that was when he stopped breathing, huh?" Narced. Sometimes these patients want something like 1.5 liters/minute of oxygen and no more. Strange but true.

68: When should I get a blood gas?

Our rule is to get a blood gas anytime we make a vent change (about 20 minutes later), or if there's a clinical change in the patient. Here's a story: not too long ago we had a patient with respiratory failure, looking kind of tenuous on 100% face mask O2 (not a CO2 retainer… even some people with COPD, just aren't) – and the intern had sent a blood gas which looked pretty good. The patient became increasingly agitated, which was treated with some Ativan, then some Haldol. He then became unresponsive, and pale, and wasn't breathing much, if at all – when we asked the intern to send another gas, (he was in the room with us), he told us that the last one had been fine – what was the problem? Audience – what was the problem? Actually, more than one person in that room had a problem.

69: Suddenly starts wheezing?

Did the patient just get a new med? Is she having an allergic reaction to something? Is she halfway through her first dose of a new antibiotic? Stop giving whatever it is she's getting, get the team, get some benadryl, maybe some IV hydrocortisone…then there are the people who "flash" in CHF and wheeze – they call this "cardiac asthma": get an EKG. It always depends on the context.

70: What if my patient is "flashing"?

This often comes under what we looked at before under the heading of the "acutely ischemic" thing. The basic rule for any acute situation always applies: get the help you need into the room right away (this always includes the resource nurse.) Try to think ahead a bit: is the patient going to need intubation in the next five minutes? Three minutes? Half hour? Try to remember "LMNOP", ekgs, blood gases, an x-ray, things like that, and suggest them at appropriate times. Then make sure they happen if they need to.

71: What is "guppy breathing"?

It doesn't a whole lot of ICU experience to figure out that a patient breathing shallowly at a rate of 60 isn't going to last very long before needing some kind of intervention: mask vent support, suctioning, diuresis, intubation – maybe all of those, depending, but guppy breathing shouldn't be allowed to go along without some kind of decision about treatment.

72: What if my patient stops breathing?

Well now that doesn't sound very good, does it? As always, it depends on what's going on. Your 92-year-old DNR patient dying of terminal whatever is probably not going to be leaped upon. A patient with too much narcotic on board might get the oral airway-mask-bag plus narcan treatment (don't forget the restraints.) Your task is to see it coming. If you can do that, then you get to wear the invisible golden badge...some of the most experienced nurses never wear extraneous pins, plates, medals, or whatever – just scrub, name and maybe school pin. They're hoping you see the invisible badge.

Note to hospital administrators: if you want your ICU to run like a swiss watch, remember that it's the experienced nurses who are the jewels in the mechanism. Hold on to them.

73: Obstructs her airway?

What with? Did her tongue obstruct? Secretions? Time for a jaw thrust? Oral airway? Nasal airway? Suctioning? All of the above?

74: Has sleep apnea?

These are the people whose tongue will obstruct their airway about 25 times an hour so that they never get any sleep. Tiring. These people often do well with the application of a CPAP mask, or a nasal bipap device – the forward pressure holds things open during the breathing cycle. Sedatives usually a bad idea.

75: Plugs?

This should be the kind of thing that you see coming – the patient who comes in with pneumonia, getting hydrated maybe, who is starting to loosen up all the dry secretions that have been hiding in his lungs for the past week or two. Remember that secretions tend to create a pattern of worsening ventilation – the O2 sat may actually be okay, but the pC02 may be rising rapidly, so the patient's excellent saturation may be fooling you. Use a nasal trumpet for frequent blind suctioning, and say you're sorry.

76: What does a pneumothorax look like?

Sometimes young people will walk into an ER someplace complaining of feeling funny, and it'll turn out that they've been walking around with a dropped lung for who knows how long. Patients in the unit tend to be in rougher shape to start with, and a pneumo is usually pretty obvious – something suddenly looks really wrong. Your main clues still come from the context – did they just get a new neck/ chest central line? How many sticks did it take? How much PEEP is your patient on (are his lung apices up around his teeth – easier to hit?)

Once you have some idea of what the problem could be, the clues will start falling into place – oxygenation worsening abruptly? Any kind of abrupt respiratory change should get a chest x-ray; then hopefully you'll really know.

Another very useful clue is the appearance of a visible pulsus paradoxus on the patient's arterial line waveform. This is easier to understand than it sounds: the patient's blood pressure will drop when the pressure in the chest rises during the breathing cycle – if the patient is intubated, that happens on inspiration; if not intubated, it happens on expiration. If there's a substantial pneumo in there (or a cardiac tamponade – anything that compresses the heart), then the small addition of added pressure during the breath compresses the heart just enough to stop effective pumping – when the pressure comes off, then the pump starts working again. It's very dramatic sometimes, and it means that the situation in the chest is really becoming critical – soon the pressures will rise high enough that the heart will be compressed all the time. Bad.

77: Should we needle the chest or not?

You wouldn't want to be wrong about this, right? (My smart-guy best friend says "I thought I was wrong once but, uh, I was wrong.") Needling the chest may produce the pneumothorax that you are hoping to treat – and that patient will be pretty much committed to a chest tube as a result. Wait for the x-ray if you can, but have your equipment on hand. If the situation approaches a code, then giving your patient a chest tube will probably hurt a whole lot less than half an hour of chest compressions…

Intubated:

78: What if my patient codes during intubation?

This may mean that you waited too long to tube him – the team may hesitate to intubate a patient who might respond to other measures. Judgment call. Patients in the middle of some really acute ARDS-like situation may need more and more oxygen over the course of even a single shift – this kind of rapid movement usually means that intubation is coming, or should be. There's often a great deal of resistance to intubation in a situation that seems crystal - clear to experienced ICU nurses – and who may even be wrong. (I know – hard to believe that ICU nurses can be wrong.) My own feeling is that you can always extubate someone, but if you wait until they're horribly hypoxic you may get into real trouble.

An example: a patient with a sat of 97 on 100% high-flow mask O2, maybe plus a nasal cannula, or maybe on a CPAP mask is not going to do well if you remove all that hardware to intubate him…as in any acutely hypoxic situation where the sat drops, say, below 70, bradycardia can result. Have atropine nearby, but see if the patient's rate comes up first after the tube gets in.

79: Bites the ET tube?

Not good. I think we talked somewhere else about patients coding, or biting through pilot lines and deflating their tube cuffs - biting your airway closed is generally not such a good idea. This patient may need sedation, reassurance, a bite block, or all three.

80: Extubates herself?

Not a good thing – the patient can do herself some vocal cord damage this way, even though the cuffs are very soft and inflated to low pressures. Confused patients can be really determined to pull their ET tubes out, and can get very inventive about getting loose from restraints. A better plan is probably to keep the patient safely sedate until she's ready to extubate. Propofol is a good choice for this situation, as it wears off quickly.

If it looks like the patient might "fly" after a self-extubation, what we do is apply 100% FM 02 (if they're not a known C02 retainer), and watch them very carefully. Clearly some people are going to do worse than others; a patient intubated for airway protection after an opiate overdose will probably do fine if he's awake enough to extubate himself, but someone with a bad pneumonia may need reintubation right away. Keep your intubation equipment handy, and make sure everyone knows that the patient may "de-tune" at any time. Set your alarm limits tight!

Jayne: We keep a bag hanging beside the vent, with a mask O2 setup ready in case this happens.

81: Extubates herself and runs down the hall extubating everyone else?

Hmm. Is she an angry respiratory therapist? Ask her to deflate the cuffs first.

82: What if I can't get the ET tube cuff to seal?

Couple of possiblities: is the tube in the right place? If the cuff is near the cords, it won't seal because it isn't big enough to seal the airway up there. Look at the cm marks on the side of the tube: in average-size people the tube is usually in good position at around 22-24 cm of depth from the lip, or teeth. Make sure the tube is secured to the patient's face and head so it can't shift in and out. No, you can't use crazy glue.

Another possibility, but rare, is that something is wrong with the pilot balloon line. Once in a while the valve cracks, which can happen from somebody inserting an inflation syringe with too much force. Another real fun event is nicking the pilot line while shaving your patient. Either way, the cuff won't hold pressure. The trick: snip the line either at the valve if that's the problem, or at the place where it's nicked. You can insert a #19 butterfly into what's left of the line (try not to poke another hole in it) - hook that to a stopcock and a syringe, inflate the cuff to seal it, tape the whole gadget to a tongue blade, and call anesthesia: the ET tube will have to be changed.

83: How do I know if she needs to be reintubated?

It really should be obvious – she'll be having trouble breathing, not clearing secretions maybe. Sat will be low, respiratory rate will be too high or too low - you'll know.

GI

84: What if my patient pulls his NG tube?

I'd probably pull mine, too. Please make sure I'm getting enough Haldol. Make that fentanyl.

Have I mentioned the DNR tattoo that I'm going to get? I wonder if the shops in New Hampshire have the radio-opaque tattoo dye that shows up on a chest film: "I am a DNR! My attorney's phone number is…". I can just see the scene at the light box.

85: Pulls his NG tube just far out enough to aspirate tube feeds?

Bad. Every now and then you'll walk into a room and say, "Well, this patient is a very short little guy - that NG tube looks way out to me." This is why you want to check the position of the NG tube at the beginning of every shift. In fact, you should keep in mind that you need to check the position of everything at the beginning of every shift (and during the shift!) – last night I noticed that my patient's central line looked like it had taken a yank; not mentioned during report. There was a blood return from all three ports, but the only thing to do was to get a film – it was okay, but who knew?

Question for the group: when do you think you should add methylene blue to the patient's tube feeds?

86: Vomits?

Did he aspirate? Why is he vomiting? Inferior ischemia? Too much tequila before he went down in the airport bar? Did I enter the room? (Why does that happen so much?)

87: Vomits tube feeds?

Did he aspirate? What was the residual last time you checked? Sometimes the end of an NG tube will tuck up into a corner of the stomach – if my patient hasn't got much in the way of bowel sounds and hasn't had much aspirate in a day, I sometimes pull the tube back a bit or advance it a bit. Sometimes you find a 600cc surprise this way.

Sometimes an NGT will get too far in. You might see a patient losing really enormous amounts of NG drainage, maybe 5 liters a day – the tube may have made it's way into the duodenum. The drainage is usually lighter and clearer than your usual gastric output, and there's really too much of it – if you think that the tube is too far in, you may find that if you pull it back while leaving it to low suction, the drainage may suddenly change color to a nice gastric green. It'll change anyhow, once the tip comes back into the stomach.

88: Vomits and aspirates?

Did he aspirate? Guess so! You were keeping the head of the bed at 45°, right? Checking aspirates, right? Has she stooled lately? Sometimes it just happens, as do many things, no matter how careful or how perfect your care is. Watch the person carefully – almost by definition they're going to have a new pneumonia to deal with. Does she need blind suctioning? Reglan? Intubation?

89: Vomits "coffee grounds"?

Did she aspirate? The classic upper GI bleed scenario. Check a crit, watch her pressure, saline lavage through an NG tube The team definitely inserts this one, esophageal varices can pop if they get poked by an NG tube going down, but how do you know ahead of time? History of previous bleeds? Cirrhosis? Is the patient getting something to block acid secretion?

90: Bright red blood?

"BRB": a little worse than coffee grounds. This person is probably going to need an endoscopy – should he be intubated for airway protection before they do it? Can the patient consent for transfusion? If no one is available for consent, they team can sign the consent themselves, indicating that they couldn't reach any "significant others", and that the situation was emergent.

91: What if he starts passing melanotic stool, or BRBPR?

Same idea, different place. Depending on the severity of the bleed, the patient can be transfused and watched, not transfused and watched, colonoscopized (how exactly do they expect a patient in the midst of an acute abdominal process to drink all that go-lytely, exactly?), or maybe even operated on. Make sure that you're in close communication with the blood bank, and have supplies set up ahead of time. We sometimes "call for the cooler" – which will have all available units of say, A-negative FFP that are due to expire in the next six hours – something like that.

92: What if my patient starts having severe abdominal pain?

This usually happens to me in the car. I need to stay out of Starbucks. Sometimes this can be a whole lot of nothing – other times, some deadly process. Assess carefully, document carefully, drag the resource nurse and the team into the room, follow up. Abdominal CT scan? RUQ ultrasound (what would that be looking for?) Does surgery need a heads-up about the patient?

93: What if he's pregnant?

This almost happened to me in a car. I never got as far as ultrasound though.

94: What does appendicitis look like?

Hurts! I understand that it can show up anywhere in the abdomen. Where is McBurney's Point? – two exits past Dennisport on the Cape, right? I know a good place for lobster rolls.

Jayne: "This whole part is stupid." (Just for the record.)

95: What does a bowel infarct look like?

This is something that we actually do see at times, unlike appendicitis, although all sorts of things are always possible. It's important to remember that hypotension can produce really serious effects in all kinds of places, especially if your patient is a vasculopath to start out with. A patient with high blood pressure at home may have kidneys that go into ATN after just an hour or two of hypotension. (They may have blood pressure like that because their renal arteries are stenosed, and the kidneys are cranking out angiotensin and all, trying to perfuse themselves.) Those renals may be stenosed just like their coronary ones are, and maybe like their carotids, and maybe their mesenteric…)

No bowel sounds, that's for sure. And what do you think their chemistries might be doing?

96: What if my patient has lost bowel sounds, has a K of 6.7 and a pH of 7.10?

See, you already knew! Dead tissue of any size in the body is going to release all the intracellular K it has, and all the poorly perfused/ dead/ almost dead tissue involved is going to go into anaerobic respiration before it dies, producing a big lactic acidosis. These people have lactate levels upwards of 10 – your basic humongous metabolic acidosis. Other things being equal, what will their ABGs look like? (A lactate of ten is high enough to make us old nurses cringe. Saw somebody in the 20's last week, but for different reasons. Your basic Real Bad Sign.)

GU

99: What if my patient stops making urine?

Remember all that stuff about pre-renal, intra-renal, and post-renal?

Pre-renal: ("dry") "Pre" meaning: what's happening in the blood <u>before</u> the kidney gets a chance to see it. <u>Ahead</u> of the kidney. The patient isn't making much urine because he's volume depleted – there's not much water component in his blood. Is his hematocrit 52? Sometimes patients arrrive in the MICU after being diuresed into renal failure from too much volume loss: the BUN will be high, but the creatinine will be normal or heading upwards, maybe something like 70/ 1.2, assuming that they were normal to start with. Some patients certainly look like they need aggressive diuresis – it's usually not wrong to treat someone for CHF if that's what seems to be the problem. Of course if it isn't CHF, or even if it is, they may get a bit too dry. These patients' will probably be making some urine, but very concentrated. One time you might see the pre-renal thing happen is in a patient receiving full-strength tube feeds as her only intake – this stuff is so concentrated that the patient may literally dry out and stop making much urine. Time to dilute that stuff to half strength, and run it at twice the speed. Watch the aspirates.

Intra-renal: In the kidney. If the patient has actually taken a "kidney hit", the problem will probably be something like ATN. This can take a long time to resolve – months, sometimes. Acutely, the scenario is usually a period of hypotension for one reason or another; sepsis maybe. The BUN may not rise right away, but the creatinine will bump up suddenly: 35/ 4.0 . Kidneys really hate to be underperfused – they become "insulted". ("Stupid kidneys!") It seems even easier to insult elderly kidneys that may be perfused by stenotic arteries – if your patient is a vasculopath everywhere else, e.g. coronary arteries, carotid bruits maybe – you can bet they may have renal artery stenosis. These folks' kidneys usually see decent perfusion only at high blood pressure levels, 'cause not a whole lot of blood gets by the stenosis – even an hour or so at a relatively low pressure may make them go into a coma. The kidneys.

Jayne: Keep the patient's MAP above 65 to try to avoid the whole problem.

Post-renal: This is what happens when nobody flushes the foley after the urine output drops. Something is stuck in the urine path <u>after</u> it's been processed by the kidney. Ureteral stone, maybe, or compression of the ureter(s) by something like lymphadenopathy, or tumor? What happens to the kidney if its drainage system is plugged? What does a renal ultrasound look for?

100: Makes too much urine?

Give a little too much lasix, did ya? Sometimes patients will do it on their own; they'll "auto-diurese" for one reason or another – often this has to do with a patient who has high baseline blood pressure and comes in hypotensive. They may not be developing renal failure, but once their pressure gets back up into their normal range they may suddenly start to produce really large hourly volumes. You might see this in a patient who gets sedation for a short period of intubation. While the sedation is on (and the BP is relatively low) the urine output may not be so great – but when the sedation is weaned off – and especially if the patient is a bit agitated (BP up), the output may suddenly become very impressive. Other auto-diuresers: patients who are a couple of days postop may suddenly start mobilizing the five liters of Ringer's that they got during the case.

Then there's diabetes insipidus – this is when you (let me think about this for a second) don't make enough ADH: anti-diuretic hormone. ADH <u>stops</u> you from peeing. <u>Anti</u> diuretic. Not enough ADH, you pee all the time, with a thirst to match. In one end, out the other. Like a siphon. Which is what "diabetes" means. Greek to me, man. Of course, you also turn into a siphon if your blood sugar is 700 for a couple of days…

SIADH is the other way: too much ADH – you don't pee hardly at all. Got something to do with holding onto sodium I think – sort of the opposite of lasix.

101: Pulls his foley out?

Ow. Was the balloon up? Call urology. Better yet – don't let this happen. (Although even with the best precautions, Houdini down the hall there may find a way.)

102: Twice?

Really ow! Where's urology? If the urethra has been injured, the foley may have to stay in for some time – a couple of weeks?- until it heals.

103: Develops hematuria?

Are you surprised? You spoke to urology, right? Time to start a saline drip through a three-way catheter – and urology put it in, right? Don't let it clot off…
104: With clots?

What did I just say? Are you even listening? Am I just talking to exercise my face? That's the problem with young nurses nowadays. In my day, we had to make our own clots! In the summer! Out of snow! Uphill! Both ways! Yadda yadda! (This doesn't work on my kids, either.)

If the clots are passing through the catheter, good! The problem is: what if they don't? This is why it is absolutely a rule that a saline infusion through a 3-way foley must never, ever be on a pump. Gravity only. Figure it out – what if the pump kept pumping in, and nothing was coming out because a clot was covering the drainage lumen…? If you think that a three-way catheter is clotted, you can try manually flushing it with 30cc of saline, but what often happens is that the clot forms a little flapper over the openings at the tip, which will let you flush into the bladder, but closes when fluid tries to drain. You're going to have to change that tube.

A word about scrotums. Yeah, I know. But somebody has to bring it up. (Maybe the wrong phrase?) We see a lot of patients who are very third-spaced – they have diffuse tissue edema, and the scrotum is not immune; they can really swell up. After getting really worried about one of my patients I checked with the surgeons – simple treatment: an ace wrap. Sometimes referred to as a "Scro-Ted". Not too tight! Works like a charm. Like a jewel. Jewels. Something like that.

105: Without clots?

You can usually prevent clots from forming if you run the saline irrigant drip quickly enough – this may involve using bag after bag of saline, but that's just what you have to do. It can be hard to measure exactly what's going in and out – just make sure that what's coming out every hour is more than what's going in! Sometimes we use the little spring measures that are used with PD bags – these tell you how much is infused by the changing weight of the bag.

It's good to have some standard to identify how bloody urine is, besides "Clots or no clots?" Over the years we've gotten comfortable with the "wine-shop" method: "Well, his urine is a nice chardonnay today, but it was definitely a merlot yesterday. Getting better." Often hematuria will be bad enough to require transfusions… what is amicar?

106: What if his BUN and creatinine are doubling every day?

Bad. Foley plugged? Did she spend eight hours hypotensive – heading into ATN? She may be in for a rough month. A useful maneuver that's come up in the past year or so: patients heading into renal failure will usually (duh!) stop making urine – but if you slap them with a big dose of diuretic while they're still on the steep part of the failure curve – just as they're heading into it – sometimes you can get them to change from oliguric ("not peeing much") to non-oliguric ("peeing pretty good") renal failure. What we do is to give some enormous dose of "synergistic diuresis" (whoa! $1.50 for that one) – something like 200mg of lasix and 500mg of diuril, one after the other. If it works, then at least the patient will get rid of water – they won't clear much BUN, but you'll be able to keep them out of CHF.

Blind Suctioning for Beginners

A couple of the newbies were really having trouble with this one, so we decided to clear things up. This is one of those procedures that people get vague about: "Did you deep suction her." "Yeah, with the Yankauer." (But Yankauer suction isn't deep suctioning.) "Uh… well, did you blind suction her?" "Yeah, like I said, with the Yankauer!" (Yeah, well, that ain't right either.) "Well, I mean, did you get into her airway?" "Yeah, in the back of her throat." (Nope, nope…)

So let's clear things up a little. As always, please remember that these articles are not meant to be official references in any way! This is just what we do, where I work, elsewhere things may be different. Always check with your local policies, procedures, and references!

1- What is suctioning all about?
2- What is "deep" suctioning"
3- Is Yankauer suctioning deep suctioning?
4- What is "blind" suctioning?
5- How do I tell if my patient needs blind suctioning?
6- How do I tell if my patient shouldn't have blind suctioning?
7- What bad things can happen from blind suctioning?
8- What is a nasal trumpet?
9- How do I place a nasal trumpet?
10- Should I pre-oxygenate my patient for blind suctioning?
11- How high should I set the suction?
12- How does Nurse Markie do it?
13- How do I collect a sputum sample during suctioning?

1- What is suctioning all about?

Lots of patients need secretion management. Pneumonia and the like. Seems simple enough – your patient has some secretions that he can't clear: he can't cough them up, maybe he's a bit weak, maybe he just has too much down there to clear on his own – what to do?

2- What is "deep" suctioning?

There's a lot of confusion about this, and as usual, using terms precisely goes a long way towards getting un-confused. Deep suctioning means going past the posterior pharynx with a catheter, through the vocal cords, down **into the patient's airway (trachea!),** and applying suction, to remove thick secretions that are making it hard for your patient to breathe.

This is a pretty serious maneuver – in essence, it's the same as intubating someone, except with a skinny catheter, and blindly - wooo…. You need to know exactly how to do this, and safely!

3- Is Yankauer suctioning deep suctioning?

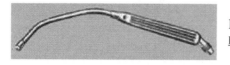

No, it isn't. It doesn't get into the trachea.
http://www.ssgfx.com/CP2020/medtech/tools/images/yankauer.jpg

4- What is "blind" suctioning"?

The idea is that you can't really see where you're going with the catheter, so you have to work "blind".

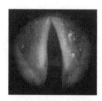

You need to get past these guys...

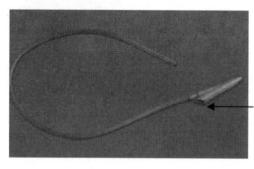

With one of these guys... a "whistle-tip" catheter. The suction only comes out of the end of the catheter when you put your finger over the opening at the proximal end...

Here...
This is a good thing, because you **don't** want the suction running while you're advancing the catheter....

http://www.medabv.ru/kendall/13-1.jpg

The catheter is lubricated with some of this stuff:

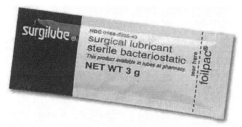

Who used to call this "kalubafax"... wow – THAT was a long time ago.

http://www.medco-school.com/images/products/88860L.jpg

126

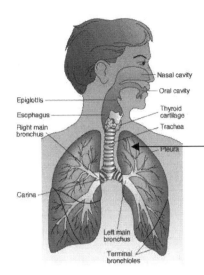

And then the catheter gets passed, up one of the nostrils, along the same path that an NG tube takes, along the curve of the nasopharynx, except not into the esophagus…

…into the trachea.

This is a pretty invasive procedure! Actually, you're intubating him…

http://connection.lww.com/Products/taylor5e/documents/Ch45/jpg/45_001.jpg

5- How do I tell if my patient needs blind suctioning?

Your assessment skill don't need to really be too advanced to notice that your patient is turning kind of blue, can't cough up the secretions he's got from his pneumonia, or aspirated ice cream or whatever. It's usually pretty clear. Was your patient extubated too soon?

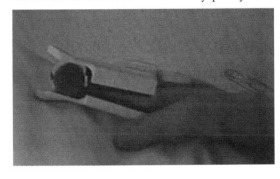

You know what this is, right?

http://www.healthsystem.virginia.edu/internet/periop/images/pacup053.jpg

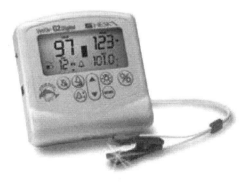

Hooked up to something like this?

And the numbers should be something like what?

http://www.heska.com/images/g2_230.jpg

6- How do I tell if my patient <u>shouldn't</u> have blind suctioning?

Assuming you would, otherwise, you mean?

- Is he on comfort measures only? Would he be more, or less comfortable if you suctioned him? Would you just have to do it again in a minute?

- Is he anticoagulated? What's he going to do if you start inserting things in his nares?

- Is he a cardiac patient? What nerve runs through the carina? What is the carina? What could happen if you stimulate your patient's vagus nerve if he's having – say, an inferior MI? What drug might you want to have at the bedside? Anyway?

7- What bad things can happen from blind suctioning?

Not too hard to figure out, but worth mentioning:

- You can make the patient seriously hypoxic.

- You can injure the patient (or get the lung biopsy the surgeons were going to get anyhow), by using suction equipment that's pulling too hard.

- You can provoke a serious bradycardia from vagal stimulation. This is pretty rare, but it does happen once in a while. Usually with inferior MI's ☺.

- You can infect the patient's lower airway.

- You can provoke nasopharyngeal bleeding, and the patient could aspirate blood.

Yup, it's all true. But if your patient's airway is almost obstructed with secretions, you need to do something! So learn to do it safely…

8- What is a nasal trumpet?

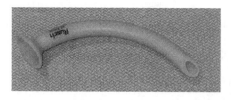 Cute! Nice and soft. Lubricate it up really well with the surgilube stuff. Passing the catheter through this, instead of the patient's bare nasopharynx, will go a long way towards preventing nasal trauma. Is your patient heparinized? Why am I asking?

http://anesthesia.uihc.uiowa.edu/proceduralsedation3/adult/images/nasalairway.jpg

9- How do I place a nasal trumpet?

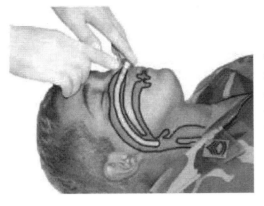

Gently! Remember that some patients have deviated nasal septa, right? One side may let the trumpet pass easily, the other may not. Never force anything, ever! If you can't pass the trumpet on either side, you may have to try passing the catheter without it. Suctioning any patient repeatedly without a trumpet is almost guaranteed to provoke bleeding…

http://www.brooksidepress.org/Products/OperationalMedicine/DATA/operationalmed/Procedures/Images/NasalAirway2.jpg

10- Should I pre-oxygenate my patient for blind suctioning?

Good question! The answer is: probably. Usually. <u>Almost</u> always. Ventilated patients <u>should</u> always get pre-oxygenated: there's a 100% Fi02 button that you can press to do this.

But a patient on prongs? Or a mask? Well… hm. Are there situations when it wouldn't be safe to give a certain patient 100% oxygen? Which patients are those? Why isn't it safe?

In those situations, you have to watch the patient like a hawk, and have mask oxygen at hand. If they desaturate

11- How high should I set the suction?

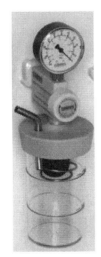

Not too high! About 140-160mm Hg negative pressure is what we use…

http://www.ecomed.com.au/cat/pimages/31.jpg

12- How does Nurse Markie do it?

Ok, the patient is drowning. Saturation is getting low. He's clearly in distress. Let's save him!

Gather your equipment: got the trumpet in? Got the catheter? The lube? Sterile gloves? Is the suction setup working? You had all this stuff ready at the bedside, right, because you knew your patient might need this…

Let's see – how do I do this? Been doing it so long…

- Make sure your patient agrees to this procedure. You are NOT allowed to attack a patient who is competent to refuse things. At the same time, you do need to keep her safe, so it's best to have things worked out in advance. Patients who aren't competent to refuse need to have proxy issues worked out…

- Apologize ahead of time. This is one of the most unpleasant things you'll ever do to a patient…

- Try to have a helper on hand to catch flying extremities. It's not nice to get punched out by an angry, confused patient that you're trying to help…

- Sit the patient up. Pillow behind the head. (Assignment for next time: look up the "sniffing position". Does she have an NG tube? I'd hook it up to suction, try to empty her stomach – if you provoke vomiting while you suction her, you KNOW what's going to happen, right?

- Apply the oxygen, in the right amount. If this patient retains carbon dioxide when she gets oxygen, I'd apply just enough for her to resaturate – it's hyperoxia that's going to make her stop breathing, right? This is rather a judgment call – what you want to do is assess her oxygenation almost continuously as you do this.

- Insert the lubricated trumpet. Slide in easily? If it doesn't, try the other side. You're watching her sat while you do this, right?

- Open the end of the catheter packaging, and tuck the catheter under your arm. Hold it there.

- Sterile gloves. I squeeze some sterile lube onto the glove paper and leave it there.

- Suction tubing handy? Set to the right negative pressure? Not too high!

- Ok – with a sterile gloved hand, reach over to your armpit and pull out the catheter. Don't get it contaminated on anything – you'll have to start over if you do, and your patient isn't breathing too well! (Jayne says: "Are you OUT of your mind? NEVER put anything, even in sterile packaging, under your ARM! Your armpit is DIRTY! Open the end of the package and leave it on the bedside table..") (Eeek! Eek! She runs an OR-based EP lab, among other things…)

- Don't hook up the suction yet.

- Position the patient's head at the midline. Start passing the catheter through the trumpet.

- Now – listen! Literally listen - put your ear to the end of the catheter that you're holding. You should be able to hear air moving through the catheter. Advance the catheter a bit, on the patient's <u>inspiration</u> (why?), listening... if it goes into the esophagus, what should you hear? If it goes into the trachea, then what should you hear? What will the patient probably do?

- In the trachea? Not too hard to tell, is it? Advance the catheter to about ¾ of it's length. <u>Now</u> attach the suction. Put your finger over the catheter button, and <u>slowly</u> withdraw the catheter, suctioning all the while. <u>Don't</u> just haul the catheter out at full speed – it needs to stay in long enough for the secretions to get suctioned out.

- Assess, assess, assess! :

    o Look at the patient: is she breathing? Vomiting? Coughing?

    o Look a the monitor: stable rhythm? Slowing? (That's bad – her airway may be occluded, or you may be poking her carina – back out the catheter while suctioning, to try to open the airway, then get it out of there...) How's her saturation doing?

    o Look at the catheter: are secretions coming out? That IS the idea, after all – are they coming up the tubing? No? Do you need to turn the suction up? You may have to turn it up to max, if the secretions are really thick, and you have to clear the patient's airway. Yup, it's dangerous – turn it back down as soon as you can. Are the secretions bloody, at all? Hmm...

    o Done? Does he need to be suctioned again? Depending, I'll repeat the process until I think the patient's really clear. If it was difficult to get into the trachea, I might even leave the catheter in place – not all the way down, but past the cords anyhow, watching the saturation the whole time.

- Now, apologize again. Wipe the tears out of your patient's eyes. Wipe your own eyes.

- Re-assess! Is he going to need it again? Is this the second time in the shift that you've had to do this? Or the twelfth? Does he need to be intubated? Re-intubated?

13- How do I collect a sputum sample during suctioning?

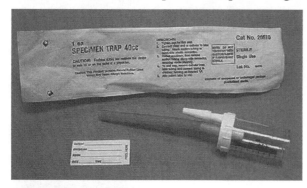

A sputum trap! The catheter plugs into the yellow part, and the suction tubing connects to the white cone thing. Applying suction with this gadget connected draws the sputum into the clear thing, which you then cap off…

http://www.trinitysterile.com/Images/L20510.jpg

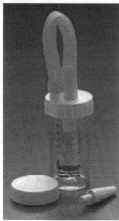

… and send to the lab.

http://www.howardmedical.com/
Merchant2/graphics/00000001/3843701.jpg

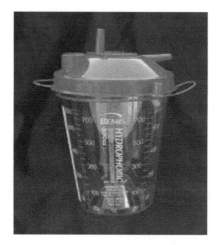

Jayne says: "Make sure you tell them that they have to use new, sterile suction tubing to the canister every time they do this, or the specimen will just get contaminated by the nasty old tubing that's just been hanging off the wall…"

Ok – change that tubing!

http://www.med-worldwide.com/media/BT-592041.jpg

Central Venous Lines

Hi all – another one! As usual, please remember that these articles are not a final reference of any kind. They are supposed to represent information given by a preceptor to a new orientee, and reflect my own understanding, which is, well…I'm getting old, you know? Please let me know what's wrong, or missing, and I'll fix it right away. Thanks!

1: What is a central line?
        1-1: How do I know if my line is in the right position?
        1-2: How do I know if my line is central or not? And what does "central" mean, anyway?

2: What are the parts of a central line?
3: What are central lines used for?
        3-1: Pressors.
        3-2: Different concentrations of meds. Central potassium.
        3-3: Volume, blood
        3-4: TPN

4: What kinds of central lines will I see in the MICU?
        4-1: Introducers
        4-2: Multilumen CVPs
        4-3: PA lines
        4-4: PICC lines
        4-5: HICKMAN® Catheters, portacaths, Tesio catheters, Quintons
        4-6: Arterial and venous cath lab sheaths.

5: Where do central lines go?
6: Who puts in central lines?
7: How should I get my patient ready for central line placement?
8: How is the insertion done?
9: What things do I need to watch for during the insertion?
10: How can I tell if any of the bad things are happening?
11: The line is in. Can I use it now?
12: What kind of dressing goes on a central line site?
13: What does "air-occlusive" mean?
14: How does the transducer setup work?
15: How often does the setup have to be changed?
16: Can I draw labs off of a central line?
17: What does a normal CVP trace look like? What does TR look like?
18: What are normal CVP numbers?
19: What does PEEP have to do with it?
20: How should I set the CVP limits?
21: What does it mean if the CVP is going up? Down? Sideways?
22: What if I lose the CVP tracing on the monitor?
23: What if the line becomes disconnected at the hub/stopcock/transducer?
24: What if the patient pulls out her central line?
25: How long do central lines stay in?

1: What is a central line?

By the time they get to the MICU, most people have a pretty good idea of what central lines are - basically great big IV lines that go into great big veins. We use central lines for all sorts of things, in all sorts of places, so it makes sense to go over the basics of what, where and why.

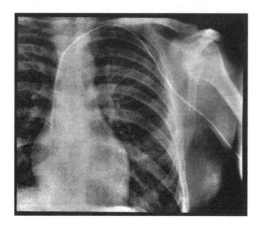

This is apparently the first central line ever, in a film from 1929. Dr. Werner Forssmann, over in Eberswald, Germany, had the sudden inspiration one day, I guess, that the thing to do was to thread a urological catheter up into his arm as far as he could, and then to run down to the x-ray room, where he had to fight his way past a couple of concerned colleagues to shoot a picture of himself…

See it there – the white line? Where's the end of the line – the tip?

So Werner – is the line in good position?

http://www.ptca.org/images/forssmann02.jpg

1-1: How do I know if my line is in the right position?

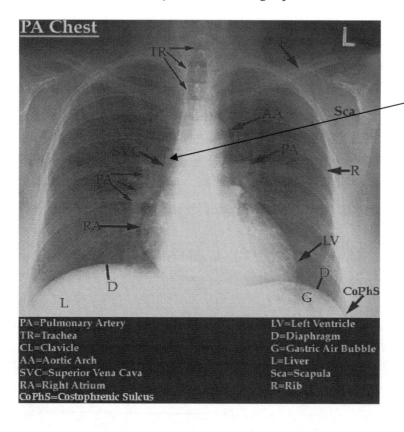

Here's how you tell. The tip is supposed to be in the SVC – if it's as far as the RA, then it's in too far.

Right about here…

No big mystery… but what if the blood in the line is really bright? Hmm…

www.vh.org

PA Chest

L

TR

AA   Sca

SVC

PA

R

RA

LV

P

D

G   CoPhS

L

PA=Pulmonary Artery
TR=Trachea
CL=Clavicle
AA=Aortic Arch
SVC=Superior Vena Cava
RA=Right Atrium
CoPhS=Costophrenic Sulcus

LV=Left Ventricle
D=Diaphragm
G=Gastric Air Bubble
L=Liver
Sca=Scapula
R=Rib

A good rule of thumb for any central line that you put into a patient, whether in the neck, the chest, or even in a femoral site – always, always transduce it before you use it. We've seen a couple of femoral arterial lines lately that were placed in hypoxic patients – so the blood return was dark, right? Wasn't venous….do you want to infuse pressors downstream from an arterial stick site towards a patient's leg? Didn't think so…

So: should we use Werner's line, or not?

1-2: How do I know if my line is central or not? And what does "central" mean, anyway?

Central means that the line is in a large enough vein, in the central circulation, that it's safe to deliver drugs that might not be safe if given through smaller peripheral ones. Pressors are a good example – it's not that giving levophed through a hand vein will immediately injure the patient, or that it won't work – but what if the IV infiltrates?

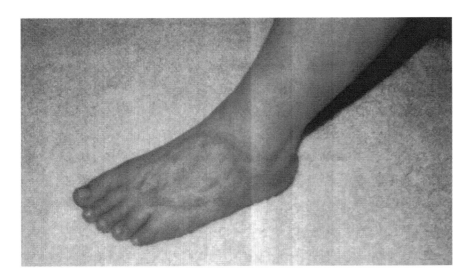

http://www.malpracticeweb.com/uch_ka.jpg

This person apparently had an IV in the foot, was getting potassium in some form or other, and wound up with skin grafting for an infiltration… now imagine if it had been levophed! Ugly.

Femoral venous lines are considered central because they go into such large vessels - as long as the team is sure they're in the vein! (It's usually easy to observe the color of the blood aspirated from the new line - dark is a good clue, but not always! What if the patient isn't breathing?)

Neck and chest lines are a little trickier - the way I was taught, the tip of the line is supposed to be beyond the third rib to be central. Take another look at the x-rays above - in our unit, the rule is that the tip of the line should be in the superior vena cava, a little above the right atrium (not in the atrium itself). <u>Every chest or neck line that's inserted in a non-coding patient must have its position verified by chest xray before it can be used</u>. (Suppose the line turned upwards on insertion, towards the patients brain? This has actually been known to happen! Do you want to be remembered as the person who infused pressors upwards towards your patients' brain?)

Update – yup, I heard that this happened not too long ago, but got caught by x-ray. (Yow!)

2: What are the parts of a central line?

This depends of course on what kind of line you're using - we use four kinds, mainly: introducers, multilumen CVPs, PICC lines, and PA lines. I'll go over each kind as we go along. The main things you want to think about though, include: how many lumens am I going to have available for what I'm probably going to need to give? How big is this line? - meaning, is it large enough bore for me to infuse volume rapidly if I need to? Where do the ports come out on the line? Which ports am I going to transduce, what should they be seeing, and what if they're not seeing what they're supposed to?

3: What are central lines used for?

3-1: Pressors

The first central-line thing that comes to the mind of the ICU nurse is the use of pressors. Pressors are vasoactive drugs - that is, they cause blood vessels to do things. (They also cause the heart and lungs to do things, but those are covered in the "Pressors and Vasoactives" FAQ file, so go over and have a look at that one sometime.) The most common effect of pressors that we're shooting for in the MICU is to cause arterial vasoconstriction: the vessels tighten up. Suppose you ran levophed through a small peripheral line and it infiltrated. That patient might wind up with a vasoconstrictive injury to the arm - maybe lose the arm, which is technically referred to as a "bad thing". Unless the patient's in a code situation, in which it might be "maybe lose the arm or certainly lose their life" - pressors must run through a central line.

Having said that, we do run dilute solutions of dopamine and phenylephrine peripherally when we have to, but only until central access becomes available. Make sure there's a good blood return in any peripheral vein you use for this purpose, and use big ones – this is why the Great Nursing Supervisor gave us antecubs.

3-2: Special concentrations of meds

Some meds come up in highly concentrated versions that are meant only for running through a central line - the one I always think of first is potassium. We give 20 meqs of potassium per hour, maximum, whether peripheral or central, but the central mix of that dose would be 50cc, while the most concentrated peripheral mix would be 80 meq in a liter of IV fluid. So that dose of 20 meqs would be what - 250cc. Is your patient "fluid sensitive"? - i.e., in CHF, or renal failure, or both? I've seen peripheral antibiotic mixes come up from pharmacy that mix one dose in 500cc - if you can't diurese your patient, what will you do when two hours of K^+, and one dose of antibiotic pushes him into failure? Lots of things to think about. Try to remember to see the forest through all those trees: keep in mind: "What is basically wrong with my patient?", and "How is this central line going to help him?"

3-3: Volume, blood

Or you may have the opposite problem. Your patient is dry - maybe hypotensive - maybe she's dehydrated, maybe dilated and shocky, maybe she's lost a lot of blood somewhere. Now you want to do the other thing - you want to give large volumes of IV fluid, or blood, or FFP, or all three - rapidly! This is also an excellent situation for a central line.

3-4: TPN.

TPN requires central access. This stuff is so concentrated that peripheral veins just can't take it for very long. Folks on long-term TPN usually wind up with some kind of long implanted line like a PICC.

4: What kinds of central lines will I see in the MICU?

4-1: Introducers:

These are the real large-bore lines - the ones that go into patients who need fluid resuscitation of one kind or another. Our introducers look like the letter "L" - one arm of the L goes into the patient, and the other arm comes off at a right angle. This second part is made of clear tubing, and you'll see right away that it's really big - this is the line that you'll transfuse your patient through when they're acutely GI bleeding. (Of course, that's only one lumen - where are you going to give the other IV fluids, the octreotide, the levophed, the FFP and the platelets at the same time? Got to think of these things!)

Another word about introducers - these are also the lines that are inserted in preparation for PA line placement. At the place where the two arms of the L come together, there is a small white cylinder that sits in line with the part going into the patient. In the top of the cylinder is a small black membrane - this is where the PA line goes in.

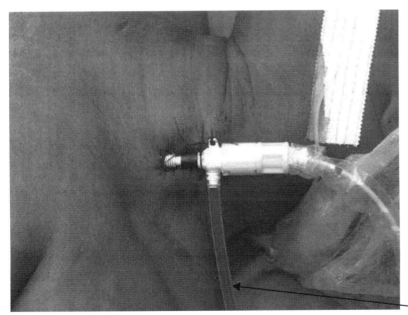

It takes a little practice to sort it all out...

The introducer is shaped like a capital "L" – one part goes into the patient, the other is the "sidearm".

A PA line has been threaded into the introducer, through the membrane, and click-locked into place – it has a clear sheath around it...

Here's the sidearm.

Oy! Put a tegaderm over that site, you dopes!

www.med.umich.edu/.../anesthesia_glossary-70.jpg

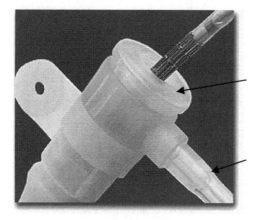

Here's the angled part, blown up.

The membrane is in here – in the picture, a line is being threaded through it…

This bit is the "sidearm", the large bore line that you can infuse through…

http://www.cardiva.biz/products/p044-7.gif

This is important: <u>the cylinder membrane will not seal up after the PA line comes out.</u> Which means that what bad thing could happen once the PA were removed? Who said "air embolus"? Very good. Either cover this membrane after it's been pierced with a tegaderm, or plug it up with an obturator - a little plastic device that slides into the line, and which screws down on the cylinder to seal it up.

4-2: Multilumen CVPs:

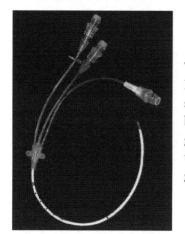

These are the most common central lines that you'll see here in the MICU. Everybody knows that "lumen" means "tube", right? For some reason we stock both 3- and 4-lumen catheters, but it would be a real mistake to pass up the chance for 4 when the team has grabbed a 3-port kit. There really is no difference in the insertion technique, and if your patient has no other access - make sure you get all the lines you can!

http://www.cc.nih.gov/vads/lines.html

A couple of things about multilumen CVPs:

The ports are described as proximal, medial and distal - these are the <u>reverse</u> of proximal and distal as regards the patient. In other words, the ports are proximal or distal in relation to the site where the line goes into the patient. So the lumen that opens up at the very tip-end of the catheter - that's the distal port, because it opens the farthest away from the insertion point. The medial port is the next one backwards, and the proximal port is the one closest to the skin. Make sure that the team has checked: you should never infuse anything through a port that doesn't have a blood return.

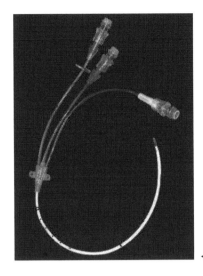

The brown port opens up distally, at the tip.

The blue port is the medial one, opening up   somewhere along here…

And the white port opens up proximally - here somewhere…

If you do use the central line for TPN - which you should! - then that lumen is tied up for good. If the patient becomes critical enough, then you can take the TPN down and use the port for something else, but you can't use the port for TPN again - the patient will need a new line. Policy.

We usually hook up the distal port to the transducer for reading CVP's, because the medial and proximal ports can snuggle up to the vessel wall and give weird waveforms. We also use the distal port for giving blood products, simply because it's big: the distal port is a 16-gauge lumen, while the other two are 18's. So plan a little - _always_ save a port - maybe one of the medial ones - on a newly placed central line for TPN (even if the patient isn't on it yet. They may be soon…)

If your patient has an introducer and you're strapped for access, you can ask the team to insert a multilumen catheter through the membrane, as if it were a PA line. This situation might come up if, for example, your postop patient went right through 3 liters of normal saline and 4 units of red cells and was still hypotensive. You still want to give blood products - where will you hang the neo that the team wants you to give?

However – think about this for a second… suppose you insert a standard triple-lumen line into an introducer. If you picture this in your head, you'll see that the proximal and medial ports open up inside the length of the introducer…hmm. That could mean that fluid infused into those ports might decide to flow backwards up into the introducer, or downwards, which is the way you'd prefer…

So – they've come up with a nice fix. There's a special version of the triple lumen catheter meant for exactly this situation: all the ports open up at the tippy end of the line. Make sure you use one of these in this situation.

4-3: PA lines:

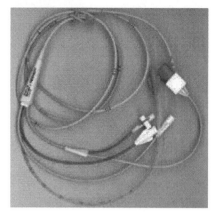

These are the "big guns" of the central line world, and they have a whole FAQ to themselves. Briefly, these lines are inserted through an introducer, and advanced through both chambers of the right side of the heart, and on into one of the pulmonary arteries. Commonly what we'll do is rig compatible vasoactive drips together, running through the introducer. This leaves a port free on the PA line - there's usually a free white port for infusions.

All of these central lines are supposed to come out within roughly a week of insertion.

4-4: PICC lines:

PICC stands for Percutaneously Inserted Central Catheter - these are very long, very thin lines that are usually inserted at the bedside by the IV team. Their distal end is also supposed to end up in the SVC, and must be confirmed by x-ray before it can be used. PICCs come in single and double-lumen varieties - try to make sure that no one goes to the trouble of placing one of these in your patient that only leaves you with a single line! Sometimes PICCs are placed by the interventional radiology team if the veins aren't accessible any other way. PICCs can stay in for a long time - months, anyhow. Anybody know, exactly?

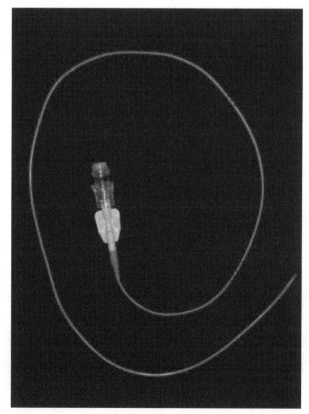

Hmm – only one line?

I guess they still make single-lumen PICC lines, which seem like a fairly dumb invention to me, since the standard is dual...

I mean, why go to all that trouble if you're only going to wind up with one access point?

http://www.cc.nih.gov/vads/lines.html

4-5: HICKMAN® Catheters, Tesio catheters, portacaths, Quintons

These are some of the rarer lines that you'll see - HICKMAN® catheters are surgically implanted lines that are designed for situations like home TPN, while Tesio catheters are put in for dialysis access.

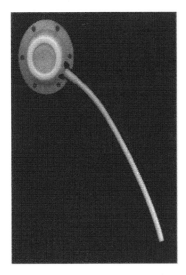

Here's what a portacath looks like… they get accessed using a gadget called a "huber needle", which goes through the skin, and into the reservoir hub of the line.

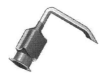

The huber needle has a luer-lock connection…

http://www.avidmedical.com/oem/Graphics/HUBER5.jpg

We usually wind up calling a nurse from one of the onc floors to place for us, since they get certified to access these lines, and we don't. Some portacaths come in double-lumen flavor (that's my kind!), and the needles have to be precisely placed, as they access the separate infusion lines. Get a pro to help you out with this.

http://www.cc.nih.gov/vads/lines.html

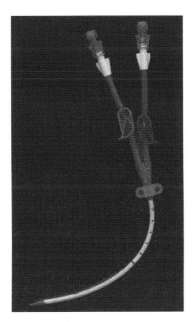

Quinton catheters (I'm not sure if this is a Quinton exactly, but it's the same idea) are short lines with two ports - the line is shaped like a Y, with the single end in either a femoral or a subclavian vein. Both access ports come out into the same vessel - sometimes people get confused and think that these are actually two separate lines. These are used mostly for short-term dialysis, like CVVH.

It's important to remember that dialysis access catheters are instilled with something to keep them from clotting after the run is done – sometimes it's a citrate solution, sometimes it's very concentrated heparin - if you need to use these lines for emergency access you can, but **don't forget to aspirate the ports first!** (And be prepared for the renal docs to be pretty upset with you…)

http://www.cc.nih.gov/vads/lines.html

4-6: Arterial and venous cath lab sheaths.

Patients will come back from cardiac cath/angioplasty/stent /IABP procedures with these lines in place. They're usually single-lumen lines, and you can certainly use them as you need to: femoral venous sheaths are considered central, and femoral arterial sheaths should be transduced, and can be used as a-lines. Intra-aortic balloon pumps are <u>very</u> central lines - but you probably shouldn't even begin to think about them until you go to balloon school...

5: Where do central lines go?

There are really only a couple of places these lines go in: neck, chest, and groin.

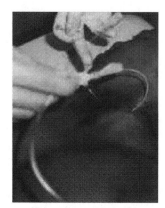

The neck sites are usually either the right or left internal jugular vein.

http://www.medstudents.com.br/proced/proced4/jugular.htm

The chest sites are the subclavians, and the last are the fems. You may see a patient come back from the cath lab with a PA line inserted femorally - in my experience these tend not to stay in place very well. Once in a really blue moon you'll see a PA line threaded brachially.

Something to remember when the team is choosing an insertion site: how much PEEP is your patient on? High levels of "forward pressure" from a vent, whether it's in the form of pressure support, pressure control, PEEP, or combinations of them can hyperinflate the lungs, and the apices will, I'm told, rise up higher in the chest. These are <u>not</u> the patients to give a subclavian line if it can be avoided - the risk of "dropping the lung" - causing a pneumothorax, which then might require a chest tube, becomes lots higher!

6: Who puts in central lines?

It depends on what kind of line it is. Introducers and multilumens are inserted by interns with a junior resident present, or by juniors on their own, or seniors likewise. PA lines are put in by the pulmonary/critical-care fellows, or by residents under their direct supervision. PICC lines - IV team, or interventional radiology. HICKMAN® and Tesio catheters are put in by surgeons, and Quintons are put in by the renal team: renal fellows or attendings.

7: How should I get my patient ready for central line placement?

There are a number of things to think about. First: how critical is the situation? Is the patient acutely hypotensive? - this person needs a femoral line, because you don't want to have to stand around until the x-ray is shot, processed, and read before you start pressors - the difference in time may make all the difference between "taking a hypotensive kidney hit" or not!

Next: is the patient oriented? Not oriented? Agitated? Will she be able to lie still, maybe with her face covered by drapes, while the line goes in? Does she need sedation? Restraint? Neither? Both? Careful, clear communication with the team, and thinking a little ahead will save you from seeing your patient abruptly sit up, fling sterile equipment everywhere, and make the resident accidentally spear you with a finder needle.

Next: labs. Is the patient anticoagulated? On heparin? Is the heparin still running? Should it be turned off? Reversed? Should the patient get FFP? Platelets?

Last: make sure that you've passed the team the right line. Try to make sure that if they're doing a multilumen placement, that they're putting in a line with four lumens instead of three - it makes no difference in the procedure, and it may make the difference between your patient getting TPN or not. Not trivial!

8: How is the insertion done?

All these line insertions are done using the ultrasound-guided Seldinger technique. The basic idea here involves a couple of steps, but the same technique is used for putting in all kinds of vascular catheters:

First: a small-gauge needle and syringe are used to find the vessel that you want to use. This is done by locating the anatomical landmarks that indicate where the site ought to be, and then carefully inserting the needle while holding back pressure in the syringe. Clearly, if bright red, pulsatile blood appears in the syringe, the needle may not be where you want it to be. Pressure may have to be applied for a while, and you're going to want to observe the patient's neck/chest/fem to make sure a hematoma isn't developing. (Did she get all her FFPs?)

Once the finder needle is in the right vessel (blood nice and dark?), a second, larger needle is inserted next to the first one, also into the vein – this one is large enough that a short sterile wire can be passed through it into the vessel. The first needle comes out.

If this is a neck or subclavian insertion, you have a specific position to take while the wire is being threaded into the vein, which is at the foot of the bed, watching the cardiac monitor. If the wire is threaded into the RV and tickles the endocardium, lots of nice ventricular arrhythmias can result – usually you'll see single or double PVCs, you may see short runs of VT, or you may see a pretty long one! Your job is to be watching for these, and to clearly call out what you see – remember that the team is looking at the insertion site, not at the monitor. At the first sign of significant ectopy, suggest that the team pull the wire back a bit, which will usually fix the problem. It's nice to know that the patient's electrolytes were optimized before this happens…

Holding the wire – if they let go of the wire, all kinds of interesting unpleasant things can happen - the team takes out the second needle. At this point a small scalpel is used to make the insertion opening just a little bit bigger – then a dilator goes over the wire, and finally the central line is threaded down over the wire. Keep watching the monitor for ectopy! Once the line is in what ought to be the right position, which varies with the size of the patient, it's sutured to the skin with a little tabbed flag thing. Now you slap a clear adhesive dressing on the site, make sure it's nice and air-occlusive, and call for a stat chest film to show if the line is in the right position or not. Remember - you cannot use the line until the film is read. Something to remember – this is a golden opportunity for blood cultures! Get the team to draw them for you off the new line.

Placing the line over the wire is simple enough if the line is a single lumen introducer, but if a multilumen line is being used, it pays to remember that the line is going to have to pass through the distal opening – the one at the tip-end of the catheter. On our lines, this is the brown port – the cap comes off, the tip of the catheter is threaded onto the wire, and the line is slid down as the wire is slid out. Make sure the caps go back on any open ports! (Air embolism – ack!)

9- What things do I need to watch for during insertion?

Putting the line into a central artery is always a big one. Sometimes it can be hard to tell which vessel you're in, if your patient is hypotensive, maybe hypoxic (why?). One trick is to transduce the line and have a look at the pressure in it: this is a legitimate move if you're not giving anything through the line yet. Hook your transducer to the distal port, zero and level the setup, and have a look. Art-line waveforms and CVP waveforms really don't look anything like each other (you need to learn to tell the difference!) Another trick is to send a blood gas spec off the line – mark the slip "?Arterial vs Venous" – venous BG's are low-O2, high-pCO2, and it shouldn't be hard to tell.

Runs of ectopy are bad. Watch carefully.

Pneumothorax happens now and again. How much PEEP did you say your patient was on? The post-insertion fil should show this developing – if this is going to occur at all, in my experience it's usually right away.

10: How can I tell if any of the bad things are happening?

If hitting a central artery is going to cause a problem you'll usually see a hematoma forming. The patient may need to have a coagulopathy treated with FFP – maybe a sandbag on the site for a while, depending on where it is. Make sure the team is aware of what you want to do and why.

Ectopy in these situations usually stops when the wire is pulled back. Sometimes the line itself may be in too far and cause tickling – ask the team how deep they think the line should go if the patient is very small. If the line isn't inserted all the way, that's okay, but make sure the team can aspirate blood from all three ports before they suture the line in place.

Pneumothorax ought to be, but isn't always, very evident. Sometimes they don't get very big, sometimes they're very dramatic. Any time your patient has a big change in respiratory status it's usually an excellent idea to ask about getting a chest film. Pneumos do unpleasant things, and it's worth the time to go over and look at the FAQ on Chest Tubes to review what they are, how to be ready for them, and what to do if you think one is occurring. The X-ray FAQ has some neat images on the subject too.

11: The line is in. Can I use it now?

The short answers: femorals, yes (assuming the placement went easily), anywhere else, no. Wait for the film. Unless it's a code.

A critical point: **always** transduce any central line before you use it – would you want to infuse pressors into a line headed towards your patient's brain? What a headache... **this goes for femoral lines too** – pressors infused towards a patient's leg can cause the loss of the limb...

12: What kind of dressing goes on a central line site?

We clean around the site working outwards with betadine and alcohol, then we apply a small sterile pad, covered by an occlusive clear sticky sheet. We tape the edges down, date the dressing, and change it every 72 hours, unless it gets wet, or displaced. (Is it 96 hours now?)

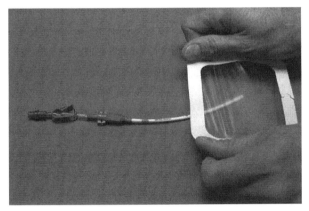

http://www.venousaccess.com/New%20Pics/sticky%20side%20down.jpg

This is almost like one of those things: "How many errors can you find?"

No cap on the line? Clamp is open? Line not sutured in place? No little sterile gauze under the tegaderm?

And what's this? – how many times have we told them: "No more practice insertions in the pool table, dammit!"

13: What does "air-occlusive" mean?

This means that the dressing won't allow air to get into the patient through the venous insertion site. Air embolism is a very unhappy thing – sometimes pressures in central vessels can actually go negative – for example during a vigorous inspiration. If the site is open to the air, a whole big hunk of atmosphere can get sucked into right into the vena cava, and get nicely pumped along through the RV into the lungs – this would be a pulmonary embolism of gas, rather than clot. The thing to try to do is to put the patient into Trendelenburg, with the right side up – the idea is to try to trap the gas bubble in the RV, from which hopefully an interventional cardiology person can remove it. I've never seen this done.

14: How does the transducer setup work?

There's a pretty detailed description of how transducers work, and how they look at the patient and talk to the monitor, in the "New In the ICU" FAQ. Briefly, the transducer is a gadget that looks at a pressure of one kind or another coming from the patient: arterial, central venous, PA, sometimes LA, sometimes urinary bladder – and translates the readings from physical to electrical. The electrical signal goes up and down just as the physical pressure does, and reads out on the monitor, going left to right, like an EKG trace does.

15: How often does the setup have to be changed?

Nowadays we change them every 96 hours – four days. Unless they get contaminated. If your patient has a CVP replaced for suspicion of infection, I would <u>not</u> use the setup connected to it even if it had been made that day – I'd make a new one.

16: Can I draw labs off of a central line?

Yes. I use a vacutainer at the stopcock site, discard a red 5cc tube, and then go on as though I was using an arterial line.

17: What does a normal CVP trace look like? What does TR look like?

I really need to buy a scanner. A CVP trace looks a lot like a wedge trace – it's wavy, and doesn't go up and down very much. There are waves in the trace that you can learn to analyze, that are generated by the chambers of the right side of the heart contracting in sequence: a-waves from the atria, v-waves from the ventricles, and there's a c-wave in there somewhere, which I forget what that one is. The main idea is that you always want to read the tracing at the end of expiration.

Here's a pretty good CVP trace – this patient is probably holding her breath, since there's no respiratory variation (meaning the whole wave goes up and down some with inspiration and expiration). What number would you put on this patient's CVP – check the scale on the left – about 10?

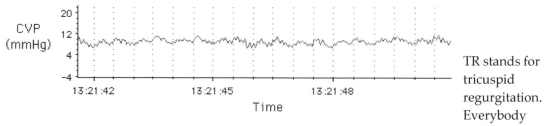

TR stands for tricuspid regurgitation. Everybody remember that the tricuspid valve is the one between the chambers on the right side of the heart? The valve is made up of several leaflets that are supposed to close up nice and tight when the RV contracts, to prevent the contraction from pumping blood backwards into the RA. If the valve leaflets don't close up properly, then the squeezing RV pumps some blood forward into the PAs, and some backwards into the RA through the opening in the valve – this is the regurgitation. Nice name. Anyhow, this has a very characteristic appearance on the CVP trace – big deflections up and down amidst an otherwise CVP-ish looking baseline. I'll try to get a scanner…

Here's a not-too-hard puzzler: you guys are all pros at PA placement waveforms now, right? You all know what RV pressures look like then, on the monitor? So, suppose you were transducing the distal port of your brand new CVP line, and you saw an RV trace? What would you think about the positioning of that line? What should probably be done to fix it?

18: What are normal CVP numbers?

I think it was in the file on arrythmias that we pointed out that "context is everything" – that's true in CVPs too. You could pick some numbers and call them normal, and you'd be right – say you put a CVP in me. I'm 46 now, but I'm pretty healthy, I don't smoke, don't drink… I swear sometimes, but that's about it. So my pulmonary pressures aren't going to be high, as in smoker's lungs. And my portal pressures aren't going to be high, as though I were a cirrhotic alcoholic. Chronically high lung pressures reflect back into the RV, raising the right-sided pressures (which is what the CVP is in the first place, right?), and high portal pressures reflect into the vena cava, also raising the CVP. So my CVP might fall in the "average normal" range of , say, 6-12 mm Hg. A high CVP might be 20, meaning maybe overhydrated, and a low one might be 2, meaning dry. Does the person with the CVP of 20 have wet lungs? Is the person with the CVP of 2 making any urine?

19: What does PEEP have to do with it?

(Didn't Tina Turner sing that song when she was a respiratory therapist?) Absolutely everybody remembers that PEEP stands for Positive End-Expiratory Pressure, right? Meaning, this patient is either on a vent, or on some kind of sealed face-mask device (I hate those – what if the patient vomits into it?) that is maintaining a positive, measured forward pressure into the lungs, even at the end of expiration. Any forward pressure like that is going to increase the intra-thoracic pressure, and is going to cause central pressure readings to <u>falsely rise</u> as a result. So the CVP will rise, the wedge pressure will rise – but this does <u>not</u> mean the patient is "fuller" of circulating volume than they were before!

In the old days they taught us a formula: for every 5cm of PEEP above the first 5, you should subtract 3 from your wedge reading. So, let's take the example of Mrs. Ventilofsky. Here she is, on the respirator, and she's got a PA line in, and she's really hypoxic, so she's on 20cm of PEEP, and her wedge pressure is 10. She's got a terrible x-ray, they think she's probably in CHF, so they want to diurese her. Should we? We need to think about her volume status.

Okay, so, let's do the PEEP calculation thing. Take away the first 5 from the 20cm that she's on, that leaves 15, right? For every 5cm of PEEP that's left, take away 3. So 15 is, uh, three units of 5, right? For each unit of 5, take away 3 from the wedge. So that would be 3 times 3, correct? Nine, to subtract from her – wait a minute, her wedge is only 10 to start with! Hmm. Maybe she is, as we say in Boston, "wicked dry" already. Has she been making urine? Maybe we need to think some more about what's really wrong with this lady's lungs before we diurese her into pre-renal ATN…

20: How should I set the CVP limits?

What you want to know in this case is not so much that the pressure is rising or falling dramatically – because as a rule CVPs don't do that too much – but that the line might disconnect. I set the low pressure limit just below the mean reading, which does the job.

21: What does it mean if the CVP is going up? Down? Sideways?

Well, the idea is that if the CVP is going up, that your patient should be getting "fuller" of circulating volume, right? So down would mean "emptier", or "more dry", and sideways would mean no change. The problem is that it's not always so simple. Remember the three parts of a blood pressure: pump, volume and arterial squeeze? Okay, try to visualize the circulation on a movie screen. See the heart there in the middle, pumping? And the arterial system all around, squeezing? You can't really visualize how full the system is of volume, so try imagining the heart with a number in it, which we'll call the CVP. We could talk about wedge this way too, obviously, but for now we'll stick with the CVP.

So your patient is hypotensive – there could be a number of reasons for that. Is she dry? Septic? Cardiogenic? Let's pick the dry scenario – say an elderly person who hasn't been feeling well, hasn't drunk much in the past week, comes in with a low pressure. The team puts in a CVP line, and you transduce it, and the number is one, maybe two.

Sounds dry. Is she making any urine? A little, maybe 20 cc per hour, very concentrated. What's her sodium? Aha, 155 – is that high or low? High, right – the normal range is what 135-145? So higher is drier, right? – the idea being that the concentration of sodium goes <u>up</u> because the amount of water that it's floating around in has gone <u>down</u>. Right? So there's more little sodium things per cc now, 'cause there's less water for them to float around in. (Sodium things?…)

Same for the red cells. Less water component in the blood, more cells per cc. So what does the hematocrit do? Goes up, right – look the lady's crit is 49! Yup, the whole picture fits together, she's dry. Consult your movie screen. What do you see? What's the heart doing? Well, what will the heart do to compensate for loss of volume? The rate rises, correct. And what will the arterial system do to try to compensate for volume loss? Tighten up, very good. So on the screen, we see a rapidly beating heart, and narrowed, tightened arteries, and the single number inside the heart is a 1, or a 2. How will you treat her? (What would she be doing differently if she had been on Lopressor at home…?)

Let's try another one. What if she were septic? CVP might indeed be low – why? Which of the three parts of the blood pressure is affected in sepsis? – the one in the example above was volume, right? So that leaves pump and arterial squeeze. Which one is affected in sepsis? – arterial squeeze, right. How come? Remember the bacterial endotoxins that are produced in sepsis: they poison the arterial muscle layer so that the whole system relaxes, dilates. (My son says that dilate means to go to heaven after midnight. And that after you dilate, you barium…) The <u>true</u> volume doesn't change, does it? No – but the relative volume sure does – look at your screen. See the nice widened arteries? Where's all the patient's circulating volume going to go? Down into their legs, if they're standing up, which they're probably not, right?, being hypotensive and all. What's the heart doing? Tachycardic, right, and for much the same reason –

148

not enough volume going around, although this time it's not because she lost any, it's because she's all dilated. She has a <u>relative</u> volume deficit. So her CVP will be low too. (And her wedge will be low as well, you PA-line guys out there…). How will you treat this situation? Take a look at the FAQs on "Pressors and Vasoactives" and "PA-lines" for more on the subject.

Here's another point worth mentioning about central pressures in general, meaning CVP and wedge pressures: pretty much anything that raises the patient's blood pressure is going to raise the central pressures too. Maybe not a whole lot, but some – this is where trending and ranges come in. If you put your patient on a Neo drip, and her pressure goes from 75 up to 140 systolic, her CVP is going to go up, probably because as you tighten up her arterial bed, the relative volume increases, right? She seems fuller, because she's tighter. Did her urine output improve with the higher pressure? The whole point here is to try to learn to think systematically about your patient's volume status in a meaningful way. What's the heart doing, and why? What are the arteries doing? What's the real volume status? Which of the three is causing the problem?

Be patient with yourself. It takes time and experience to learn how to assess this stuff. We're talking a couple of years here, probably. And even then you can run into mixed situations that get really hard to figure out, such as a cardiogenic patient on a balloon pump who develops hardware sepsis…Learn to use all the tools you have available: from high tech - PA-lines are really helpful in figuring out volume situations - to low-tech: is she peeing? If there's no renal failure, then urine output is a really good clue. (They used to call a foley catheter the "poor man's PA-line".)

One more point about volume assessment – is the patient hot, or cold? Did he just come up from spending five hours in the OR with an open abdomen? His arterial bed will certainly be nice and tight, right? (High SVR, you PA-line guys.) As he warms up, what will happen? Right – he may lose pressure. Or a previously "normothermic" (whoa!) patient with a decent pressure might spike a fever and dilate – does he need volume? It's a lot to think about…get help!

22: What if I lose the CVP tracing on the monitor?

First off, make sure the line is still in the patient! If the line is okay, then you need to start troubleshooting. Here's how I do it – starting from the patient, work backwards along the line. Make sure everything is connected, make sure the stopcocks aren't closed, make sure the cable is still plugged into the transducer and the monitor. Is the scale on the monitor right? If the scale is set at 0-300 on a 2-inch hunk of monitor screen, a CVP of 8 won't show up at all. Whole setup is okay? Does the line maybe have a clot at the end? Are you going to forcibly irrigate it to find out? (Someone once called this "giving it a Canadian.")

No you should not! If you suspect that there's a clot at the end of a catheter, the only thing to do is to try to aspirate it back up the line, which sometimes you can actually do. Use careful sterile technique, and try this: unscrew the stopcock cap, screw on a small syringe, and gently aspirate. If you can't clear the line this way, clamp it, flag it "? clotted", and talk to the team…try transducing another lumen and see if you get a decent tracing.

23: What if the line becomes disconnected at the hub/stopcock/transducer?

This is why you tighten up the transducer setup when you first put it together – this really shouldn't happen. If someone else makes the setup for you, check it yourself again before it goes up.

This is also why you must remember, at the beginning of every shift, to **make sure that you have meaningful alarm limits set.** There is no reason to ever, ever forget this. Even if your patient is, say, someone who is being allowed to pass away, **you must check the alarm limits**, if only to lower them. I usually set the CVP "low" limit at zero, or a little higher – this will readily detect a line disconnect.

If the line does disconnect, assess quickly for the possibility of an air embolus. Is the patient bleeding outwards from the disconnected lumen? – definitely better than pulling air inwards! Has the lumen connector gotten contaminated? Cap it, flag it, don't use it, inform the team. If the line becomes disconnected farther away from the patient, you'll probably get blood backing up along the line – close the stopcock at the lumen connector, and make a new transducer setup. Has the patient lost much blood? Send a hematocrit…

24: What if the patient pulls out her central line?

The same concern about air embolism applies, as well as bleeding. In practice, this really happens very rarely. Use your assessment skills at all times to figure out if your patient needs safety measures applied. There's lots of discussion about sedation, restraints, and how to use them in the "Sedation and Paralysis" FAQ.

Slap an air-occlusive dressing on the site. (Don't really slap it!) Put the patient on their left side so that any air that may have been sucked into the circulation will rise to the right atrium and not go into the patient's circulation. Notify the team right away. Assess for blood loss, air embolus, local injury to the site if they've pulled their sutures…

25: How long do central lines stay in?

Like everything else, this is a topic of ongoing debate. I'm pretty sure that the current rules say that a percutaneous stick-at-the-bedside line is supposed to be changed after 7 days. Maybe ten days? Of course if it looks like the line has gotten contaminated, or if the insertion site looks infected, or even if the patient is just spiking fevers for otherwise unclear reasons, the line should come out sooner. You really don't want to leave this nice germ conduit going into the central circulation if you think it isn't clean.

You also need to think about where the line is: a femoral line that was put in emergently during some sort of near-code situation should probably come out as soon as more access can be put in – the fem is not the cleanest place in the world. Then again, I've had the teams tell me that a really well-prepped femoral line is just as clean as one in the neck or chest – things to keep in mind.

26: How do I know if the line should come out?

How long has it been in? How does the site look? Does the patient still need central access? Has she been spiking temps? Has the line been contaminated?

27: How do I take the line out? How do I culture the tip?

Nurses do take out central lines in our ICU, but if there's anything unusual about the situation – coagulopathy, pneumothorax, anything out of the ordinary, I'll usually ask the team to do it. In practice, it's simple enough: first, take out the stitches. I usually have a helper at this point. Have a sterile tube ready to put the catheter tip in. I put a sterile 4x4 on the sticky side of a clear adhesive dressing, which I hold over the line site with my left hand (not touching the site yet). Then - at end-expiration - with my right hand, I do a smooth pull to remove the line, and as the tip comes out of the site, the left hand slaps (!) the dressing over the site opening, and holds it down. The right hand is now holding the catheter up in the air, tip downwards. Your helper now holds the sterile tube up, slides the tip of the catheter into the tube, and uses sterile scissors to snip the end,remember to use a second sterile scissors, letting that end drop down. Cap the tube, hold the site for several minutes. (there is some data that it makes more sense to send a sample about an inch up from the tip for culture, as the tip has a great deal fo blood flowing past it.)

Assess the site. Any bleeding? Hold pressure for another 5 minutes. Still bleeding? Ask the team to come and have a look. You checked the coags before you pulled the line, right? Does the site need a sandbag? Is a hematoma forming?

28: What kind of dressing goes on the site after the line is out?

I use a large clear adhesive dressing over a gauze 4x4 for the site. If no bad things are happening, make sure the dressing is firmly in place, and come back and check it once or twice in the next half hour, then again maybe an hour later.

*HICKMAN is a registered trademark of C. R. Bard, Inc., and its related company, BCR, Inc.

Chest Tubes

1- What are chest tubes used for?

2- Where exactly is a chest tube placed?

3- How does the three-chamber system work?

4- Can suction be bad for the patient?

5- What is the difference between exudate and transudate, and why do we care?

6- What is an effusion?

7- How are effusions treated?

8- When should a chest tube for effusions be removed?

9- What is pleurodesis?

10- How are malignant effusions treated?

11- What is streptokinase used for when it is given through a chest tube?

12- What is empyema?

13- What exactly is an air leak?

14- How can you tell if the chest tube port is out of the chest?

15- How can this be fixed?

16- Are air leaks good or bad?

17- Would that be a bad situation?

18- What is the black button on top of the pleurevac for?

19- What is tube "stripping"?

20- How could I tell if a patient were developing a tension situation in her chest?

21- What is a pulsus paradoxus?

22- Should you ever clamp a chest tube?

23- What if the chest tube gets pulled out by mistake?

24- What is "water seal"?

25- What is subcutaneous emphysema, and what does it have to do with chest tubes?

Please keep the following in mind as you read this FAQ: the information written here is meant to reflect the knowledge and experience gained over "too many" years of ICU nursing at the "trenches" level. My idea is to provide useful information for the newer nurse at the bedside, the kind of information that a preceptor would pass on to a newer staff member in orientation on the unit. It is not meant to be any kind of "official" reference, and it is certainly not meant to be the final word on any question of any kind! The goal is comprehension. If you see an error, or think something isn't clear, let me know, and we'll change it right away. I think that these files will be much more useful if everybody gets to contribute. Thanks!

Thanks Iowa! ("Is this heaven?", "No, it's Virtual Iowa...").

1- What are chest tubes used for?

Chest tubes are long, semi-stiff, clear plastic tubes that are inserted into the chest, so that they can drain collections of fluids or air from the space between the pleura. If the lung has been compressed because of this collection, the lung can then re-expand.

Some reasons for inserting a chest tube:

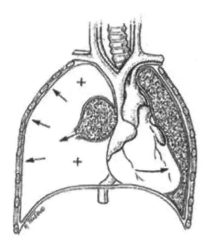

http://www.uib.no/akuttmedisin/spesielle-prosedyrer/thorax-punksjon/pneumothorax.jpg

Pneumothorax: a collection of <u>air</u> in the pleural space. These can happen spontaneously: I saw a young man walk into the ER once, who "just didn't feel right" - he had a nearly completely collapsed right lung. Pneumos can occur after central line insertion, after chest surgery, after trauma to the chest, or after a traumatic airway intubation. Important to remember: if the air continues to collect in the chest, the pressure in that collection can rise, and push the whole mediastinum over to the other side - this is called a "<u>tension pneumothorax</u>", and is definitely life-threatening. Call the surgeon.

Hemothorax: a collection of <u>blood</u> in the pleural space, maybe from surgery, maybe from a traumatic injury.

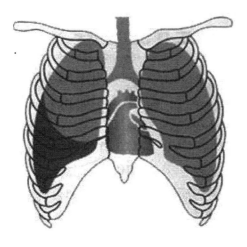

http://www.chgranby.qc.ca/images/hemothorax.jpg

Here's a really nice picture from the University of Iowa's Virtual Hospital, used with permission. See the shifted mediastinum? – the trachea's shoved over to the right.

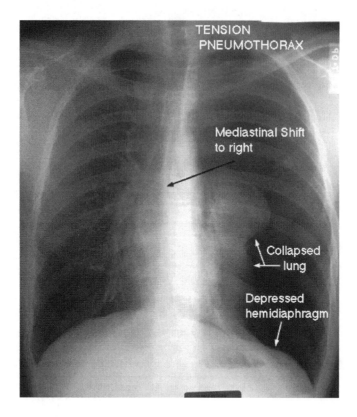

Pus can collect in the pleural space - "**empyema**".

Fluid, usually serous, maybe from CHF, sometimes from a tumor process, will collect between the pleura - "**pleural effusion**".

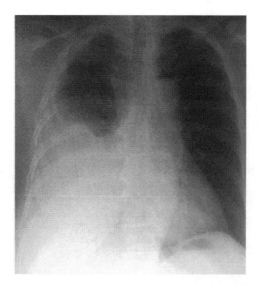

Another nice picture from Iowa – big effusion there on the right! (No, Ralph – the patient's right!)

2- Where exactly is a chest tube placed?

The chest tube is inserted by a surgeon, usually thoracic, but sometimes someone from the general surgical service. The entry point is the fourth or fifth intercostal space, on the mid-axillary line, which is pretty close to the point at which you level a line transducer. The tube is inserted towards the collection: sometimes up and in front, or up and in back, or wherever the collection lies.

3- How does the three-chamber system work?

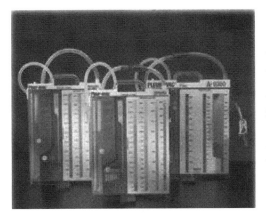

We use a device called a pleurevac, a large plastic box with what seems like fourteen separate compartments in it - actually the ideas behind it are not hard to grasp. The box actually imitates an old system that was invented to drain chest tubes, which used three chambers - they were actually glass bottles held by a metal rack - in series. (I remember those glass setups - I must be getting really old.)

http://www.proasepsis.com/productos.html

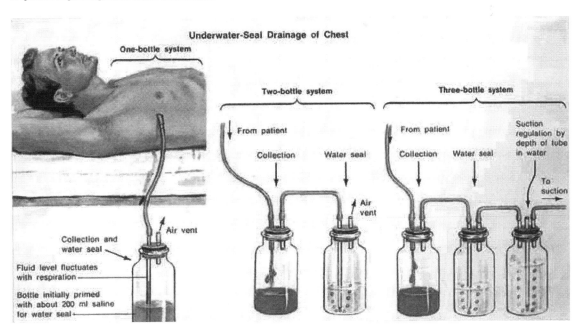

http://home.ewha.ac.kr/~chestsg/dong/poster/99/2-08.jpg

Wow – look what you can find if you hunt around on the web…the patient's looking very relaxed! "Chest tube placement in tanning booth…"

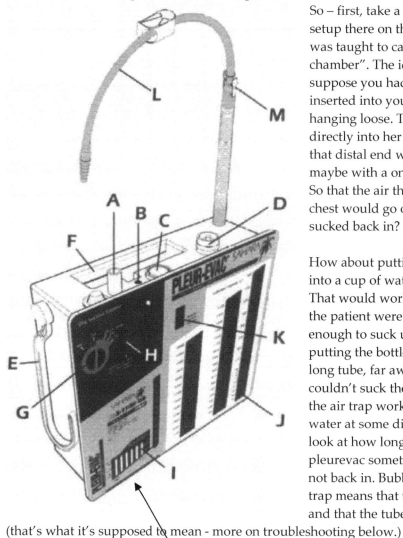

So – first, take a look at the single-bottle setup there on the left of the picture.. what I was taught to call an "air trap", or "air leak chamber". The idea here is pretty simple: suppose you had a chest tube freshly inserted into your patient, with the end hanging loose. The patient could suck air directly into her chest through the tube if that distal end wasn't controlled somehow - maybe with a one-way flapper on the end? So that the air the patient pushed out of her chest would go out, but none would get sucked back in?

How about putting the distal end of the tube into a cup of water? Or **a bottle** of water? That would work as a one-way valve, unless the patient were able to breathe in hard enough to suck up the water - how about putting the bottle of water at the end of a long tube, far away from the patient - so she couldn't suck the water back? That's how the air trap works. The trap is filled with water at some distance from the patient - look at how long the drainage tube is on a pleurevac sometime - and only lets air out, not back in. Bubbles moving through the trap means that the patient has an "air leak", and that the tube is draining air properly (that's what it's supposed to mean - more on troubleshooting below.)

This isn't quite the one we use, but it's close enough to point arrows at:

Air coming out of the patient will bubble out here, which is the defninition of an "**air leak**". No bubbles, no leak. First bottle.

Here's where the drainage comes out. Second bottle.

Here's where the water column goes. Third bottle.

http://www.auh.dk/akh/afd/afd-n/intensiv/procedurer/bilag/bil11.htm

So a single-chamber setup would work if the only thing comng out of the patient's chest was air – what if there's fluid in there that needs draining, too? Time for a **second bottle**.

In the multi-bottle setups above, the second chamber is the air trap, while the first collects fluid drained from the patient: blood, or serous fluid from the pleural space. You may be surprised at how rapidly these can fill up in certain situations - for example, tumor-related effusions can drain more that a liter - or two liters – in a day. You'll have to change the pleurevac when it's full. **This is the only time that we routinely clamp a chest tube** - remove the clamp after the boxes are switched. Don't forget!

Hey – here's an idea: what about adding suction to this arrangement? It only makes sense that it would help drain the patient's chest if you could <u>gently</u> suck air and fluid out of her pleural space, right? But if you hook up suction from the wall, even with a regulator, you might pull too hard…now you need the **third bottle**. To deliver very precise suction, we use the weight of a measured column of water, which shouldn't change as long is it's topped up now and then. The regulated wall suction is applied to a partly-water-filled plastic column in the pleurevac box, above the water level - and the weight of the water acts as a suction limiter. No matter how hard the wall suction pulls, the actual suction delivered to the patient is only as hard as the amount required to pull air out past that fixed weight of water. Any suction above that just pulls in air from outside the box, through a vent. The incoming air bubbles through the column, which is what makes all the noise you hear when the box is hooked up to the wall suction. All you need to apply is enough to make it bubble – more than that just makes noise, and makes the water evaporate.
Oh yes: fill a pleuevac up with sterile water instead of normal saline. As saline evaporates, it will actually (a surgeon told me once), leave salt crud on the sides of the box chambers…

4- Can suction be bad for the patient?

Obviously, you need to control the amount of suction applied to the patient. Make sure you have your pleurevac set up correctly. The surgeon who inserts the tube should order a specific water level in the control column - we usually fill it to 20 cm, but sometimes they order less.

5- What is the difference between transudate and exudate, and why do we care?

"Transudates" and "exudates" are descriptive names for types of fluids that can collect in the pleural space. Transudates you might think of as "thinner" - they often result from CHF, and you might think of them as more "watery", being "sweated" into the pleural space when a patient is "wet". Exudates might be thought of as "thicker" - they contain more protein, and usually result from some kind of inflammatory process. They can also be a result of tumor processes - patients with lung Ca or pleural mets often show up with exudative fluid collections. You tell the difference by sending thoracentesis specs to the lab.

6- What is an effusion?

Transudates and exudates are types of effusions - the idea being that the collections of fluid are "sweated" from the lung. Recurrent effusions can be a real problem for a patient who is dealing with a long-term illness, but as long as the patient has a reasonable hope for living a while yet, there is good reason to treat the effusion, either with treatment for underlying CHF, or for an underlying tumor process, or for whatever else is causing the problem.

7- How are effusions treated?

In the short term, with a chest-tube. Some effusions related to CHF can be treated with diuresis - the idea is that decreasing the amount of the water component in the blood will cause the effusion to be re-absorbed. If the effusion is large enough to produce respiratory distress, or tension symptoms, you obviously would think more about inserting a chest tube.

8- When should a chest tube for effusions be removed?

"When it's safe to to do so." This sounds stupid until you stop and think about the underlying reason why the tube was inserted in the first place. Is the effusion just going to re-collect after the original one is drained? Maybe something needs to be done to stop the effusion from recurring, like "pleurodesis".

9- What is pleurodesis?

Pleurodesis is a technique of instilling some substance or other into the pleural space through the chest tube, which is then supposed to "weld" the pleura together by scarring them, preventing the re-collection of fluid between them. This doesn't sound like it would be a very pleasant idea, but it works pretty well for some situations. I remember the old days, when the scarring agents used to cause a lot of pain - I'm sure that they weren't chosen to be painful, but they were - let's forget about those... Nowadays they use sterile talcum powder, which comes up from the pharmacy in large sterile syringes and looks strange - apparently it works very well.

10- How are malignant effusions treated?

Talcum powder is instilled into the pleural space, right through the chest tube. Then the patient gets rolled around into different positions every whichy-way so that the scarifying agent gets distributed everywhere.

11- What is streptokinase used for when it is given through a chest tube?

Sometimes you'll see narrow-gauge chest tubes inserted instead of the large clear ones, and because they're narrow, they get can plugged up with fibrin, which stops the drainage. The tube in this case is usually rigged with a stopcock between the end of the tube and the connector to the pleurevac - the team will instill a dose of streptokinase through the stopcock and into the patient through the chest tube, let it sit for half an hour, and then turn the stopcock back to drain. The dose I see given is 250,000 units.

Strepto is also injected if the patient has a "loculated" effusion, which means that it's managed to become surrounded by a fibrin membrane. The drug breaks up the membrane and lets the effusion get to the tube for drainage.

12- What is empyema?

This is a collection of pus in the pleural space, or in a big abscess space in the lung tissue itself.

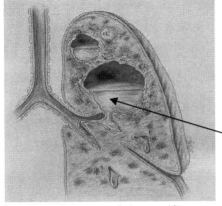

Feh! Pus can collect in large enough quantities to compress the lung, and certainly will act as a septic "focus" until it's drained. Empyema can result from chest trauma - say, a gunshot or knife wound - or necrotizing pneumonia, or any other process that puts bacteria into the chest.

And you were wondering why your patient was on pressors? Actually, that's a good question: new ICU nurses, why might this situation make your patient need pressors? Look one paragraph up for the hint.

http://www.koreacna.or.kr/cuecom/diseasecare/respiratory/07.respiration-empyema.htm

13- What exactly is an "air leak"?

The idea of using chest tubes to remove air from the pleural cavity means that there has to be some way to tell that air is actually coming out. The smaller bubble chamber in the pleurevac shows an air leak very simply - if there are bubbles coming through it, then air is coming down the tube and being evacuated. It's important to remember that this does <u>not</u> mean automatically that air is coming out of the chest. If there's a leak in the tubing, or if a chest tube suction port (the openings along the lumen of the tube inside the chest that draw in the air and fluid for drainage) is outside of the chest wall, then air will be sucked in there - instead of being pulled out of the chest. So bubbles are a good sign, but you have to check everything else too.

14- How can you tell if the chest tube port is out of the chest?

Sometimes you'll suddenly hear a new sound in your room. Hunting around, you may find that your patient's chest tube has inadvertently taken a yank - and it's whistling at the insertion site. A port has come outside the skin, and it's continuously sucking in air from the atmosphere around it. You can put your stethoscope on the dressing over the site if you're suspicious, and you'll hear it clearly there.

Take a look at this picture – one of these chest tubes isn't quite right. See the radio-opaque lines going along the tubes? Look at the one on the patient's left. See the break in the line? That's the drainage opening. Nicely inside the chest? So what about the one on the other side?

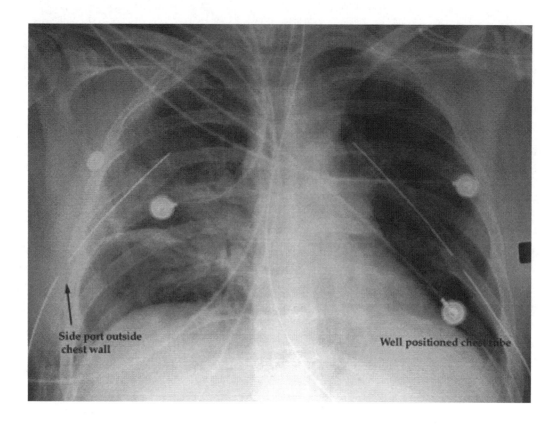

Side port outside
chest wall

Well positioned chest tube

15- How can this be fixed?

If you take the site dressing down, you can wrap the port with sterile vaseline gauze and apply an occlusive dressing, but usually this situation means that the tube will need to be replaced. You'll also need a stat x-ray - air may be dangerously re-accumulating in the chest!

16- Are air leaks good or bad?

It depends on the situation. (Everything always depends on the situation!) If a patient has a chest tube put in for a pneumothorax, then at least initially an air leak is a very good thing - because you certainly want that air out of there. If you don't see bubbles coming out through the air leak chamber after a tube is placed for a pneumo - then you may have a non-functioning chest tube on your hands; it might not be in the right place. Get a look with the team at the followup x-ray immediately to see if the pneumo has shrunk at all - if not, the patient may need another tube put in. Same thing is true for a number of postop situations involving chest surgery: open lung biopsies, lobectomies, pneumonectomies - all these leave an area of lung tissue that will leak air into the pleural space until they heal, and so require chest tubes to get rid of that air. So air leaks in those cases are also good. But say a patient still had an air leak two weeks after an open lung biopsy - what then?

17- Would that be a bad situation?

Probably - either the chest tube is leaking and sucking air in around itself somewhere - which means it isn't working, and ought to be pulled anyhow, or it means that the patient is continuing to leak air into her chest - at this distance from the operation, this would mean that the tissue leaking the air into the pleural space isn't healing - and in fact the patient may have developed a broncho-pleural fistula - meaning a semi-permanent tract connecting a bronchus and the pleural space.

This happens a lot with patients who need a lot of inspiratory pressure from the vent - say, pressure control of 25cm, and peep of 10cm, adding up to 35cm of forward pressure, being pushed into stiff, noncompliant lungs. That's a lot. That much pressure means that air is being pushed pretty hard into those stiff lungs, and that air will be pushed out into the pleural space too, preventing it from healing closed. That healing won't occur until that pressure can be mostly reduced, but the patient will lose a lot of ventilation because of the loss of volume through the fistula. A tough spot to be in. Time for permissive hypercapnia? Class – look that one up and get back to me…there will be no quiz, however. You are safe here in the FAQ!

18- What is the black button on top of the pleurevac for?

This is actually pretty important. Go back to the picture on page 5, and look at item D. See that button? The air leak chamber of a pleurevac, just like the first bottle of a drainage set, needs to be partly filled with water – that's how the bubble-trap idea works, like putting the end of the chest tube in a cup of water, like a one-way valve. You put that water into that chamber when you set up the pleurevac, through a filling column that has an opening on the top of the box.

If you remember to look at the air leak chamber at various times during the course of your shift, you'll notice that the water in it can sometimes rise up the filling column towards the top of the box. This usually happens if the patient is "pulling" very hard with inspiration - what they call "excess negative pressure". Kind of like what high school teachers do…in other words, not only is the patient trying to pull in air through his airway, but also from the pleurevac itself, which actually he can't, because that's what the air leak chamber prevents, right? But the water in the trap chamber will rise up in the filling column after a while, and the air that's trying to escape from the chest won't be able to get out because of the increased weight of that column.

The resistance of the air trap, or leak chamber filled with water to the proper level, is only supposed to be tiny - about 2cm of water - not like the 20cm in the control column. So what you have to do is lower that column of water back down to the level indicated on the chamber - there's a line marked on the box. Holding down the black button is the thing to do - hold the button down, and the column will slowly sink down towards the correct level - let go when it gets there. This problem also happens very often with tube "stripping".

19- What is tube "stripping"?

Stripping is something people argue about a lot. The idea is that if a chest tube is "milked" every couple of hours after, say, a surgical procedure, then it won't get plugged up by clots, which only makes sense, since if the tube gets plugged, then the air and fluid that it's supposed to remove will not get removed, and a tension situation could develop in the chest. Definitely a bad thing.

But stripping and milking can pull too hard suction-wise on the chest cavity, possibly causing tissue injuries to the lung. Also a bad thing. So the only thing to do is to ask the surgeon what she wants done. If you're instructed not to strip, watch carefully for signs that the chest tube is still working properly: draining air, fluid, or blood. If air were to stop coming out three hours postop a lobectomy - I'd page that surgeon right away.

20- How could I tell if a patient were developing a tension situation in her chest?

Sometimes the signs and symptoms are obvious, sometimes not. The first thing to do if you suspect this is to get the team to order a stat chest film - and then get it promptly read! Observing the patient, you might see hypotension, cyanosis, general signs of respiratory distress - maybe even tracheal deviation to the opposite side as the mediastinum gets pushed across the chest. If the patient has an arterial line, look for a pulsus paradoxus.

21- What is a pulsus paradoxus?

The idea here is that blood pressure varies as the patient inhales and exhales: literally goes up and down, maybe by 50 points, systolic. Maybe more. There are three main situations where you see this: tension pneumothorax, pericardial tamponade, and (maybe) severe hypovolemia.

Let's take the first one, which is the relevant one here: what happens is that as the patient gets a breath, the intrathoracic pressure rises. The tension gets worse - maybe there's already some mediastinal compression. The heart is squeezed tightly, and compressed, and literally doesn't have room in the chest to pump.

This makes sense if you think about tension pneumothorax - a lung may go all the way down, and as the pressure in the chest continues to rise and rise, with every breath, the mediastinum gets pushed over harder and harder. So now when the patient gets a breath, the small addition of positive pressure (assuming they're vented - in which case positive pressure happens on inspiration because the vent is <u>pushing</u> the air in) the heart gets squeezed just a little more, is able to move just a little less - can't pump well - and the blood pressure drops.

When the patient exhales (on the vent, this is when intrathoracic pressure is released - after the breath is pushed in) - then the intrathoracic pressure drops again, and the heart is un-squeezed a bit, the heart can move just a little better, and the blood pressure rises again. This can sometimes be clearly seen if the patient has an arterial line - watch the tops of the blood pressure waves on the A-line as the breaths go in and out - if they drop more than 15-20 points per breath, you've got a "clinically significant" pulsus paradoxus - often a very clear classic sign of pneumothorax. Think about it - did the patient just have a central line put in…?

You can measure this by using the arterial line cursor - there is one there, although we hardly ever use it. Chase the wave tops up and down, measuring the distance between the tops at inspiration and the tops at expiration, and find the difference. You might see a dramatic change – in a severe situation, maybe a systolic of 150 dropping to 80.

Here's a nice sample of a pulsus paradoxus showing up on an arterial-line waveform:

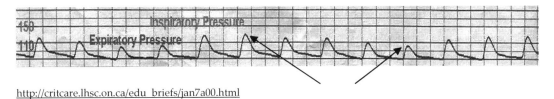

http://critcare.lhsc.on.ca/edu_briefs/jan7a00.html

See the pressures going upand down? ICU nurses: is this patient vented, or not? Try to calculate: is this pulsus greater than 20 points?

22- Should you ever clamp a chest tube?

Aside from changing the pleurevac, it sounds like a bad idea to me. If the pleurevac tubing comes disconnected from the chest tube itself, then I would clamp the tube only long enough to hook up another one, to prevent air from being sucked back into the chest. But only that long! Did the tube get contaminated?

23- What if the chest tube gets pulled out by mistake?

That's what you keep vaseline gauze at the bedside for. You would slap that gauze right onto the site, (don't really slap the patient, right?) and occlude the opening - you don't want air going back into the patient's chest – for the same reason why you'd (briefly!) clamp a chest tube in the question above. Again, you'd want to stat page a surgeon if the patient needed the tube back in, and get a CXR ordered right away.

24- What is "water seal"?

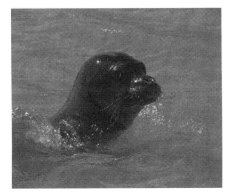

"Water seal" means that you've disconnected the wall suction line from the pleurevac (on purpose). Usually this is ordered when the air and/or fluid draining from the patient is assumed to be pretty much over and done with - several days after surgery - maybe not in the case of recurrent effusion - maybe a day or so after pleurodesis when you'd expect the drainage to have stopped. You'd want to watch carefully for signs of re-accumulating air or fluid in the chest - daily, or sometimes twice-daily x-rays will help determine this. It's done as a maneuver when you're thinking about pulling the tube after it's served its' purpose.

163

25- What is subcutaneous emphysema, and what does it have to do with chest tubes?

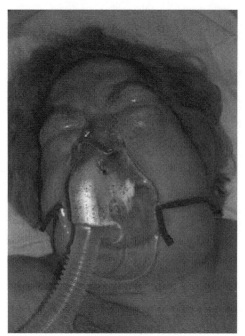

Subcutaneous emphysema is the collection of air in the tissues just under the skin – once you feel it, you'll never forget it: as though Rice Krispies had been spread around under the patient's skin. If a chest tube isn't properly placed, or maybe if the site dressing isn't airtight, air can leak into the tissue around the insertion site. Eventually it can track up and down the body, sometimes causing the neck and face to swell, sometimes threatening the airway. In that case the patient should be <u>immediately</u> assessed for intubation - there may be no time to waste! Correcting the position of the chest tube usually stops the leakage of air into the tissues, and the air itself is almost always very rapidly reabsorbed - a matter of several days at most, in my experience.

http://www.aic.cuhk.edu.hk/web8/chest_injuries.htm

Hard to tell which side it's coming from – both eyes are certainly swollen, aren't they? Is this patient really a little heavy-set, or is that air in her facial tissue? Actually, if her eyes look like that, it's probably the second…

CVVH

Another one! As usual, please remember that the preceptor is not the final authority on anything in any way – just old, beat-up, and over-experienced. (What is that noise I make, anyway? Probably going to need a new transmission soon. Might not be worth it.)

These qualifications do **not** equal "correct" – check with your own references, and let us know when you find things wrong. This time there will probably be lots! Also – this article was written with our current machine in mind. If that changes, we'll update it.

Basic Ideas

1- What is CVVH?
2- What is "renal replacement therapy"?
3- Why do kidneys shut down?

- Pre-renal
- Intra-renal
- Post-renal

4- What is dialysis?
5- What is dialysate?
6- What is ultrafiltration? Hemofiltration?
7- What is SCUF?
8- Is CVVH the same as hemodialysis?
9- Why use CVVH instead of hemodialysis?
10- What is creatinine clearance?
11- What is the "filtration spectrum"?
12- What will CVVH clear from a patient's blood, and what won't it clear?
13- What are the main reasons for starting a patient on CVVH?

Hardware

14- What is the basic hardware setup?
15- What is the blood path?
16- What is the ultrafiltrate path?
17- What is the fluid replacement path?
18- Which machine do we use?
19- What is a Prisma?
20- What is a Quinton catheter?
21- Does it matter where the Quinton is placed?
22- What is the catheter flushed with?
23- What is the hemofilter?
24- What are the two spaces in the filter?
25- What is the membrane?

26- What is the transmembrane pressure?
27- What is the "blood flow rate"?
28- What is the "turnover"?
29- What is the air detector for?
30- What is the blood leak detector?
31- What are all the transducers for?
32- What does the arterial transducer tell me?
33- The venous transducer?
34- What about the other two transducers?
35- What is the circuit heater for?
36- How do I prime the circuit?
37- Why would I prime with heparin or without it?
38- How do I make sure that the circuit is ready to run?

Choices of Treatment

39- Why would my patient get citrate replacement fluid?
40- What is "citrate toxicity"?
41- Why would she get bicarb replacement?
42- If I'm running heparin into the circuit, am I anticoagulating the machine, the patient, or both?
43- What if the patient is already on heparin?
44- How do they figure out how much fluid to give or take off every hour?
45- How do the patient's CVP, PCW and hematocrit come into that decision?

Up and Running

46- How do I prep the catheter before starting up the machine?
47- How do I get things started up?
48- How do I calculate the first hour's fluid removal?
49- How do I calculate the TBB up to the point where the CVVH started?
50- How do I figure out what rate to start the calcium drip at?
51- How should I take care of the Quinton?
52- How long can a system stay up?
53- What is specific to running a citrate system?
54- A bicarb system?
55- What can I infuse through the circuit, and what can't I?

Labs

56- What labs do I need to look at before I start my patient on CVVH?
57- What about labs while the system is up and running?
58- What about hemes?

59- Why would the machine "go down"?

60- Are there ways that can be prevented?

61- What if the machine goes down, and I can't figure out what's wrong?

62- Where are clots likely to form in the circuit?

63- What does it mean if the arterial pressure starts getting very low?

64- What if the venous pressure starts getting very high?

65- What if blood backs up into one of the transducers?

66- Both transducers?

67- Could something be wrong with the Quinton?

68- What does it mean if the filter pressures start getting very high?

69- What if the air detector stops the machine?

70- What if the blood leak detector goes off?

71- What if the heater alarm goes off?

72- When should I start thinking about taking the system down?

73- What should I do if I think the system is going to crash?

74- Could something on the machine pop, and spray?

Basic Ideas

1- What is CVVH?

"Continuous Veno-Venous Hemofiltration" is a <u>substitute</u> for hemodialysis that runs continuously on a machine that stands at the bedside. There are different kinds, all coming under the general heading of "renal replacment therapy".

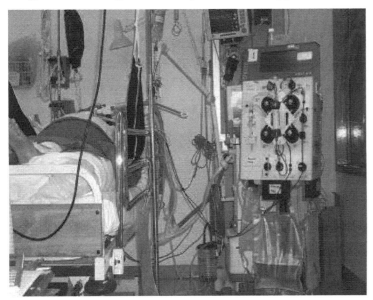

That's it there, on the right side of the bed.

http://www.aic.cuhk.edu.hk/web8/cvvh.JPG

2- What is "continuous renal replacement therapy?"?

I guess that hemodialysis and peritoneal dialysis were the only games in town for a long time, but nowadays we're ever so much more modern than that, and there are several methods around for doing what the kidneys would ordinarily do.

We only use one of them at the bedside in our unit: CVVH; it's called "V-V" because it runs from vein-to-vein. Systems that we don't use: an "arterio-venous" method (CAVH), meaning that the circuit of blood runs from an artery, to the machine, and back into the patient through a vein, and a third treatment called "SCUF": "Slow Continuous Ultrafiltration", which doesn't use a blood pump they way our system does – it's driven instead by the patients' own blood pressure.

It's important to point out that what we're doing with this system isn't dialysis exactly; it's actually "hemofiltration", also called "ultrafiltration". Dialysis and filtration work on different principles, and we'll look at those briefly in a bit. Suffice to say, we've found that our system works quite well to clear uremic wastes in patients whose kidneys have quit for one reason or another.

3- Why do kidneys shut down?

Remember all that stuff about pre-renal, intra-renal, and post-renal? They describe the three main ways that kidneys get hurt. The fourth way is toxicity, but we'll leave that for the tox FAQ that ought to come together someday.

Once again, (and as always, "with a lot of lies thrown in"), this stuff isn't that hard Just think of where the urine comes from, and where it goes:

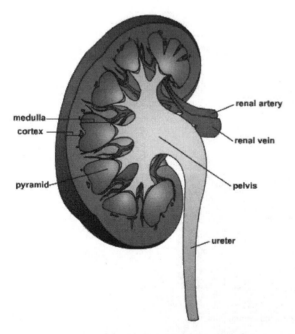

Pre-renal stuff has to do with the blood supply arriving to the kidney, here… at the artery.

Intra-renal: bad things are happening <u>within</u> the structure of the kidney – ATN, that kind of thing.

Post renal stuff happens here, where the urine is trying to flow out towards the outside world…

http://www.talktransplant.com/images/Kidney/kidney_cross_sectionL.gif

168

Pre-renal:

In front of the kidney.The urine is coming from the bloodstream – before it reaches the kidney. Most often the problem is simply that there isn't enough blood volume in front of the kidney – reaching it. The patient is dry. Remember the BUN/creatinine ratio thing? Not too hard. Put the BUN over the creatinine, like so: 10 /1.0 – so you could call that ten to one.

Now try this one: 100 /1.0 – a hundred to one. This one is "way" dry – the patient's kidneys are working, you know that because the creatinine is still normal (won't be for long!). But the BUN is, as we say in MA, wicked high – meaning not an excess of BUN so much as a loss of water. This patient might have a hematocrit of 50 – it's not that she has too many red cells, but that she's lost a lot of the water that they should be floating around in.

Intra-renal:

Inside the kidney, where the urine is being made. The kidney itself has "taken a hit" – in our patients this usually the evil ATN: Acute Tubular Necrosis, usually from hypotension. I hate it when that happens. It turns out that kidneys are very sensitive creatures; they don't tolerate being insulted ("Stupid kidney!"), and they fail if they're underperfused for any serious length of time. It varies, but sometimes it seems that an elderly patient who becomes hypotensive for 20 minutes will develop kidney failure.

Probably related: it seems as though some patients with hypertension at baseline don't make much urine at what we would consider normal MAPs, but turn into Niagara Falls when their pressure rises – maybe for the hour when you were doing their bath. The interpretation put on this is usually that these people are the ones with renal artery stenosis: their kidneys are used to seeing a higher perfusion pressure most of the time, and even though they're not failing yet, exactly, they're still not doing their stuff at what they think are hypotensive pressures. Makes sense, in that a vasculopath with bad coronaries may have bad renes for the same reason. I think it was in "The Tennis Partner" that I read Abraham Verghese's description of feeling a patient's radial arterial pulse, and trying to intuit how much diffuse vasculopathy she might have from the feel of the radial's stiffness. That's real doctoring!

Post Renal:

After the kidney – enough blood got there, the urine got made okay, but now it's having trouble getting out, after the kidney. Maybe a ureter is blocked (oof – I know about that one!), maybe the urethra is blocked. Flush the foley!

4- What is dialysis?

It's an interesting thing about molecules – they're adventurous. They want to go places. But – and they're very serious about this - it's really important for them to spread themselves around evenly; they want to travel with their friends, or not at all. If they see a place where they're under-represented, over across yonder semi-permeable membrane for example, (Montana, maybe), well, off they're gonna go, until there's just as many over there across the border in

Montana as there are over here in Idaho. Wyoming maybe. Nice, compulsive little ICU-personality molecules – so cute.

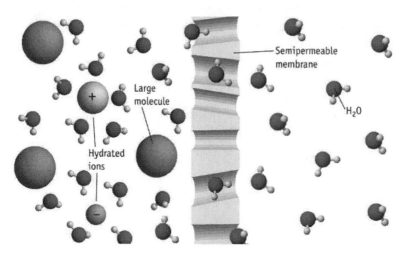

That's the basic idea behind "diffusion across a concentration gradient". Why can't these people just speak English? If there's too much molecules over here on this side, and not hardly none of 'em over on that side, why then, they're just gonna get up and go over across there – it's what they do, as the Great Physicist decreed, way back there in the Bang.

Of course the membrane has to have holes in it to let 'em through, right? Just the right size holes too, 'cause ya don't wanna be losing your albumins and all, or your red cells, know what I'm sayin', yo?

5- What is dialysate?

So - when you dialyze someone, you put <u>their</u> blood (hypertonic – very full of stuff that needs removing) on one side of a membrane – and put some hypotonic solution on the other side (that's the dialysate), and off the little critters go a-running over the membrane border there, from where they get washed away and sent back into the Great Pond, or wherever. And the number of BUN and creatinine molecules in the blood decreases, along with a bunch of even smaller ones like the electrolytes, which is why we spend so much time worrying about giving them back.

However – you haven't removed any fluid yet…

6- What is ultrafiltration? Hemofiltration?

These appear to be the same thing: fluid (in the form of water molecules) can pass through the semipermeable filter membrane, and by applying a suction pump on the far side of the membrane, you can suck water out of the patient, through the filter, at apparently whatever rate you'd like. This is called "creating a transmembrane pressure gradient", for those of you who like the big words.

It turns out that when you do this, small solute molecules get dragged out through the membrane pores along with the water – this is what they mean by "convective transport", or "solvent drag". Solvent drag turns out to have nothing whatever to do with concentration gradients – the molecules just get swept along out through the filter pores. In the process, a lot of fluid gets removed from the patient (as "ultrafiltrate") – and so we have to give some back. The movement of solutes through the membrane ("convective flux") is calculatable using all sorts of horrid renal mathematics, but happily we can leave that to the engineers; we just run the machine, which is tricky enough.

7- What is SCUF?

Slow Continuous UltraFiltration: we haven't seen this in our unit, but I understand it used to be done a lot in postop heart situations. This is a patient-driven system (no pump) that gets hooked to an artery: the patient's MAP sends the blood through a filter, and the arterial pressure is enough to push water molecules across the membrane in large amounts; one reference said 14 liters a day can come off this way. Apparently it doesn't work well to clear BUN or creatinine. Karen the CVVH goddess says that SCUF doesn't get used much anymore.

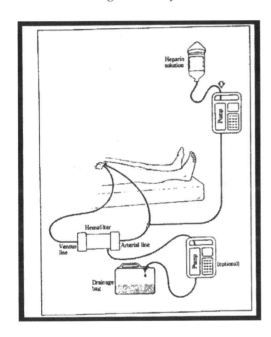

http://dric.sookmyung.ac.kr/NEWS/apr97/fig2.jpg

8- Is CVVH the same as hemodialysis?

No. CVVH is a form of "hemofiltration", aka "ultrafiltration", and isn't really dialysis.

9- Why use CVVH instead of hemodialysis?

The basic idea is that hemodialysis treatments produce really enormous changes in the patient's body over a pretty short time: they can pull off volume very quickly, change electrolyte and BUN/cr concentrations quickly – that kind of thing, and patients with hemodynamic problems just don't like that very much. I mean, if your patient's kidneys have "taken a hit" because of a hypotensive episode, does it make sense to do it again, hauling off large volumes with a hemodialysis treatment while they're on pressors?

CVVH is apparently much more gentle. The whole circuit holds only about 150cc, compared to a lot more for an HD circuit, and even though the device processes blood rapidly, (200cc/minute is <u>fast</u> – what is that?: 12,000cc = 12 liters an hour! Hoo-wah!), fluid is replaced by the machine as fast as it is being pulled off, plus or minus some every hour, depending on what you want to do. It can also run 24/7 – it's a pretty stable form of treatment. HD doesn't routinely replace anything, although you can give volume back while it's run.

CVVH also apparently is effective in removing septic materials: cytokines and endotoxins, and there may be a more routine role for it coming in the management of septic patients.

One last point is that CVVH avoids "disequilibrium syndrome" (I have that one all the time), which involves the patient developing acute cerebral edema after rapid HD. Making the blood suddenly hypotonic encourages water to soak into the hypertonic brain cells.

10- What is creatinine clearance?

Simple enough – how well are the kidneys getting rid of the creatinine in the blood? The level in the blood is compared to the level in the urine. There are all sorts of calculations and formulas to help predict what the clearance rate ought to be – all I want to know at the bedside is: are the BUN and creatinine going down? Just call me stupid…

11- What is the "filtration spectrum"?

This has to do with the size of the molecules that can pass through the pores of the filter in the circuit. The spectrum is size: molecules up to "this" big and no bigger will pass through the pores.

Things that will pass through:

- Little ions like sodium, potassium – no sweat.
- A little bigger: ammonia, glucose, bicarb.
- A little bigger even: some meds: heparin, some antibiotics.

Too big: protein, and therefore anything that binds to it: dilantin, etc.

12- What will CVVH clear from a patient's blood, and what won't it clear?

This is the filtration spectrum thing again – you want to be thinking about how big things are when you wonder about what will clear and what won't. In the meantime, I ask the renal people. If they don't know, I ask Karen the CVVH queen.

13- What are the main reasons for starting a MICU patient on CVVH?

Given that the patient is probably on pressors, and unable to handle HD, the three main ones are easy: in the presence of renal failure, the patient has to be any combination of hypoxic (from fluid overload), hyperkalemic, or acidotic – which we're mostly looking at metabolic acidosis's here, right?

Hardware

14- What is the basic hardware setup?

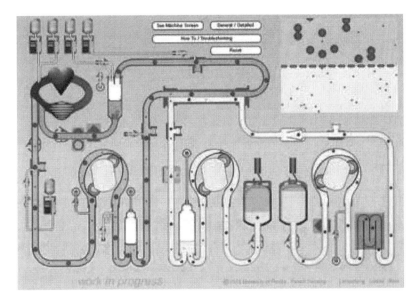

Well that's godawful looking, isn't it?

But if you look for a second... see the three colors? Red for blood, yellow for pee, and green for replacement fluid?

Three parts.

http://vam.anest.ufl.edu/dialysis/images/screenshot.jpg

http://vam.anest.ufl.edu/dialysis

15- What is the blood path?

There are three parts of the CVVH circuit: tubing paths for the blood, the ultrafiltrate, and the replacement fluid. The blood path is simple: from the patient ("arterial" catheter port), pulled out by the blood pump, to the filter, back out of the filter, to the air/clot/debris trap/detector, then back into the patient.

16- What is the ultrafiltrate path?

The ultrafiltrate is the stuff you're removing from the patient's blood: water, solutes, BUN, creatinine, all that stuff. Technically known as "pee". Ultrafiltrate gets pulled off from the outer space of the filter by a pump, applying a negative pressure – aka "suction". It passes through a blood-leak detector, which tells you if blood has gotten out of the filter tubules into the ultrafiltrate – bad, because it means your filter has ruptured. Bummer. Take the system down. After that it goes to a collection bag. Should be nice and yellow. So cool.

17- What is the fluid replacement path?

This is what you're giving the patient back. See the big bags hanging down under there? Fluid is drawn from them by a third pump, warmed up, and simply pumped along back into the circuit ahead of the filter. (Karen my queen – why <u>ahead</u> of the filter? Something to do with diluting the blood flow?) Update: it helps keep the filter from clotting.

18- Which machine do we use?

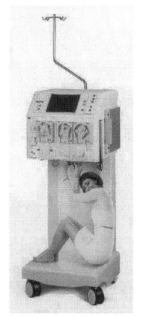

We use a machine made by Braun – here it is. Pretty good machine. It's fussy though, and you really have to stay in practice with it.

Hm.. some kind of symbolism going on here…

http://www.bbraun.cz/braunoviny/reportaz/images/mefa03.jpg

19- What is a Prisma?

Apparently the Prisma is the main competition for the Braun machine. Different company.

20- What is a Quinton catheter?

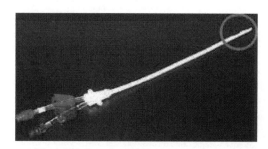

I don't think this is a Quinton exactly, but it's the same basic idea: two lumens going into one larger one, which sits in a big vein: one lumen for blood outflow, the other for return.

http://www.cfdrc.com/serv_prod/biomed_dev/images/catheter1.jpg

174

I wish this pictures showed the ports better: there are openings in the side of the catheter that lead to the two lumens. Or is there one at the tip and one at the side? Anyhow – the point is that a port open at the side of the catheter may find itself up against the vessel wall. If you hook up the "pull" line from the machine to that port, will it be able to suck out 200cc/min of blood from the patient? No way, man – it'll just suck up tight against that vessel wall, and you'll get bupkes. The "arterial" transducer will yell at you: "I'm pulling too hard!" - (the suction will reach the set limit of negative pressure), and the machine will shut down.This is why they teach us to "swap the ports": hooking up the return line to that port will probably be just fine – blood will go back into the patient through that port with no problem. Make sense?

Or you could rotate the catheter – it's the holder that's stitched in place, and the tube itself will turn – turn it over, and now the port that was against the wall should be facing into the bloodstream; a trick a renal fellow showed me.

21- Does it matter where the Quinton is placed?

Does it ever! We see catheters placed in the fems, subclavians, the IJ's – a bigger vessel is usually better, but problems can always pop up, especially in heavier patients – a catheter may bend where it goes into the skin, even though it followed Harry Seldinger's nice wire right in there, and you may have all sorts of trouble positioning the patient so that the machine will be able to pull and push blood in and out of her. Him. Them.

22- What is the catheter flushed with?

Actually the catheter is flushed with saline, but we instill heparin or Acid Citrate Dextrose solution afterwards to keep it from clotting off. Make sure that your coagulopathic patient doesn't get orders for heparin catheter flush, and make sure that you don't prime his system with heparinized saline unless specifically ordered (and even then you should probably argue about it).

Also make sure that you **ASPIRATE THE CATHETER PORTS BEFORE USING THEM!** The heparin solution we use is pretty concentrated – 5000 units per cc. You want to give all of that to your patient at once? I didn't think so.

23- What is the hemofilter?

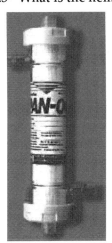

This is where the action happens. Take a look at the filter: see that big white clump of bitsy tubes going along it, inside, lengthwise? The blood flows through those. You'll notice that there's some space around the clump of tubes between them and the clear plastic wall of the filter itself.

http://www.cablon.nl/nederland/images/asahi-1.jpg

24- What are the two spaces in the filter?

The first space is where the blood is: inside the bundle of little white tubes. The second space is the one <u>outside</u> the bundle of tubules. Imagine cutting off one of the ends of the filter, crossways. Now pick up the part that's left, and look down into it, as if you were looking down a cardboard tube. See the thick outer plastic wall of the filter? Now see the bundle of little tubes, cut off? And see how there's a space around the bundle, between the wall and the bunch of tubes? That's the second space – the space on the outside of the membrane. Make sense?

25- What is the membrane?

Another way: all of those little tubes have walls, right? Take another look at the picture up in question 4. Those walls are full of carefully engineered little tiny holes that let molecules pass through, but only up to a certain size. Semi-permeable. My son's head is semipermeable: anything to do with motorcycles goes right in, but chemistry – bounces right off. Maybe I need to change his filter.

Added up together, all those walls form a large area for water and solutes to pass out of the blood, and that whole area is the "filtration membrane".

26- What is the transmembrane pressure?

How hard is it for the water and the solutes to get across that membrane? Too hard? The little holes in the tiny tubes may be getting clotted up. Too low – you sure you're hooked up to the patient?

27- What is the "blood flow rate"?

This is the speed at which blood is pulled through the main blood path: it's measured as the number of cc's passing through the blood path each minute. It's different for the two replacement fluids that we use: for citrate the machine is set at 120cc/min, for bicarb it's 200.

28- What is the "turnover"?

This is how much volume you're going to <u>pull out of the patient and replace every hour</u>: how much the ultrafiltrate circuit pulls off, and how much replacement fluid gets poured back in every hour. We usually set this at 1.6 liters/hour. This is the determines the total volume of blood that gets run through the filter, but it doesn't reflect fluid removal or addition – left untouched, this would run the patient "even". If you want the patient negative, say 100cc per hour, then you dial that in, and the machine will replace only 1500cc that hour. Make sense? It pulls 1600 off, and puts 1500 back in? Negative 100.

If you wanted to <u>give</u> the patient 100cc that hour, how much would the replacement amount be?

29- What is the air detector for?

This is part of the main blood path. The air detector is the last part of the machine that monitors the main blood path, looking through the blood going by before it goes back into the patient. It's just below the big venous trap that collects debris, clots, and (hopefully) any air in the tubing. Would you like to have your machine keep on nicely pumping along if no blood was in the tubing? Sort of a bad idea. If the detector sees air – the machine stops.

The thing is, this whole machine setup really sort of is the octopus from hell, the "thing with a thousand arms". (Maybe we should call Roger Corman. Wes Craven?) If something is clamped wrong, then one of the 138 and a half screw connectors may start to suck air into the system, and that air will make its way along through the system towards the patient – the air detector sees it and stops the machine. It does take time, but eventually you can get comfortable with the setup. I always run along the three tubing paths before I start the thing up, making sure that things are tight, and that clamps are open and closed as they ought to be.

It is possible to save an air-contaminated system sometimes, depending on how much got in there – but this is a hands-on maneuver that you have to learn with a preceptor. The other problem is that air in the filter will tend to clot it up.

An important point: this machine does **not** turn on the air detector while it is in priming mode, which is why you **NEVER RUN THE MACHINE IN PRIMING MODE WHEN IT IS CONNECTED TO A PATIENT.** Everybody got that?

30- What is the blood leak detector?

This is part of the ultrafiltrate path. Remember that the ultrafiltrate is pulled out of the little tubules – if they break, then red cells start showing up in the ultrafiltrate path. Not good – this translates as "filter rupture" – time for a new circuit.

Some people will just change out the filter, which I think is a terrible idea. For one thing, the circuit is at least moderately pressurized, right? You want Hep B pressurized blood spraying around in you local area? Not to mention sterility issues. Just change the whole damn thing.

31- What are all the transducers for?

The transducers are telling you what the pressures are in the system. As with transducers everywhere, the trick is to try to remember what they're "looking at". An art-line transducer for example is looking at the pressure in the radial artery, through the stiff tubing that connects the transducer to whatever vessel you're trying to measure the pressure of. These machine transducers are doing the same kind of thing: they're watching something, and the trick is to try to visualize what it is.

32- What does the arterial transducer tell me?

There are five transducers built into our sytem, and the first two are easy – they're looking at the blood flows in and out of the patient: one is looking at the flow coming out (the "arterial" side), and the other looks at the flow going back in ("venous").

Interpreting the arterial transducer number is a little trickier than usual, because it's measuring a negative pressure. You need to remember that transducers measure pressures that rise and fall. Positive and negative. In this case, the pump is pulling blood out of the patient through the "artierial" port of the Quinton – and pulling is measured as a negative number. Like a "NIF" – the negative inspiratory force that you measure when you're trying to see if your patient is ready to extubate, which is also measured as a negative number. Wall suction is measured negatively. My brain is often measured negatively – actually my son's brain…but I promised I wouldn't yell any more.

Anyhow. Suppose your arterial catheter pressure is a nice "low" number – meaning only about, say, negative 20mmHG - everything is good, and your patient decides to sit up, or curl up, flip over, or leap out of the bed and do a pirate dance – if the catheter kinks, the machine will continue pulling, harder and harder, but only up to a limit. The number indicators on our machine help you here, because as the negative pressure gets "higher and higher" – meaning "greater and greater", except it's negative, right? – then the numbers will change and tell you what's happening. And when it reaches it's limit, the machine will stop and alarm, to the effect of "Uh, excuse me, you want to come over here? I think I'm kinked!" This can also happen if the arterial port is up against the vessel wall, something you'll usually discover when you aspirate the ports manually at startup – try switching.

33- The venous transducer?

This one's a little easier – the venous side is going back into the patient, and it has to be pushed back in, so the venous side transducer is looking at a positive pressure. Higher numbers mean that the machine is having to work harder to push – if the catheter isn't kinked, this usually means that clot debris is building up in the venous trap, plugging up the works. If the pressure gets too high, the system may have to be changed – again some people try changing out only part of the circuit, but I think that's just a rotten idea.

34- What about the other transducers?

Instead of looking at the catheter flows, two of these are looking at the pressures on one side or the other of the filtration membrane. One is looking at the pressure of the blood as it's going into the filter. Remember, the blood on the inside of the little filter tubules is on the **inside** of the membrane, and the ultrafiltrate is on the **outside**. Another transducer is looking at the pressure coming from the blood leak detector, which is full of ultrafiltrate ("pee") – which is on the other side of the membrane.

If the pressure across the membrane – the "trans-membrane" pressure – rises, it means what?: that the fluid is having a harder time getting across, probably because some of the openings in the tubules are getting plugged up with clot. If the pressures get really high – time to change to blood path and filter. Or preferably, the whole system.

A last transducer looks at the pressures involved in the replacement fluid circuit. If something is clamped, this will honk at you.

Jennifer M. points out that even though the transducers can be temporarily clamped, it's really unsafe to leave them that way, since pressures can go off the scale on one end or the other, and you really do need to know if the machine is becoming unhappy, and why.

35- What is the circuit heater for?

Those replacement fluid bags hanging there under the machine are at room temperature, and they're infusing into the patient at 1.6 liters an hour. Cold. Even with the heater running, your patient may get really cold on CVVH – use the Bair Hugger®.

If the intern came around and wanted to know if this patient had spiked a temp overnight, what would you say? What if your CVVH patient had a temp of, say, 100.4? Remember, the machine cools your patient VERY rapidly... so if they spike while they're ON the machine... hm.

36- How do I prime the circuit?

At this point we do machine prime: meaning, we set up all three tubing sets on the machine, and let the pumps prime it up with whatever solution is ordered; either NS or NS with a bit of heparin per liter, which helps keep the filter from clotting.

There are all sorts of steps in the priming dance that you have to learn – really, after the first hundred times, it's lots easier.

37- Why would I prime with heparin or without it?

Lots of our patients are anticoagulated for one reason or another – sometimes they're doing it all by themselves as a result of being "hepatorenal". These people really don't need any help from extra heparin, and they often do a good job of keeping their machine circuits free of clots. Pretty nice of them. Not to mention the problems of HIT...

38- How do I make sure that the circuit is ready to run?

Once you've gotten the whole entire enormous thing set up, the machine primes itself. I takes about 20 minutes, and may need some tweaking as you go. Once it's done, you're all set – you can let the system just sit now, and it will be ready to go when you need it.

Choices of Treatment

39- Why would my patient get citrate replacement fluid?

Citrate has a couple of advantages – besides being pretty much physically tolerable, the citrate has the effect of anticoagulating the CVVH system itself, hopefully without anticoagulating the patient as well. This works the same way that the citrate does in stored blood, interrupting the clotting cascade by soaking up (chelating) free ionized calcium. Everybody remembers the role of calcium in the clotting thing, right? Yeah – me too.

If the patient's liver is in reasonable condition and the stars are right, the citrate is cooked off (metabolized) into the form of bicarb – a safe result, especially if your patient has some degree of acidosis.

40- What is "citrate toxicity"?

Some patients – usually liver failure patients, but also a certain percentage of non-liver folks – don't cook off citrate in a normal way, and it collects in the serum, doing its anticoagulant thing by chelating the free, ionized calcium.

The citrate toxicity comes from the resulting hypocalcemia – the ionized number drops drastically, and the patient is at risk for hypocalcemic tetany and the like. I <u>hate</u> it when that happens.

Interestingly, the total, or serum calcium number RISES in this situation. The citrate, bound to the ionized calcium, forms a "citrate/calcium complex", that <u>adds</u> to the serum total in the assay, so the total serum number rises, even as the ionized number falls.

Be alert for this situation – we make a point of watching our patient's ionized and serum calcium numbers anyway, because the machine pulls it off so rapidly that they get continuous infusions of Ca gluconate while they're on.

41- Why would she get bicarb replacement?

This is the one to use when your patient is severely acidotic, horribly pressor-dependent – that kind of thing. A patient in multi-system failure is often going to have a humongous acidosis going on, maybe partly from acute renal failure (there are at least two "renal tubular" acidosis's), and probably in large part from doing the lactate thing whilst in the grip of hypotension.

The bicarb systems are the ones that get heparin infused pre-filter, to try to prevent clotting. If your patient can't tolerate citrate, bicarb may be the way to go – this may be a liver failure patient, right? – can't metabolize bicarb? – and so they may do you the favor of anticoagulating your system for you.

42- If I'm running heparin into the circuit, am I anticoagulating the machine, the patient, or both?

Probably both – check with the renal fellow for goal numbers to shoot for. According to one source, about 75% of the heparin infused into the system will be ultrafiltrated off, with a suggested dose range of 500-1000 units/hour. In practice, we hardly ever use heparinized systems.

43- What if the patient is on already on heparin?

Hey – you're golden!

44- How do they figure out how much fluid to give or take off every hour?

This has more to do with the overall condition of your patient than just pulling off nitrogenous wastes – is the patient horribly fluid-overloaded? Take some off. Hypotensive? You may have to give some back. Hypotensive but still fluid overloaded? (grin!) Fairly stable but severely uremic? Run 'em even. Things like that. If you're doing serious hemodynamic monitoring, make sure that you get a consistent set of goal numbers for CVP (and wedge, if you've got a swan) from both the medical team and the renal people. Of course, the <u>patient</u> may not be happy when he gets there….! Evaluate! ☺

45- How do the patient's CVP, PCW and hematocrit come into that decision?

See the discussion just above. Weren't you listening?

Up and Running

46- How do I prep the catheter before starting up the machine?

Our policy is to soak the catheter ends between two 4x4's saturated with alcohol for several minutes. We use sterile gloves and an OR mask when we work with the catheter connections.

47- How do I get things started up?

Machine's all set, right? Out of priming mode, final check, turnover and pump rates all correct, all that good stuff? At this point set the business ends of the tubing down near the catheter tips, usually on a chux, still connected to the priming bags.

- Keep things clean.

- Mask, gloves.

- **Don't forget to aspirate 10cc from each of the catheter lumens!** Sometimes – not always - these lines are inserted and flushed with concentrated heparin, which your liver-failure patient does NOT need to have injected! You also want to aspirate any little clots in the ports.

- See if both sides of the line draw rapidly – whichever one draws the easiest is going to be the "arterial" side, regardless of whether it's blue or red. **Be very aware of what you're doing with the line clamps** as you do the hookup.

Give a moment's thought: do you want to give the patient the volume in the circuit? Yes? Hook up both lines and go. No? Hook up the arterial side, turn on the machine, and let the patient's blood displace the priming fluid up into the priming bag on the venous end. Then hook up the venous connector and go. In practice, we usually give them the volume in the circuit – supposedly no more than a couple hundred cc's.

48- How do I calculate the first hour's fluid removal?

You should get plenty of practice in figuring this out when you get precepted on the machine, but it's the same as any other "run": add up all the "ins" for the hour, and adjust the machine to run even, positive, or negative. I usually do the first run "even" to see how the patient is tolerating the whole procedure.

49- How do I calculate the TBB up to the point where the CVVH started?

Just calculate it up the way you would at any other time: add up the "ins", add up the "outs", figure out where you are, and go on from there. "She was positive two liters at 3pm, which is when the system went up, so wherever she is at the end of the shift, add the two liters to that." If you'd removed two liters by then, the patient would be even.

50- How do I figure out what rate to start the calcium drip at?

This is usually the renal fellow's call. They pretty much use a standard scale, and leave orders for an ionized calcium check <u>before</u> things get going – we're supposed to replace calcium with "x", for a result of "whatever", and repeat if necessary, then start up the drip. This means that if you can reliably assume that you're going to put your system up in an hour or so, you can go ahead and use that order. Just make sure the team knows that you're doing it.

51- How should I take care of the Quinton?

Carefully. They're pretty flexible, so patients can roll around with them in, but the blood won't flow through them rapidly if they kink – always a problem in one way or another. Make sure the connections stay sterile, the site dressing is clean/dry/intact and all that good stuff.

52- How long can a system stay up?

There's definitely a voodoo aspect to this. I've seen systems stay up for 3-4 days at a time, which is when IV tubings and things get changed anyway where we work. Other times the systems will crash after an hour or two, usually because the catheter isn't in a good place, or because the system managed to suck in some air during priming. Air in your system equals clotting, by definition, so this kind of priming problem almost guarantees difficulties with the system when it goes up. Citrate systems will often go quite a while, but the bicarb systems can be a real bear to keep going – they clot, crash, and get into trouble more frequently.

53- What is specific to runnng a citrate system?

The pump rates are different, depending on the fluid used. Citrate is almost always much preferable – the pump runs at a rate of 120cc/min.

54- A bicarb system?

Besides being a major pain in the butt, you mean? They need to be heparinized if possible. You can certainly get your assembly skills in good shape when you're running one of these and it goes down twice a day… the pump runs at 200cc/min. Both fluid systems turn over 1.6 liters per hour, unless the renal people want to fool around with "high flux" systems – meaning faster. More exposure to ultrafiltration through the circuit, aiming for better clearance – there are studies going all the time.

55- What can I infuse through the circuit and what can't I?

We use three sites on the circuit to infuse: we put a stopcock manifold at the end of the return line, and that's where we usually infuse the replacement calcium, although there's no reason that you can't give it through another central port or peripheral line. Other things that are compatible can run there as well.

However – bear in mind that these infusions are bypassing the final air filter detector, right? This is a big deal, because the flow rate of the blood through the CVVH circuit is **really fast**. Actually, it's always true that air can get sucked into your patient through a loose connector. So there's always a risk, especially at central venous sites, right? So imagine what could happen at an infusion site when the system flow is 200cc per minute, instead of, say 50cc an hour! Without an air detector, a really impressive air embolus could occur. Be very aware of your connections.

The other infusion sites are on the venous return line: one above the air trap, and one further back. Karen the CVVH goddess points out that while giving red cells through the trap is usually fine, it's probably not a good idea to run FFP there, since the clotting factors may go to work within the filter in the trap.

Labs

56- What labs to I need to look at before I start my patient on CVVH?

You really want to have a good look at the basic everything: for example, is the hematocrit okay? The system holds 150cc of blood, which isn't a stupendous amount, but if the patient's crit is 19, you might want to transfuse. What if the system goes down, and you can't give that blood volume back?

Coags okay? – high? Low? Potassium low? (Probably not, right?) Baseline BUN/creatinine, and what are they now? Calcium for sure, both serum and ionized. Magnesium, and phosphorus, definitely. And oh yeah, is the patient acidotic, and why?

57- What about labs while the system is up and running?

Calcium again, obviously – is it obvious by now that the system pulls off tons of small electrolytes? Potassium tends to drop quickly as well – we usually have a prn order to replace it (no faster than 20meq/hour) to keep the level around 4.0. Some patients need it infusing almost constantly.

58- What about "hemes"?

Which way is the hematocrit going? PTT? I think CVVH does something to platelets – sequesters them in the filter, maybe? Is Karen around?

Problems

59- Why would the machine "go down"?

Usually this is a kink somewhere, probably the catheter, or a clot, probably in the venous trap. You want to keep an eye on the trap – give the machine a 200cc NS flush to get a look if you can't see clearly. (And remember that that bolus <u>does</u> go into the patient.) A growing clot may suddenly just drop to the bottom of the trap and occlude the line. If you're lucky, it won't be completely blocked, and you'll be able to give the patient her blood back from the system – if not, she may need a packed cell. Much more common in bicarb system situations.

60- Are there ways that can be prevented?

Keeping the system nicely anticoagulated is the whole key, along with keeping the catheter flows nice and smooth. Kinky catheter flows are apparently hemolytic, and the debris forms clots in the system, not to mention destroying lots of your patient's red cells.

61- What if the machine goes down, and I can't figure out what's wrong?

The system in general is a fussy, unpredictable beast. Did the patient cough, briefly drive up the arterial pressure and get the arterial transducer wet? Did just enough air get into the system somewhere to set off the air detector, even though you might not be able to see it in the line? Arrggh! This is one of those situations where two heads are definitely better than one (or half of one in my case) – you'll see the senior nurses rending their garments and calling each other for help sometimes.

62- Where are clots likely to form in the circuit?

The arterial and venous traps are the most visible places, but actually the filter is the place where I understand most of the clotting problems go on – all those little tubes, y'know. Sometimes you can look at the ends of the filter and see some clots forming there – gives you a clue as to what's going on in the filter as a whole. What will the transmembrane pressure be doing?

63- What does it mean if the arterial pressure starts getting very low?

"Low"? You mean: "more lower than before", which is to say, "a greater negative pressure"? Or "not quite as low as it was before", meaning "higher towards zero", and therefore "less"? Ack!

If the arterial pressure zips downwards towards -100, the machine is pulling too hard; it's having to work too hard to pull blood out of the patient, and it'll stop and alarm. The catheter may be kinked – did you turn the patient over in bed? Did he flex his leg? Or maybe you need to switch ports. If a clot is growing in the trap filter – you may need to plan for a tubing change.

64- What if the venous pressure starts getting very high?

This means the machine is pushing too hard – remember? But the transducer isn't looking directly at the catheter lumen that goes back into the patient – it's actually looking at the pressure in the venous trap. If the flow through the trap and it's filter is smooth and quick, then the pressure will be in a nice range. If the catheter kinks anywhere along the venous line, the machine will have to push harder to get the blood to move – the pressure will rise.

65- What if blood backs up into one of the transducers?

If a patient coughs, bears down, valsalvas, or otherwise briefly hypertenses, the pressure going into the arterial side of the system will rise as the patient's does, and it may back up into the arterial transducer. The machine will stop, but it's an easy fix: take a 10cc syringe (use a new one every time), take off the wet transducer, push the blood column back down, screw on a new transducer, plug it back in, and off you go. The trick is learning to see it happen.

The venous transducer can do the same thing, but it usually means that things may be clotting up in the venous trap. Be careful pushing the blood back down in the transducer tubing – you may dislodge a big clot and get into serious problems – although if this is happening with any frequency, it's sort of your clue that a crash may be coming.

66- Both transducers?

Both things can be going on - you need to try and figure out what you need to fix first…

67- Could something be wrong with the Quinton?

Besides being kinked? The ports might need switching. Sometimes the site is just no good – if a patient is heavy the catheter may stay bent, and you may just have to struggle along until the docs are convinced that they have to try another site. Sometimes several sites.

68- What does it mean if the filter pressures start getting very high?

The filter is probably getting clotted up. This means that you may not be able to get good amounts of ultrafiltrate out of it – time to change the setup.

69- What if the air detector stops the machine?

Air get into the line somewhere? The detector is pretty sensitive, so that even if there's only "micro" air in the line it will shut down the pump. There's a procedure for pulling back on a syringe attached to the venous trap, while running the pump at slow speed, but you need to get someone to do this with you about 300 times before you're comfortable with it. The first 290 are the hardest...

70- What if the blood leak detector goes off?

This one looks at the ultrafiltrate – blood here means that some of the little tubules in the filter have ruptured. Not good – time to change the blood path and filter. How high was the TMP, anyway?

71- What if the heater alarm goes off?

This one can be confusing – it can alarm because there's high pressure in the replacement line, or if the heater itself is unhappy. Make sure that the line clamps are all open when you start things up – if the replacement fluid clamp is closed, the heater circuit will become very unhappy.

72- When should I start thinking about taking the system down?

If you see big clots forming in the traps or on the ends of the filter, that would be a clue. A really high and rising TMP would be another one.

73- What should I do if I think the system is going to crash?

Get your catheter flushes ready: two 10cc syringes of NS, and two of whatever catheter flush your patient needs: either heparin or ACD solution. If it looks like an imminent crash, slow the pump rate down, give the patient her blood back, and go ahead and take it down.

74- Could something on the machine pop, and spray?

I don't think this has happened lately – I haven't heard of it, although if the TMP pressures were high enough I guess it could. Unpleasant idea – who thinks up these questions, anyhow?

Defibrillation and Cardioversion

Hi all. Another one! As usual, please remember that this is not an "official" reference in any way at all – it's what a preceptor would teach to a new orientee at the shop-floor level. Please let me know when you find mistakes – I'll fix them right away. Thanks!

1- What is fibrillation?
    1-1: What is atrial fibrillation?
    1-2: What is ventricular fibrillation?
2- What is de-fibrillation?
3- What is cardioversion?
4- What is a defibrillator?
    4-1: the monitor
    4-2: the capacitor
    4-3: the numbered buttons 1,2,3; output dials
    4-4: the paddles and the pads
5- How do defibrillators work?
    5-1: What is depolarization?
    5-2: What does electricity have to do with it?
    5-3: What is a joule?
    5-4: What is monophasic defibrillation?
    5-5: What is biphasic defibrillation?
    5-6: What is "transthoracic impedance"?
6- How do I cardiovert someone?
    6-1: Cardioverting a-fib.
    6-2: Cardioverting VT-with-a-pressure.
7- How do I defibrillate someone?
    7-1: Defibrillating VT
    7-2: Defibrillating VF
8- What bad things do I have to watch for during cardioversion or defibrillation?
    8-1: Using synchronization correctly.
    8-2: Keeping the process orderly.
    8-3: Clearing the bed.
    8-4: Using contact gel properly – contact burns.
9- What things should I do after the cardioversion/defibrillation?

1- What is fibrillation?

Fibrillation is an arrhythmia that affects either the atria as a pair, or the ventricles as a pair, producing "a-fib", or "v-fib", respectively. (Come to think of it, if a person is in VF, do their atria fibrillate as well? Does it matter?) Most cardiac rhythms are organized – they're regular in some way, producing some sort of regular (as opposed to disorganized), rhythmic motion of the chambers, hopefully producing a blood pressure. In fibrillation, the cardiac tissue of the chambers involved wiggles about like (classic phrase) "a bag of worms". Does a chamber wiggling like a bag of worms pump any blood, produce a cardiac output, eject any fraction of its contents? No, it does not!

As I always try to point out, all the waves that you see on EKG strips actually represent some kind of physical motion of one or the other set of cardiac chambers, and the trick is to try to visualize what those chambers are doing in any given rhythm situation. Let's see if a quick review of some strips helps the visualization process. Can I have the first slide please?

Here we are: look familiar? Sinus rhythm. Organized, rhythmic, producing stable contraction of the chambers – first the atria, then the ventricles. So - visualizing on the mental screen, that's what I see: nice orderly motion, first above, then below.

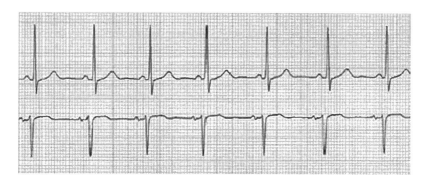

Okay so far? Right – next slide, please. OK: atrial flutter. Still organized: the atria are contracting rapidly, sure, at about 300 bpm, and the ventricles are responding to every third or fourth impulse, slowly enough that the ventricular chambers have time to fill up nicely between beats, fast enough to probably maintain a good blood pressure. So I visualize the atria clipping along, with the ventricles contracting every third or fourth time.

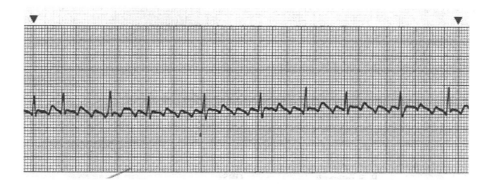

This one? Well – is it organized? Actually it is: see the pattern of doubles? It's a little easier to figure out by looking at the lower part of the strip – this is a sinus rhythm, and after every sinus beat comes a PAC, followed by a compensatory pause. So yes, still organized. "Regularly irregular".

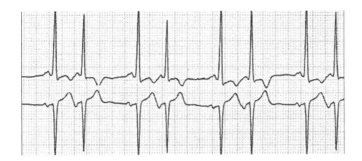

How about this one? Yup, VT. Ugly, scary, but still organized, regular – the chambers (which ones?) are moving in a steady manner. On your mental screen you should see the ventricular walls contracting very rapidly – do they have time to fill? Should we shock this rhythm? It depends…

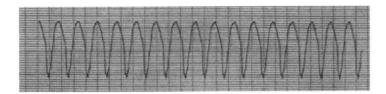

1-1: What is atrial fibrillation?

How about this one? Not organized? Should we shock this rhythm? A-fib for sure can be a shockable rhythm, but look at the QRS rate – in the 70's. What would have to be happening to make this a shockable situation? What do you visualize here? Atria: bag of worms. Ventricles – occasional, but normally conducted QRS's. Are they too slow or too fast to make a blood pressure? How do you tell?

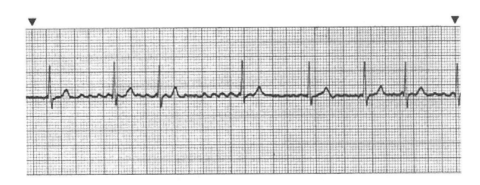

1-2: What is ventricular fibrillation?

Here's an ugly one - you probably recognize this one right off. Doesn't look organized to me! What rhythm is this? Visualize the ventricles – everybody see the worms? What should we do?

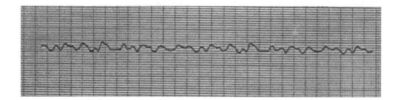

2- What is de-fibrillation?

So: all set on organized, and not organized? The treatment for nasty arrhythmias is often electical, right? The point is: one type of treatment: cardioversion - is for the organized kind of rhythm, and the other is, uh…for the other kind! <u>Defibrillation</u> is for <u>dis</u>organized rhythms.

What you want to do is to send a fixed amount of electrical energy along the normal conduction path of the heart: along the Lead II pathway. Next slide, please?

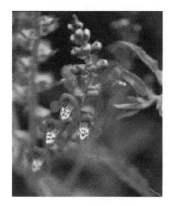

(What's this one? Oh yeah...)

Audience, this is the foxglove plant, the one that digitalis comes from. (The Chief Review Editor likes flowers…)

Here's a diagram of the normal lead II: the positive electrode is down near the apex of the ventricles, the negative one is at the atrial end. Everybody remembers that the normal direction that the cardiac impulse takes is from the SA node at the northwest corner, up near Oregon, down and towards the southeast in Florida, where the positive electrode lives? And that the signal moves along the pathway as the cells depolarize, in sequence, along that pathway?

Negative electrode goes here (Oregon)

(here)   (Ground electrode goes here…)

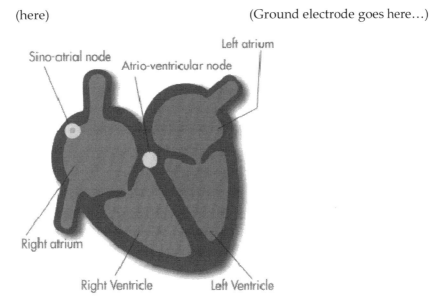

(here)
Positive electrode here (Florida)

www.arrhythmia.org/ general/whatis/

The idea is that applying an electrical impulse - of a specified amount of power - along the conduction pathway should depolarize all the rhythm-generating-and-transmitting cells at once. Bam! (Emeril? That you?) Now, hopefully, one of the normal, built-in, "intrinsic" pacemakers will take over – and in fact, often enough, they do! Remember: **D**efibrillation is the method to use in **d**isorganized rhythms like VF, as in "Go **d**efibrillate that **d**isorganized rhythm, you **d**oofus!" (Got to watch your language in those emergency situations.)

3-What is cardioversion?

This is the other one. Cardioversion is the electrical maneuver that you use for <u>organized</u> rhythms.The difference between cardioversion and defibrillation is pretty simple – the secret lies in timing the shock correctly. If you're treating an organized rhythm, and if the electricity you give the patient happens to arrive during the "vulnerable" period of the T-wave, then the unhappy "R-on-T" thing may occur. Everybody remember what that is?- an ectopic beat, (or a jolt of external electricity – in either case a stimulating electrical signal) landing in the conduction system during the vulnerable period can trigger VF. Bad!

So – how to prevent this ugly thing? The defibrillator/cardioverter has the ability to track the QRS's, and to stick a visible marker on each one. This lets the machine figure out when it's safe to deliver the jolt. All too well do I remember seeing a patient once, cardioverted out of an a-fib with the machine in defib mode – that's to say, <u>not</u> synchronized (forget to push the "Sync" button, did ya?) – and who immediately went into VF, which responded to a defib shock. Fortunately.

The three situations where I've seen cardioversions occur are:

- Decompensated, rapid atrial fibrillation (afib with "RVR": rapid ventricular response) – this means that the ventricular response rate to the a-fib is so fast that the chambers can't fill with blood between the beats. No filling, no blood pressure. Generally if a patient is in rapid a-fib and still has a blood pressure, the team will try meds first: verapamil, beta-blockers, etc.

- VT-with-a-pressure (as opposed to VT- with-no-pressure; what ACLS calls "pulseless VT"). More on how to actually do a cardioversion below.

- SVTs: narrow-complex rhythms, which are usually really bloody fast – up in the 200's. Can your ventricles fill and empty properly at that rate? Mine can't, mate!

All organized rhythms. "Organized" is of course pretty relative: AF is a sort of "just-about-organized-enough" rhythm.

4-   What is a defibrillator?

The goal here is to try to understand what the machine is trying to do. Let's say your patient pops into a nasty rhythm – not handling it very well, not making much of a blood pressure; and you want to deliver electricity – what do you need?

4-1: The monitor.

First: you need to be able to see what's going on. This is of course one of the reasons why our patients are monitored at the bedside: so you can see what rhythm your patient is in. Defibrillators are built to travel– so they have a monitor screen built in.

Second: suppose you want to cardiovert instead of defibrillate – in other words, deliver a timed shock rather than a blind one. The machine is going to need to see the rhythm to do this, and you need to be able to make sure it's seeing the right thing. This is a useful concept: lots of the devices in the unit are trying to "see" the patient in one way or the other – your job is to make sure they do, and that you learn how to interpret what they're trying to tell you.

Anyhow, the machine needs to see the patient. You're either going to have to put sensing wires on the patient that go back into the defibrillator (which may not have time for), or use the paddles as sensors. Our machines have a paddle-monitor mode called "quick look" – the procedure is to gel up the paddles, make sure the monitor is in paddle mode (the word 'paddle' appears on our monitors' screens). Hold the paddles firmly against the skin in the defib position (with gel!) and get a good look at the patient's rhythm. I bet that the newer defib pads do the same thing. I should know this…

4-2: The capacitor.

Unless you have a <u>really</u> long electric cord, you'll need a battery to run any transportable medical device. Rechargeable batteries are why all these devices are so flippin' heavy, and the defibrillator is no exception, so we keep ours on rolling carts that we can whip up and down the unit.

The battery stores electricity, but only if the machine is plugged in when you're not using it. You do <u>not</u> want to arrive on the scene with a dead defibrillator! The battery feeds electricity into a capacitor – this I think of as a black box that holds whatever amount of electricity you choose, for a fixed amount of time. The capacitor fills up with electricity when you push the button that selects the charge you want to give. Our machines charge up with sounds that let you know what's happening: once you push the button, you hear a rising whine as the charge collects - that turns into a steady, high-pitched whistle when the machine is ready to discharge. Loud, but effective. Practice this.

4-3: Numbered buttons: 1,2,3: output dials

Here the goal is to try to keep things very simple: there are three things you need to do when operating the defibrillator, and the people who make these machines are trying to help you do them when you may be, let us say, a bit distracted by the situation. I'm going by the machines in our institution here – make sure you know what to do with your own, although the three moves are probably the same:

> **1: Button number one** (actually on our machines it's a dial, but it has a big number one next to it) turns the machine on, and sets the machine with the joules (the amount of electrical energy) you want to give.

> **2: Button number two** charges the capacitor to the level you picked. At this point we hear the rising tones that tell you that the capacitor is charging up, and then the steady tone that says that it's ready to go.

> **3: Button number three** lives on the paddles (there are actually two "number three" buttons, so you don't squeeze just one by mistake and fire the device before you're ready) and discharges them.

4-4: The paddles and the pads:

I hear that (rather like myself), paddles are considered "old-tech" – nowadays the thing to do is to slap on sticky defibrillation pads that hook up to the machine – the same ones as external pacing pads – then stand back, charge and discharge the machine from a few feet away. I have seen this done, but most times in our unit we make one quick defib move or two – there's much less defibrillating going on since clotbusters came along and fewer people complete their MI's.

In the MICU, I think that the pads are more for the elective cardioversion kind of maneuver rather than the emergent defibrillation thing. The critical point is that you really want to just jump in there and shock that rhythm – you don't want to futz around with the pad packaging, the wires, changing the cable connectors so the pads are hooked up instead of the paddles... get the job done quickly. If the paddles are hooked up and ready, use them – don't waste time; you can hook up the pads later and leave them on the patient for use if the problem happens again.

5- How do defibrillators work?

5-1: What is depolarization?

(I have to stick this in: my son pointed out a while ago that when a white bear is captured, and taken from his iceberg to the zoo, he becomes "de-polarized". Excellent!)

Here's how I understand it. Cardiac pacing and conduction cells work by a sort of magic ion pump dance: the concentrated ions on the outside of the cells all flow inwards at once, then outwards again. Swoosh, swoosh. The charges around the cell reverse as the ions flow in, or out, and the polarity flips: the cells are de-polarized – then re-polarized. Is that clever engineering, or what?

In the process of the depolarization dance along the cardiac conduction pathway, a measurable electrical energy is generated: (P-wave for atria, QRS for ventricles – remember?) Then re-polarized. (T-wave.) The conduction cells do this dance in sequence, along the conduction route from the SA node to the AV node, along through the bundle of His, (hey - where's Her bundle?) and on downwards through the bundle branches into the contractile tissues in the ventricles.

Fine so far. But what happens in a lethal arrythmia? The big sign hanging on the inside of the walls of the ventricles says: "whosoever shall paceth these walls the fastest, shall captureth." Right?- the fastest pacemaker always captures the heart. So what to do when a rapid, excitable, unpleasant little terrorist pacemaker down in the ventricles somewhere has taken over the rhythm, and generates VT?

5-2: What does electricity have to do with it?

As we saw, it turns out that applying a jolt of electricity along the conduction pathway makes all the cells depolarize at once, interrupting the sequence. In sinus rhythm the conduction cells do their sequential dance along the normal route. In VT, they establish some other route – backwards along the normal conduction path? (Anybody know who the EPS fellow is this month?) Depolarizing all the cells at once interrupts the sequence as it's travelling – in whatever direction - and hopefully lets one of the intrinsic pacemakers take over. Which hopefully it does - but sometimes doesn't...what can you do then?

5-3: What is a joule?

(I always tell my family that they're my joules.)

Well. This is so incredibly simple that no one should have any trouble with it. Ready? Here's the encyclopedia: "Joule: unit of work or energy...equal to the work done by a force of one newton acting through one metre....it equals 10^7 ergs, or approximately 0.7377 foot-pounds. In electrical terms, the joule equals one watt-second – i.e. the energy released in one second by a current of one ampere through a resistance of one ohm."

I can't understand why I even had to mention this subject. I mean, really!

Here's the way I think of it. A joule is a hunk of electricity. You need a certain amount of electricity to cardiovert or defibrillate. That electricity is measured in joules. Fortunately for us, the medical engineering folks have done all the worrying about this, and made nice machines that fill themselves up with the right amount of joules when we ask them to.

Let us never forget that we know about these amounts through the generosity of many, many selfless dogs, who went to heaven with frisbees and bones awaiting them (only beef, not chicken), never knowing that they gave their lives for us...thanks, dogs.

Another way to think of it: I remember being told once that 360 joules is about the same amount of power that's required to start a big diesel truck engine. (!)

5-4: What is monophasic defibrillation?

"Monophasic" means that the current delivered by the machine travels in only one direction between the paddles. This has been the standard way of doing things for many years, but is now (like your preceptor) seen as out of date, and is being replaced with a newer method, called "biphasic" defibrillation.

5-5: What is biphasic defibrillation?

Biphasic means that the current initially moves towards the positive paddle, then reverses direction and heads the other way. (My daughter used to drive this way.) The difference for us at the bedside is that biphasic shocks seem to be just as effective as the monophasic ones, but at lower power levels. This is a good thing for a couple of reasons: first, less power applied means less trauma to the patient. Second, less power required means longer battery life, and apparently all implanted defibrillators now use biphasic shocks for this reason – they can also be made smaller. I remember seeing patients come in with what looked like a small brick implanted under the skin of their chests...

5-6: What is transthoracic impedance?

This is the electrical resistance that the patient's chest creates between the paddles. If it's high, then more electricity will be needed to successfully shock the patient. Apparently the new automatic external defibrillators that are being put in airports, phone booths and lunchboxes practically are able to automatically measure a patient's impedance, and adjust the amount of electricity they deliver to match: less for a small person, more for a large one – just the right amount. Nice trick!

6- How do I cardiovert someone?

Okay – let's cardiovert somebody. Any volunteers from the audience?

Many of the moves that you will make in either cardioversion or defibrillation are the same – so let's go over the basics first, and then we'll get to the specifics.

Let's remember that the decision to cardiovert means that your patient is not-quite-in-a-code-yet. As in every critical situation, remember: there's time - more time than you think - available for you to make sure of your plan. How long until anoxic brain injury – 3 to 6 minutes, right? Five minutes times sixty, that's 360 seconds – a lot of seconds! <u>There is always all the time you need.</u> Let's take a little of that time now to look at what needs to be set up:

<u>Make sure that you have everybody you need.</u> In our hospital, elective cardioversions are supposed to include the presence of anesthesia, in case the patient codes and needs intubation. You certainly want to have the team coming if you start a non-elective electrical maneuver!

<u>Make sure your patient has IV access.</u> More is better. If my patient were being intubated (this situation might turn into an intubation), I'd have a gravity bag dripping slowly. Make sure your line isn't infiltrated. (How?)

<u>Make sure your patient is unconscious, or appropriately sedated</u>. This is not a procedure to do on someone who's awake.

<u>Make sure your patient is oxygenated.</u> Why is your patient doing this rhythm in the first place? Ischemia? Or is the rhythm itself creating ischemia, because the heart is using up all the oxygen it's getting, going so fast, but still needs more? (That's what they mean by "rate-related ischemia".) Anyhow, more oxygen to the myocardium is usually better than less, so apply some! (Does your patient have COPD? Why am I asking?)

The Buttons:

Button One: Turn the machine on, and pick the amount of energy you want to give. The ranges vary for different situations, but the general rules seem to be: for cardioversion start low – usually 50 joules for example, for elective cardioversion out of a "relatively" stable, a-fib with RVR. For VT/VF, ACLS says to start with 200 joules. (That's the monophasic machine number – with the biphasic machine you start with 150 joules.) Usually you turn a twisty dial control to set the joules level. The numbers are clear, and there's a simple arrow pointer that you line up with the number that you want.

Make it a practice, every now and then, to go over to the machine and make sure you know how to work it. Familiarity comes with time, so do this a couple of times every week - at least when you're starting out in the units. Obviously, you don't want to have to stand there trying to figure out how the machine works in the middle of some busy situation.

<u>At this point, make sure your patient's rhythm is clearly visible</u> on the defibrillator monitor. Cardioversion is by definition elective, so you should have time to do these things, or you'd be defibrillating, right? In this situation, take the time to connect the patient to the defibrillator's sensing cable. External pacing boxes use the same method – generally, they have to see the patient somehow. Three sticky electrodes set up a standard lead II. Three wires go to a thicker cable, the cable plugs into a socket on the machine, and you should see the rhythm clearly.

The monitor should let you choose between leads I, II , III (or paddle view –but that's for quick-look, usually in defib) – choose the one that gives the clearest upright QRS waveform,

Now comes the "synch" button. This is what makes cardioversion different from defibrillation, and you absolutely <u>must use this properly</u>. Luckily, it's not hard at all. Push the button. You should see a blip, or a dot of some kind that the machine puts on each QRS – this shows you that the machine clearly sees the QRS, and knows when to deliver the shock – remember that cardioversion has to be properly timed to avoid the T-wave.

Here's an important point about the difference between cardioversion and defibrillation: with the synchronization on, the machine will <u>wait</u> after you hit the discharge buttons to make sure of it's timing, and it won't discharge until it's ready. So be prepared to hold those paddles down, hit those buttons, and <u>wait</u> – it might only be a second or two, but if you're not ready for what the machine is doing, you may decide that it's not working.

Button Two: Charge the machine. Listen for the charging tones.

Button Three: This discharges the electricity from the paddles, so make sure that everything is quite ready before you do this. Several things need to happen:

<u>Make sure the paddles have conduction gel on them</u>. The electricity will not be properly transmitted to the chest wall without it. Also, even with the gel these paddles will often cause a second-degree skin burn – imagine what would happen without the gel!

<u>Make sure that you've cleared the bed</u>. This means that just before defibrillating, you take a quick but careful look around to make sure that no one is holding onto the bed, or leaning on it. You should not be leaning against the bed either – you should get the rails down, and then lean over the patient with the paddles in your hands. Yes, it's true that modern beds are electrically designed so well that any stray electricity should go into the grounding system, but would you want to be wrong and have to shock your friend the pharmacist who was leaning over the bottom of the bed, after you put <u>him</u> into VT?

Bed's clear? Steady tone from the machine? Place the paddles on the chest – here's an image from the web…

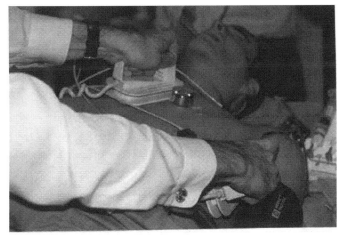

I know – if it's elective, we're supposed to be using the pads. What if you don't got no pads? What if you're in the CT scanner? Or MRI? Should you go running into the scanner room with the defibrillator? (**NO!**) What should you do?

Who knows what the round silver thing is? Has to do with implanted pacemakers…
http://www.usuhs.mil/psl/images/defib.JPG

The idea is that the paddles are sending current from one end of the heart to the other: see that? The upper paddle sits where the negative lead II electrode lives, and the lower one sits where the positive electrode lives, so the current travels along the normal conduction path, and so depolarizes the whole system at once. (I know: I repeat myself a lot – my kids remind me all the time. Those stupid ginkgo pills – I can never remember to take them…)

Hold the paddles down firmly – the book says 25 pounds of pressure – which is more than you might think. My wife brings a scale to her ACLS classes, and has the student press the paddles down on the scale until it reads 25 pounds. (Is she smart or what?) It turns out to be a lot of pressure.

Clear the bed. Yes, apparently it is quite true that the current can be transmitted to someone leaning on, or holding onto the patient's bed. "One, I'm clear! Two – you're clear! Three – everybody's clear!"

Push the third button. Our paddles have a button number three on each of them, so that you don't mistake: you have to hit both, deliberately, to discharge the paddles. Remember now: are you defibrillating or cardioverting here? Will the paddles discharge right away, or will they wait – and should you?

Watch the patient and the monitor at the same time – this is why you have two eyes, right?, to watch two things at once? Ask an old ICU nurse how many things he can watch at once… did the rhythm convert to normal sinus? Or VT? Or worse? Or was there no change at all? What's the patient's pressure like? What's the sat like? What's your pressure like?

Ok – let's do the pads. There's some discussion about where they should go:

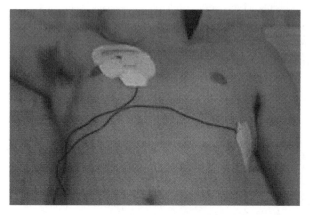

This way, they take the same positions as the paddles would, right?

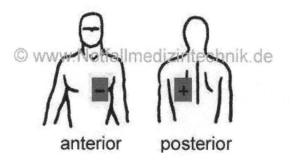

anterior   posterior

This is the other way: "antero-posterior" pad placement.

There's all sorts of learned argument about which way works better – but we've recently gone with this one.

This pad arrangement does seem to work better for transcutaneous pacing…

All other things being equal, the pads really are a nice development. They're larger in area than the paddles, and much stickier, which means less chance of burns, better transmission of the electricity…just make sure you know which method to use, and when.

6-1: Cardioverting A-fib:

Here's a nice strip of a not really too rapid a-fib, followed by artifact from the shock, and then – what? It's a little fuzzy - I've blown it up a bit too big on purpose so you can really see. See the shock artifact – the big ugly bloopy thing there?

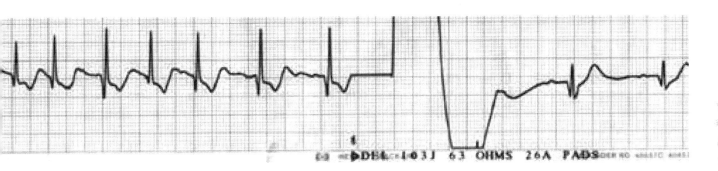

How about this next one?

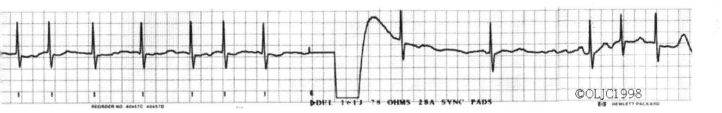

Did it work? What's the rhythm after the shock?

My wife the ACLS instructor says that you should start with low monophasic discharge settings, 50 joules, followed by 100, then 200, then 300 if the patient doesn't convert. A chart out on the web says that the equivalent biphasic shocks would be: 70, 120, 150, and 170 joules. After that, you might have to try chemical maneuvers again.

Then again, it does pay to think a little about why your patient is doing this rhythm in the first place. Is she septic? Does the rapid rhythm mean that her heart is trying to keep the her pressure up in the face of a totally dilated arterial bed? Maybe she's dry. Maybe ischemic. Maybe all of the above. Maybe she's being totally stressed because of vent-weaning trials that she's not ready for – how does the rhythm fit into the whole picture? It always pays to think about these things…

6-2: Cardioverting VT-with-a-pressure:

As opposed to VT-with-no-pressure, right? This scenario is a little closer to a real code situation than the a-fib one, because these folks are very likely to lose whatever pressure they've got, at any time. Jayne says that you should set up for an elective cardioversion if you've got the time, but be ready to defibrillate pulseless VT at a moment's notice. In practice, if your patient is sitting there smiling at you while in VT on the monitor, the team will try chemical cardioversion first. Up until recently this involved a lidocaine bolus, followed by a drip, then maybe procainamide – nowadays I understand that the first drug to try is amiodarone, 300mg IV over ten minutes, followed by a drip, and then maybe the procaine. Would someone please find out and let me know?

7- How do I defibrillate someone?

7-1: Defibrillating pulseless VT
7-2: Defibrillating VF

This is by definition a code. In this situation the ACLS is very clear: shock them first. I would just add – establish unresponsiveness, right? Could be embarrassing if the rhythm turned out to be monitor artifact of some kind. (Ask me how I learned that.) It also helps to remember if your patient is a DNR…

Here's a pretty good strip, probably from an electrophysiology lab: the official description says that what's happening here is first sinus rhythm, then pacing impulses to induce VT – then a defibrillation shock, and then – what?

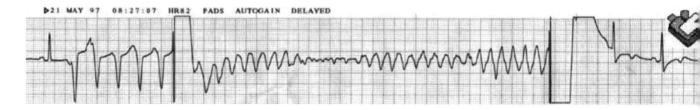

CCU nurses: what rhythm does that look like, there in the middle? Anybody got some mag in her pocket?

Defibrillation is obviously not an elective procedure – the studies show that the most effective thing to do in both pulseless VT and VF is go right on in there and shock them, starting with 200, then 300, then 360 joules (or 150/150/150 when using a biphasic device.) In this situation you don't wait for the paddles to see the patient's rhythm, you don't wait for anything. One thing you should do is to <u>keep the paddles on the patient's chest between the shocks</u> ("Shock shock shock!") – they may be the only system you have running to monitor the patient's rhythm. The monitor should be set to "paddle view" when defibbing – there's a button marked "lead" – push it a couple of times to cycle through views until the monitor screen says "paddles" – but do that <u>after</u> you've shocked the patient!

8- What bad things do I have to watch for during cardioversion or defibrillation?

We've covered a lot of them already:

- Don't shock a patient who's awake!
- Don't forget to synchronize when cardioverting – a-fib can be turned into v-fib this way.
- Don't forget the conduction gel.
- Don't forget to clear the bed.
- Try to keep the process orderly. This means keeping yourself calm and deliberate when you're not really sure you can. Set up systematically. Set up communication with the appropriate team member for orders – don't take orders from two doctors at once! Do your best.
- Remember that no matter what situation you're in, you may shortly be in a full-fledged code – make sure that backup help is on the way.

9- What things should I do after cardioversion/defibrillation?

- Monitor the patient carefully – is the patient staying in the converted rhythm?
- Keep the patient well-oxygenated. This is not the time to wean your patient's oxygen! I would aim for a sat no lower than 98%. Remember however, about COPD patients and oxygen treatment...
- Check up on your patient's labs – does she need K^+, or magnesium? Is she acidotic? – not a helpful thing.
- Get a 12-lead after the cardioversion for documentation- was the patient having chest pain? Does she still? Is it gone now? Can she tell?
- Talk to the team about cycling CPK's and troponin studies.
- Assess the patient's skin – does he need treatment for skin burns?

Foleys For Beginners

This is the second article of a series that we hope to bring out on subjects for new grads in the ICU - topics that seem simple, but which actually aren't. Lots of things in the ICU will suddenly sit up and bite your head right off if you don't use them correctly, and the humble foley catheter is absolutely one of them. As with NG tubes, they have to go in the right way, to the right place, stay in for a certain amount of time, have problems that you do need to think about, and complications that do happen. As always, please remember that these articles are not the final word on anything! They are only meant to reflect the experience of a couple of very elderly ICU nurses ☺. Always check with your own resources and authorities on ANY question you might have. And when you find errors, omissions, or anything else just wrong – let us know? Thanks!

Special thanks for an editorial review go out on this one to our newest consulting "recent-grad-wizardess", Nurse Ruthie, our own oldest child. What a world ☺

1- What is a Foley catheter?
2- Is a Foley sterile or not?
3- How do I know if my patient should have one?
4- What size catheter should I put in my patient?
5- What if my patient is latex allergic?
6- What are the lumens for?
7- What is the balloon for?
8- How is a Foley catheter inserted in a male?
9- In a female?
10- What if it won't go in?
11- How do I know if it's in the right place, and I can inflate the balloon? Something **INCREDIBLY** important…
12- What is a coudé catheter?
13- What is a suprapubic catheter?
14- How do I attach the outside part of the catheter to the patient?
15- How do I work the urine-measuring thing?
16- What if I'm giving my patient Lasix?
17- How long can a Foley catheter stay in?
18- Should they be routinely changed?
19- What is "catheter care"?
20- What is a Texas (condom) catheter?
    a. Our invention…
21- What is a 3-way Foley catheter?
22- What are bladder irrigant drips all about?
23- What is a Murphy drip?
24- Can bladder irrigant drips go on a pump?
25- What can I do if the catheter causes the patient pain in the urethra?
26- What if it causes bladder spasms?
    a. ditropan
    b. B&O suppositories

27- What if the catheter gets plugged up?
    a.   With a clot?
    b.   With a fungal plug?
28- How do I keep my patient's catheter from becoming infected?
29- Should a Foley catheter ever be clamped?
30- What is a neurogenic bladder?
31- How can I monitor my patients' temperature with a Foley catheter?
32- What is a bladder scanner?
33- What are bladder pressures all about?

1- What is a Foley catheter?

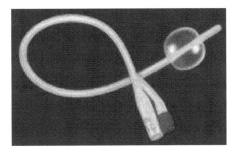

They seem simple enough: soft tube, goes into the bladder, drains the urine, with a little balloon towards the end, inflated inside the bladder to keep it from slipping out.

http://www.medproducts.com/pictures/50130-Foley-Balloon-Catheter.jpg

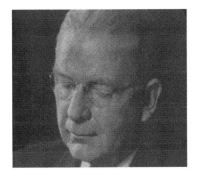

The man! Dr. Frederick Foley... invented the catheter in the 1930's.

http://www.auanet.org/museum/content/collections/uropeople/foley/p2.cfm

2- Is a Foley sterile or not?

Yes, they absolutely are. Remember all that about how urine is sterile? – the whole urinary path is sterile. On the inside, anyhow, and with normal urine flow, it stays that way. The kidneys make urine, it collects in the bladder, it gets drained out promptly, and nothing gets back in through the urethra... no problem. So what happens when you put in a tube?

3- How do I know if my patient should have one?

There are lots of things that a foley can tell you about your patient:

- **What's her volume status?** Enough to make urine, anyhow? Lots of estimations about a patients' volume status - whether a patient is "wet" or "dry", start with the question: "Is she peeing?"

In fact, there's an old saying that the foley catheter is the "poor-man's PA-line". You need to know about your patient's volume status? – there you go.

- **Are her kidneys actually working?** This is always a relative question – we see a lot of patients in renal failure: acute, chronic, acute-on-chronic… someone may be very "wet" indeed, but if her kidneys don't work, the urine output won't be a good indicator. The kidneys are also dependent on the blood pressure reaching them to make urine – a hypotensive patient won't make much urine, even if her kidney function is still ok…

Which raises another question: have you seen patients make enormous amounts of urine with a high blood pressure, and virtually none with a lower one – maybe a "normal" one? Does that say something about their renal arteries? Narrowed, maybe?

- **Is her urine clean?** Got bugs? Sediment? Crud floating around? A person with a fungal urine infection is probably at serious risk for a systemic fungal blood infection, huh? "Fungemia." Very bad. What should we do about that?

- **The only way to accurately measure hourly**, and total urine output, is with a foley, connected to a urimeter.

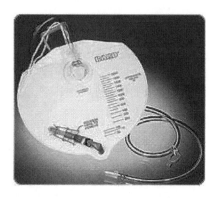

Not this one.

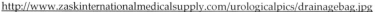

http://www.zaskinternationalmedicalsupply.com/urologicalpics/drainagebag.jpg

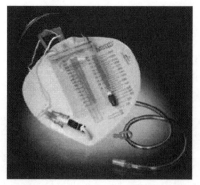

That's the one – the plastic thing in front of the bag measures the urine output every hour. And so should you!

Just can't do it any other way. I hear that in the pedi ICUs they weigh the wet diapers on a scale, and subtract the weight of dry ones? Not really practical with the grownups…
Oh yes – and make sure the tubing leads downhill!

http://www.bardmedical.com/urology/metertour2/bag.html

4- What size catheter should I put in my patient?

I've never quite understood where the French catheter sizes come from – anybody know? Smaller is smaller, and bigger is bigger, unlike IV catheters, in which bigger is smaller – right? I mean, a higher number means a smaller bore IV catheter, but a bigger foley. Goofy.

Anyhow – after a little looking, it turns out (as if life wasn't complicated enough), that the French scale corresponds to diameter in millimiters, divided by three. Say what? It means a size 3 French tube has an outer diameter of 1mm. An 18 French has a diameter of 6mm. Oh! Well why don't they just call it a six then? Jeeze!

Usually a 14 gauge foley is the smallest we'll put in – they drain pretty slowly, and they probably plug more easily, being so narrow. Most of the catheters I place are 16's, occasionally an 18 if the smaller ones are leaking along the urethral path. Doesn't happen often. They do get bigger – but that stuff we leave to urology...

5- What if my patient is latex allergic?

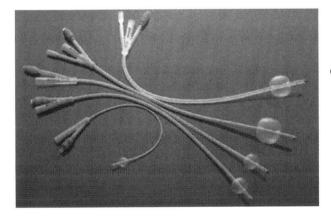

Get out the silicone ones! Nice colors!

6- What are the lumens for?

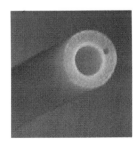

"Lumen" is a big ICU word – it simply means "tube". Lots of devices that we use have multiple tubes in them, so they're "multi-lumen" thingys...

Here we see two, right? One to drain the urine, the other for the balloon.

7-   What is the balloon for?

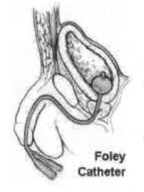

Not too hard to see that the inflated balloon snugs up against the neck of the urethra, and keeps the tube from just sliding out.

http://www.uroport-tbc.org/Tube%20drainage.html

Foley Catheter

8-   How is a Foley catheter inserted in a male?

Here's a link: http://teach.lanecc.edu/nursingskills/cath/cathMale.htm

A couple of thoughts: if you have any reason to think that the catheter isn't going to pass smoothly, grab one of these ahead of time:

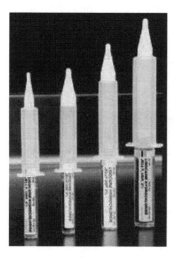

"Uro-jets". These are great – they're lubricating goo mixed with lidocaine. Before even trying to place a foley in a patient with, maybe, BPH (go look that one up), you inject this stuff upwards, backwards, through the urethra, into the bladder. Then let it sit for a minute. Lubes things up, numbs things up... a wonderful trick. I want one!

Just be careful. If the catheter doesn't want to go, don't make it go! A little steady forward pressure, along with a pre-lubed urethra, may allow the catheter to sort of wriggle it's way into the bladder past a swollen prostate, but no more! You may be creating a "false tract" – yow! Time to call urology!

http://www.ims-limited.com/images/URO-JET.jpg

9-   In a female?

Another link: http://teach.lanecc.edu/nursingskills/cath/cathFemale.htm

The preceptor doesn't put catheters in females, nor does he give vaginal meds. I ask my female peers to do these tasks for me. That's just the way it is. Got questions not covered here? Ask the peers. I understand flashlights are involved...

A couple of female-foley tips from our nurse consultant Amy:

- For women – for inexperienced nurses – have another nurse or nursing tech help to hold the patient's legs so that when you insert the foley and if the patient jumps – which happens frequently – they won't close their legs on the sterile field. Otherwise – placing foley catheters in women takes some practice…

- Insert the foley until you obtain urine and then go in another inch or two. Inflate the balloon slowly and ask the patient if they feel any pain or discomfort with the inflation. If so… deflate the balloon and push the catheter in another inch or two and try to inflate again.

10- What if it won't go in?

Don't force it! The Great Nursing Supervisor created urologists for a good reason! A foley catheter that won't pass is NOT a job for a medical intern, or even a junior. ALL of these situations should be referred to the urology person on call.

A story of genius: unfortunately, the team docs don't always agree to this, despite the best arguments from nursing. A story I heard once: a young doc, I think an intern at the time, was making her way through a first rotation in the MICU… she was one of the occasional geniuses that go through the residency program from time to time. Published in Cell… MD, PhD, this, that, the other… and apparently had become something of a legend in her own mind. A nurse got stuck trying to pass a foley in her male patient… suggested calling urology. Genius girl decided that she wasn't get let any nurse tell her what to do with something as simple as a foley catheter… she went in, went ahead, and inflated the balloon… apparently it was rather the blood bath. The patient went to the OR… turned out ok in the end. Sigh. Sadly, **this is the common error with foleys**. Happens every once in a while, and is **totally avoidable!**

11- How do I know it's in the right place, and I can inflate the balloon?

There are a couple of basic clues:

- The catheter has gone in smoothly.

- Urine starts draining through the tube.

Once you're in the bladder, you're **almost** ready to inflate the balloon. Look at this picture again…

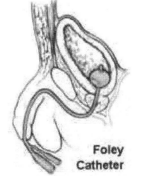

Foley
Catheter

See how far in the catheter is? Almost all the way to the Y – where the two lumen connectors separate – see that?

THAT's how far you should insert a foley – in a male patient, anyhow, **before** you inflate the balloon.

This is **SO** important! And **SO** simple! And yet, even <u>geniuses</u> don't grasp this!

Tells you something, right there…

For women – I'll have to check!

12- What is a coudé catheter?

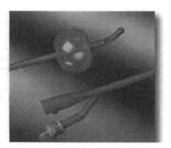

Little curve in the end of the catheter, a bit stiffer, lets it slip past urethral obstructions, etc. Urologists put these in for us.

http://www.allegromedical.com/images/products/0102L16.jpg

13- What is a suprapubic catheter?

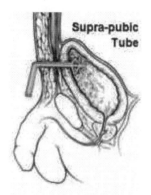

Sometimes, no matter what, the darned tube just won't go into the darned bladder, urologist or no urologist. So they have to go in through the abdominal wall, and drain the bladder that way.

http://www.uroport-tbc.org/Tube%20drainage.html

14- How do I attach the outside part of the catheter to the patient?

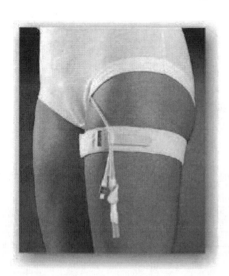

Stylin'! Do they come in colors? Can I get one that lights up?

Well, again, you don't want the catheter getting pulled on by accident – urethral injuries are not trivial, and your patient can be seriously hurt.

I always flag my patients' catheter to a leg. Usually theirs…

http://www.sslaustralia.com.au/medical/images/foleycatheter.jpg

15- How do I work the urine-measuring thing?

Easy enough – read the level by the numbers, and empty it into the bag every hour.

16- What if I'm giving my patient Lasix?

Good thinking! If you're diuresing your patient, then the hourly drainage will probably overflow the hourly measuring thing… so what should you do with the bag, whenever you give your patient a dose of a diuretic? And maybe for an hour or two after that, until they're done dumping 700cc/ hour?

A question for the group: suppose you give your patient a dose of lasix, and they're going great guns… and the team asks for a UA specimen. Or urine lytes? What should you do? Send it? How about 24 hour urine collections?

17- How long can a Foley catheter stay in?

We often leave them in as long as they seem clean. We don't do routine survey cultures, although they're frequently cultured anyhow when our patients spike fevers…

18- Should they be routinely changed?

It looks like people with long-term catheter needs have them changed every month.

19- What is "catheter care"?

An awful lot of our patients are incontinent of stool, which is something like 1/3 to 2/3 germulous material, right? So – suppose that stuff gets into contact with the catheter? Where are those germs going to go, that normally they wouldn't be able to?

Back in the Little Ice Age, this was a sterile procedure – we were taught to cleanse the catheter at the meatus with normal-saline-soaked gauze sponge, then to apply to iodine goo around the catheter where it entered. Nowadays, we wash the meatus with soap and water, and the iodine has gone the way of the woolly Nurse Mammoth…

20- What is a Texas (condom) catheter?

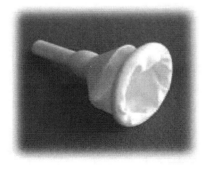

Simple idea, but they don't work so well. Some gentlemen are not very well… suited?, for this device. (Guess they're not the ones from Texas.) These things fall off a lot. But the advantage is clear – there's no direct path for infection backwards up into the bladder.

(I wonder if they make glow-in-the-dark ones… the night nurses need all the help they can get.)

http://www.mkandrew.com/surgT.jpg

209

Nurse Ruthie says that she's seen some folks using these for longer periods of time, and that they use ostomy cement to make them stay on. I just wonder – how sore do they get doing this?

a. Our invention…

We do have the occasional brainstorm in the MICU, and a couple of our senior ICU nurses came up with the really neat idea of combining the condom cath with the oxygen sat probe. Brilliant! You know – for the male patient with cold fingers? The Condosat! The problem of keeping it in place is easily solved by coating the inside with Viagra gel… we're looking for investors!

21- What is a 3-way Foley catheter?

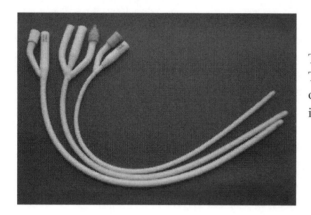

That would be the one in the middle there. Three ports – see 'em? One for the balloon, one to drain the urine, and the third for irrigating the bladder with… what?

http://www.elimedical.com/img/bag%20and%20tube/latex%20foley%20catheter.jpg

22- What are bladder irrigant drips all about?

Sometimes patients have infections growing inside the bladder. Some of these can be severe, and can migrate back up towards the kidneys: pyelonephritis. Not knowing enough about the ID medicine involved, I can tell you that we treat patients with fungal bladder infections using drip irrigants of nystatin or Amphotericin B. The mixes come up from pharmacy in a bag, and they're connected – **sterilely** – to the irrigant lumen of the 3-way. The mix is run using a standard infusion pump, at whatever rate the gods of pharmacy, urology, and ID decree. Other urinary tract infections seem to do just fine with IV antibiotics and bladder drainage.

23- What is a Murphy drip?

This is what they call a saline bladder irrigation system at my hospital. We use these mostly for hematuria – did your patients' foley get yanked on? How'd that happen? Some patients on chemotherapy get hematuria: "hemorrhagic cystitis".

This is a bit tricky – the idea is to keep the bladder clear of clots, because they'll block the foley drain for sure – and what will happen to the bladder then? Sooner, or later?

So the trick is to run the saline rapidly. Really rapidly. We use really big, heavy bags of saline, 3 liters, and there's special tubing, really big gauge, and just run that sucker wide open through the infusion port of the three way, trying to keep clots from forming. Make sense?

Measuring the patient's own urine output while this is going on can get really tricky – what we do is to use one of those scales that you hang peritoneal dialysis fluid from? We hang the infusion bag from that, and read that for the amount that's gone in over an hour. Then subtract that from the total hourly output, which has to be emptied every hour. Make sense? It's still really hard.

A point of aesthetics – we put some thought into describing our patients' hematuria by color: "Well, it started out like a merlot, but it's come down to a sort of nice rosé by now… no clots." "Ah, you think that's a rosé? Dat's a zinfandel!" "No way, you ignorant slob! Didn't you watch 'Sideways'? Sheesh!"

24- Can bladder irrigant drips go on a pump?

Think about this for a second: if you were irrigating someone's bladder at high speed, say a liter or more an hour, and that fluid was on a pump… and the foley managed to clot off… yow! We do put the therapeutic irriigants on pumps – they usually run at a fixed rate of something like 50cc/hour. So you have to do a bit of addition and subtraction every hour to get the true hourly urine output, which is the total minus the irrigant volume, right?

For those terrified of numbers, it's like this – you have a couple of columns, thus:

Time:	Irrigant In	Total Urine Out	True Urine	Cumulative Urine Total
12am-1am:	50cc	52cc	2cc	2cc
1am – 2am:	50cc	950cc	900cc	902cc

Um… was the patient lying on the foley for a while?

25- What can I do if the catheter causes the patient pain in the urethra?

Some people don't tolerate catheters very well – it's rare, since usually people usually have the most discomfort while the catheter is going in – even that can be minimized with a good lube job. But some folks are sensitive, and the catheter just hurts like crazy – for them there's a nice med called pyridium (phenazopyridine): oral med, which as I recall gets loaded with 300mg for the first dose, and then given 100mg po tid. Turns the urine a lovely orangeade color. Rifampin do that too? Something does…

26- What if it causes bladder spasms?

Couple things you can do for this, which is pretty painful:

a. Ditropan (oxybutynin): this is the stuff they advertise all the time on daytime TV... gotta go right now? I suppose it works – I don't really know. You see it ordered sometimes.

b. B&O suppositories: My my... belladonna and opium... this IS an old one. (All the ancient nurses are grinning now.) We still stock these guys, and we count them in the narcotic count every shift. This is an ancient med, going back probably a couple of hundred years, like DTO (deodorized tincture of opium, aka laudanum, the seaman's favorite drug in the Napoleonic Wars... colchicine is even older, going back to ancient Greece I think. Around the time I graduated school.) Haven't seen one actually given in a while, but Cathie F. and I always think of this at the same time when the issue comes up – we grin at each other and feel like old wise guys ☺.

c. Of course, you could always take the catheter out and replace it with a smaller one...

d. And no caffeine! (And maybe no chocolate? Doesn't seem worth it....)

27- What if the catheter gets plugged up?

Absolutely happens – in fact, if your patient's urine output drops off, the first thing you want to do – after making sure it's not kinked – is to give it a gentle manual flush. This is a sterile procedure!

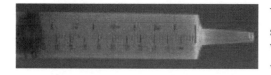 You take one of these guys, and draw up 30cc of sterile saline, and GENTLY inject it into the Foley. Why gently? If your patient can't speak, try watching his face as you do this...

http://www.vetmed.wsu.edu/ClientED/images/dog_meds/syringes.jpg

Now let the irrigant drain, or try gently aspirating. <u>You should get all the volume back that you instilled</u>. Sometimes plugs form on the drain openings, and will let you instill, but won't let anything back out. Like a flap valve.

a.   With a clot?

Yup, could be a clot. Has the patient had hematuria? No?

b.   With a fungal plug?

Could be a fungal plug. Has the patient had funguria?

It could also just be a little fibrinous plug, mucoid plug - these happen too. You'd be absolutely amazed at how much urine a patient may drain once you've irrigated his foley. In fact I've seen patients admitted from outside facilities with hydronephrosis – usually both kidneys, all swollen up – why? "Well, the patient hasn't made much urine for the past couple of days... what do you mean, did we change the foley?"

28- How do I keep my patients' catheter from becoming infected?

Looks like you can't: apparently all urinary catheters become "colonized" with bacteria after two weeks.

Right – but it's commonly said in the MICU that every patient with a foley catheter becomes uroseptic in the end… the same article cited above says that 3 times as many nursing home patients die if they have an indwelling foley, as opposed to those who don't.

(Colleagues, please remember, the author is a registered DNF!)

29- Should a Foley catheter ever be clamped?

The only time I ever do this is when I'm trying to get a sterile urine spec out of the sampling port, or for measuring a bladder pressure – more on that a bit later.

30- What is a neurogenic bladder?

This is a bad thing. In the context of foley catheters, I understand that severe overdistention of the bladder causes the nervous structures to stretch, become damaged, and the patients' bladder never works properly again. Foley get plugged?

31- How can I monitor my patient's temperature with a foley catheter?

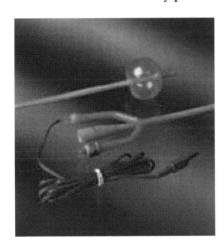

Cute gadget, this. Has a little digital thermometer built into it, that plugs into the bedside monitor console we bought. Used mostly for continuous core temperature monitoring, when we do the aggressive post-cardiac-arrest cooling protocol – the one that apparently improves brain death outcomes after anoxic events? I'd better be pretty darned anoxic before they put a foley in me…

http://www.bardmedical.com/urology/cathtour/array.html

32- What is a bladder scanner?

Neat device, which only urology floor nurses know how to work. This is a kind of ultrasound machine, which can tell you if your patients' bladder is empty or not. This could be pretty useful if someone's urine output fell off, and, say, the catheter had been very hard to place initially, maybe in a very large person, or a person with an unusual anatomy, and would be difficult to change.

33- What are bladder pressures all about?

This is pretty interesting. It turns out that there are situations in which the pressure inside the abdomen can rise to the point where they actually threaten organ perfusion – this is called "abdominal compartment syndrome", taking its name from the compartment syndrome that can threaten a severely swollen arm or leg. Or head, in my case… a person passes out, for whatever reason, and lies on his arm, on a concrete floor, for a day. Or two. The arm suffers diffuse muscle crushing, swells severely, loses perfusion - and produces all sorts of secondary problems like rhabdomyolysis, renal failure…

Anyhow – really high intra-abdominal pressures can literally squish the organs, reduce their perfusion, and produce injuries – patients with lots of ascites are at risk for this. Hepatic failure patients often become hepato-renal failure patients, and it's possible that high intra-abdominal pressures squishing the kidneys are the reason. Anyhow, you can actually measure the intra-abdominal pressures by measuring the pressure in the bladder, and you do it through the Foley.

Here's how:

-    First thing, you want to make sure that the Foley is patent, and the bladder is empty.

-    Next, you're going to set up a regular pressure transducer set, with a stopcock at the end of the stiff transducer tubing, and a blunt needle connector at the end of the stopcock, pointing straight along the lumen of the line.

-    What you do is, you clamp the Foley tubing downstream from the sampling port with something really tight, like a Kelly clamp. Then you swab the port, and poke the blunt needle into the port. Now you're going to instill a fixed volume – we use 100cc – of normal saline into the bladder. Drip it in using regular gravity tubing screwed into the stopcock, which is connected to the blunt. Turn the stopcock such that the saline instills, and when it's done, turn the stopcock so the transducer can "see" through the blunt into the saline – which is partly in the bladder, partly in the catheter. Now you'll get a waveform on your monitor, which should vary with the patient's respirations. As with all these measurements, you want to read the number at end-expiration.

A tricky point – make sure that the tip of the blunt isn't up against the tubing wall, but right in the middle of the fluid column in the catheter. If the fluid doesn't reach the blunt because there's air in the tubing, unclamp the foley a little until the saline – draining out of the bladder – reaches the blunt. Then reclamp.

This making sense? You're using the transducer to feel the pressure, through the saline, into the bladder. Normal bladder pressures are pretty low – the docs usually want to hear about it when they're above 20mm of mercury. I've seen a patient undergo a big paracentesis for this, and start making lots more urine afterward. Cool!

Hi all. Yet another one, which occurred to me that I should do about two weeks ago, when a patient was doing some pretty strange things on the monitor. As usual, please remember that this is not meant to be an official reference, but is supposed to represent the information that a preceptor would pass on to a new orientee in the unit. Please get back to me if things aren't clear, have been left out, or are just plain wrong, and I'll fix them up right away. Thanks!

1- What is a heart block?
2- What exactly is being "blocked" in heart block?
     2-1- The key idea: all of the time, some of the time, none of the time…
     2-2- It can <u>not</u> be that simple…
3- Why do heart blocks happen?
4- What are the three types, or degrees of heart block? What is a "dropped beat"?
     4-1- A normal rhythm for reference.
     4-2- First degree heart block.
     4-3- Second degree heart block.
          4-3-1- Second degree, type 1: Wenckebach/ Mobitz 1
          4-3-2- Second degree, type 2: Mobitz 2
     4-4- How I tell them apart?
     4-5- Third degree (complete) heart block.
5- A puzzler…
6- What is the treatment for heart block?
7- Where can I learn more about pacemakers?

1- What is a heart block?

Heart block is a kind of arrhythmia, usually caused by ischemia or an MI. There are three kinds, or degrees of heart block, and although sometimes people get confused about them, actually they're pretty simple to understand.

2- What exactly is being "blocked" in heart block?

The signal from the SA node is trying to get to the AV node, and it's being slowed down, or blocked altogether – it's having a hard time getting through. The result is that the SA signal going through the atria makes a normal P wave, but if that signal doesn't trigger a response from the AV node, no QRS gets produced – so you'll see **a P wave that isn't followed by a QRS**. The QRS represents ventricular depolarization – so what? So what is: no depolarization, no contraction, no blood pressure!

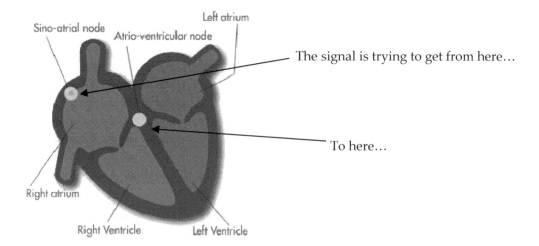

2-1- Here's the key idea - the signal is either getting through:

1- <u>All</u> the time (but taking a little longer than usual).
2- <u>Some</u> of the time.
3- <u>None</u> of the time.

Got that? All, some, or none of the time. And see, those are the three kinds, or degrees of heart block: first, second, and third degree. All, some, or none.

2-2- It can <u>not</u> be that simple...

Sure it can. This is one of those things that people get scared of, and they build it up in their heads as if it were this enormous mysterious thing, like running a nuclear reactor. (When she learns about something new, Jayne always says: "Well, is it easier or harder than a ventilator?")

3- Why do heart blocks happen?

Heart blocks usually happen when the patient is having ischemia, or an MI. The blood supply to the nodes is interrupted, or reduced, and they become unhappy – but at least in this regard, they do it in recognizable ways.

CCU nurses – what kind of MI or ischemia commonly produces heart blocks?

4- What are the three types, or degrees of heart block? What is a "dropped beat"?

4-1- First of all, here's a normal strip for reference:

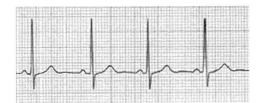

Right – a quick bit of review. See the P wave? Now, see where it meets the QRS? Actually, that first upright part of the QRS is the R wave - there's no Q-wave here. (There's more about Q waves and what they mean in the faq on "Reading 12-lead EKGs" – basically you don't want to see them, because they mean the patient has gotten into the tissue necrosis stage of an MI.)

So – no Q waves here. Ok... so the first, upright move of the QRS complex is the R wave, right? So the measurement from the beginning of the P wave, until it hits the R wave, is called (surprise) the P-R interval. A normal PR interval is supposed to be no more than .20 seconds – which is five little boxes, or one big box on the EKG paper. Calipers definitely help here.

Now. Remember what the PR interval actually is? That's to say, not how long it is, but what it actually means? It shows the movement of an electrical depolarization signal along the path through the atria, from the SA node in the right atrium, to the AV node at the atrioventricular junction.

Say what?

Remember, the signal is trying to travel from the SA node to the AV node, and from there it goes on southward to make the QRS complex as it goes through the ventricles.

If the PR interval is normal, then the signal is travelling from the SA node to the AV node in a normal amount of time.

Okay so far? Onwards...

4-2- <u>First degree heart block</u>.

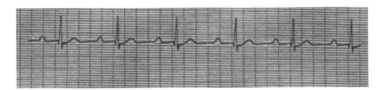

Right – here we are in first-degree heart block. Look at the PR interval now – see how long it is? Longer than .20 seconds, anyway. So that means that it's taking a longer-than-normal time for the signal to go from node to node: SA to AV. It gets there <u>every time</u>, and goes on through the AV node to make a QRS – and therefore a ventricular contraction - but it takes longer than it's supposed to.

4-3- <u>Second degree heart blocks:</u>

This is where a lot of the confusion comes in. It really isn't all that hard. Look at the P-waves in the wenckebach strip below. Some of them have **no QRS** after them. **This is what's meant by a "dropped beat".** The SA node fires off a signal down the conduction path to the AV node, but the AV node doesn't respond by starting a QRS – in fact, nothing happens. The SA node just continues shooting off signals at it's own rate, and some of the time the signals get through the AV, and some of the time they don't. If you're lucky, enough of the beats are conducted to the ventricles that your patient can still make a blood pressure. If you're not lucky...what would you do for that patient?

Next confusing bit: there are two kinds of second degree heart block. And just to make things really interesting, <u>the first of the two kinds has two different names</u>. But only the first. Just in case it wasn't complicated enough already.

4-3-1- Second Degree Heart Block, Type 1: Wenckebach/Mobitz 1

Here's the first kind. This rhythm is called Wenckebach. It's also called Mobitz 1. Why it should have these two names, I have no idea – anybody know? Co-discovered, probably.

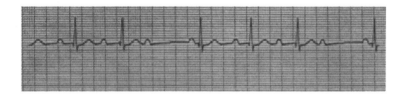

See the dropped beats? The signal is getting through to the AV node <u>some of the time.</u> Mobitz 1 is actually considered pretty benign – you see it in some patients in and around the time that they're having an MI, but it turns out that the rhythm usually disappears after the event, and doesn't cause much problem. Not the one to worry about. (I worry anyway, but hey, I'm old.)

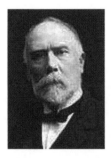

Here's Karel Wenckebach himself. Doesn't look very happy. Missed out on Mobitz 2... poor guy. Still, one out of two isn't bad.

4-3-2- Second Degree Heart Block, Type 2/ Mobitz 2

Now, here we are in second degree, type 2, "Mobitz 2". This one only has one name. Where was Dr. Wenckebach for this one? I bet his kids are really jealous of those Mobitz kids – they have two named after dad! Or was it mom?

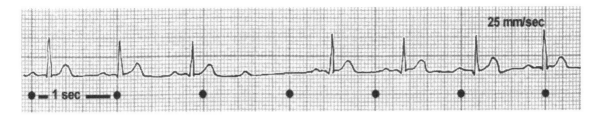

http://www.grundkurs-ekg.de/rhythmus/e_av_block_2_mobitz.jpg

This is the kind of second degree that you <u>don't</u> want to see – it turns out that
<u>Mobitz 2 frequently progresses to the big bad heart block</u> – namely: complete, or third degree
heart block.

So – if the first kind is (relatively) good, and the second kind is bad, (really bad) – it becomes
pretty important to be able to tell them apart.

4-4- How do I tell them apart?

It's all about the PRs... look at the PR intervals of the beats leading up to the dropped one. In
Mobitz 1, the PRs do what? - they get longer, longer, longer, and then there's a dropped beat.

Now look at Mobitz 2. What do those PRs do? They stay the same, the same, then a beat gets
dropped.

See? Not so hard. It's either: "longer longer longer, drop" – or, "the same, the same, the same,
drop".

"Longer" comes first, so that's type 1.

"The same" is second – that's type 2.

If you say "Longer, longer, longer, drop", and then "The same, the same, the same, drop", in the
car, or the shower a few times, you'll never forget it again. What were we talking about? My wife
looks at me strangely in the car…

4-5- Third degree – complete heart block.

This is the big bad one. This time, <u>none</u> of the P-waves are conducted to the AV node. Once
again, luck and the condition of the patient come into it – if the patient still has a functioning AV
node, and if the goddesses are smiling, the AV node will generate a rate by itself : a "nodal", or
"junctional" rhythm – remember the intrinsic rates? SA node is what?: 60 to 100 beats per minute,
AV node is 40 to 60. But – you wouldn't be having a heart block problem if the AV node were still
functioning reasonably, would you? So the AV node may just sit there, probably ischemic, either
unable to do anything or only generating an occasional beat. In that case, you wind up with
something like this:

219

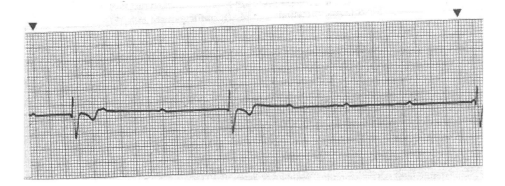

Ack! Can this patient generate a blood pressure? Nuh-uh! And the P-waves are only coming at a rate of about 60 – this is a very bad situation. But of course you were ready – what would you do in this situation?

5- A Puzzler:

Here's a puzzler: what's this one?

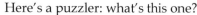

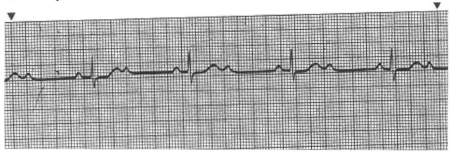

Well, are the P-waves being conducted? <u>Some</u> of them are, right?- not every P is followed by a QRS - so this has to be a type 2; a second -degree heart block. What kind is it? (Do you see that this was a trick question?)

You <u>can't tell</u> what kind of second-degree this is. **You need a series of PR intervals** to look at to be able to tell, remember? – either "longer, longer, longer", or "the same, the same, the same" before a dropped beat. There are certainly dropped beats here – lots of P-waves with no QRS's after them. But there's no series of PRs to look at that will tell you which of the Mobitzes this is. So it could be the nice one, or it could be the bad one – you can't tell. So which do you prepare for?

6- What is the treatment for heart block?

Again, it depends on which degree your patient is having. First degree I've never seen treated just because it's there – but if it's there because of something like a high digoxin level, or because the patient has been started on a combination of cardiac meds that might combine to block conduction – then maybe you need to think about those meds. Combining blockades can definitely produce these rhythms.

Second degree – still depends. Type one – watch it carefully, because it's probably associated with an MI process. Type 2- watch it <u>really</u> carefully, because that's the one that progresses to third degree. Have atropine nearby, have a Zoll/external pacemaker nearby… I'd go ahead and put the pacing pads on the patient, and you would actually do well to go ahead and figure out what the capture threshold is for the patient. Notify the team, and make sure that someone is thinking about taking the patient to the cath lab for a temporary pacing wire.

Third degree – emergently, you may have to call a code. You probably will have to call a code. If you even think that the patient has a chance of going into third degree/complete heart block, get the equipment ready as in Mobitz 2, make sure the team is well aware, have the transvenous pacing kit ready at the bedside along with the external pacer. Test the external pacer, make sure it's capturing, and leave it on in demand mode. Get the code cart into the room, and make sure that the cardiology people are coming, either to place the wire at the bedside, or in the cath lab if the situation allows for it.

7- Where can I learn more about pacemakers?

There's lots more on pacers, both internal and external, in the "Pacemakers" FAQ.

Intra-Aortic Balloon Pump Review

Hello all – here's the latest topic FAQ. As usual, please remember that these documents are not meant to replace reference texts, and they are certainly not meant to be the last word on anything! The idea here is to present information that passes on the experience of a preceptor to the newer ICU nurse, gathered over "too many" years of ICU experience at the "trenches" level. I do try to fill in the gaps with reference sources, usually from the web, and I'll list them at the end.

I've tried to organize the questions so that different topics are clearly separated, so that people can quickly find the answers that they need. As usual, please feel free to write all over this document, point out mistakes (there are probably lots), and add questions, criticisms, etc.

1- What is an intra-aortic balloon pump?

2- Why is an IABP inserted?

> Inflation: perfusing tight lesions..

> > 2-1 What is diastolic augmentation?
> > 2-2 How much volume does the balloon hold?
> > 2-3 Why do they use helium?
> > 2-4 What are tight lesions?
> > 2-5 What is stable angina? Unstable angina?
> > 2-6 What is LMNOP? What if LMNOP doesn't work?
> > 2-7 How do I know if the balloon is working?
> > 2-8 What if the balloon goes in, and they're still having symptoms?
> > 2-9 What are V-waves? Why do they come and go?

> Deflation: treating cardiogenic shock.

> > 2-10 What is cardiogenic shock?
> > 2-11   What is afterload?
> > 2-12   What is "afterload reduction"?
> > 2-13 Why can't we just use pressors?
> > 2-14 How can I tell if the balloon is working?
> > 2-15 What happens to the CVP, PCW, urine output?
> > 2-16 How do I know if the patient is balloon dependent?
> > 2-17 What is the "chemical balloon"?

3- How is a balloon inserted? Who does the procedure?
4- What is balloon timing?

> Inflation timing

> > 4-1 Why does the balloon inflate at the dicrotic notch?
> > 4-2 Why do we use the arterial wave for timing?

4-3 But there's also the "balloon pressure waveform". What is that for?

4-4 What is a dicrotic notch, and why do they call it dicrotic?

4-5 What is diastolic augmentation?

4-6 How does inflation help?

4-7 What are all those initials pointing to the different parts of the timing waveforms?

4-8 How do I make sure my inflation timing is right?

Deflation timing

4-9 What is the "point of isovolumetric contraction"?

4-10 What is "myocardial stroke work"?

4-11 How does deflation help?

4-12 How do I make sure my deflation timing is right?

4-13 Which way do I turn the knobs on the console?

Timing Problems

4-14 I know that there are two big bad timing errors – what are they, why are they so bad, and how do I make sure I don't make them?

4-15 What is early inflation?

4-16 What is late deflation?

4-17 Are there "good" timing errors?

4-18 Can the EKG be used for timing?

4-19 What if the patient is being paced?

4-20 What if the patient is having ectopy? Or A-fib?

4-21 What is "triggering"?

4-22 What is "trigger mode"?

4-23 How often do I need to check my balloon timing?

5- What bad things do I have to watch for when caring for a patient with a balloon?

5-1 What if they bleed at the insertion site?

5-2 What about platelets?

5-3 Why do we use two sets of monitoring wires?

5-4 What do I do if the patient rips off all the wires?

5-5 What if the patient codes?

5-6 What if I have to shock the patient?

5-7 What if I find the patient standing at the bedside?

5-8 With the balloon still in?

5-9 Holding his balloon in his hand?

5-10 What if they're bleeding at the insertion site?

5-11 Should they be transfused?

5-12 What if the balloon gets pulled out just a little bit (or a lot)?

5-13 What if it gets pushed in just a little bit (or a lot)?

5-14 What is balloon rupture, and how can I tell if it happens?

5-15 What do I do for a balloon rupture?

5-16 Why can't the patient sit up?

5-17 Can the head of the bed be raised at all?

5-18 Why can't they bend the leg that has the balloon?

5-19 What about the left radial pulse?

5-20 What about obstructing the renal arteries?

5-21 What should the x-ray of the balloon tip show?

5-22 What about the distal pulses?

5-23 Should I document the pulses in both legs/feet?

5-24 How should I document the pulses?

5-25 What if the leg/foot goes cold?

5-26 What if I can't even doppler the pulses any more?

5-27 What is an embolectomy?

5-28 What is a PVR machine? Do we have one? Where do I get one? How do I use it?

5-29 What about retroperitoneal bleeding?

5-30 How can I tell if my patient is having a retroperitoneal bleed?

5-31   What if the patient becomes confused or agitated?

5-32   What if the nurse becomes confused or agitated?

5-33 What is "hardware sepsis"?

5-34 What are prophylactic antibiotics?

5-35 Why do the ballooned patients have to be anticoagulated?

5-36 What about heparin, or reopro (abciximab), or integrilin (eptifibitide)?

5-37 What are the new platelet drugs all about?

5-38 What is Plavix?

5-39 What are stents?

6- Which balloon console do we use?

6-1 What is the purpose of the "balloon pressure waveform"?

6-2 How often should I check it?

6-3 Can I assume that the balloon pressure waveform is okay if my arterial-line timing waveforms are okay too?

6-4 When do I have to worry?

6-5 What should I do if something is seems wrong with the balloon pressure waveform?

6-6 How is the entire setup connected to the patient and the bedside monitor?

6-7 What is the "root line"?

6-8 Why does the root line transducer need to be air-filtered?

6-9 Why do we mark the root line "No Fast Flush"?

6-10 Why can't I draw bloods from the root line?

6-11 Can I ever?

6-12 There seem to be eight arterial blood pressure waves coming from this patient. Which one do I believe?

6-13 Why do I need to transduce all of them?

6-14 How do I check the helium level? How do I change the helium tank?

6-15 What is purging? Should I purge the balloon?

6-16 What do I do if the console quits?

6-17 Why can't I run the console with the gas alarms off?

6-18 How do I reset the console if it alarms?

6-19 What do I do if the console says "gas leak"?

6-20 Or "kinked line"?

6-20 Or "no trigger"?

6-21 What if I have to travel with the patient?

6-22 What if there's a lot of water in the balloon line?

6-23 Should I ever turn the console off?

6-24 When should I call the balloon tech for help?

6-25 How do I page the balloon tech?

6-26 How do I know if the helium is getting low? How do I change the helium tank?

7 - What about documentation?

7-1 Which pressures do we document?

7-2 How do I document pulses?

7-3 Should I paste in the PVR strips?

7-4 What about the weaning ratio?

7-5 What goes on the flow sheet, and what goes in my note?

8- What is balloon weaning?

8-1 Is there a weaning protocol?

8-2 When should we start weaning the balloon? What is "stunned myocardium"?

8-3 How do I know the patient is tolerating the balloon wean?

8-4 How do I know if they're not?

8-5 Should I stop weaning if the patient is having trouble?

8-6 How long can a balloon stay in?

8-7 Who pulls the balloon?

8-8 When should I turn off the heparin before a balloon gets pulled?

8-9 What should I worry about after the balloon gets pulled?

Intra-aortic Balloon Pump Refresher FAQ

1- What is an intra-aortic balloon pump?

An intra-aortic balloon pump is a device that basically does two good things for a heart in trouble. These two effects correspond to the two movements that the balloon makes, namely: inflation and deflation. The balloon itself looks like a wire coat-hanger with a transparent plastic hotdog on the end, which inflates and deflates in careful timing with certain parts of the cardiac cycle of systole and diastole. The balloon is inserted into the femoral artery, threaded up, and the tip is placed so that it sits just below the aortic arch – this is usually done in the cath lab under fluoro, but can be done at the bedside in an emergency.

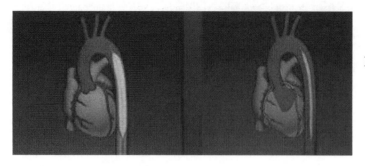

Inflated, on the left…

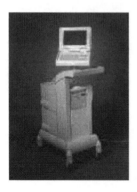

The balloon is "driven" to inflate and deflate by this device, the console. The helium does the inflation lives in a small (very small) tank, and the timing of the movements is controlled in careful synch with the rate and rhythm of the heart. It has to be VERY precise, for reasons we'll get into.

2- Why is an IABP inserted?

Two reasons: first, to help perfuse the coronary arteries, when they are nearly closed by tight lesions. If you try to visualize the cardiac cycle, think of the heart during diastole: the chamber walls open up, and on the left side of the heart, the valve leading from the LV to the aorta – the aortic valve – flips shut. The aorta has just been filled by the previous systolic contraction, and now with the aortic valve closed, it rebounds a little, like a garden hose with a pulse of water going through it – the walls stretch a bit with each systole, and then spring back a bit, creating a small backwards pressure towards the heart. The openings leading to the coronary arteries are actually in the wall of the aorta, just above the aortic valve, and the arteries fill <u>passively</u> during diastole. The balloon is timed to inflate at the end of diastole, creating a <u>forcible</u> pressure backwards along the aortic arch, pushing blood actively through the coronary arteries.

The second reason is for the management of acute cardiogenic shock. This is what the deflation movement does.

Inflation: perfusing tight lesions, treating ischemia that won't go away.

2-1 What is diastolic augmentation?

Because this occurs during the diastolic part of the cycle, and because it "augments" the normal coronary blood flow, this is called "diastolic augmentation".

2-2 How much volume does the balloon hold?

The balloon itself can hold different volumes, but usually is set to an inflation volume of 40cc.

2-3 Why do they use helium?

"The advantage of helium is its lower density and therefore a better rapid diffusion coefficient." What I think this means is that helium, being very light, and not very dense, is easier to push and pull in and out of the balloon through the line tubing. I'm not sure what happens if the helium gets into the patient – I remember being told that it's physiologically inert – maybe the patient talks funny?

NB: Balloon Tech Gary says that the "rapid diffusion coefficient" means that the helium will dissolve very quickly in the blood if the balloon were to leak some into the circulation. Hopefully not a whole lot of helium: if the balloon were to rupture, a bolus of helium would act just like any other gas/air embolus in the circulation – for any sign of balloon rupture (like blood in the balloon line), the console must be shut down immediately, and the balloon removed.

2-4 What are tight lesions?

Tight lesions are the narrow spots along the lumens of the coronary arteries that make for all the trouble – if they're nearly closed, say >95%, then the patient may develop spontaneous angina ("unstable angina").

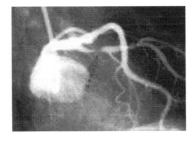

See the tight spot? That's an LAD lesion. Not much blood getting through, huh? To which part of the heart? Pretty important vessel, this…

http://www.hgcardio.com/preplad.jpg

2-5 What is stable angina? Unstable angina?

<u>Stable</u> angina is the ischemic chest pain that a patient gets early in the development of their coronary lesions – they get the pain under stable, predictable conditions, like climbing a flight of stairs. <u>Unstable</u> angina is the pain the patients get as the coronary lesions get tighter. This angina can strike spontaneously, without any exertion, and represents worsening CAD.

Now – which kind of EKG changes are you going to see in episodes like this?

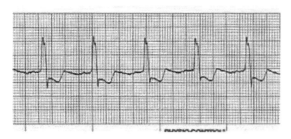 This kind? What is this kind?

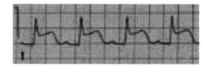 How about this kind? Which is this? Is your treatment going to be the same for these two? Different?

2-6   What is LMNOP? What if LMNOP doesn't work?

LMNOP are the initials that some people use to remember the maneuvers to make for cardiac ischemia: Lasix (assuming they're "wet"), Morphine, Nitrates, Oxygen, and Position (sit them up if they're short of breath – unless they're hypotensive!). If LMNOP doesn't work, then you have to think about putting in a balloon pump to forcibly perfuse the coronaries.

2-7   How do I know if the balloon is working?

You know that the balloon is working if the patient's chest pain goes away! You also want to look at their EKG to see if their ischemic changes, if any, have resolved – remember, some diabetic patients, and we see lots of them - don't have chest pain with ischemia, so you have to be careful. There are "anginal equivalents" – meaning, the patient becomes ischemic, but instead of having pain, does something else – breaks into a sweat maybe, becomes short of breath…

2-8   What if the balloon goes in, and they're still having symptoms?

If the ischemia isn't controlled with IABP insertion, they probably need to go for an emergent CABG or stent procedure, since something is probably about to infarct.

2-9   What are V-waves? Why do they come and go?

V-waves are a sign of ischemia – they can show up as part of a PCW waveform, and in this context it means that the patient has developed "ischemic MR" – mitral regurgitation. The idea is that the ischemia has affected the papillary muscles that control the mitral valve.

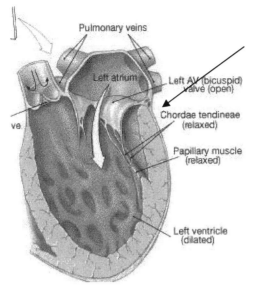

Pulmonary veins

Left atrium

Left AV (bicuspid) valve (open)

Chordae tendineae (relaxed)

ve

Papillary muscle (relaxed)

Left ventricle (dilated)

That's these guys.

They've stopped working properly, and the valve starts leaking. You can use the presence of V-waves as an indicator that the patient is still in ischemic trouble – sometimes this is useful if a patient is intubated and can't tell you they're having pain, or in people who don't have pain, like diabetics with neuropathy sometimes. The goal would be the same as treating someone with ischemic changes on their 12-lead – you want to see the v-waves go away. Look for the oxygenation to worsen with v-waves, since the valve is letting blood flow backwards towards the lungs – look for it to improve once the valve is working again.

http://www.biosbcc.net/b100cardio/images/FG21_07A.jpg

<u>Acute</u> backflow of blood into the lungs... what's the other name for that?

This is the definition of a "flash". You hear lot of people say – "Mr. So-and-So flashed today." – meaning what, <u>exactly</u>? People throw terms around with no clear idea of what they mean...did he have ischemic MR? Did he plug? Be precise...

Deflation: treating cardiogenic shock:

2-10   What is cardiogenic shock?

"Cardiogenic" means that the shock state is being caused by heart failure: the pump isn't pumping. Why not?

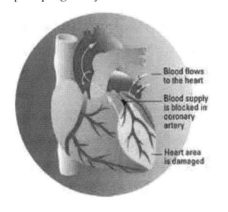

Blood flows to the heart

Blood supply is blocked in coronary artery

Heart area is damaged

This is actually a pretty good image – the yellow bit representing infarcted area is in just the right area for producing cardiogenic shock. Why?

http://www.aspirin.ca/English/CardiovascularDisease/HeartAttack.asp

Remember that there are three parts of a blood pressure, and the common kinds of shock are caused by bad things happening to one of those: pump, volume, and arterial squeeze. Which one is this?

2-11   What is afterload?

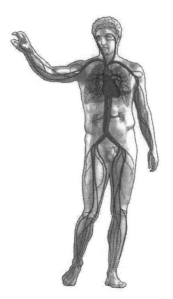

Afterload is the <u>resistance</u> that the heart is looking at, as it tries to pump blood out into the <u>entire arterial system</u>.

(Preload is the <u>volume</u> arriving in the LV, measured as the wedge pressure. What number would tell you the preload of the RV?)

Remember that the arterial bed <u>as a whole</u> can squeeze, and loosen. If the arterial squeeze is high, then the heart has a harder time pushing blood into the tight vessels – so looser is better! Not too loose! Afterload corresponds to the SVR number – normal is around 1000, septic would be low, and cardiogenic would be high. Remember – high is tight, low is loose.

SVR <u>rises</u> in cardiogenic shock, the arteries tighten, trying to keep blood pressure up… is this a good thing?

http://en.wikipedia.org/wiki/Image:Grafik_blutkreislauf.jpg

2-12   What is afterload reduction?

Since a high afterload makes it <u>harder</u> for the LV to empty itself, it <u>adds</u> to the work that the failing heart has to do – bad! So the goal is to lower the afterload – to dilate the arterial "bed" - to lower the SVR. You can do this with drugs, like NTG or nipride, but if the patient has a systolic pressure of 90 – probably not a good idea!

So now comes the IABP. The balloon, deflating just at the beginning of systole, creates an area of lower pressure in the aorta – which helps the LV empty itself, and takes a lot of the workload off it – <u>mechanical</u> afterload reduction. Almost everyone with cardiogenic shock died of it before the IABP came along for this purpose.

2-13   Why can't we just use pressors?

Well – you could, and sometimes you have to, even with the balloon pump working. But do you really want to add a pressor to failing heart muscle? Probably not – you want to <u>avoid</u> things that make the heart work harder, things that increase "MV02" – myocardial oxygen consumption. Do**b**utamine - the **b**eta pressor - would be the drug of choice. You sure you want to use it?

What about the other pressors? Remember, the **a**lpha receptors are in the **a**rteries, and pressorizing the arteries in this situation would be **bad** – it <u>increases</u> afterload resistance, and those arteries are probably <u>already</u> quite tightened up – that's the reflex response the body uses to try to maintain blood pressure if cardiac output falls. These people already have bad peripheral perfusion – they're so tight that they may not have detectable pulses – add an alpha pressor and they might lose their fingers!

Now – see? This is the mirror, the opposite of the reflex response that the body uses to compensate in sepsis, in which the patient has a <u>loose</u> arterial bed, and the compensation is really <u>elevated</u> cardiac output. SVR in sepsis would be… high or low? Low – correct. See that? Two reflex responses available for two different situations.

So - what might happen if the balloon insertion went "dirty"?

2-14   How can I tell if the balloon is working?

Simple: if the balloon goes in for chest pain/ischemia, you look for the patient's pain and EKG changes to go away. Those nasty v-waves should go away too, if they were there before, and MR going away should improve oxygenation quickly. "Un-flash"…

If the balloon goes in for cardiogenic shock, then blood pressure should improve as the cardiac output comes up. The SVR should come down, and you should be able to wean some on the dobutamine.

2-15   What should happen to the urine output, and the wedge pressure?

The PCW should go down for two reasons – the balloon should improve the blood supply to a hurting LV and help it pump better – empty itself better. Afterload reduction from deflation should help PCW go down because of the mechanical advantage the balloon gives to the LV. With better cardiac output, urine output should improve – remember that somebody needs to check the X-ray to make sure the the tip of the balloon is in the right position – too low and it can obstruct the renal arteries, which tends to be bad for the kidneys.

2-16   How do I know if the patient is balloon dependent?

"Balloon dependent" describes a patient who is cardiogenic, and whose heart depends on the mechanical assistance from the IABP to keep blood pressure up. Pause the IABP – their BP falls. This patient is obviously not ready to wean from the balloon yet. A patient with a big MI producing cardiogenic shock may recover enough function in about a week's time to wean.

2-17 What is the "chemical balloon"?

The phrase "chemical balloon" refers to using a combination of vasoactive drugs to mimic the effect of the IABP – usually this is tried in an outside hospital to stabilize a patient before they can be moved somewhere that a balloon can be placed. Dobutamine is used to increase cardiac output, and IV NTG or sometimes nipride is <u>very</u> carefully added to decrease afterload resistance

– remember that nipride dilates the arterial bed, and dobutamine can too! This is a very tricky road to go down, and is obviously dangerous, since the dobutamine can produce tachyarrhythmias, and the nipride can produce really stupendous hypotension. Never forget to take ridiculous care using nipride, running it alone, never flushing the line, etc.

3- How is a balloon inserted? Who does the procedure?

An IABP is inserted by an interventional cardiologist, usually in the cath lab under fluoroscopy, using much the same technique as any central line placement. Very rarely the balloon is put in at the bedside, but this is usually in a near-code situation – it's been many years since I've seen this done. Careful placement is needed to avoid placing the balloon too high or low, and the patient **must** have an x-ray to confirm proper placement of the balloon tip. This can be read by the balloon techs, but has to be confirmed by a knowledgeable doc.

4- What is balloon timing?

Timing is everything in life, and the IABP is no exception. If you think about it even for a moment, you'll realize that if the balloon is still inflated in the aorta, when the heart is trying to pump blood into that aorta – well, that would be a bad thing. So the timing of both inflation and deflation must be carefully looked after. **This is the responsibility of the nurse caring for the patient.** You can **not** avoid this – you can not rely on the timing set by the balloon techs, because timing needs can change frequently. If you feel uncomfortable with timing, that's probably a good thing, because that means you care about your practice. I'll try to cover this as best I can – and we may be getting a simulator into the unit that we can connect to a console. Then I'll run the staff by it on the night shift until everyone is more comfortable with this. Meanwhile, you should feel free to call the balloon techs at night, or call the RNs in the CCU or the cardiothoracic ICU for advice.

One more word about timing before going into the details: remember that there are "safe" positions for each timing knob, or slider. On our machine, turning the knobs inwards, towards the center of the console, puts them in a position where the timing can not hurt the patient. It won't help them either, but at least no damage will be done. When I trained on the old console, they taught us to remember that it's like during a storm: "safe inside", and "dangerous outside" – the old consoles had two timing sliders instead of knobs, but the idea was the same: moving the sliders **inwards** was always safe if you were worried, and moving the sliders **outwards** was moving first into treatment, and then if you went too far, danger. So if you're not sure where you are with the timing, turn the knobs inwards – left-hand knob towards the right, clockwise – right-hand knob towards the left, counterclockwise, always towards the center of the console. Then work the left knob carefully back towards the dicrotic notch to set inflation, and then work the right knob to the right to set deflation.

Timing Basics

Right! Finally got a scanner. (All strips come from documentation by the Datascope Corporation, and are used with permission). Okay, here's a nice strip of a balloon that's just about perfectly timed, with the console set at a ratio of 1:2 – meaning, it's "ballooning" every other beat. Let's see if I can remember how to do arrows…

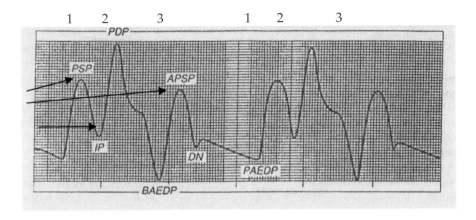

www.datascope.com/ca/pdf/preinservice_self_study_guide.pdf Used by permission.

Okay, what have we got here? First off, see the groups of three? Three peaks? Look for the groups to help you orient yourself. Now - everybody see the first arrow on the top left, pointing at "PSP"? Number 1? That's the patient's peak systolic blood pressure. Now look at the next arrow down, "APSP", number 3. See how the peak that it's pointing to is <u>lower</u> than the first one? You can see the same thing happening clearly in the beats that follow – this is important – see how the second arterial peak is lower than the first one? (The really high waveform in the middle, number 2, is the balloon doing its thing, but we'll get to that in a minute.) The first waveform, the PSP, is the "patient's systolic pressure", and number 3, after the balloon wave, is the "assisted patient's systolic pressure", which reflects "unloading".

Why is this such a good thing? Let's remember that in cardiogenic shock, the heart is trying to pump against a really tight arterial system – it tightens up to try to maintain blood pressure when the heart loses pumping power. Is this a good thing? It ought to be – it's the only thing the body can do in this situation. But does a weakened LV enjoy pumping against a really tight set of arterial vessels? No it does not! Remember, this is what "afterload" means – the resistance that the LV is facing as it tries to pump blood out into the arteries. Anybody know what number we use to measure afterload? Who said SVR? Very good! Higher is tighter, lower is looser, and if your patient's heart is failing, looser is better. <u>So the first goal of proper timing is to make sure that the assisted systole is lower than the patient's own systole.</u>

This is where the difference in arterial pressures comes in – the balloon, by deflating, lowers the arterial pressure in the aorta – that's part of the "assist". The other part of the assist is that the deflation helps the LV empty itself – more on that below.

After the dicrotic notch – this is the point at which the balloon inflates – see the waveform shoot upwards? Number 2? This is the pressure generated in the aorta as the balloon inflates, and since this inflation is happening during – which phase of contraction? – diastole – this really high part of the wave is called the "augmented diastolic" pressure. (On the diagram it says "PDP" – I have no idea what they mean.) Since this is the highest pressure generated in your patient's arteries,

233

your transducer setup is going to display this number as the patient's own systolic – which it ain't. We follow the MAP in this situation anyhow. But it is perfusion pressure – that inflation pressure does help perfuse tissues, so maybe it doesn't matter so much, as long as you know the difference. I usually write "augmented diastolic" over my hourly BP checks on the flow sheet to indicate what the transduced systolic number really means.

Now look at the place where the pressure in the aorta is lowest, at the end of balloon deflation – this is called the BAEDP: the "Ballooned Aortic End-Diastolic Pressure". Say <u>that</u> three times fast. This point should always be **lower** than the patient's own diastolic pressure – which on the diagram is the bottom arrow on the left. See how the one is lower than the other? <u>This is the second goal of proper timing – to lower the diastolic resistance in the arteries.</u> Both pressure components are lowered, decreasing the SVR.

Now take a look at the group of three peaks on the right side of the diagram. This should be the pattern you want to get with proper timing. With the machine set at a ratio of 1:2, you should see the assisted systole lower than the patient's, and the BAEDP lower than the patient's diastolic. See the pattern? Systolic peaks lower, diastolic bottoms lower. You'll see people standing, scrutinizing the monitor, saying, "Okay, this should be lower than that, and this should be lower than that."

Inflation Timing

4-1 Why does the balloon inflate at the dicrotic notch?

The balloon is supposed to inflate towards the end of diastole. So - the walls of the heart open up, the chambers fill, and the aortic valve flips shut. It turns out that the anatomical openings - the ostea - leading to the coronary arteries are in the wall of the aorta, just above the valve, and at the end of diastole the aorta rebounds a little bit, and the coronaries perfuse – passively. Now, if your ischemic patient needed <u>more</u> than just passive perfusion – what could you do? Inflate the balloon. How do you know when to inflate? It turns out that the dicrotic notch, coming at the end of diastole, indicates exactly the event we want – the closure of the aortic valve. Once the valve is closed, the balloon inflates, and blood is forcibly pushed backwards along the aortic arch, and into the coronary arteries <u>under pressure,</u> improving perfusion.

4-2   Why do we use the arterial wave for timing?

Simple: we use the arterial wave to look for the dicrotic notch, to use as the marker for inflating the balloon. Use the inflation knob to move the inflation wave leftwards, until it meets the dicrotic notch.

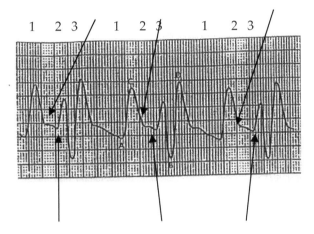

Arrows again. This time, the arrows from above are pointing to the dicrotic notches. The arrows from below are pointing to the inflation waves of the balloon. (The inflation wave is a lot smaller in this picture than it usually is. Bad diastolic augmentation…) Is it anywhere near where it ought to be? At the notch? No – it needs to be moved leftwards. Move it to the left with the inflation knob, turning away from the center of the console. If you do it slowly, you'll see the inflation wave actually move over until it intersects with the dicrotic notch. Don't go too far! Bingo! Can you see how the arrows coming later in the strip point to the same things? The augmentation should improve as you fix the inflation timing.

4-3   But there's also the "balloon pressure waveform".   What's that for?

The arterial wave comes from the patient, so it doesn't tell you anything about the balloon itself. The balloon pressure wave tells you if the balloon is inflating or deflating properly. Usually in my experience if the balloon is timing well and producing a good-looking waveform, then the balloon waveform is taking care of itself. You are still responsible for knowing what the wave is supposed to look like, and you should keep a copy of the IABP waveform card to check. Here's an example of a properly timed waveform:

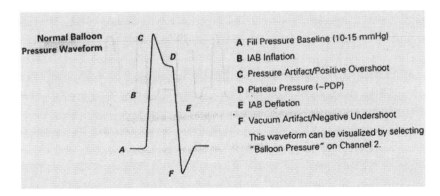

4-4   What is a dicrotic notch, and why do they call it dicrotic?

The notch indicates closure of the aortic valve, and comes at the end of diastole, as the pressure falls. Why **is** it called dicrotic?

4-5 What is diastolic augmentation?

Remember that the balloon inflates at the end of diastole, just after the aortic valve closes – the rapid inflation is what augments the perfusion of the coronary arteries through the ostea. This rapid inflation can produce a pressure wave that's actually higher than the patient's systolic pressure, and that high pressure wave is referred to as diastolic augmentation. That's the high waveform in the middle of the three peaks.

4-6 How does inflation help?

Inflation helps by forcibly perfusing the coronary arteries, instead of letting them be perfused passively. Look at the "PDP" point in the diagram below – that's the pressure perfusing the coronaries generated by the inflation of the balloon. A lot of pressure! This is often enough to control angina/ischemia along with ischemic symptoms, and can stabilize an ischemic patient until they can go to either the cath lab or the OR.

4-7 What are all those initials pointing to the different parts of the timing waveforms?

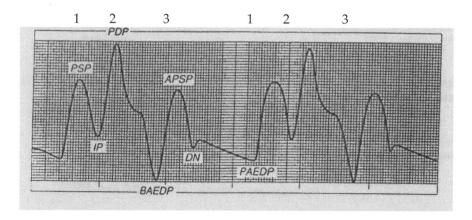

Everybody has their own system for labelling the important points on a balloon timing waveform, but they refer to the same events. Starting at the left:

- PSP: meaning the "patient's systolic pressure".
- Next is IP – here I think they mean "inflation point", which of course is also what?- correct, the dicrotic notch.
- Next? What do they mean by PDP? I have no idea. I would call this the "augmented diastolic peak".
- After that? BAEDP – that's what I call it as well.
- Then – APSP: this I think means "assisted patient systolic pressure". Close enough – I call this "assisted systole".

- <u>DN</u> – okay, this one they call the dicrotic notch.
- <u>PAEDP</u>: probably "patient's aortic end-diastolic pressure". Which is to say, the patient's diastolic, unassisted.

4-8   How do I make sure my inflation timing is right?

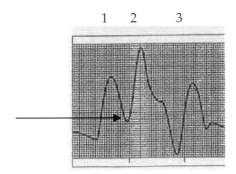

The safe position for the control knobs is always inwards towards the center – the inflation knob is the left-hand one on the console, and turning it to the left, counterclockwise – outwards from the center – will move the inflation wave to the left (earlier) as you watch on the arterial line trace. The inflation wave should coincide with the dicrotic notch. See the arrow?

As a note: you want the angle there where the inflation wave goes up from the notch to be nice and sharp. "Crisp", I think is the word they use.

Deflation Timing

4-9   What is the "point of isovolumic contraction"?

This refers to the point in the cardiac cycle when the chambers have filled with blood at the end of diastole – the chamber walls are building up pressure to start systolic contraction, and this is the point at which the heart is working the hardest.

4-10   What is "myocardial stroke work"?

Myocardial stroke work is the effort that the heart puts out with each systolic contraction. In cardiogenic shock, the pump is having a hard time pumping – so stroke work is something you want to try to reduce – which is exactly what balloon deflation does.

4-11 How does deflation help?

Rapid deflation of the balloon creates an area of lowered pressure in the aorta just ahead of the emptying left ventricle. Sort of like suction. The suction helps empty the ventricle with each beat, and takes some of the workload off of the cardiogenic heart. Almost everyone with cardiogenic shock died before the invention of the IABP because there was no way to assist the failing LV – now the survival numbers are pretty good.

4-11   How do I make sure my deflation timing is right?

The deflation knob is the right-hand one on the console. Turning the knob clockwise, to the right, moves the deflation wave to the right (later). Move the knob to the right until the BAEDP looks sharpened, and lower than the patients' diastolic, but not so far that it begins to rise – check the diagram to help you remember which points are supposed to be lower than which.

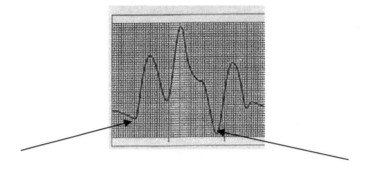

See how the second diastolic (the assisted one) is lower than the first one (the patient's)? Like the inflation point, the point at the BAEDP (the point of the arrow on the right) should be nice and sharp. If this point begins to rise, you need to reset the timing to correct it.

4-12   Which way do I turn the knobs on the console?

This is worth repeating – the safe positions of the knobs are turned "inwards" towards the center of the console. You time inflation by moving the left-hand knob counterclockwise, or to the left, away from the center. Deflation is timed with the right-knob, again, starting from the center, towards the right, away from the center.

Timing Problems

4-14 I know that there are two big bad timing errors – what are they, why are they so bad, and how do I make sure I don't make them?

The two big bad timing errors are <u>early inflation</u> and <u>late deflation</u>.

They both come from moving the timing knobs too far away from center.

4-15 What is early inflation?

Early inflation is just that – the inflation knob is turned too far to the left, and the inflation wave actually comes before the dicrotic notch. To the **left** of it. This means that the balloon is inflating before the aortic valve closes, pumping backwards into the LV, which is already having a hard time emptying itself…

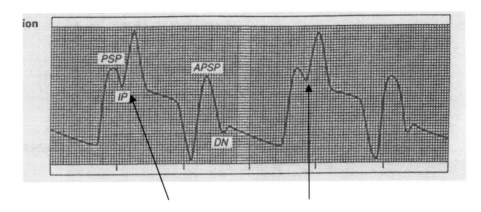

More arrows. Here they're pointing to the inflation wave, which is way out ahead of where it ought to be. (IP I guess stands for "inflation point".) See where it says DN? That's where the inflation wave should be. (Why?) Ack! I have to say, just looking at this wave is enough to give me chest tightness…

4-16 What is late deflation?

Late deflation is when the balloon remains inflated too long – the heart is trying now to pump against an inflated balloon. Bad! The deflation knob has been turned too far to the right – move it back towards the center, make sure the BAEDP is lower than the patient's diastolic pressure on the waveform, and start over.

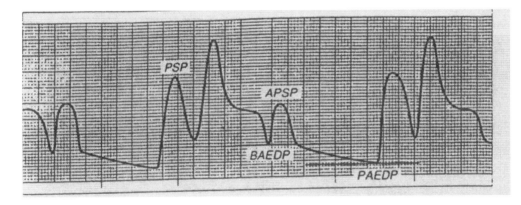

See the BAEDP all the way up there? The patient's end-diastolic pressure is that PAEDP that you see down lower – this is also a certified Big Bad timing error – <u>don't</u> let this happen.

4-17 Are there "good" timing errors?

Sure - if the knobs are too far inwards, then the balloon is safely inflating and deflating – it's just not really helping much. Here's the opposite of early inflation: what can it be but "late inflation"? Duh. See the inflation point? Which way will you turn the inflation knob to fix this? How does the deflation look?

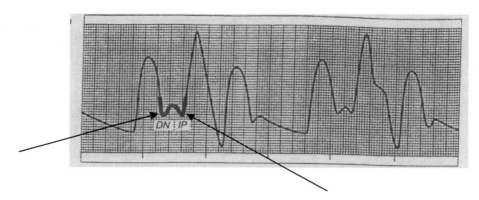

Here's the other one. This is the opposite of late deflation – has to be "early deflation". Won't hurt the patient, but doesn't help either. How would you fix this one? How does the inflation look?

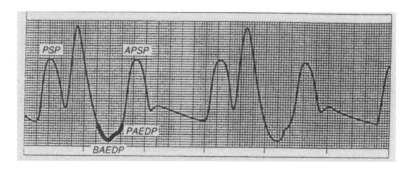

4-18   Can the EKG be used for timing?

Yes – there are timing markers that you can use to time by EKG, and the Transact console that we use does this automatically. Actually in practice, we never do this, because we never, ever, balloon people in our ICU without an arterial wave – if only because we transduce the "root line" that's built into the balloon to give us one.

4-19   What if the patient is being paced?

In practice – yes, you can balloon a paced patient. I haven't done this myself in a while, but I remember that there used to be a "pacer reject" mode on the older IABP consoles – we should put this question to the balloon techs for a better answer.

Balloon Tech Gary says: If the patient is A-pacing, use the R-wave trigger mode, (see a couple questions down), and decrease the gain to make the QRS smaller – that way the balloon will trigger off of the A-spike. With V-pacing, use the same R-wave trigger mode, and the balloon will trigger off the V-spike.

4-20   What if the patient is having ectopy? Or a-fib?

Balloon pump consoles really don't like irregular rhythms. There are lots of claims by companies that make the consoles that their machines track a-fib with good timing – I haven't seen it yet. Likewise ectopy – balloons become unhappy with FLBs (funny looking beats) of any kind – seriously consider having the team try to abolish ventricular ectopy in the patient if they're balloon dependent. Amio – whatever. Watch their electrolytes: K+, Mag... Likewise it might be a good idea to try to convert a person from a-fib to sinus rhythm, for the same reason.

4-21   What is "triggering"?

The console needs some way to know where it should start – we can adjust the timing from there, but the machine needs to see some signal from the patient to tell it when to start inflation and deflation.

4-22– What is "trigger mode"?

The console can use several ways to recognize trigger signals – the most commonly used is "R-wave". The balloon techs will work with you to figure out which mode to use. On the Transact console, sometimes "peaks" mode works well – I don't know enough about this. There are pacemaker trigger modes too – we need to look into this.

4-23- How often do I need to check my balloon timing?

You certainly want to check the balloon timing as soon as you get into the patient's room. I usually take a quick look at the patient, the monitor, and then the console. I set the IABP ratio to 1:2, and I make sure that the timing is as good as I can get it. Then I print a timing strip and stick it on the back of the flow sheet. The timing may change as the patient's condition does: changes in heart rate, blood pressure, arrythmias (obviously) – all can make differences in they way the timing will need to be set. Be alert!

5-   What "bad things" do I have to watch out for when caring for a patient with a balloon?

5-1 What if they bleed at the insertion site?

IABP patients always have to be anticoagulated. The balloon itself is a very convenient place for clots to form, which of course would tend to break off and float downstream to unhappy places, producing infarcts. This certainly qualifies as a "bad thing". With anticoagulation, whether with heparin or one of the newer anti-platelet aggregation meds, comes the risk of bleeding, and since the balloon is inserted into a large, pressurized artery, some bleeding at the insertion site is common. I wouldn't worry about having to change the site dressing once or twice in a shift, as long as I knew that the PTT was in range and not too high. Obviously, big bleeding would mean a call to the interventional people to come and look.

There's also some risk, as always with femoral sticks, of puncturing, and bleeding out the back of the vessel, retroperitoneally. Watch for crit drops, and later, hematomas forming on the patient's back, or flank, starting on the same side that the IABP is on. Try to think ahead, be vigilant for signs that things like this might even possibly be coming. The fewer surprises, the better.

5-2 What about platelets?

Balloon pumps eat platelets – these patients often show falling platelet counts. I haven't actually seen anyone need platelet transfusion, but you definitely see drops in the counts. Anybody know why this is?

Balloon Tech Gary: "the platelet count drops because the balloon physically injures them as it operates."

Travelling Dawn points out: "make sure that this heparinized patient doesn't have HIT!" Excellent point. The patient might need argatroban instead of heparin.

5-3 Why do we use two sets of monitoring wires?

The balloon console needs a trigger of some kind – it can be from the patient's ecg, or their arterial line. If the console is set, as usually, on ekg trigger, and the patient loses a wire, it can't see the EKG, and it won't run – in a patient who is balloon dependent, this can be very bad unless you have a backup system in place – which we always do. One set of skin electrode wires goes as usual to the bedside monitor, and a cable goes from there to the balloon console, which triggers off the R-waves it sees. The second set of wires goes from the patient's skin using another set of 3 electrodes in a lead II pattern straight to the console without going through the bedside monitor – these are called the "skin wires" – and you'll see the choice shown on the console: "monitor" and "skin". If you lose one, switch right away to the other.

5-4 What do I do if the patient rips off all the wires?

A neat thing about the Transact console is that if you lose all your wires altogether, you can still trigger and time off the patient's arterial waveform – there's a button to select it. Patients on balloon pumps are famous for becoming confused – as I'm sure I would be if someone stuck a harpoon in my groin and didn't let me out of bed for a couple of weeks! Again, this definitely comes under the heading of "things to anticipate" – try to have a plan ready with the team if the patient should even start becoming disoriented. Remember that if this patient sits up straight, the IABP can migrate inwards, upwards, and literally poke up through the aortic arch. ("Bad thing".)

5-5 What if the patient codes?

There used to be an mode called "internal 80" built into most of the consoles that you were supposed to activate in case of a code – this was supposed to inflate and deflate the balloon "blindly" at a rate of 80 bpm, and possibly generate some blood pressure. More recent material I've found on the web suggests switching to "pressure triggering" – which makes sense, since the balloon would inflate and deflate in sync with compressions. We need to follow up with the balloon techs on this question.

5-6 What if I have to shock the patient?

The documentation says that the Transact console is safely grounded to allow the patient to be shocked.

5-7 What if I find the patient standing at the bedside?

Actually, there was a famous story about a patient, years ago, who apparently managed to get out of bed and tried to take off down the hall with the IABP still in place. I don't know if the story is true, but if it was true I don't think he would've gotten too far. This would actually be an awful scenario, since even sitting up too far in the bed can make the stiff balloon catheter migrate inwards to the point where it can poke a hole in the aortic arch. The nurse that let this happen would probably have to claim to have been temporarily comatose. The point of course is to stay very alert to the fact that ballooned patients get very confused, very frequently, sometimes to the point of requiring intubation so that they can be kept safely sedated until the balloon can come out. Other people do just fine on the balloon. Be vigilant.

5-8 With the balloon still in?

Don't let this happen! If it did happen: you would try to physically secure the patient. Get lots of help, alert every physician concerned, call in the interventional doctors, get stat films to check the position of the balloon tip, assess the patient continuously for signs that the aorta might be perforated: chest pain, hematocrit drops, widening mediastinum on chest x-ray, awful hemodynamic instability… Follow up closely – would the patient need to return immediately to the cath lab to have the IABP inspected, removed, or changed under fluoro?, follow hematocrits, blood gases, PT/PTT, chemistries – the lot.

5-9 Holding his balloon in his hand?

Don't let this one happen either, although this might actually be preferable to number 5-8. Maybe not. The point is that the IABP is about as invasive a device as there is, and it is **your responsibility to keep the patient safe** – you need to stay way ahead of events, and be ready to head off surprises. Work with the team, and with your peers, and have a plan ready if the patient should become agitated – don't wait until it happens!

5-10 What if they're bleeding at the insertion site?

Remember that IABP patients have to be anticoagulated, because the balloon itself is very thrombogenic – that is, clots will form on it, and get shot downstream to unpleasant places causing the death of, say, a kidney, or a foot. So since the insertion site connects to the anticoagulated femoral artery, some small leakage is common, and easily dealt with by changing dressings. More than minor bleeding obviously should be seen by the docs – is the patient bleeding into the tissue around the site? Has the back of the artery been poked during insertion – could there be retroperitoneal bleeding there? Sometimes there'll be bleeding at the little suture sites more than where the catheter goes in – holding pressure usually works, and then some gelfoam.

5-11 Should they be transfused?

Transfusion goes in and out of fashion, but in general it seems that keeping a hematocrit greater than 30 is the rule in cardiac patients, to keep up oxygen delivery to myocardium that's at risk.

5-12 What if the balloon gets pulled out just a little bit (or a lot) ?

Not good. The tip of the balloon is supposed to sit in the aorta just below the left subclavian artery. If the balloon gets pulled downwards, it could obstruct flow from the main aortic lumen into the renal arteries. Any time a ballooned patient suddenly loses urine output volume, along with everything else you want to check and see if the balloon itself has come loose or taken a yank downwards. Nowadays the balloon is stitched to the skin – along with that it's a good idea to magic-mark the skin next to the stitches, or flag the balloon with a bit of red tape at the stitch site – anything to make it clear that the balloon has changed position.

5-13 What if the balloon gets pushed in just a little bit (or a lot) ?

Also not good. Obviously, and as can't be mentioned too often, the balloon can poke upwards through the aortic arch.

5-14 What is balloon rupture, and how can I tell if it happens?

Balloons break sometimes – I've never seen it myself. Sometimes patients have severely calcified aortas, and the roughened surfaces rub against the balloon with every inflation until finally a hole gets worn into it. The clues are loss of inflation volume – normally set at 40cc, sometimes 30cc, or blood in the balloon line.

5-15 What do I do for a balloon rupture?

Shut the console down – you do NOT want to be pumping helium into the patient's arterial circulation. This balloon needs to come out promptly – notify the appropriate people immediately. At this point of course, if the patient is balloon dependent, you may have real trouble. Think about what to do to support them in the period of time until the balloon can be replaced - the "chemical balloon" might be something to think about. Remember how it works?

5-16 Why can't the patient sit up?

Because the stiff IABP line will migrate inwards, and upwards.

5-17 Can the head of the bed be raised at all?

Usually to about 25-30 degrees, no more.

5-18 Why can't they bend the leg that has the balloon?

The balloon will migrate inwards if the leg flexes too sharply, and the balloon won't work properly if it bent or kinked, which usually happens just inside the insertion site. Keep a soft restraint on the affected ankle to help the patient remember not to flex the leg.

5-19 What about the left radial pulse?

If the balloon moves upwards, the patient may lose perfusion to the left arm, because the left subclavian artery will be occluded. **This means that the tip of the balloon is moving towards the**

aortic arch! Check this once in a while, even if you're sure nothing is wrong with the balloon's position.

5-20 What about obstructing the renal arteries?

Same problem but in the opposite direction – if the balloon is too low, the renal arteries can be occluded – urine output will fall dramatically, and the patient will be at risk for kidney injury.

5-21 What should the x-ray of the balloon tip show?

"The balloon is threaded over the guide wire into the descending aorta just below the left subclavian artery."

5-22 What about the distal pulses?

Definitely a critical point to watch. Any time that an artery is "hardware-ized", you want to be very careful that there's still good perfusion downstream from that artery – the easiest check for this is the pulse. You also want to monitor all those good perfusion things: temperature of the affected leg/foot compared to the other, CSM, etc.

5-23 Should I document the pulses in both legs/ feet?

Yes. Check both the DP's and the PT's. Mark them with magic marker. The policy when I learned it was to check the distal pulses hourly.

5-24 How should I document the pulses?

What I do is to make two columns on the flow sheet using the "stat meds/treatments" column – left and right, each marked DP/PT. Under that I note "palp", or "dop", or (hopefully rarely) "absent". On the sides of the columns I write "warm" or "cool". Be sure to notify the team of any significant change.

5-25 What if the leg/foot goes cold?

Bad thing. Let the team know right away. Document the change carefully. This is obviously not something to sit on until the morning! (The preceptor is a night nurse.) The balloon may have to come out, sooner rather than later.

5-26 What if I can't even doppler the pulses any more?

Big bad thing. Same procedures as above. Sometimes vascular surgery is paged to come and assess the limb. Balloon probably should come out in a short period of time– I've seen times when another one was immediately put in on the other side.

5-27 What is an embolectomy?

Surgical removal of a clot plugging an artery. Did your patient throw a clot from the balloon? Is your patient properly anticoagulated? Very very important. Follow your labs without fail.

5-28 What is a PVR machine? Do we have one? Where do I get one? How do I use it?

PVR stands for pulse volume recorder – this is basically a blood pressure cuff that prints a visual graph of the pulse in a limb. Any time that you can't easily palpate or doppler all four pulses distally, or any time there's a change in pulses or the temperature/perfusion of a leg or foot, you need to get the machine from the CCU – I believe the vascular floors have one, the SICU may have one too. The folks a the desk can get it for you, and the other units are used to us asking for it. You need to get someone to show you how to work it – it's not difficult, but it can be tricky.

Basically what you're doing is putting a blood pressure cuff around the affected limb, usually at mid-thigh or calf, and inflating to about 80mm. Leaving the cuff inflated, you turn on the recorder, which looks like one of the old single-channel EKG printers, and the machine records upward blips on the paper. The blips should match the heart rate, and the higher they blip on the paper, the better the perfusion. If the signal is weak, you can increase the "gain" to make the machine more sensitive, but then you'll have to use the pen control to chase the printer line up and down on the paper - get someone to help you out with this the first couple of times.

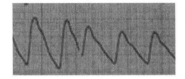 Nice pulsatile flow.

Print a strip for each leg to document the difference – the vascular people will be very interested in these, and will probably want to do a set for themselves. I tape the strips to the back of the flow sheet.

Bear in mind that a change in pulses may be the early signal of something threatening the foot, or the leg. Any significant change, say from palpable pulse to dopplerable pulse should start you thinking, and communicating with the team. Some people think that all IABP patients should have baseline and followup PVRs – I think that a patient with a warm extremity and with stable pulses probably doesn't need them, since they only tell you what you already know. It's the pulses that you can't feel that should worry you. Any time you think you need a PVR, get one.

5-29 What about retroperitoneal bleeding?

Any time the femoral artery gets stuck there's a risk of bleeding internally, towards the back as the patient is lying in the bed – especially when they're anticoagulated.

5-30 How can I tell if my patient is having a retroperitoneal bleed?

Watch for crit drops, watch for bleeding or ecchymosis at the site, or elsewhere, check the patient's back and flanks for hematomas that can signal a retroperitoneal bleed. (That's Somebody's Sign – I don't know who…) In other situations the patient could have an abdominal CT scan - but travelling with a balloon, while possible, is a hairy proposition, and only done once in a while. Sometimes this kind of bleeding means that the patient will need a vascular repair at the site, along with having the balloon removed.

Here are some numbers from a study we found on the subject of IABP complications. Of 580 patients, here are some of the things that went wrong:

- Vascular complications (ischemia, mostly) happened in about 12% of the patients (72).
- Of these, 21 got better by having the balloon removed.
- Another 21 had to have an embolectomy.
- 13 had to have vascular repair.
- 2 had a fasciotomy (that doesn't sound so good – compartment syndrome in the leg? Yow.)
- 4 required amputation (I've never seen either this or fasciotomy happen).
- There were three aortic perforations. **All were fatal. Do not let these patients sit up!**

5-31 What if the patient becomes confused, or agitated?

Watch carefully for any change in alertness or orientation. Patients on balloon pumps very often get **very** confused, probably as the natural result of being restrained, kept flat, and not allowed to move around much for a long period of time. The goal is to keep the patient safe. Provide appropriate reassurance and re-orientation, but sedation may be necessary – try to have a plan in place ahead of time. I find it's always best to bring the team into the room and have them observe the patient themselves, rather than trying to describe their mental state. Haldol is often useful – it depresses respiration the least, but can have bad cardiac effects by lengthening the QT interval and producing arrhythmias. Don't be afraid to pester the team if you think the patient isn't safe. Restraints may have to be used – remember to document why, how, how much, how long, and when you got them ordered.

I've think myself that the confusion often comes from lack of sleep and being uncomfortable all the time, day after day. These patients often get very sore in the back – sometimes an order for a Percocet every 4 hours can get them enough comfort and sleep to keep them oriented. Sometimes not.

5-32 What if the nurse becomes confused or agitated?

Very common! (But can you tell if you're confused, when you're confused?) Seriously, sometimes life in the ICU can really get a newer nurse's head in a whirl, or even an experienced nurse's head in a whirl. The point is, don't let yourself get lost or isolated enough in your assignment that you feel like you're having to deal with frustrations alone. Likewise, don't get caught up in the feeling that you "have to prove to yourself" – or anyone else – that you really can do this job, that you really are up to the task of taking care of this or that person who's probably the sickest person in the state right now, all by yourself. **ICU care is by its' nature a team effort**. This is not philosophy – it's reality. A doctor couldn't do what you do – and you couldn't place an IABP or a pacemaker. You can't change ventilator modes, and respiratory can't shoot cardiac outputs. If you are feeling stressed, or isolated, or frustrated – extremely common and natural feelings for staff in the ICU at every level – reach out and get help. **This is not optional**. It is a critical part of your ability to work in the unit. Swallow your pride, make humility your goal, and team up.

5-33 What is "hardware sepsis"?

This is what happens when bad germs get into your patient along the routes created by the devices stuck into him: the balloon pump, PA line, or whatever. It's the same as any other septic picture: the patient gets hot, tachy, dilated, hypotensive, and it's treated like any other septic situation: fill the tank, squeeze the tank, kill the bugs. It's also a good idea to try to remove the piece of equipment that's causing the problem: swan, IABP – sometimes it can be hard to tell where the problem is coming from, so you'll see the team go in and pull every line the patient has, and replace them.

Just make sure that you have pressor access if you need it, which may mean that a new central line will have to go in before the old ones come out. It can be helpful to remind the team that a femoral line can be placed and used quickly, without an x-ray – even though they're considered the "dirtiest" of the central lines, they can save a situation from going from "mildly stressful" to "call a code". **Ensuring that the patient has the right kind of IV access is your job.**

5-34 What are prophylactic antibiotics?

Nowadays they'll start ballooned patients on Ancef as soon as they come back from the cath lab. Come to think of it, I don't think I've seen IABP hardware sepsis in a while.

5-35 Why do the ballooned patients have to be anticoagulated?

The balloon itself is very thrombogenic – clots like to form on it – and remember, clots in the arterial circulation float downstream and can plug any vessel that they wind up in – whatever tissue is beyond the plug, infarcts. "Bad thing". Keeping patients therapeutic on heparin prevents this pretty well, but not always, so you have to stay alert and monitor the perfusion to the leg downstream from the balloon.

5-36 What about heparin, or reopro (abciximab), or integrilin (eptifibitide)?

Heparin is the traditional drug that we use to anticoagulate cardiac patients with – we have a lot of experience with it, and we know how to use it pretty well. But it turns out that it's the formation of clots out of platelets that causes the trouble inside the coronary arteries. A new group of drugs, like reopro and integrilin has been developed that specifically works on platelet-clumping, and apparently they work very well. Sometimes you'll see patients run on both for a while.

5-37 What are the new platelet drugs all about?

Stopping the platelets from clumping up and forming clots apparently is incredibly helpful in preventing thrombosis, which you really don't want to happen in your brand new stents! Apparently the new drugs are so helpful in this regard that they stopped the studies and released the data early.

5-38 What is Plavix?

Plavix is a platelet-aggregation inhibitor that comes in pill form.

5-39- What are stents?

Stents look like the little springs that come inside ballpoint pens.

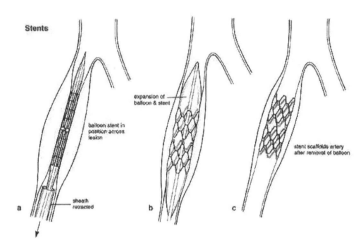

Little metal mesh tubes that are put into place in the cath lab – they are placed inside the coronary artery, and then clicked open, so that they hold the lumen of the artery open wide just where the tight spots are. Easier than bypass surgery. I don't know how long they last, but I do know that patients with them need to take something like Plavix, because platelets love to stick to things like stents – anything irregular – and they'd clot off as a result.

http://www.surgery.usc.edu/divisions/vas/graphics/stents.jpg

Obviously there's been a lot of progress in the stent world since this article was written. Wow – six years ago already? Nowadays stents are coated with some kind of drug-releasing material that inhibits clot formation – pretty smart! Jayne says that the patients still take Plavix for a while after the stents go in – not sure for how long.

Update – the stent wars go on. As so often, the studies point in different directions. What does seem clear though is that patients probably need to stay on Plavix or something like it for good, after the stents go in.

6-   Which balloon console do we use?

We use the Bard company's Transact IABP console. The console drives and controls the balloon: it holds the helium tank, which nowadays is a little gold thing the size of your fist. It has a pretty good computerized brain that helps you with timing – in fact it will try to time the balloon all by itself, and sometimes can do a good job. The control panel is divided into fairly obvious groups:

Power (AC or battery – the balloon will work for a time on battery – a couple of hours? – but we only do this when we're transporting to and from the cath lab or the OR, and the balloon techs usually handle this.)

Choice of either skin wires, monitor signal, or arterial wave for trigger signal. The two wire systems back each other up – the console needs some way to see what they patient's rhythm is. The neat thing about the Transact is that if the patient loses all her wires, you can time the machine off of the arterial line waveform – you always have one of these because there's one built into the balloon itself.

Choice of triggers: R-wave, peaks, pacer – there's lots of choices. Consult with the balloon techs about this – about 90% of the time we run on R-wave trigger.

Controls to stop and start the balloon: off, standby, purge, run, automatic. Bear in mind that the balloon will run in non-automatic mode, but the gas alarms will be off – meaning that if the line kinks, or leaks, or for any reason the balloon loses volume or gas you won't know it. Be careful.

Weaning controls: to set the ratio of ballooned beats to the patient's own beats: 1 to 1, 2 to 1, 4 or 8 to 1. Remember that timing is always checked with the balloon set to a ratio of 2 to 1. You'll see the balloon techs time the console at 1 to 1 – I don't know how they do this, but hey, it's much more their thing than mine – I don't argue with the pros.

Monitor screen – this can be set to see the patient's arterial waveform or the waveform that sees the balloon itself inflating and deflating. You have to know what both are supposed to look like. More on these later on. You can set the monitor to either waveform, change the scale, freeze the screen, all those things. There's a printer as well – I print a strip of the patient's arterial waveform with the ratio set at 2 to 1, to show how well the balloon is working, and stick it on the back of the flow sheet. It can be hard to see the waves clearly on the console monitor, so for timing what I do sometimes is set the scale on the bedside monitor so that the art-line waveform is really enormous and clear, and then do my timing.

6-1- What is the purpose of the "balloon pressure waveform"?

Remember that all these waveforms are coming from transducers, which are hooked up to lines, that are connected to and "looking at" something – either a vessel or cardiac chamber in the patient, or in this case the balloon that's going into the patient. This is the waveform coming from a transducer built into the console – it looks at how the balloon is working as it inflates and deflates, and the wave is supposed to look a certain way. Changes in the waveform can tell you different things.

Lately, our main problem has been that we don't get enough balloons in our unit, and lots of people go to the class and then don't see one for 4 months. Stressful. Hopefully soon we may be able to get a simulator that will stay on the unit, hooked up to a console, and we'll play with it to the point where everyone will be more comfortable.

6-2- How often should I check it?

Certainly switch back and forth from both waveforms on the console at the beginning of the shift and every hour or so after that.

6-3- Can I assume that the balloon pressure waveform is okay if my arterial-line timing waveforms are okay too?

My experience is that if the patients' arterial waveforms are clear and correct, that means that the balloon is working the way it ought to be, and that the balloon waveform will be okay as well.

6-4- When do I have to worry?

I always worry.

6-5- What should I do if something seems wrong with the balloon pressure waveform?

Check this over at the beginning of the shift with the nurse you're following – get some idea of what things look like at the start of your shift. Likewise, check with the balloon techs when they bring the patient to you. There are times when the balloon just won't run right – maybe it's kinked inside the patient, or the balloon can't be inflated to it's full volume for some reason. The balloon may need to be purged, because it may have lost some helium – not into the patient, but through the machine line somewhere. If you notice a change during the shift that looks significant in any way, you can call the balloon techs to look. Check the reference card for hints – is the line kinked outside the patient, is there a gas leak along the line somewhere? I've had to run the length of the pump tubing through an emesis basin of water looking for a leak sometimes. Don't hesitate to call for help.

6-6- How is the entire setup connected to the patient and the bedside monitor?

There's a cable that jacks out of our monitor that plugs into the balloon console – that's how the balloon sees the patient's rhythm one way. Then there are the skin wires – second way. Then a transducer is hooked up to an arterial line that runs along the whole length of the balloon inside the patient, opening at the tip-end. (This is the 'root line') – that's one arterial wave. Hopefully, but not always, there's a radial art-line – second arterial wave. Sometimes there's an arterial arm to the sheaths that stay in the patient after cath lab procedures – that needs to be hooked up too- that's three arterial waves. Lot of waves! Important: any pressurized line that goes into a patient needs to be connected to the monitor, if only so you'll know if it comes disconnected. Once you have a chance to work with the machine a couple of times, the setup will make more sense – expect to be confused at first.

6-7- What is the "root line"?

The root line is the arterial line built into the balloon. It runs along the length of the device, opens up at the end, and reads the pressure in the aorta where the balloon tip is.

6-8- Why does the root line transducer need to be air-filtered?

We go to a lot of trouble to make sure that air doesn't get into the patient's arterial circulation. (Venous too.) If a pressurized transducer bag began for some dumb reason to pump air into a patient's aorta, the result would be an air embolus – just as bad as any other embolus, like a clot, travelling along in the artery, eventually causing an infarct somewhere.

6-9- Why do we mark the root line "No Fast Flush"?

Again, to prevent air in the line from going into the patient. If for any reason you need to aspirate or flush the root line, you don't want to hit the flusher and push several inches of air that might happen to be in the tubing along into the patient. The idea is that you're supposed to do all these moves manually, using a ten cc syringe, watching for air the whole time.

6-10- Why can't I draw bloods from the root line?

What if it became clotted? And you had no radial line? Could you time the balloon without an arterial wave? Not properly, anyhow.

6-11- Can I ever?

You really should not. If you're in an extreme situation, you do what you have to, but it's not a good idea. Insist on a radial line if you think the patient needs one.

6-12- There seem to be eight arterial blood pressure waves coming from this patient. Which one do I believe?

People argue about this one. I usually believe the highest pressure I see. Remember though that the highest pressure that the monitor reports is usually not the patient's systolic pressure – it's the augmented diastolic pressure, which is often higher than the patient's when the balloon is working right. MAPs are usually a better guide.

6-13- Why do I need to transduce all of them?

If a pressurized arterial line were to come disconnected, the alarms would let you know. Remember to set and check alarm limits for everything.

6-14- How do I check the helium level? How do I change the helium tank?

There's a gauge on the side of the console – the helium tank for the transact console is supposed to last a very long time – months? I've never had to change one, but there's always a spare in the equipment bags that some with the machine, and I'll make sure that we have some manuals available.

6-15- What is purging? Should I purge the balloon?

The balloon and the long clear tubing that connects it to the console are only supposed to contain helium, which is lots lighter than air, and therefore lots easier to pump in and out of the balloon. If air were to get into the line or the balloon, it wouldn't work properly – purging empties the balloon and refills it from the helium tank. I learned that usually the only time you need to purge the balloon is if you drain water from the line – sometimes water condenses in the clear balloon line and needs to be drained out. In that case air would get into the system, and it would need to be purged. Once in a while an unclear root line tracing will clear up with a purge.

6-16- What do I do if the console quits?

I've never seen it happen, but it's always good to have a plan. The CCU, and possibly the cardiothoracic ICU are supposed to have an extra console on hand – send for it right away.

Meantime, here's what one online hospital reference suggested:

- Get another console immediately. (Uh, I think we knew that one.)

- Manually inflate and deflate the balloon if the console is going to be down for more than 15 minutes. Use a big catheter-tip syringe (we call these "GU guns" for some reason), and use about 10cc less than the balloon's volume, inflating about 10 times a minute. The idea is to prevent the formation of clots on the balloon – don't worry about trying to time it to the patient. (That would be a neat trick! "Hey guys, watch this!")

- Don't **ever** put air into the root line. (Jeepers, why would you?)

- Tell the cardiology people what's going on right away.

6-17 Why can't I run the console with the gas alarms off?

You can, but it's not a good idea because it's not really safe. The gas alarms are what tell you if something has changed about the inflation or deflation of the balloon – if the line is kinked, you won't know, if the line leaks, you won't know, and so on. There are times when you do have to run with the gas alarms off – recently I took care of a man whose balloon was kinked just inside the insertion site – the decision had been made to leave it in place, so we ran it with lots of advice from the balloon techs, who agreed that it might only run that way if the gas alarms were left off.

6-18 How do I reset the console if it alarms?

It depends on why it alarmed. If the patient rolled over and the line is kinked, then resetting the machine won't work. The console actually is pretty good at telling you what's wrong – read the messages at the top of the screen. Make sure the line is clear, then hit standby, then auto – that will restart at 1 to 1, with gas alarms on.

6-19 What do I do if the console says "gas leak"?

Make sure the clear balloon line is tightly connected at both ends to the patient and the console, then restart the console. If you get the message again, you might have to run the length of the tubing through a pan of water to see if there's a pinhole leak. Or you can listen along the length of the line with a stethoscope. Most of the time there's no detectable leak, and the machine does make message mistakes sometimes. Be alert to the possibility of balloon rupture though – inspect the line for blood. If you see any at all, the console must be shut off, and the balloon has to come out.

6-20 Or "no trigger"?

This means that the console can't see the patient – either the skin wires or the monitor wires have come off. Try switching to the other system from whatever it is you're using, and see if the console will work. If neither wire system works, change to the arterial trigger – there's a button for it, and the machine will trigger pretty well off of the root line waveform until you get electrodes and wires re-connected to the patient.

6-21 What if I have to travel with the patient?

The only travelling that you'll do with a ballooned patient is either to or from the cath lab, or rarely to the CT scanner. If the patient goes to the OR, they'll be moved by anesthesia and a balloon tech. Either way, if you have to go anywhere, ALWAYS call in the balloon tech to go with you. The console has a set of inputs on one side for running when the patient is connected to a bedside monitor – on the other side is a set of inputs for travel cables. The equipment bag has an ECG cable for triggering, and an arterial cable for the root line.

6-22 What if there's a lot of water in the balloon line?

If there's a lot of condensate in the line it can make the console unhappy. I was taught that we were supposed to stop the console (standby), disconnect the tubing from the console and drain it downwards towards the floor onto a chux or something, reconnect, purge, and then restart. I've seen very little condensate with the newer console – we should check with the balloon techs about this.

Balloon Tech Gary: the machine purges itself every 3-4 hours, and removes any water in the line when it does.

6-23 Should I ever turn the console off?

The only time that I'd shut the console off would be if I thought that there was a balloon rupture, with blood in the balloon line. To stop the console temporarily, push the standby button. Sometimes house officers will ask you to do this so they can assess heart sounds, or bowel sounds. This is okay very briefly, but remember that a balloon-dependent patient may not handle this well.

6-24 When should I call the balloon tech for help?

Any time you think you need it. Most problems can be solved by a little group thinking among the nurses in the unit, and a call to the nurses in the CCU might be useful, but if you think you have a problem you can't fix – that's why the techs are there.

6-25 How do I page the balloon tech?

During the day they carry in-house pagers that you can call through the regular page operators. At night they have a different paging number – if the page operator doesn't have it, the CCU or the SICU will. Sometimes the techs do stay in-house overnight if there are a lot of consoles running, or if there are unstable patients in the units.

6-26 How do I know if the helium is getting low? How do I change the helium tank?

There's a pressure gauge on the right side of the console that shows the current pressure in the tank – if it gets too low, a message will flash on the screen that the tank will need changing soon. Changing the tank turns out to be pretty easy – according to the balloon tech who talked us through it on the phone one night:

- a- leave the console running
- b- find the big black lever on the right side of the console, and pull it outwards, away from the machine until it stops
- c- grasp the helium tank (a rubber glove will help, because it's a little hard to grab), and unscrew it
- d- screw in the new tank firmly
- e- push the black lever back down, which spikes the new tank
- f- the gauge should show a nice high pressure.

7- What about documentation?

Do it carefully.

7-1 Which pressures do we document?

In the space on the flow sheet where we put the blood pressure, we still write the systolic and diastolic numbers from the monitor, but you have to remember that the higher number will be the highest pressure peak that the transducer sees – which is usually the augmented diastolic when we're ballooning.

7-2 How do I document pulses?

I make two columns marked left and right, and mark "palp", or "dop", or "absent" for each DP and PT. On each side I write "cool" or "warm", underlined if there's been a change.

7-3 Should I paste in the PVR strips?

Definitely. I sometimes take one of the sticky sheets that we use for blood product slips and stick them on that – that stays with the flow sheet so that people can find them quickly.

7-4 What about the weaning ratio?

We use a split column to mark the ratio every hour, and to document that we've observed the waveform: ratio on top, like 1:1, and a check mark below.

7-5 What goes on the flow sheet, and what goes in my note?

I try to cover the basics in my note and leave the details to the sheet. For example, I might say:

CV: Pt. in stable sinus rhythm, no ectopy, Lido at 1, NTG at 200, heparin titrated to scale with am result 68.8. No c/o SSCP or SOB. IABP fx well at 1:1, site dressing changed x1 for sm amt sang drainage, site clean. See timing strips on flow sheet for details. Distal pulses: L (IABP) DP and PT doppelerable only, foot cool but CMS intact; R DP and PT palpable, foot warm. PVRs taped to flow sheet, showing good waveforms for both legs. UO qs, > 50cc/ hour over night. Hematocrit am 32 (unchanged 32.4).

Resp: Pt. on 4liters nasal cannula O2, ABG 4am: 126 - 41 - 7.42, RR 20's, BBS grossly clear, afebrile, denies SOB

GI: tolerating diet with no difficulty, BM x1 soft formed guiac neg, am glucose 112

Stuff like that.

Now – documentation people? You'll notice, right off, that I don't use nursing diagnoses. Alteration in reality? Potential versus actual? As evidenced by the doodah doodah day of the eelang badoodang baday? Are you serious?

I consider this a crucial point, actually, although it makes me a subversive in my own profession – or would, if I hadn't been doing it so long. I know that my attitude gives the people at the Joint Commission the conniptions, but the point is that what's wrong with your patient is NOT an "Alteration in Cardiac Output" . Actually, of course, it IS an alteration, but that stuff is all so much window dressing – what's **really** wrong with your patient? He's having a ruddy huge MI, is what! The more time you spend worrying about your nursing diagnoses – in fact, in Ancient Nurse Markie's opinion, ANY time you spend doing that is **time taken away from thinking about your patient.** Instead of that junk, watch her electrolytes! Jeepers…

Or put it this way: if one of the Joint Commissioners came into your ICU with a ruddy huge MI, what do you think they'd want you to be worrying about?

8-   What is balloon weaning?

The balloon does have to come out of the patient at some point. Weaning is the process of changing the ratio so that the balloon supports at first every other beat (1:2), and then every fourth, or eighth beat, and observing how well the patient tolerates the wean.

8-1 Is there a weaning protocol?

Yes. What you're trying to do is to see if the patient gets into trouble if you try to wean the balloon. So the first thing is to get a baseline EKG with the balloon at 1 to 1, along with a set of numbers: CVP, PCW, output, index, SVR, SV, all that good stuff. Then you set the IABP at 2 to 1, and try to go for two hours, at the end of which you do another EKG, and shoot the numbers again, looking for ischemic changes on the EKG, and anything that might indicate that the patient isn't tolerating the wean, like a rising wedge pressure, dropping output, rising SVR. Chest pain… If nothing bad occurs, you try two hours at 1 to 4, again followed by EKG and numbers, and finally 1 to 8 with EKG, etc., followed by a return to 1 to 1 when the weaning is done.

8-2 When should we start weaning the balloon? What is "stunned myocardium"?

It depends on why the balloon went in. Remember that there are two main reasons for an IABP – to help keep tight lesions open in the coronary arteries (inflation), or to help a failing LV in cardiogenic shock (deflation). The first reason includes ballooning a patient for just a day or two after stent placement, after which hopefully they'd tolerate a rapid wean and removal. In that situation, anticoagulation is really of critical importance – do you want to be the one that let the patient clot off her brand new stents?

The second situation is more difficult, but hopefully somewhat predictable. The idea is that a heart that's been hit by cardiogenic shock will need a certain amount of time to recover. What is there **to** recover? It turns out that around the area of infarct (you don't have acute cardiogenic shock without a big infarct) is an area that is still alive, still ready to pump, but dazed, or as they say "stunned". This area of "stunned myocardium" will eventually come back to work, but not for a given period of time, usually about a week. So the person who may have an EF of 12% right after an enormous MI may have a **much** better EF a week later, after the stunned areas come back and start to work. The goal of ballooning this patient is to get them through that period of time, with the balloon functioning as an LVAD – a left-ventricular assist-device.

So – the answer to the question? In the second case? About a week.

8-3 How do I know if the patient is tolerating the balloon wean?

The patient will remain stable according to all the things you're following: EKGs, cardiac output, central pressures will all stay stable.

8-4 How do I know if they're not?

They become symptomatic. Chest pain, ischemia on EKG, blood pressure drops, wedge pressure rises, oxygenation gets worse. (Think about sending blood gases if you think the patient's condition may be changing.)

8-5 Should I stop weaning if the patient is having trouble?

Absolutely stop the wean. Go to the house officers and show them your numbers, your EKGs, and your blood gases. The game plan may have to be changed. In the case of cardiogenic shock, you may have to briefly try a wean for several days in a row until the stunned part of the heart starts working again.

8-6 How long can a balloon stay in?

It's variable. I've heard of patients being ballooned for longer than a month when they're waiting for transplant. Ten days is the usual rough limit.

8-7 Who pulls the balloon?

The interventional fellow comes to the unit, or, in some cases, the techs can pull the balloon.

8-8 When should I turn off the heparin before a balloon gets pulled?

The medical team should speak with the interventional people to determine this, or sometimes the fellow will call you in the unit to plan things. You should try to get a specific time, and be very clear. One source said that heparin can be stopped four hours before the balloon comes out, with the console running at 1:1 to prevent clot formation.

8-9 What should I worry about after the balloon gets pulled?

Your concern is the site and the perfusion to the leg. Provide site care as it's ordered – cardiology still likes sandbags, although it seems that angiography doesn't. Check the site for drainage, ecchymosis, swelling, anything that might mean that there was bleeding into the tissue around the site. Check the pulses in the affected leg, and compare with previously – is the leg and foot warmer now? Are the pulses stronger? Document properly. Keep the patient flat for the ordered amount of time. Get clear orders about when, or if, the patient is to be re-anticoagulated, or started on oral anticoagulation, or not anticoagulated at all. When's the Plavix due?

<u>Some sources:</u>

www.rxlist.com (a very useful site for finding pharmaceutical info)

http://critcare.lhsc.on.ca – the website of the London (Ontario) Health Sciences Centre, Critical Care Division

www.ispub.com/journals/IJTCVS/Vol2N2/iabp.html – The Internet Journal of Thoracic and Cardiovascular Surgery

www.cardio-info.com/_disc6/0000007e.htm the Johns Hopkins protocol cited in the CV Talk Educators and Professionals Discussion Group

www.datascope.com/ca/abstract_1.html "Vascular Complications from Intraaortic Balloons: Risk Analysis

www.datascope.com/ca/pdf/preinservice_self_study_guide.pdf "Pre-Inservice Self-Study Guide To Intra-Aortic Balloon Counterpulsation.

ICP Monitoring

1- What is intra-cranial pressure monitoring?
2- What is the ICP?
3- What is the "Modified Monro-Kellie Doctrine"?
4- Why does ICP rise or fall?
5- What is the normal range for ICP?
6- Why is elevated ICP so bad?
7- What does a patient look like when she has a rising ICP?
   - A story that illustrates the point.
8- What is the CPP?
9- What is the CCCP?
10- How is ICP measured?
11- What is a "bolt"?
   - ventriculostomy
   - subarachnoid screw
   - fiberoptic monitors
   - epidural sensors
   - noninvasive ICP monitoring
12- How long can a bolt stay in?
13- How do I take care of a bolt?
   - ventriculostomies
       i. levelling
       ii. the foramen of Monro
       iii. drainage
   - subarachnoid bolts
   - the fiberoptic cable
14- What is a bolt waveform supposed to look like?
15- What is it not supposed to look like?
16- What if the waveform is dampened, or goes away?
17- How is a high ICP treated?
   - Drainage
   - Positioning and treatments: do's and don'ts
   - Hyperventilation, or not
   - Mannitol – "drying out the brain"
   - **A Very Important Point!**
   - Steroids
   - Anticonvulsants
   - Barbiturate "coma"
   - Other sedatives
   - Cooling
   - Oxygenation
   - Hypertensive therapy

This one is definitely a little different. This time the preceptor really has only the most basic idea of what is going on, since we see these things only once or twice in a year. So this time the project involved going out into the field, looking around, writing stuff down, and coming back to tell the rest of the tribe what I saw. So - please correct things in this file that are not the way they should be. This is serious stuff, as always, and we need to get it right every time. Do not use this article as a primary reference or substitute for in-house training on this subject! If one of these devices should show up, <u>call the neuro ICU RNs</u>; they are always happy to come down, inspect the setup, and give advice.

References: We're getting better at this – wherever possible we're including website sources as embedded hyperlinks in the text. If you're reading this text on a machine that's hooked up to the web, clicking the blue link should take you to the site that we got the material from.

1- What is intra-cranial pressure monitoring?

A little more than a third of all victims of traumatic brain injury develop enough cerebral swelling to threaten their lives – if it can be adequately treated, then they may recover their function. It's all about the pressure in the head. Normal is good, high is bad. For a number of reasons, the brain can swell up – treat it right away, and maybe the patient can be saved from death, or maybe worse, from a life of severe disability.

2- What is the ICP?

The ICP is the number that represents the pressure inside the head, which is the reflection of the total of not too many components and facts:

- Cranial size is fixed. Sounds right.

- The volume of blood in the head. (I definitely don't get enough. Or maybe it's too much. Maybe both.)

- The volume of csf in the head.

- The constriction or dilation of the vessels in the head. (Hmm. What do migraines do to ICP? What's that migraine stuff they give nowadays – opens up the constricted vessels? - could that be used for ICP? Quick look at the web – um, Imitrex, yeah, sumatriptan, uh-huh, works by producing vasoconstriction? Oh. Forget that, then.)

- Anything else that's taking up space inside the head: edema, tumors, etc. (Or as my mother-in-law would say: "A big hunk of something stupid!")

3- What is the "Modified Monro-Kellie Doctrine"?

Look back up a paragraph: the Monro-Kellie doctrine is the mathematical way of expressing the total of the items in the list. Now look down – here comes an equation. No panic, okay? - an easy one – just addition. Remember this important thing, which we might call Rule # 3 of the ICU: "A lot of this stuff really is easier than it looks."

(For those of you with elevated ICP, here are rules 1 and 2:

- **"There are no stupid questions in the ICU."**
- "Refer to question number one.")

Okay: the Monro-Kellie doctrine, "modified". (What was it before it was "modified"? "Monro-Kellie and P.Diddy vs. Godzilla and Mothra"?):

"v.intracranial (constant) = v.brain + v.CSF + v.blood + v.mass lesion"

It's just a matter of adding them up - we won't even do the numbers – just trying to get the idea across.

The "v" stands for volume. Each of the separate, smaller volumes adds up to the total volume of what there is inside the head.

So: if one part of the total contents of the brain increases in size, then something else is going to have to shrink, or the pressure inside the head is going to rise.

(Well, no kiddin'! Can I have a Nobel Prize too? I seem to recall that one guy won the prize for being the first to thread a catheter along the veins in his arm, and then running downstairs to get an x-ray of himself, thus inventing central lines, or central Foley catheters, or central something…I hope the money paid for his hospitalization afterwards, 'cause I don't remember reading if he took it out again or not. For a short and maybe a little more accurate story about someone who thought up a Nobel Prize idea - in a Honda - take a look at the FAQ article on "Labs". They didn't <u>give</u> it to him in the Honda…)

Where were we? Actually, and here's another example of the skills of the Great BioMedical Engineer – the brain turns out to have a neat autoregulatory maneuver that it performs, trying to keep its perfusion (the Cerebral Perfusion Pressure) nice and steady. Let's see if I have this right:

- If the systemic blood pressure **rises**, then the cerebral vessels will **tighten** up, to maintain a nice even perfusion pressure.

- If the systemic pressure **falls**, then the vessels will **dilate** to allow better flow, with the same goal in mind. (In mind! Ha!) This is a pretty effective mechanism – apparently it can keep the CPP fairly even, despite really wide swings in the patient's systemic blood pressure. The mechanism can fail however, after a traumatic injury.

4- Why does ICP rise or fall?

Remember Monro and Kellie? The whole point was what? – that there's basically not a whole lot of room in the closed box of the head, and that only one of the separate volumes has to change - just a little - for the pressure inside the box to rise. If something else can shrink – maybe the size of the vessels – that helps.

Some of the main causes of rising ICP:

- Something blocks the normal drainage of csf
- Bleeding inside the head
- Edema (there are a couple of kinds, but both will make the affected tissue swell)
- "Mass effect" – something's in there that shouldn't be, and it's taking up space where there isn't any. If it's big enough it can shove the brain over to one side, producing a "shift".

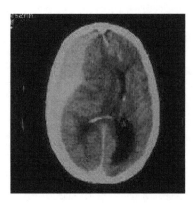

Shifted over to the right...

"Subdural haematoma, significant midline shift, intraventricular haemorrhage."

http://www.trauma.org/imagebank/imagebank.html

Didn't wear his bike helmet, huh?

- Rising pC02 will make the cerebral vessels dilate, taking up more space. (Here comes a question: it seems to me that they order nipride a lot in cases of increasing blood pressure stemming from rising ICP. Nipride dilates blood vessels – should we be using this? Just a question...)

- Valsalva maneuvers, coughing, suctioning, noxious stimuli ("You moron!"), seizure activity, and even putting the patient in the wrong position will cause the ICP to rise. Driving in traffic? Definitely.

Reasons for ICP to drop:

- Anything, basically, that reverses one of the processes just listed: csf not draining? – drain some off! Bleeding inside the head? Take out the clot! Got edema? Do the mannitol thing, and so on. Obviously the treatment is going to vary with the cause.

5- What is the normal range for ICP?

The normal is 0-10 mm Hg. Greater than 20 is bad, and often seems to be the treatment threshold: call the team, open the drain, both, etc. Greater than 40 is usually super bad.

6- Why is elevated ICP so bad?

It's all about perfusion, what they call the **CBF** – cerebral blood flow. If the parenchyma ($1.29 please!) gets squeezed, then the perfusion is going to get worse. Cerebral ischemia. I hate it when that happens!

The worst thing of course is **herniation** –

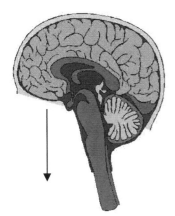

- the brain tries to escape downwards through the foramen magnum, which I think was named by Dr. Tom Selleck. Maybe it was Dr. Eastwood. Herniation pretty much equals death, and the name of the whole game is: try to prevent it.

http://www.fsm.ac.fj/pws/lnbp/img11.jpg

7- What does a patient look like when she has a rising ICP?

The first sign is a **change in mentation**. People learn all about Cushing's triad: dropping heart rate, dropping respiratory rate, widening pulse pressure – that stuff all shows up <u>late</u>; you definitely do not want to wait for that stuff to appear!

A story that illustrates this point: I was working in a medical CCU, this is back in the middle 1980's, long before I was anybody's preceptor, on the night shift, and the word came that I, as the owner of the only open ICU bed in the entire hospital, was going to receive a patient from the OR, status post craniotomy, **20 something years old**, evacuation of a head bleed. Did I have an anxiety attack?! Did I have elevated ICP? Are you kidding?

Patient comes up, extubated, sleepy, but speaking. Holy cow – along with what was ordered, I thought of absolutely every neuro thing I'd ever seen or heard of to document what this kid was doing, and I did it every five minutes, then every ten minutes, then every 20, then every half hour – I did his vital signs, I looked at his pupils, I checked his grasps, I had him "step on the gas" with either foot, I asked him who the President was, what year it was, what size shoes I had on – I had him stick his tongue out (it's supposed to be at the midline), I asked him to grin (supposed to be symmetrical), I did everything I could think of, created a little chart, checked it all off with times and all.

The surgeons did a postop check about two hours along, looked at my little chart – the kid was doing fine. Then word came again from on high: the patient was to be transferred to the floor, so that a crash bed (mine) could be opened. Thanks a lot – I already had my crash for the evening, thanks! Off he went.

So what happens? I get a call from the floor – this is not 20 minutes after he left – had the kid been **unresponsive** when he left the CCU? What!?.... he had re-bled into his head.

Lessons we learn from this:

- **Change in mental status** (for the worse) is the first sign of bad things happening inside the head. (Yours <u>or</u> the patient's!)

- Know what to look for.

- Document everything very carefully.

Other changes that may signal problems are the ones you know about: changes in pupil sizes:

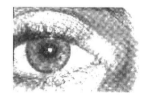 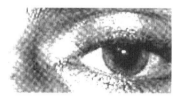 "Anisocoria". (Why can't they just say: "Whoa! Blown pupil!"?)

Stat CT scan!

- Change in the strength of an extremity (or two), recurrent or worsening headache (I <u>definitely</u> get a worsening headache in a situation like this), nausea and/or emesis – **don't** wait for Dr. Cushing to show up! – you should be on a hair trigger in these circumstances.

Another scary symptom that can show up is a truly frightening fever – what they used to call a "cone fever" back in the ancient days, "coning" being the sort of crude term for describing the form the brain would take as it tried to squeeze it's way through into the spinal column. Temps up to 108 degrees F, usually taken to mean that – is it the hypothalamus? – is being squeezed. Ack!

8-   What is the CPP?

Cerebral Perfusion Pressure: this is what you're trying to preserve, and **within the proper range**; the pressure pushing blood through the brain. The brain uses something like 20% of all the available oxygen taken up by the lungs, and can definitely use all that it gets. Like myocardium, right? Like the feet, nose, liver – perfusion is the thing. I wonder if ENT people watch the NPP …nah. Actually, we <u>were</u> dopplering some poor patient's tongue pulses a while back, after one of those head/neck/tongue tumor resection/grafting procedures…

Numerically, **the definition of the CPP** is the patient's MAP, minus her ICP. The patient we had just recently with the subarachnoid fiberoptic device, had a monitor hooked up separately from ours, which calculated the CPP continously. The usual goal is 70 – 80mm Hg; some say 80 – 100mm Hg, with the goal of preserving the CBF.

That nice autoregulatory trick that the brain uses to keep the CPP constant – remember that? Dilating, constricting? It often loses this ability after a traumatic injury – so the brain is at the mercy of changes in BP – and ischemia can result. Try to avoid wide swings in BP for these patients – smooth perfusion at the right pressure is the goal. (Ha – try that when the patient is on two pressors, and propofol, and a vent, and going for CT scans every eight freakin' hours…).

9- What is the CCCP?

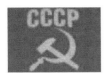

There ain't one any more. Where you been comrade, under a rock?

http://users.tkk.fi/~mtanttar/wap/kuvia/cccp.jpg

10- How is ICP measured?

There are a several devices that are used:

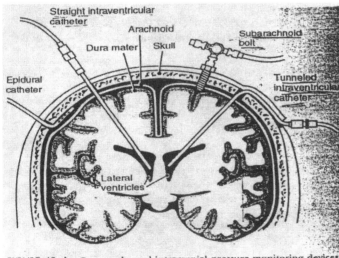

FIGURE 42–1 Commonly used intracranial pressure monitoring devices

Of the ones in the picture, we usually only see (infrequently) the fiberobptic subarachnoid bolt and the intraventricular catheter.

Thanks for this image to Mary B. P.!

11- What is a "bolt"?

In the MICU we call anything that gets put into someone's head a "bolt", but actually there are several kinds of devices that are placed. Let's listen to a short audio on this subject:
(Theme plays from: "The Dating Game" Meets "World-Neuro-Federation Wrestling")
Bob: And heeeere they are! Johnny, tell the guests what's behind each of the curtains! Remember, contestants, you only get to pick one out of all of these choices, so make sure it's the right one!

Johnny: Bob, let's get ready to rummmbbblllle! Behind curtain number one is the device we know the best. Yes contestants, this is the one that's really going to tell you and your neurosurgeon what you want to know – it's the <u>most</u> invasive, the <u>most</u> terrifying, yet the <u>most</u> versatile, the <u>most</u> useful of all the monitoring/drainage devices: the one, the only, the infamous:

- **(a) ventriculostomy draaaiiinnn!** From Neu-Ronco, maker of the famous Pocket Burr-holer! (Wild applause from the neurosurgical residents in the audience, waving sterile drills. Audience chanting: "Drill, drill, drill, drill!")

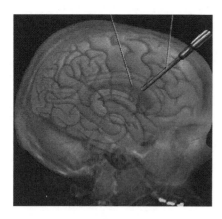

(Johnny continues): "The intraventricular catheter is a soft tube placed through a burr hole into the lateral ventricle (audience: "Burr hole! Burr hole!"), and allows for both monitoring and for therapeutic drainage of CSF to reduce the ICP. It can be inserted in either the OR or in the ICU (groups of nurses from the OR and from the ICU throwing folding chairs at each other, neurosurgeons running down the aisles to drill burrholes for the head injuries), and connects to a standard transducer set, which is never pressurized. ("Pressurize! Pressurize!")

There is a greater risk for infection with this device (boos from the audience, a shout of "culture this!"), since it is the most invasive ("Invasive! Invasive!"). It can also cause bleeding ("O neg! O neg!"), and must be carefully leveled to the Foramen of Monro. ("Leveling is for wimps!" More chair-throwing.)

Fluid drained must be monitored for amount, color, and clarity at hourly intervals, ("Measure this!"), and drainage can be either constant or intermittent. ("Constant!" "Intermittent!" – chairs fly.)

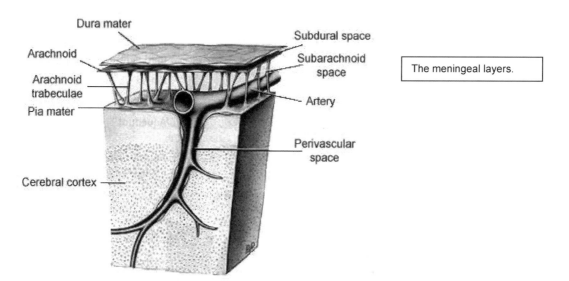

The meningeal layers.

http://www.psychology.psych.ndsu.nodak.edu/mccourt/website/htdocs/HomePage/Psy486/System%20Neuroanatomy/meninges.JPG

Bob: "That is just fabulous, Johnny! Now tell our guests what's behind curtain number two!"

Johnny: "Well Bob, we certainly don't screw around on this show! (laughter from the audience), because we wouldn't want our audience to bolt on us, now would we? (Boos.) Behind curtain number two is the true screw of the bunch, the second choice of champions after the ventriculostomy drain, the one we all want to thread our way toward, the:

-(b) subarachnoid screw!" (The crowd goes wild!) The subarachnoid screw (or **"bolt"**) is considered the **second choice** of devices placed by neurosurgeons for monitoring ICP. They are relatively easy to install, but their accuracy is apparently significantly less than the more direct ventriculostomy drain.

(In a soft, rapid voice: "Members of the neurology and neurosurgery departments and their families are not eligible. Void where prohibited by law. Your mileage may vary.")

Anyone need more of Bob and Johnny? Didn't think so...

c- **Fiberoptic Monitors**: Pretty much what they sound like, I guess. The fiberoptic device has a pressure sensor at the tip, and it can be placed into the ventricle, the subarachnoid space, etc. I think we got one of these a while back and it was hooked up to some kind of neat self-contained monitoring device instead of using our usual transducer-to-monitor setup. Very cool.

An update: apparently fiberoptic monitors don't have to be leveled and recalibrated – the transducer is built into the tip of the device, and gets calibrated once just before insertion.

d- **Epidural sensor:** this device is less invasive – I'm not sure we've ever seen one. CSF can't be removed through this one.

e- **Noninvasive ICP monitoring:** This is the one I want. It turns out that NASA is working on a monitor that doesn't require drilling. (McCoy: " You mean you're actually going to <u>drill</u> into that man's <u>head</u>!? Is this the Middle Ages?") Apparently the skull moves a bit, hard as it may be, and the fluctuations can be measured, etc. Here's a reference:

http://nesb.larc.nasa.gov/NNWG/VOL8.2/TASKS/ARC/arc82_1.html

12- How long a bolt stay in?

We had a neuro ICU nurse come down recently to take a look at the subarachnoid bolt that one of our patients had – he'd fallen off the train platform onto the tracks and hit his head. He had an impressive tox screen too – anyway, she said these things usually stay in for about two weeks.

One source we looked at said that ventricular drains have an infection rate of about 5%.

13- How do I take care of a bolt?

The nurse told us that the site itself is dressed the same way a central line is, every four days unless the dressing gets gnarly. You also have to make sure that the system is patent – it **never**

gets flushed into the patient, but sometimes gets flushed "backwards", towards the transducer. I never did it, so I really need to ask around and find out what that means; when in doubt, I don't do <u>anything</u> to one of these devices without getting the specialty nurses down to show us how.

Ventriculostomies:

Levelling: make sure that the transducer is levelled properly. The patient above had the fiberoptic device in – no leveling - but we had someone else a while back who had an intraventricular catheter that had to be levelled just so. It also had a drainage bag arrangement that had to be at the proper level. According to the NIH source we looked at, the patient should be consistently head up at 30-45 degrees for the measurement. So the patient has to be up at the right angle, the transducer has to be level, the bag has to be level, the whole thing is complicated. The transducer is supposed to be leveled at the part of the patient's face that corresponds to the Foramen of Monro – a document at the NIH website says this should be the outer canthus of the eye.

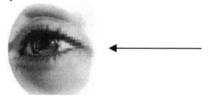

http://www.cc.nih.gov/ccmd/pdf_doc/Clinical%20Monitoring/04-Intracranial%20Pressure%20Mo.pdf

Another sources says the level should be halfway between the outer canthus of the eye and the tragus of the ear.

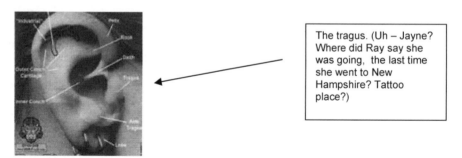

The tragus. (Uh – Jayne? Where did Ray say she was going, the last time she went to New Hampshire? Tattoo place?)

The point that is always stressed: just as we do with PA-lines and the like, the transducer must always be leveled to the same point on the patient. So pick one, mark it, and stick with it.

Drainage: with a ventriculostomy, there need to be specific orders for the height of the drainage bag. The bag has a scale of cm on the side, and it has to be hung at just the right point. The way I understand the source text that I used, the height of the bag relative to the patient's head determines whether CSF is going to flow outwards or not. Too high – won't flow out. Too low, and <u>too much</u> flows out. Just right – the fluid will only drain if the pressure in the head is above the prescribed limit. There should be orders for specific ICP numbers that will be the "threshold" for drainage.

We also had to measure and record the hourly drainage, and check the waveform to make sure it was still clear. If not, the system might need backflushing towards the transducer. What would you do if the drain suddenly stopped draining?

An apparently important point: **the system has to be filled with normal saline that has no bacteriostatic preservative in it**, which is <u>not</u> the usual stuff we keep at hand.

Subarachnoid bolts:

These are a lot less invasive than the ventriculostomies, and it's usually one of the fiberoptic gadgets that gets put through them, so there's none of the levelling and zeroing going on. A couple of things to watch for:

- the fiberoptic cable itself is fragile, and can break if twisted, stretched, or tightly bent.

- apparently it's possible for brain tissue to herniate upwards into the bolt if the ICP rises uncontrolllably. ("Uh, Ralph? You want to come and take a look at this?")

14- What is a bolt waveform supposed to look like?

Here's one off the web - a normal tracing:

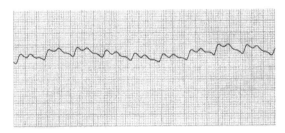

http://www.son.washington.edu/courses/nurs405/lecturedocs/icp.doc

This is a pretty clear trace. Each of the waves is made up of three smaller waves: P1, P2, and P3. It's hard to see all three – here's the same image blown up:

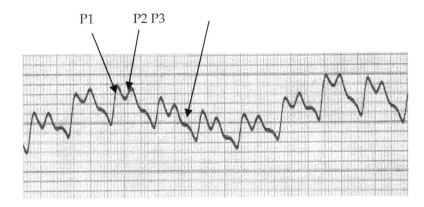

I couldn't really see the third one until I enlarged the image. Getting old. There does seem to be some respiratory variation – see how the whole wave system goes up and down?
Here's another one:

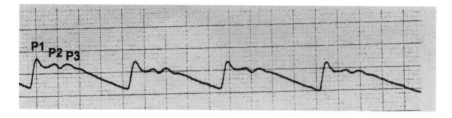

15- What is it not supposed to look like?

A tracing showing "badness":

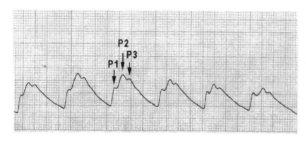

http://www.son.washington.edu/courses/nurs405/lecturedocs/icp.doc

Hey, how about putting a numeric scale on the strips, you guys? See how P2 is higher than her sister waves? P1 is supposed to be the highest. Also the entire amplitude of the wave is greater – that's to say, it goes up and down more. It's bigger - higher. Not a good thing – this means that overall the ICP is rising, right? – higher wave, higher pressure. The waves are interpreted according to the rules of the mystical cult of neurological astrology (which is how they probably look at balloon pumps) – the image reference says that the elevated P2 means that the intracranial compliance is probably decreasing, as the pressure is rising. Makes sense – pressure rises, things get less compliant, more rigid. (Now what the heck does that remind me of…? It'll come to me.)

Here's another bad one. Looks pretty high to me. It's doing that P2 thing again too:

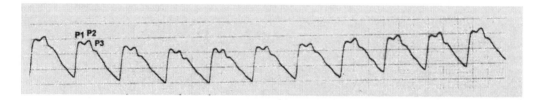

16- What if the waveform is dampened, or goes away?

It's not supposed to get dampened or flattened out – this usually means that the transducer system is getting plugged up in some way. Check the system for air in the tubing; air doesn't conduct pressure waves along the tube system the way water does. Check for leaks, disconnections, correct level, problems at the insertion site. Call the neuro nurses, or the neurosurg person on call (I'd think about calling both.)

A dampened trace:

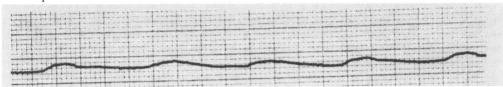

17- How is a high ICP treated?

- **Drainage**: The gold standard treatment is apparently the drainage of some of the CSF through a ventriculostomy device.

- **Positioning and Treatments**:

    i. <u>Sit the patient up</u> - It helps lower the ICP. There's argument about this one – I guess there are studies pointing in different directions. (Why do I imagine two guys – always guys – getting really angry, waving their studies in each others' faces, then rolling them up and smacking each other upside the head? Do the studies say they should get mannitol?)

    ii. <u>Lie the patient down</u>. It helps the cerebral perfusion. Hey, what do I know? They say sit 'em up, I sit 'em up; they say lie 'em down, I lie 'em down.

- **Don'ts** in relation to positioning and treatment:

    i.   don't lift the patient's legs up unnecessarily
    ii. don't position the patient on her side
    iii. don't flex her neck
    iv. don't repeatedly go at the patient with tasks to be done

- <u>**Do's:**</u>

    i.   touch and massage the patient – but monitor the effects.
    ii. let family visit and speak to the patient – but monitor the effects.
    iii. try to get things done and then let the patient rest.

Apparently there are all sorts of studies that point in all sorts of directions about all of these maneuvers. Ask the docs what they want, figure out what works best for your patient, then communicate the plan.

- **Hyperventilation**, or not: I remember this one - this used to be a standard move, overbreathing the patient on the vent to get her $pCO2$ down to about 25;

271

apparently not any more. The idea is that lowering the pCO2 has the effect of lowering the ICP, but in a bad way? – it works by constricting the cerebral blood vessels – a bad thing to do if perfusion is what you want. Apparently this maneuver only works for a short while anyway, and the ICP can pop back up suddenly if discontinued.

- **Mannitol**: more arguments. Back in cave-woman days we were taught to practically keep a bag of mannitol in our hand, and that at the first sign of increasing ICP (which is what, you guys?), up it went. Now we give something like 100Gm IV q 4hours to keep the serum osm up – which means drying out their brain, right?

Osmosis

Let's go really quickly over the drying-out-the-brain thing. Everyone remembers osmosis? (No, it's not what you do after drinking too late at Chuck's Pub, and adding extra salt to the margaritas does <u>not</u> help.)

Start with a semi-permeable membrane, like a net. Some stuff will pass through it, some stuff won't. Water molecules will. Proteins, blood cells, big things - won't.

Now - take a bathtub. Pour some salt into the water, stir it up, dissolve it up good. Well. Properly. Yeah. Halfway along the length of the tub, divide the water with a film of the membrane, from the surface down to the bottom. Got that? Now dump some more salt into side – what does the water do?

When she was inventing chemistry, the Great Biomedical Engineer made a commandment unto the water: "When thou art nearby to a semipermeable membrane, thou shalt goeth to where the more Dissolved Stuff is, and where the lesser of the Dissolved Stuff is, shalt thou not remaineth, except until thou hast tried to make the Stuff equally diluted on both sides of ye membrane."

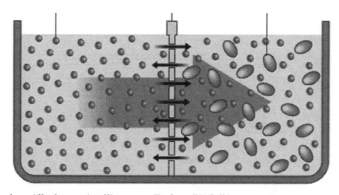

See the big arrow? That's the water, heading over across the membrane, towards where the green Stuff is… so the water level on the left should be going down…

The water moves – some of it, anyway, across the membrane, towards where there is more dissolved Stuff, trying to make the concentration equal on both sides. The water level on the dilute side of the membrane should go <u>down</u>. Where's Bill Nye when I need him?

Now - take a brain. See all the little brain cells? See how they have "water" in them?, and see how they're surrounded by blood vessels, which also have "water" in them? The coverings of those cells are the membranes this time, and the other side of the bathtub is the blood serum in all the zillions of little capillaries surrounding all the cells. See that? Make sense? Now if you dump something concentrated into the blood side – say, by infusing something really concentrated, oh, let's just say by chance, hmm – how about mannitol? Mannitol is, as we say up here in MA, "wicked hyperosmotic".

"Osmotic-ness" , meaning: "How much stuff is dissolved in this solution, anyhow?", is measured by a number – "osmolality". "Yo Jeannie, check off an osm on that blood gas, okay?" The normal range is something like 280 – 300 mOsm/kg. Higher is more concentrated – either you've added more stuff, or you've removed some water. Lower is more dilute – told you not to drink all that tap water! Gatorade much better – water is hypo-osmotic, otherwise known as hypo-tonic. Gatorade is closer to iso-osmotic, or iso-tonic.

So okay – patient's got brain cells swelling up – becoming edematous. You want to shrink those cells back down if you can, right? Give the patient an IV dose of that nice, hyperosmotic mannitol. What happens? – the **serum** osm goes way up – the goal is high, around 310, but not too high; you want to keep it <320. The water molecules inside the brain cells say: "Yo! Time to cross the membrane towards that greater concentration thing over across there!" And so they do, according to the Engineer's Design – each and every one of those little brain cells sends water out of itself, through its membrane, out into the surrounding blood vessels, where it stays, and mannitol having a diuretic effect, then gets peed out.

Result – the brain cells, losing some of their water, shrink down. All of them. And the tissue edema shrinks down. And the ICP goes down. And the brain avoids herniation. A life is saved. Woo-hoo! (But you'd better know when to give it.)

! - A very important point goes here. Patients with cerebral edema issues should only get hypertonic or isotonic IV fluids. If hypotonic fluids were given, **they would do the osmotic thing the wrong way**, and go **into** the cells, **making the edema worse**. Examples we've seen of appropriate fluids are normal saline, Ringer's lactate, albumin (5% or 25%? – probably 25%, since it's more osmotic, right?)

Another point: even if you're diuresing your patient with mannitol, the sources all say that it's just as important to re-hydrate the patient, to keep her euvolemic, rather than total-body dry. You're trying to shrink the brain and keep it perfused, all at the same time. Which IV fluid are you going to give to do this?

- **Steroids**: apparently a big hairy no-no in head trauma or in either kind of stroke, (what are the two kinds?) I think they do still use them for brain mets – I remember when my mom got them…I think they helped, for a while. She missed out on Zofran. And grandchildren. Don't smoke, you guys.

- **Anticonvulsants**: apparently meds like dilantin and tegretol are useful in treating seizures that occur soon after a brain injury, but preventing those seizures doesn't seem to help in the ultimate outcome. I'm pretty sure that all of our acute neuro patients get dilantin-loaded – although most of our patients aren't traumatic injuries; we get the subdural hematomas, it seems like. Do the same rules apply for bleeds and traumas?

- **Barbiturate "coma":** I want to say that the young female children of America are in a Barbie coma... maybe I shouldn't.

  (Whoa! Brain wave! How about "Burr-hole Barbie"? I mean, girls grow up to neurosurgeons too, don't they? Whoa! Another one!: "Oy mate, throw another Barbie on the... never mind.)

  Anyhow, the idea here is that the barbs (usually pentobarbital – seems like we've used phenobarbital too) have two effects: they lower the ICP, and they also lower the rates of the body's metabolic processes – which should take some of the strain off the brain while it tries to recover.

  But – bad things can happen with barbs. One study compared the use of barbs against the use of mannitol in head injury (the one or the other only, I guess) – the barb people did much worse. The other thing is that the barbs produce systemic hypotension. With the recent emphasis on keeping these patients a bit hypertensive, this would seem to be your basic Bad Thing. Not really sure when I saw them used last.

- **Other sedatives:** the sources list 'em all: opiates, benzos, propofol – even paralysis is on the list, apparently also with lowered metabolic demands in mind.

- **Cooling:** Apparently a change of one degree in temperature produces something like a 7% decrease change in the overall metabolic demand. Cooling blankets work better <u>under</u> the patient. Don't set it lower than 60 degrees. I find that making the patient nakey (we still watch Rugrats in our house), and covering him with a few carefully placed wet towels helps cool things down very well. Tepid water – they'll get cool fast enough! Lately we've started seeing the cooling protocol used for the post-anoxic-event patients... supposed to help.

- **Oxygenation:** Keep the sat greater than 95% - maintain good oxygen delivery to the brain.

- **Hypertensive therapy:** this seems to be one of the more recent strategies in improving CBF – shrink the brain, keep them euvolemic, keep up the MAP, keep up the perfusion. Lately the MAP and SBP goal ranges have been rising on these patients. The texts say that pressors can be used – hey guys, most of those alpha pressors <u>vasoconstrict</u>, y'know! Dobutamine might be the way to go. They also say that pressures can get too high: a MAP of greater than 130 should probably be brought back down. Don't want to pop anything in there... labetolol was cited as the drug to use in that case, along with oral calcium channel blockers. Hmm... not nipride?

Intubations

The Tube

1- What is intubation?
2- What are some reasons why a patient might need to be intubated?
3- What is an endotracheal tube?
4- What is the balloon thing at the end of the tube?
5- What is the thing that hangs out of the patient's mouth?
6- Why do ET tubes come in different sizes?
7- What are the numbers along the side of the tube?

Getting Ready

8- What do I need to do to get my patient ready for intubation? (IV, NGT), box.
9- What if they're very agitated, or confused, or anxious?
10- Who does the intubation?
11- Can the medical team intubate the patient?
12- What is the role of the respiratory therapist?
13- What is the role of the nurse?

Intubating the Patient

14- What meds are used during intubation?
15- What is rapid-sequence induction?
16- What is the laryngoscope for?
17- What is the stylet for?
18- What is the surgilube for?
19- What is "cricoid pressure"?
20- What is the gadget that turns from purple-to-yellow, that they put on the end of the ET tube after it goes in?
21- How do we know if the ET tube is in the right position after intubation?
22- Why does the patient need a stat x-ray after intubation?
23- What if the tube goes into the esophagus?
24- What do they mean by "intubated in the right main stem"?
25- How do I make sure the tube stays in place and doesn't move around?
26- What if the patient bites on the tube?
27- Why do so many patients lose blood pressure after they've been intubated?
28- What kind of vent settings should the patient start out on?
29- What if the patient extubates herself?

As usual, please remember that these articles are not meant to be the final word on anything – instead, they're supposed to reflect the information that an experienced preceptor might pass along to a new RN orienting in the MICU. When (not if!) you find errors, please let us know, and we'll fix them right away.

A note about the images: if you're reading these articles on-line, try clicking on an picture, then grabbing its edges with your mouse. You'll find that you can change their size, and get a better look at things, depending on their resolution. Very cool.

The Tube

1-What is intubation?

Intubation is the placement of a tube into a patient's trachea. This is a tricky maneuver, requiring skilled assessment and performance, so in our institution it's usually left in the hands of the on - call anesthesiology resident. Even they have trouble at times and can wind up calling their attending to the unit for help. Not as simple as it looks.

2- What are some reasons why a patient might need to be intubated?

Usually it's because they can't breathe, for one reason or another. CHF, pneumonia, ARDS, BOOP (paging Dr. Betty!), we see a lot of respiratory failure in the MICU. Opiate overdoses – nothing wrong with their lungs – they're just not breathing, is all. Once in a while a severely agitated or confused patient will need to be intubated, so that he can be safely sedated for some procedure – balloon pumping prior to CABG, maybe. I remember one man who had to get a femoral, intra-arterial infusion of streptokinase overnight and was frantically, confusedly climbing out of the bed, risking his limb, and maybe his life. He was intubated, sedated with propofol for the infusion, extubated, and once he wasn't confused anymore, went off to the floors.

3- What is an endotracheal tube?

The tube itself, otherwise called the ET tube - a silicone/plastic tube about 10 inches long.

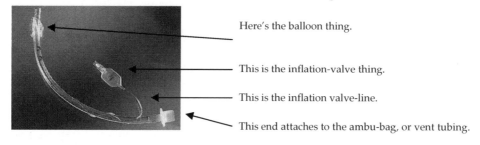

Here's the balloon thing.

This is the inflation-valve thing.

This is the inflation valve-line.

This end attaches to the ambu-bag, or vent tubing.

www.pahsco.com.tw/5anesthsia/10.html

4- What is the balloon thing at the end of the tube?

The balloon is inflated after the tube is put in – it seals up against the walls of the trachea to prevent air from leaking in or out of the patient's lungs. The pressure in the balloon is supposed to be checked several times a shift by Respiratory, and should not be higher than 20cm – the RRTs have little manometers that they check this with. If the pressure is too high, the trachea can be permanently damaged. This happened sometimes back in the Punic Wars, when they used to use red rubber ET tubes.

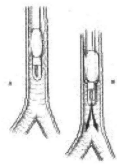

Over on the left there, the cuff isn't inflated. What would happen if you sent a breath down the tube? Would the air go into the patient's lungs, or take the easy way out and wiffle back upwards towards his mouth?

In fact, this is a really useful trick to use: if your patient can tolerate it breathing-wise, you can drop the cuff, ambu the patient, and let them talk to you as you squeeze the bag. Suction them first: airway, mouth and oropharynx. With a little practice you can make repeated short squeezes and keep a fairly steady forward flow, letting them tell you all the things they've desperately been trying to say…

On the right the cuff has been inflated, so that air sent into the patient pretty much has to go to the lungs.

http://www.mtsinai.org/pulmonary/books/physiology/images/fig10-1small.gif

5- What is the thing that hangs out of the patient's mouth?

Besides the other end of the ETT, you mean? The thin little tube is the inflation line for the cuff. It has a little plastic valve on it, where you can inject air with a ten-cc syringe. If your patient is "leaking", as we say, it means that the cuff isn't full enough, and probably needs some air added. Usually 0.5 –1 cc of air will do the trick. Let respiratory know, so that they can recheck the cuff pressures with their manometer. Cuff pressures higher than something like 20cm can hurt the trachea, and respiratory checks them once or twice a shift.

Something to remember: once in a while someone gets enthusiastic about shaving a patient and nicks the cuff inflation line with a razor. Besides being terminally embarrassing for you, this obviously puts the patient at risk because the cuff won't hold pressure any more. The tube will have to be replaced by anesthesia, but what to do in the meantime? Try to find the nick in the line visually – you can try putting a small tegaderm doubled tightly around the nick, and see if the line will hold pressure. If that doesn't work, you can snip the line at the nick, <u>gently</u> insert a 19-gauge butterfly into the remainder of the line, and join to a ten cc syringe with a stopcock attached. You should be able to get the cuff to seal. Tape the whole thing down to a tongue blade to keep it stable until anesthesia arrives.

6- Why do ET tubes come in different sizes?

Basically, because people do. It does pay to think a little about what size tube to use. Most people wind up with a 7.0 or 7.5 mm tube – the number means the width of the tube lumen in millimeters, not the length of the tube. I believe that if a patient is going to need a bronchoscopy, then they'll need an 8.0 mm tube.

7- What are the numbers along the side of the tube?

The numbers tell the distance along the tube from the cuffed end in centimeters. You want to know how deep the tube is into the patient, so you check what number is showing at the teeth, or the lip at the time they're intubated – that way if the tube should come out somewhat, you'll know where to replace it to. It's a good idea to mark the number on the tape that goes on the patient's face: "22 cm at lip", or something like that.

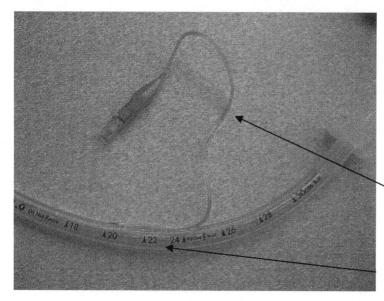

Most of the time the tube will wind up at something like 20 or 22 cm "at the lip". Make sure that the tube can't shift inwards or out – too far in and the tube can poke the carina, which is never fun, or end up in one of the main stem bronchi. Too far out, and the patient isn't intubated any more!

This is the part not to nick when shaving your patient.

About 23 cm from the distal end of the tube.

www.whoshootsthesegoofypicturesanyhow?.org

8- What do I need to do to get my patient ready for intubation?

The single most important thing to do is to have really good IV access. If the patient has no central line, then make sure a good heplock is in place (two or even three is always better). There really should be a visible blood return in the vein – this is no time to futz around with an infiltrated IV. You'll want to hang a gravity bag of NS that runs well, so that the meds that get pushed during the intubation get right into the patient. The anesthesia people often depend on the rapid effects of these drugs, such as:

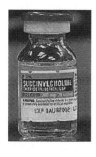 or 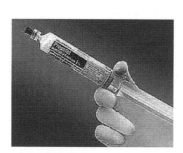 and/or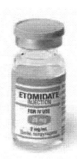

http://www.healthdigest.org/images/cat/succsuttsuccinylcholineinjectioninjectable.jpg

http://www.vbphoto.com/Ad%20Frames/pages/Propofol%20Revised.htm

http://www.bedfordlabs.com/products/762-10.html

And you'll need to have a reliable line to give them through. Using as large a peripheral vein as possible is always a good idea – try the antecubitals.

A moment for a couple of quick questions:

- What is succinylcholine? What really horrible scary thing can happen (very rarely, thank goodness) with this drug, but which if it happens you will never, ever forget?

- What is propofol, and why do they call it "Milk of Amnesia"? What is the single most dangerous thing about this drug?

- What is etomidate? Why the heck don't I know anything about this drug?

Another excellent idea is to try and prevent the aspiration of stomach contents - try to make sure the patient's stomach is empty. Obviously this isn't always possible, but if she has an NG/OG tube – flush it clear, and hook it up to low suction.

You'll need a couple of other things – make sure the suction is all set up in the room with a tonsil tip attached. Get the intubation box open, and locate:

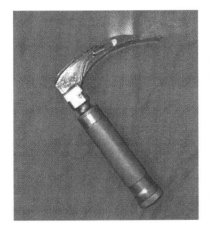

This guy: the laryngoscope handle and blades – test them to make sure the lights work. See the light glowing? Make sure you know how to check the bulb, the batteries…just like a flashlight.

http://www.med.umich.edu/anes/tcpub/glossary/anesthesia_glossary-14.htm

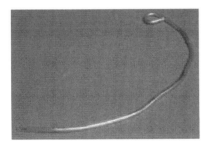

And this guy: a stylet – the bendable wire thing in sterile wrap. This goes inside the ET tube to make it stiffer when it's being placed in the trachea – otherwise the tube will be too soft and floppy to pass properly.

Remember, after intubation…take the stylet out!

http://www.icc.cc.il.us/HAPS/respiratory/equipment/equip-ami.asp

Find an appropriately-sized ET tube.

Make sure someone checks that the ET tube cuff works properly with a syringe – not that they fail often, but it would be a real bummer to go through intubation and find that the cuff wasn't working. You'll want your trach tape stuff ready too. Certainly not last or least – make sure that all your monitor equipment is working properly – you must have a decent EKG trace, a clear O2 sat probe wave, and some kind of blood pressure monitoring. If you're using the non-invasive cuff, set it to cycle once a minute.

A question for the newbie group goes here: (you just got a clue) - what other situation might develop, maybe after the patient's been intubated, that you're going to want to be ready for? What drug, or drug mix might you want to have on hand? We'll get to this a bit later on – but any nurse who's seen more than two intubations will know this one…can't wait? See question 27.

You're going to need one of these, too:

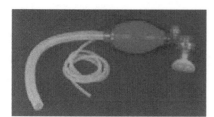

After the tube is placed, you're going to need an ambu bag to ventilate your very-sedated patient until the vent is set up and ready. The face mask comes off, and the bag fitting slides onto the end of the ET tube. Make sure that the oxygen line is hooked up, and that there's good flow through the line.

http://www.helixindia.com/images/ambu_bag.jpg

9- What if they're very agitated, confused, or anxious?

Wouldn't you be? I'm going to be a handful, I'll tell ya! This is managed by anesthesia. Depending on their judgment, I've seen them use propofol alone, sometimes versed, sometimes etomidate, sometimes combinations of meds. Successfully intubating a patient often depends on careful, appropriately timed sedation – this is why you must have proper IV access. After intubation nowadays, we've found that propofol alone is usually enough to help a patient remain in sync with the vent. They're going to need a whole lot of it for me!

10- Who does the intubation?

The intubation is supposed to be either done by, or supervised by the anesthesia doc on call. The medical team can go ahead with intubation in an emergency while the anesthesia person has been paged and is coming.

A word about supervised intubations – often a situation that is rapidly deteriorating can become really stressful while the anesthesiologist and the medical team member are both trying to look at the patient's vocal cords. Your position during intubation is facing the both the monitor and the patient. You may be the only person looking at the monitor, and noticing that the patient's O2 sat has gone to 60, and that the heart rate is dropping, and it may be you that has to point this out! Don't hesitate!

11- Can the medical team intubate the patient?

Yes, but if possible they should wait for anesthesia.

12- What is the role of the respiratory therapist?

Respiratory is the assistant to the person doing the intubation. They make sure that all the equipment is at hand, assist with bagging, and advise during the procedure. They are also responsible for having a vent ready and in the room.

13- What is the role of the nurse?

First – make sure that respiratory knows that an intubation is going to happen! This is <u>not</u> a happy surprise for them if they don't have a chance to get ready.

Next- collect your equipment, and make sure it all works.

Then – stand in the room so that you can see the patient, the people intubating, and the monitor. You also probably will be in charge of the IV meds. Let's say it again: make sure that the IV is running freely throughout the procedure, with a good blood return, so that all meds given get into the patient quickly. This is probably the most important aspect of intubation besides passing the tube itself, and <u>it is your responsibility</u>.

<u>Intubating the Patient</u>

14- What meds are used during intubation?

Anesthesia will choose. Depending on size, weight, medical history, empty or full stomach – there are a lot of considerations – they will choose from a number of drugs available. Lately I've seen more intubations done using pushes of propofol alone. In the past I've seen them use pentothal, etomidate, (sedatives) sometimes with small doses of succinylcholine (a paralytic).

15- What is rapid-sequence induction?

Here the idea is that the patient is getting a couple of different meds at just about the same time: a sedative, and sometimes some kind of paralyzing agent, although they use paralytics less and less lately. Lots of intubations nowadays are done just with propofol boluses, although the anesthesia people still carry around an enormous bag full of all sorts of stuff. There's a new version of etomidate nowadays, I hear, with hardly any respiratory suppression. I want that one.

16- What is the laryngoscope for?

The laryngoscope holds the tongue out of the way, helps the anesthesiologist move the jaw downwards, and has a lightbulb to act light a flashlight – it lights up the inside of the mouth so that the vocal cords can be seen – then ET tube is passed through the cords into the trachea.

It's important (but not always possible) that the ET tube is passed into the trachea under "direct vision" – otherwise it may go into the esophagus. Bad.

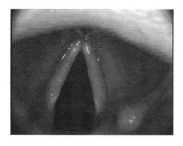

Grab this image and drag it bigger – see the tracheal rings starting below the cords?

http://www-scf.usc.edu/~susannam/healthycords3.jpg

17- What is the stylet for?

The stylet is the copper-colored long bendy piece of wire thing that comes in a sterile wrapper in the intubation box. You put the stylet into the ET tube to stiffen it as it goes into the patient – the ET tube is fairly soft, and may just curl up or bend if you try to place it without the stylet, which comes out after the tube has been placed beyond the cords.

18- What is the surgilube for?

The surgilube helps the ET tube slide into place – just like for an NG or OG tube, or a Foley catheter. Anybody else remember that back in cave-nurse days they used to call this stuff "Kalubafax"? Wasn't there an eskimo by that name? A bear?

19- What is "cricoid pressure"?

I didn't learn what this actually was for until I took ACLS (a very useful thing to do): pushing downwards (straight down, towards the bed) on the patient's adam's apple pushes the opening of the trachea backwards so that the intubating person can see it.

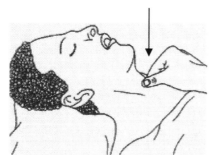

We got an email awhile back from a CRNA, who pointed out that cricoid pressure also closes the esophagus at the moment of intubation, hopefully preventing the patient from vomiting and aspirating as the tube is passed into the trachea. Aspirating stomach contents – all that acid and all? Never a happy thing.

http://www.nda.ox.ac.uk/wfsa/html/u02/u02c_t03.gif

20- What is the gadget that turns from purple-to-yellow, that they put on the end of the ET tube after it goes in?

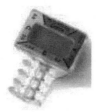

This is an end-tidal CO_2 detector – it tests the air passing through the ET tube that it's attached to. If the detector changes color with exhalation, that means that the patient is intubated in the trachea – CO_2 is coming out of the patient.

If it's not changing color...well, where else could that tube have gone?
www.life-assist.com/ac01.html

21- How do we know if the ET tube is in the right position after intubation?

Right after the tube goes in, the anesthesiologist checks the CO_2 detector. If that looks right, and if the tube is in to the right average depth (usually around 22 - 24cm at the lips), then they check for bilateral breath sounds with ambu-bagged breaths. Watching the O2 sat is also usually your basic clue.

22- Why does the patient need a stat x-ray after intubation?

You can never really tell if the tube is in the right position without an x-ray. Sometimes lung sounds can definitely fool you, and you may hear them on both sides even if the patient is intubated in the right main stem. The tip of the tube should be 2-3cm above the carina.

23- What if the tube goes into the esophagus?

Take it the heck back out!

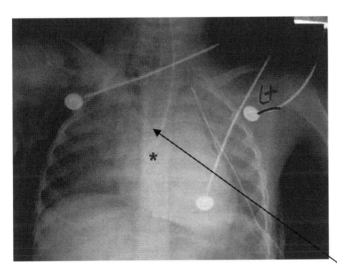

This was a pretty hard image to find, so I thought I'd put it in, even though it's not the kind of thing most nurses look at, much. (That should change.)

The little star marks the end of the ET tube (see the white radio-opaque line on it?), which is really not where it ought to be if it were in the trachea, or either the right or left main stem. Too far down, and in the middle? What's up with that? I played with the brightness a little bit to highlight what I think is the trachea, the shadow that the arrow is pointing at. And hey – what's that on our right? A chest tube? Think it's in far enough? Whoa! And hey – why's this guy's heart as big as his head? And hey…(grin!)

Uh, guys? Trachea's over here?

http://www.caep.ca/004.cjem-jcmu/004-00.cjem/vol-4.2002/v41-041.htm

If the CO_2 detector doesn't change color, then no CO_2 is coming out, which means that the tube is in the esophagus. At this point it needs to be pulled back out immediately, and intubation needs to be tried again. Esophageal intubation did indeed happen once in a while before these devices came along, despite the best efforts at visually placing the tube, and auscultation after placement. It's definitely saved many lives.

24- What do they mean by "intubated in the right main stem"?

The trachea divides into two main branches, right and left. The right branch, or main stem, is in nearly a straight line with the trachea itself, so if the ET tube goes in too far, that's where it usually goes. (That's also why most aspiration pneumonias go to the RLL.) In that position, with the cuff inflated, the patient is only getting one lungful of air with each breath instead of two.

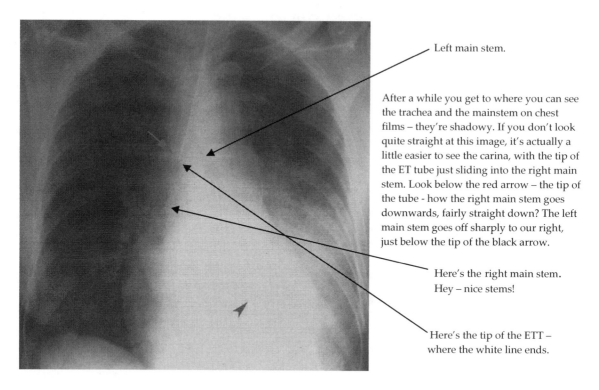

Left main stem.

After a while you get to where you can see the trachea and the mainstem on chest films – they're shadowy. If you don't look quite straight at this image, it's actually a little easier to see the carina, with the tip of the ET tube just sliding into the right main stem. Look below the red arrow – the tip of the tube - how the right main stem goes downwards, fairly straight down? The left main stem goes off sharply to our right, just below the tip of the black arrow.

Here's the right main stem. Hey – nice stems!

Here's the tip of the ETT – where the white line ends.

http://www.med.virginia.edu/med-ed/rad/chest/lines_ett5.htm

25- How do I make sure the tube stays in place and doesn't move around?

What we do in this ICU is to prep the upper lip and one cheek with benzoin, and use a piece of cloth tape about six inches long, that we split for 3-4 inches. The unsplit part goes on the cheek, the top of the split goes on the lip, over the skin where a mustache would be, and the bottom of the split wraps around the ETT. Try to leave a flag on the part wrapped around the tube, or no one will be able to get it off when it needs changing. After the cloth tape is on we use a trach tie string, doubled in a loop around the tape wrap, which passes around the back of the patient's head, and gets tied on one side. This should be loose enough to allow at least one finger to slip underneath – too tight and you'll definitely cut the patient somewhere.

26- What if the patient bites on the tube?

Definitely a bad thing - I've seen people arrest doing this: no oxygen, no gas exchange – a bad thing. Some people are just too agitated sometimes to understand explanations about this (or much else), and need some sedation. Other people may need to have a bite block. Or both. There's always an oral airway in the room – this can go in for a while, but I was taught that they shouldn't stay in place for more than a day, because they can cause pressure injuries to the tongue and the palate. Sometimes we cut the oral airways down to leave only about one-half to one inch left – that can work well for longer periods, but you have to make sure it's properly in place – good mouth care is still essential.

Another thing we've seen recently is a patient who chews through the pilot balloon line – there's no quick way to fix this since the break is right at the teeth. These patients need to have the ET tube changed right away, because the cuff won't seal anymore. Use a bite block .

27- Why do so many patients lose blood pressure after they've been intubated?

Remember what we said about having good IV access – a visible blood return in your peripheral lines, all that?

Consider this common scenario: your patient has been working hard to breathe, maybe for the past day or so, and he's getting tired. pCO2 is rising – maybe getting a bit of respiratory acidosis. Maybe the team has been diuresing him for several days, hoping that his problem is CHF and not something worse – now he's dry as a bone; dry as a doggy-biscuit, we used to say.

So he's working hard to breathe, he's anxious, he's got a pressure of, maybe, 110 systolic, he's dry. Now the anesthesiologist gives him a slug of propofol to sedate him for intubation. The only thing that's been keeping his pressure up has been his agitation – he's been secreting his own pressors, right? Endogenous catecholamines, all like that? Mediated by his excitement?

Lots of patients lose blood pressure after being sedated for intubation – you may want to give a fluid bolus or two. You can run the peripheral neo mix in these situations sometimes – large-bore peripheral veins are really mandatory for that stuff. You do <u>not</u> want to learn what it looks like when a peripherally administered pressor extravasates in someones arm! (What would you do if you thought that was happening? Look up "local regitine infiltration").

28- What kind of vent settings should the patient start out on?

This will depend on all sorts of things – does the patient need a rate? Maybe once she wakes up some, she'll only need pressure support ventilation without a rate. Maybe she'll need something else – discuss the plan with the team and respiratory.

29- What if the patient extubates herself?

Depends. Obviously, some people will need to be immediately re-intubated, and some people may be able to "fly" on mask O2. The first move we usually make is to put the patient on 100% mask O2, and observe carefully. (What if the patient had severe COPD? Would you put her on that much oxygen?) Send blood gases to document how the patient tolerates the change. Be ready for quick re-intubation, and remember that when the patient gets ready for (planned) extubation later on, that she might have injured or inflamed her vocal cords – is there cord edema? A good way to check – is there an active air leak when the cuff is dropped? Check while giving the patient breaths with an ambu-bag. No leak? Let the team know, and remind them of the possible trauma. (This goes for traumatic intubations as well.) The patient may be at risk for a bad airway situation after extubation – think about having racemic epinephrine nearby to deal with stridor and swelling. You know how to give it? (1:1000 epi, 2cc, with 2cc NS, in a nebulizer.)

Know where the trach kits are?

Quiz Questions

1- Intubation means:

    a- placing a tube in the esophagus
    b- placing a tube in the esophagus, and another tube in the trachea
    c- placing a tube in the esophagus, or the trachea, or anywhere else that sounds good
    d- placing a tube in the trachea

2- The tip of the tube should be:

    a- two centimeters below the carina
    b- two or three centimeters above the carina
    c- docked next to the cigarette boat at the marina
    d- in the stomach, below the diaphragm

3- The cuff at the end of the tube should be:

    a- Inflated to about 20mm hg
    b- deflated
    c- hyperinflated, then deflated every four hours
    d- there is no cuff at the end of the tube

4- The cuff at the end of the tube:

    a- holds the tube in place
    b- should be removed before the tube is put in
    c- should be filled with water
    d- seals the trachea so air, sent to the lungs, through the tube, doesn't rush back up out of the patients mouth

5- The numbers along the side of the tube:

    a- tell how long the tube is
    b- tell how far the tube has been advanced into the esophagus

c- tell how far the tube has been advanced into the trachea

d- I don't know what they're for, and I ignore them

6- Personnel allowed to intubate in our hospital include:

a- Condoleezza Rice

b- the anesthesia resident, the medical residents, occasionally the critical care attendings

c- Anastasia, the sleepy Russian princess of gas

d- the nurses and the respiratory therapists

7- True or false: succinylcholine is a completely safe drug with no side effects, such as collapsed airway from paralysis, and the rare but terrifying episode of hyperkalemia.

8- The end-tidal C02 detector is used to:

a- check if carbon dioxide is coming out of wherever the tube has gone

b- make sure enough carbon dioxide is going into the patient

c- check the level of carbon dioxide at low tide

d- end-tidal C02 detectors are useless, and we shouldn't bother with them

9- If the tube has gone into the esophagus:

a- a clue will be that the patient's sat will not improve with bagging

b- the end-tidal C02 detector won't change color

c- the abdomen below the diaphragm may swell with bagged breaths

d- it doesn't matter – don't worry about it

e- all of the above except d

10- A question about responsibility: if the patient extubates herself:

a- she may need re-intubation quickly

b- the nurse is at fault

c- the patient is at fault

d- this just proves that all intubated patients should be restrained, sedated, and probably paralyzed

e- a is probably the only correct answer to this question

<u>Labs</u>

I must be out of my mind. Am I confused? Would I know? Who in their right mind sits down and writes things like this for the fun of it? Did I get all my meds for today? Can I at least have one hand loose?

This one took a while to put together, as it required a lot of looking-up on the part of the preceptor. Got to love the web!

As usual, <u>please</u> remember that this article is <u>not meant to be the final word on anything</u>, or even comprehensive in any way. Nurses at the bedside have to work on the fly, and the things that they need to keep in their heads have to be practical and brief – not that this article is very brief, but hopefully the items are. This information is supposed to reflect what a preceptor might teach a new orientee, or maybe to answer some of the questions that the orientee might come up with. Each item in this article is backed up by (apparently) an average of not less than eight thousand pages of reference material in 37 different languages – I just tell what I know! **Please make sure that you check your own references to verify lab/drug and toxic ranges!**

Let us know when you find errors, and we'll fix them up right away. Thanks!

Update note: holy cow, this one was torture. **Useful tip**: remember that if you're reading this article online, or on your computer, you can click on any of the images, grab a corner, and pull to make the image bigger, easier to see.

What are some of the labs that we follow on our patients in the MICU?

1- Chemistries

1-1- The basics: "Chem 10"

1-1-1: Sodium, including Free Water Deficits, and an **Extremely Important Thing**
1-1-2: Potassium
     i. What does "hemolyzed" mean?
     ii. A hemolyzed potassium story…
1-1-3: Magnesium
1-1-4: Chloride
1-1-5: Bicarb
1-1-6: BUN
1-1-7: Creatinine
1-1-8: Glucose
     i. Acetone
     ii. HbA1C
1-1-9: Calcium
     i. Ionized Calcium
     ii. Corrected Calcium
     iii. Calcium and Citrate Toxicity

1-1-10: Phosphorus
1-2- Some other basic chems:
    1-2-1: Lactate
    1-2-2: Osmolality
    1-2-3: Amylase
    1-2-4: Lipase
    1-2-5: Ammonia
    1-2-6: Albumin

1-3: Renal Labs

    1-3-1: Creatinine Clearance
    1-3-2: Uric Acid
    1-3-3: Myoglobin
    1-3-4: Urinalysis
    1-3-5: 24-hour urine collections
    1-3-6: urine electrolytes

1-4: Drug Levels

    1-4-1: Dilantin
    1-4-2: Valproate
    1-4-3: Tegretol
    1-4-4:Lithium
    1-4-5:Theophylline
    1-4-6:Thiocyanate
    1-4-7: Vancomycin
    1-4-8: Gentamicin
    1-4-9: Digoxin
    1-4-10: Tacrolimus, cyclosporine
    1-4-11: Peaks, Troughs, and Random Levels

1-5: Tox Screen Panel Meds

    1-5-1: Tylenol
    1-5-2: Salicylates
    1-5-3: Opiates
    1-5-4: Cocaine
    1-5-5: Benzodiazepines
    1-5-6: Ethanol
    1-5-7: Methanol
    1-5-8: Ethylene glycol
    1-5-9: Miscellaneous
    1-5-10: A really cool thing.
    1-5-11: A scary story…

1-6: Cardiac Labs

- Electrolytes

    1-6-1: Potassium
    1-6-2: Magnesium

- Cardiac Enzymes

    1-6-3: What are cardiac enzymes?
    1-6-4: Which cardiac enzymes do we follow on our patients?
    1-6-5: Can a patient have elevated enzymes without having an MI?
    1-6-6: Can a patient have an MI without having elevated enzymes?
    1-6-7: What is CPK again?
    1-6-8: What is the reference range for CPK?
    1-6-9: What are isoenzymes?
    1-6-10: What is the "MB fraction"?
    1-6-11: What are MM and BB?
    1-6-12: Does a higher CPK mean a larger MI?
    1-6-13: How many CPKs should be drawn, and how far apart?
    1-6-14: What is troponin?
    1-6-15: What is the reference range for troponin?
    1-6-16: How often should troponins be drawn, and how far apart?
    1-6-17: What is "washout"?
    1-6-18: Can cardiac enzymes go up if a patient is ischemic, but not having an MI?
    1-6-19: What is hBNP all about?
    1-6-20: What is C-reactive protein all about?

1-7: Lipids

    1-7-1: Total Cholesterol
    1-7-2: HDL
    1-7-3: LDL
    1-7-4: Triglycerides

2- Respiratory Labs:

2-1: ABGs:

    2-1-1: pO2
    2-1-2: pCO2
    2-1-3: pH
    2-1-4: bicarb

4-4: Coagulation Studies

    4-4-1: PT
    4-4-2: PTT
    4-4-3: INR

4-5: D-dimer
4-6: DIC screen
4-7: Fibrin Split Products
4-8: Fibrinogen
4-9: ESR
4-10: Coombs test

5- ID

5-1: Cultures
5-2: Sensitivity Reports
5-3: Some specific tests:

    5-3-1: TB/ AFB's
    5-3-2: Influenza
    5-3-3: H5N1 Avian Flu
    5-3-4: HIV testing/ CD4 count
    5-3-5: Viral Load
    5-3-6: CMV
    5-3-7: RSV
    5-3-8: Herpes testing
    5-3-9: Branch-chain DNA and PCR
    5-3-10: Kary Mullis
    5-3-11: Lyme Disease and Babesia

5-4: CSF

    5-4-1: Which kind of infection?
    5-4-2: Some normal values for CSF

5-5: Opportunistic Infections in the MICU

    5-5-1: MRSA
    5-5-2: VRE
    5-5-3: What are survey swab studies all about?
    5-5-4: C.difficile
    5-5-5: A suggestion for a study – should ICU nurses be routinely screened to see if they're carriers of opportunistic infections? Anyone doing a Master's?

12-4- Stool specimens

  12-4-1: stool for O&P
  12-4-2: stool for C.diff
  12-4-3: stool for occult blood

What are some of the labs that we follow on our patients in the MICU?

There are a lot of labs out there, and they come in a wide variety of flavors. If you never got comfortable with frequently looking up lab results on the floors, you're probably going to have to get over that one quickly, since watching trends of one kind or another is about 90% of what we do in the ICU: labs, vital signs, effects of meds, transfusions – it all makes a dynamic picture that you have to learn to grasp, and follow as it changes.

The basic idea is often really easy: if some lab value is way out of line, then something having to do with the patient probably is too. Doh! You don't want to be wrong about this, which is why the team will sometimes ask you to re-send a spec. Which of course is frustrating when you think that your GI-bleed patient **isn't** losing his blood pressure because he forgot to drink his Gatorade this morning or something...

Remember that basic physiology thing about how the body is made up of subsystems? That sort of basic sort of thing? The labs reflect those systems and how they're doing (or not doing) at whatever it is that they're meant to do. Simple example: if the kidneys aren't clearing nitrogenous wastes from the blood, then the levels of those wastes will rise – makes sense to interpret that as kidney failure, right?

But nothing is ever as simple as you'd like it to be. My son and I just bought an elderly motorcycle...(What? What do you mean, "Don't talk about the motorcycle"?... What do you mean, "it has nothing to do with the topic"?... It's got <u>plenty</u> to do with the topic...you're just jealous, 'cause... What do you mean, you "wouldn't get on that thing even if"?… so we <u>had</u> two quads in the unit last month, so what?!)

Anyway, for the ICU newbie there's lots to learn, as usual, and also as usual the best thing is just to try to get some idea of what you're looking for, and then to accumulate mileage and experience – then the things that you learn by reading will make lots more sense. This is a pretty important point: **don't try to memorize it all at once** – come back and re-read this article a year from now. This is especially true when it comes to motorcycles. See, the float bowl in the carburetor... ow!

<u>**1- Chemistries:**</u>

There's lots of chemistries out there, but the basic ones are always easy to get, and can give you lots of clues about what you're looking for. Maybe I can get one of the kids to draw the little diagram thingy.

Now here's the thing – every day these kids come home from school:
"Hey kids, whad'ya learn at school today?"

"Nothing." And man, you can sit there and ask them about school until your jaw just drops right off, but they just won't tell you a thing. Then later, daughter # 2 wanders by where I'm struggling to do some (probably) really easy thing with the word processor, and she says: "Dad!! Use a text box!"

The preceptor: "What's a text box?"

D # 2: "Here, just get up and let me show you." Eight lightning moves follow, a nice box or line drawing (as below) appears, and I'm still in the dark. Nice drawing, but still in the dark. I never did that to my parents, not once. Except that time with the cable box.

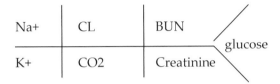

 Right – this is the little electrolyte drawing gatsy, which makes it easy to remember the values that you want to write down someplace quickly, like on your scrub pants. This is one of those doctor-ish things that nurses hate, but actually (like lots of other things) it isn't hard to learn at all – seven items? And you use them all the time anyhow, or most of them anyway – and it makes things easy to write down.

Let's take these guys one at a time, and please remember that all this info is strictly "from the hip" - I mean, you can keep on going and going with this stuff, and pretty soon you're an endocrine fellow or something. So all this stuff is "with a lot of lies thrown in", as they say.

1-1- the basics: "Chem 10"

1-1-1: Sodium/ Na+ (135 - 145 meq/l):

Sodium is confusing – like lots of things in the physiology world, it doesn't always do what you think it's going to do, or what you want it to do. I guess lots of things are like that. In fact, the motorcycle ...ow!

The basic idea is that sodium is a solute, floating around in the serum solvent. If Izzy Shmulewitz has a TIA, and lies on his bed for three days before his no-good bum of a son-in-law comes to check on him, he's going to get very – what? Very dry – dehydrated, mostly from "insensible loss" - I think that you lose something like a liter and a half every day this way, mostly through breathing and sweating. And that's when things are normal – imagine what happens to marathon runners. No wonder they don't look so good at the end. "Pruned."

Anyway, if some of the solvent goes away, that leaves more solute in what remains, correct? So if you measured Izzy's sodium before his TIA, it might've been something like 138. After three days of not drinking anything, it might be in the 150's. Too high! All sorts of unpleasant things can happen – seizures, drain bamage, renal failure (why?), and so on.

Here's a formula for figuring out exactly how dry they are (the water they should have, but don't have, is the "Free Water Deficit". No screaming now – I know it's math, but it's not so bad.

Free Water Deficit = (0.6 x pt's weight in kg) x [(pt's sodium / 140) –1.0]

So let's try it in steps: say the patient weighs 70 kg, and his sodium is 160 (oof – he's dry!)

First step: 0.6 x 70kg = <u>42</u>

Step two: His sodium is 160, divide that by 140, that gives 1.14. Subtract 1.0 from that, you get <u>.14</u>

Last step: 42 x .14 = 5.9 liters. Call it six liters. That's about 13 pounds.

That's a lot of liters, in case anybody's counting. Try it sometime.

What about other way? What if Shmulewitz turns out to be one of those people, (like my dad), who insists on drinking eight glasses of water a day? And what if his doctor puts him on a diuretic, say twice a day for his swollen ankles, because he won't stop drinking them ("Gotta flush the kidneys!")?

(This next part is probably mostly lies, but it was explained to me this way once): it turns out that the loop diuretics make you dump not just potassium, but all the other cations that float around dissolved in the serum : sodium and hydrogen come to mind. (In fact, whenever you hear the word "diuretic", you should immediately respond in your head with "K^+!". Check the patient's creatinine before you give any. Why?)

Apparently people dump enough sodium in urine in response to diuretics to cause a significant drop – actually, I was told that you pee half-normal saline. What if you now replace the lost volume with pure water – tap water, or bottled? No electrolytes in it at all. You can see what's coming, right? - having dumped lots of sodium, Izzy now takes in lots of solute, and both of these maneuvers make his sodium drop a whole lot. If the solute levels get too low, water may start moving into the third space ("Head for the third space, Mr. Spock." One eyebrow goes up: "Um, captain, can I pee first?"). Gatorade! (Who is that Picard guy, anyhow?)

(Losing a lot of hydrogen can produce bad things too – several days of diuresis will usually produce an alkalosis, because it leaves a lot of bicarb floating around with no hydrogen dancing partners – they all got peed out. Because the patient's fluid volume has "contracted", they call this a "contraction alkalosis". Easier to call it a "diuretic alkalosis", but no…)

"Third - spacing" of fluid into the brain tissue in response to hyponatremia can result in a rising intracranial pressure. I hate it when that happens – all sorts of unpleasant things can result, right? Including, possibly, herniation. Ack! Quick now – what's the first sign of rising intracranial pressure?

Back to the patient. So – what to do? <u>Hyper</u>natremia usually means that a lot of circulating volume has been lost – give some back! <u>Hypo</u>natremia? - got too much volume going around? Restrict fluid intake for a few days and the patient should straighten out. Might want to give some hypertonic saline, usually as 3% saline, in case overdiuresis or something has caused too much sodium loss.

Now comes an extremely important thing. Try very hard to remember this. Can anybody pronounce the following?: **"Central Pontine Myelinolysis"**. This is a truly awful result of **too rapidly correcting a hyponatremia**, in which crucial parts of the pons (in the midbrain, is it?) **become de-myelinated**. Stripped. Leaving the patient possibly quadriplegic, possibly comatose, possibly (shudder) "locked-in". Oh yeah, and maybe dead. Possibly preferable.

Let's say that again: **central pontine myelinolysis happens when hyponatremia is corrected too quickly.** Apparently it is **entirely avoidable**. The way we do it nowadays is: treat the patient **cautiously** with IV fluids. The team will have all sorts of groovy calculations to do here involving weight, renal function, age, and probably the color of the socks the patient was wearing on admission - but the main thing is that the **sodium must not be corrected faster than one mEQ per hour.** Or maybe **half** that. Which means **sending electrolytes every hour**. Make out those slips!

1-1-2: Potassium/ K (3.5- 5.0):

Critically important, especially for the heart. Take a look at the section below on "cardiac labs" for more on the subject of electrolyte repletion.

Remember a couple of things:

- Potassium can be tricky to give. It's very irritating to the stomach – nauseated patients will not be able to take it po. A conversation I heard once involving a young doc:

    1- Nurse: "I'm not sure you want to give this patient potassium by mouth y'know, he's got an empty stomach and doesn't feel too well."

    2- Doc: "How else could we give it?"

    3- RN: "Well, he's only got peripheral IV access, so we can only give him 10 meq per hour in a dilute mix of eighty in a liter – that's 125cc/hour. You could put in a central line to give less volume."

    4- Doc: (appalled) "But we have to diurese him! He's in CHF, and the fluid overload is causing increased hydrostatic pressure to progress retrograde from the LV into the pulmonary circulation of the whangbang kabam and the elang badoodang doodah day!"

    5- Outcome: the patient vomited his potassium. Got a bed bath and a central line.

    - IV potassium can only be given at fixed rates. Peripherally (try to avoid this, since you can really injure someone's arm if this stuff infiltrates) we can give it as described above. Centrally we can give 20meq per hour. Take a look at the article on "Peripheral IVs for Beginners" to see a really unpleasant example of a peripheral infiltration injury…

- IV potassium <u>must</u> be delivered on a pump. No exceptions. If it goes in too quickly, as with many drugs, **disaster may result**.

- Keep an eye on the patient's creatinine – a failing kidney will not excrete potassium at a normal rate, and your patient may end up with a K way higher than you wanted. And if it looks like your patient is heading into renal failure, you might not even want to replete a low K at all.

i- What does "hemolyzed" mean?

When you draw a blood spec, it's important to try and remember that you're actually sending off a bunch of red cells that are swimming around in serum. Often we get our lab specs from arterial lines - if you were to manually pull really hard on a blood gas syringe, pulling the red cells through the stopcock, lots of the red cells would break, or burst. Hemolysis. Poor little red cells. Anybody remember the phrase "chief intracellular cation"? Everyone still asleep? This is actually important – the most prevalent positive ion inside the cell is what – anybody remember? Potassium.

When you send off a blood spec for chems, the result you get is actually from the serum (which is why they call them, um, serum chemistries. Doh!) Not from <u>within</u> the red cells. A normal serum potassium level will be something like 3.5 to 5, right? What if all the little red cells get busted – hemolyzed - as the blood spec is drawn? All their intracellular potassium gets to come out and mix with the K that was already in the serum, maybe doubling the result that you get. I'm not sure how they know it, but the chem lab will often mark the results as "hemolyzed" so that you don't jump out of your skin when you see a K of 8.3... Sometimes I think a spec gets "sort of" hemolyzed, although it won't say so on the results – maybe the stat chem result will be 5, and the one from a blood gas will be 3.2 . I think this is probably because people draw the gas specs more gently (the only way, right?) than the suction does in the vacuum tubes.

ii- A Hemolyzed Potassium Story…

Here's a quick "hemolyzed K" story, which is also an example of How Things Are Not Supposed To Be Done… it's also a bit gossipy… anyhow: I follow this nurse I don't know, who's given me report on her patient… and it's immediately clear that this is one of those people who just aren't doing things right. The transducers are both a foot too high, the patient is a mess, the IV lines are every whichy way with tubing still plugged in from meds given 6 hours before… and the patient is having a LOT of ectopy. The counter is saying 40+ pvc's a minute, couplets… and yes, the nurse mentioned seeing them. She also mentioned diuresing the patient a couple of times during the day, but that his K was "fine – it was 4.1". Doesn't sound right. I look in the computer – the result is clearly marked as hemolyzed…

Now I'm pretty mad. Not only is the patient a mess, not very well cared for, not only are the transducers totally out of whack, giving totally wrong cvp numbers – and she was diuresing the patient based on them? But the K result from the computer is CLEARLY marked as hemolyzed. Which means what? That the TRUE potassium is what? A LOT lower! And look at all that ectopy, and couplets and stuff! Holy smokes … with ears steaming, I send a repeat spec, drawn gently, manually, from the patient's arterial line (why?)… any bets on the result? **Two point seven**… why was I so angry?

1-1-3: Magnesium: Just as important as potassium in keeping the heart happy. Skip down to the section on cardiac labs, at **1-6-2** for more on this.

1-1-4: Chloride (95 – 105 meq/l):

Reader, sadly here your preceptor fails you. I don't know hardly nothing about chloride, except that if a patient is fluid resuscitated with many liters of normal saline, (and each of those Na's carries a little Cl along with it), the patient can develop "hyperchloremic acidosis". Of course there's a zillion and a half other things that I'm sure you ought to know about this ion, including the fact that hyperchloremia seems to show up in most metabolic acidosis's, but your preceptor has totally dropped the ball on this one. (Hangs head in shame. Then - remembers motorcycle. Happy again!)

1-1-5: Bicarb (22 – 29 meq/l):

This is a confusing one for those of us who only remember biochemistry as a bad memory. And I have a really bad memory in general. Bicarb is also described as carbon dioxide, probably because they associate with each other in the carbonic acid reaction – I seem to remember arrows pointing both ways, indicating that the reaction could go forwards and backwards. (At the same time? I had a car like that in nursing school.)

The important thing is that this number, whether expressed as serum bicarb or as serum C02 (<u>not</u> **pCO2**, which is something else), indicates the amount of bicarb present in the blood, available as "buffer".

This gets into acid-base balance, which I think is going to require an article of it's own! Meantime, take a look at the section below on "Anion Gap" – yeah, like I understand that stuff – under "Respiratory Labs".

1-1-6: BUN (10- 26 mg/dl):

"Blood Urea Nitrogen" represents the amount of nitrogenous waste in the blood, which is supposed to be cleared by the kidneys. The BUN number always travels accompanied by its partner **1-1-7: creatinine (0.6 – 1.3 mg/dl),** but it's the creatinine number that is actually telling you directly how well the kidneys are working, since a rising BUN by itself can just indicate dehydration, just like a high sodium can. (A high admission hematocrit can be a clue too. Also the prunelike appearance. Then, again, some of us just look that way at baseline. Sigh.)

The thing to remember is that it's the **creatinine** that indicates if the kidneys are in trouble or not. High is bad. Someone told me once that if the creatinine increases by one whole number, it represents the loss of a third of the patient's kidney function, which means you can't do that very often!

So look at the BUN and creatinine as a ratio: normal would look like 12/ 1.0, right? A high BUN with a normal creatinine means a dry patient whose kidneys are still okay – if she gets hypotensively dry, her kidneys may become unhappy as a result of being under-perfused. Something like BUN of 70 with a creatinine of 1. High ratio. If the creatinine starts to rise, then real trouble is coming, because the kidneys are getting into trouble at the tissue level, maybe in the form of acute tubular necrosis, never a picnic. Might look like 70 / 3.0 – higher numbers, lower ratio. Comparison is everything, so take a look at a couple days' worth of chems and see if the creatinine has been going up, down or sideways.

Something we've noticed over the years: it seems as though alcoholic patients come in with very low BUN numbers, like 4 or 6. Somebody's opinion was that alcoholics will often drink instead of eating, so their muscle mass isn't very good, so they don't make as much BUN as the rest of us. Something to think about when your patient comes in unconscious and you're waiting for the tox screen to come back…

1-1-8: Blood glucose (70 – 115 mg/dl):

This is where I hope I don't get into trouble – I was diagnosed with Type 2 DM a couple of years ago, and I'd really like to keep my kidneys, if it's all the same to everyone else. This has given my kids an excuse for pulling various kinds of food right out of my hands, with the look of a teacher catching a kid eating, uh… candy? I wonder where they learned that?

Tight glucose management has gotten a whole lot of recognition lately as critically important in managing really sick people. It turns out from the studies that all sorts of things happen for the better if a patient's glucose is kept under tight control – as a result we've started to use insulin drips a whole lot in our MICU. Apparently everything is affected, from wound healing to recovery from septic infection, to length of stay, etc. We run insulin drips at rates of something like one to ten units an hour, checking glucose with either chems to the lab or glucometers every two hours, with a goal range of 80 to 130.

Sometimes, despite the closest monitoring, insulin-drip patients get low. Hard to know why, maybe their tube feeds didn't absorb when you turned them in the bed or something. The drip gets shut off, and the patient either gets a half or a whole amp of D50…

DKA patients obviously come under the frequent-glucose-check category. These people often require changes in IV fluid treatment every couple of hours, and we check their electrolytes every two hours. We don't use the same protocol though – DKA people get NPH somewhere along the line, while the others may or may not.

i. Acetone (positive or negative):

A DKA patient's need for insulin does <u>not</u> go away once her blood glucose comes down. Ketoacids can hang around for a long time afterwards – maybe another 12-24 hours, I think, and the acidemia they produce is NOT a happy thing. Continued insulin treatment is what will help the patient cook off the ketoacids, so once the glucose gets down to a reasonable level, the IV hydration fluid usually changes from something like normal saline with some K to something like 5% glucose with K – the glucose keeps the blood sugar <u>up</u> now, while the ketoacids get fixed by the insulin drip, <u>which continues to run</u>. Lately they've started using NPH when the glucose numbers get down towards normal. I wonder if the whole setup could be simplified by giving the patient a dose of lantus insulin on the way in the door… someone want to do a study?

We check the acetone level every four hours until it goes negative. You'll (hopefully) know that the situation is improving anyway, since the serum **pH (7.35 – 7.45)** will be improving. We had a DKA patient come in a day or so ago with an initial pH of 6.90 – yow!

The serum CO_2 / bicarb will improve, too – these patients come in sometimes with bicarb numbers less than ten.

ii. HbA1C (3-6%):

This is a nice test to know about – otherwise known as glycosylated hemoglobin, it actually indicates the overall trend of a person's glucose over the three month period before the spec gets drawn. They can also work out a mean glucose value for that period – with a value of 6.0%, my mean glucose came out as something like 108 – not too bad. Nice to know that the pills are working… we'll see what my kidneys have to say ten years from now. We don't use these much for acute management in the ICU, but it's good to know how the patient has been doing.

1-1-9: Serum Calcium (8.5 – 10.5mg/dl):

Let's see if I can get this right. Calcium binds tightly to proteins that are floating around in the serum, so the serum calcium number reflects that, and varies as the protein level (measured as albumin) goes up and down. There are formulas to figure out the "corrected" calcium - they factor in the numbers that your patient may show if she comes in, say, malnourished. A person's serum albumin can drop drastically in the first couple of days after admission to an ICU, and since proteins are what holds "water" in the vasculature, peripheral edema and third-spacing will start to develop. Start those tube feeds early.

i. **Ionized Calcium: (1.0 – 1.3)** This is the calcium that isn't bound to protein – it floats about in the serum. We follow these a lot with patients on CVVH, which rapidly sucks electrolytes out of the blood – these patients usually have a calcium drip running.

ii. **Corrected Calcium:** Since serum calcium measurements are affected by the patient's albumin level, you have to figure in a correction if the albumin is off. So – for every drop of 1gm/dl of albumin, you need to add 0.8 to the serum calcium number that comes back from the lab. The point is that your patient's calcium may higher than the uncorrected number would make you think. This is the kind of thing that gets very important when you have a patient whose calcium comes back high in the first place, like people with bone mets.

iii. Calcium changes in citrate toxicity:

This one comes into the picture with CVVH. Let's see if I can get my head around this one. It turns out that calcium – in this case we're talking about free, ionized, unbound calcium, is critical to several steps in the coagulation cascade. Who knew? Think I remember that stuff from nursing school, back in the early Cretaceous Era? No way! Dinosaurs – now those, I remember! One of them taught OB.

Citrate in solution **chelates** free ionized calcium – soaks it up, binds it up, removes it from activity – you get the idea. Citrate mix is used more and more often nowadays to keep the CVVH machine from clotting itself up – they call this "regional anticoagulation".

So - citrate is normally rapidly cooked off by the liver, also the kidneys. The end product is apparently bicarbonate.

If the liver and/or kidneys don't, or can't metabolize the citrate, then it hangs around, binding up the free, loose calcium. The ionized calcium number goes down. Hypocalcemia. Dangerous. Citrate toxicity. Bummer. Strangely enough, the <u>total</u> serum calcium number <u>rises</u> in this situation – citrate binds to calcium, right? It forms a citrate/calcium "complex", apparently taking the ionized stuff and binding it up. So the total number may rise, while the ionized number falls.

Anyhow - what to do? Patients in liver failure – maybe hepato-renal failure - sometimes can't metabolize the citrate, and the clue will be that rapidly falling ionized calcium number. At this point we would probably change to a different replacement fluid, usually bicarb based. Bicarb-replaced systems are infamous for clotting up, but if your patient is in enough liver failure to produce citrate toxicity, she's probably auto-anticoagulated enough that she'll anticoagulate the machine as well! Otherwise we might use a low-dose heparin drip into the machine circuit.

1-1-9: Phosphorus (2.6 – 4.5 mg/dl):

Pretty important stuff, phosphorus – remember ATP, ADP, those guys? Renal failure patients often get very high phos numbers, since they can't clear it, and they take meds like calcium acetate ("Phos-lo"), or Renagel to bring it down.

Sometimes patients with poor nutrition will come in with really low phos's, maybe less than 1.0, which we replace with 10 – 30 millimoles of either sodium or potassium phosphate IV, which has to be given slowly on a pump over the better part of a day. There's an oral form too ("Nutra-Phos"). Maybe we could come up with a new product: "Nutra-Phos-Lo" – that would either replace or remove itself, depending.

(What's that supposed to mean: "Husbands should be like that…"?)

Turns out that a low phos can severely affect the strength of the diaphragm. Apparently absolutely true. So that's why Mr. So and So can't wean from the vent!

1-2: Some other basic chems:

1-2-1: Lactate (0.6 – 2.2 mmol/l):

Okay – everybody remember the definition of a shock state? I mean besides how you feel after work. Three parts to a blood pressure: pump, volume and squeeze - three shock states: cardiogenic, hypovolemic and septic. Right? All three produce low blood pressure. Low perfusion to the peripheral tissues, which switch from aerobic to anaerobic respiration. The byproduct (the "exhaust") is what? Lactic acid. More is bad. This lab helps you figure out why your hypotensive patient is so acidotic, although you should probably be able to guess. Higher is worse. Nurses with a year or so's experience in the unit will look at each other in real worry when they see a lactate of 10.

A high lactate and a high potassium can be a clue that something has died inside your patient. Bowel-infarct patients do this – it's classic, and a critical early sign. (Why does the K rise when this happens?)

1-2-2: Osmolality (280 – 295 mOsm/kg H20):

Cute units, huh? ("Yo Einstein! Nice units!") Almost as good as "dynes/sec/cm^5", which is what measures SVR and PVR and the like. This lab becomes very important in the case of increased intracranial pressure – the whole point is to try to keep the brain from swelling up, and treatment is with mannitol, which pulls fluid out of the vascular, fluidy brain by osmosis. Remember, making the blood hyperosmotic means that water will move out of the cells, right? – and into the bloodstream, from where it gets diuresed out. The goal for mannitol treatment is usually to keep the serum osm above something like 310. Dry.

Used to be we'd mannitolize them, and sit them up in a high Fowler's postion, which we called "keeping them high and dry" – nowadays I don't think they do that any more. Ask! You never cross the same river twice… practice changes all the time.

1-2-3: Amylase (23 – 85 units/l):

Units of what? Amylase usually rises with it's cousin **1-2-4: lipase (0 – 160 u/l)** when patients develop pancreatitis. Painful. It seems that in recent years the numbers of these patients going to the OR has really dropped – I guess many of them do better if left alone for a period of time. There's a whole staging process for pancreatitis that I don't know much about. Ranson's scale?

1-2-5: Ammonia (11 – 35 mcmol/l):

(All the experienced ICU nurses give a big sigh when they see this one.) Ammonia is one of the nasty substances that accumulates in the blood when the liver doesn't work – makes people encephalopathic. Some of us are like that even without the ammonia. These folks often have a level in the 200's or higher, and treatment involves inducing lots of diarrhea with lactulose. (It really does seem like karmic revenge…)

Make sure that you warm up the duoderm on the rectal bag before you put it on, and it'll stick much better – I put it under my arm while prepping the patient's, um, "area". Use a razor if you need to. Remember that benzoin really hurts on sore skin.

1-2-6: Albumin (3.7 – 5.0 gm/dl):

Very important for a couple of reasons – first, albumin is a main indicator of your patients' nutritional state: low is bad, normal is good, too high – never heard of. An elderly person can get into albumin trouble in a couple of days without sufficient nutrition, so get the tube feeds going as soon as possible.

Second: albumin is a main constituent of blood protein, right? This is what maintains oncotic pressure in the blood vessels – if this drops, then the patient will start third-spacing all that nice IV fluid you've been giving her to keep her pressure up. And if all that fluid leaks out of the vessels, will it help her pressure?

1-3: Renal Labs

1-3-1: Creatinine Clearance (90 - 130ml/min):

This is another name for the glomerular filtration rate – the normal rate at which blood is filtered through the kidneys. Low is bad – the kidneys are unhappy. Creatinine clearance can also be calculated and predicted when patients are on hemodialysis or CVVH. Higher is better, although the numbers are probably different for machine filtration.

1-3-2: Uric Acid (4.1 – 8.8 mg/dl):

Too much of this gives you gout, and also accounts for some kidney stones. Holy smokes – mine wasn't much fun last year, although I did get my first-ever IV morphine. Wow – worked really well. They tried IV ketorolac first, which did squat.

1-3-3: Myoglobin:

You don't want to see this show up – it's an indicator for muscle damage, much the way CPK is, except that it's **extremely** nephrotoxic, and is what damages the kidneys in rhabdomyolysis. Turns the urine an interesting color. Think about a bicarb drip, which helps protect them. Anybody know how that works?

1-3-4: Urinalysis:

We send off tons of these – and they give back a lot of information. Some of the main points:

- Color: "straw colored" is always nice. Blood – not so nice, but we have fun with the descriptions: "Oh, it's a nice rose today, but it was definitely merlot yesterday." Drugs like rifampin and pyridium can produce a really nice orange Gatorade color. Methylene blue can make urine a nice teal green. ("Ya tink dat's teal? Nah, you dope, dat's like, aqua! Totally! Ha! Hey Ralphie, dis guy tinks dis color heah is teal, ha ha!")

- Turbidity: is there stuff floating around in it? Casts maybe? Fungal clumps? – time to ask about an Ampho-B irrigant even before the culture comes back. (You sent both UA and C&S, didn't you?)

- pH: very important sometimes, as in rhabdomyolysis, where large-scale muscle destruction releases lots and lots of myoglobin, which will show up in the urine, assuming the patient is making any, since the stuff is so nephrotoxic. The pH of the urine is kept above 7 with a bicarb drip.

- Specific Gravity: higher means more concentrated, lower means more dilute.

- Sediment: any there? Any idea why?

- Blood: shouldn't be any.

- Bacteria: 0 - 1/ml
- WBCs: 0 – 3/ml

- Glucose: none. (Yes, I take my glucophage, and no, I don't check my blood sugars often enough. Grrr.)

- Ketones: also none.

- Nitrite (indicates that bacteria are present): shouldn't be any.

1-3-5: 24 hour urine collections

We do these sometimes to evaluate creatinine clearance, and sometimes to measure the excretion of metanephrines – I think that's right. When your patient is hypertensive, tachycardic, and there's just no clear answer why, they'll want to rule out a pheochromocytoma – a functional adrenal tumor, that sits there secreting pressors. (How do you think they invented pressors, anyhow?) Some of these have to be collected in iced bottles, sometimes with acid in them – the smell is rather impressive.

1-3-6: Urines for electrolytes

I can't say that I know how to interpret these very well, but the point of sending these is to try to figure out how well the nephrons are working. Let's see… if the urine sodium is low, that means the kidneys are holding on to sodium… so that means… the patient is dry? And the kidneys are holding onto water with the sodium? Which all assumes the kidneys are working…

Correspondents? Anyone want to look into this one for us?

1-4: Drug Levels

These definitely come under the heading of "chems", and we follow a lot of levels in the unit. We do a lot of dose adjustment for renal failure – digoxin and vancomycin are good examples. The list below was created using the most sophisticated technique available: "Oy Kathleen! What do we send levels on?"

1-4-1: Dilantin (Total: 10 – 20mcg/ml):

You should definitely know this one. Dilantin turns out to be one of the drugs that floats around in two forms like calcium does: free and albumin bound, the free drug being the active part. In general, it seems that following the total number is usually okay, but changes in the serum albumin will change the bound levels of the drug, making more or less of the free stuff, um, free, or actively available, as in renal or liver disease states. Nurses tend to let the physicians worry about calculating corrected levels – it's seems strange though to come across some dosage that they calculated, that comes out to something like 27.32 mg IV q 41 hours. Or something like that. **Free dilantin** is supposed to run around **1.0 – 2.0 mcg/ml.**

1-4-2: Valproic acid (50-100mg/l) We don't do these too often.

1-4-3: Tegretol Also not too often.

1-4-4: Lithium Rarely, we'll see an OD. Does it need to be dialyzed? I forget…

1-4-5: Theophylline Hardly ever any more, but this was a real big mover "back in the day".

1-4-6: Thiocyanate (goal: < 30 mcg/ml) This is a cyanide byproduct of nipride – anyone on a drip for more than a day should probably have these levels followed. Nasty.

1-4-7: Vancomycin (30 – 40mcg/ml) Watch the BUN and creatinine.

1-4-8: Gentamicin (4 – 10mcg/ml) Also watch the BUN and creatinine.

1-4-9: Digoxin (0.8 – 2.0ng/ml) A range you should know. That's <u>nanograms/ml</u>. Got to hurt to do that one in the lab…a digitalized patient with acute-onset renal failure may show up with a level up around 5 or 6 - dangerously high. Go look up "Digibind".

1-4-10: Tacrolimus (10-20ng/ml) and Cyclosporine (100-300ng/ml)

Tacrolimus is apparently something like a hundred times more powerful than cyclosporine. Nice! Both these drugs can become toxic in renal failure (uh… transplant working?) – so they need adjustment based on weight and BUN/creatinine… apparently the dosages also vary somewhat depending on which organ has been transplanted. MICU nurses probably have a pretty unrealistic view of transplantation – most of the patients we see with them have come in because they're failing…

1-4-11: Peaks, Troughs, and Randoms:

There seems to be some confusion about peak and trough levels. Here's the way we do it: the <u>trough</u> gets drawn <u>first</u>, just <u>before</u> a scheduled dose, when the level should be <u>lowest</u> (the trough of the drug-level graph.)

The <u>peak</u> gets drawn about 45 minutes <u>after</u> a scheduled dose ends, when the level should be <u>highest</u>.

<u>Random</u> levels are just that – they're drawn without any relation to the timing of the doses. We follow a lot of random vancomycin levels, because we have a lot of renal patients who can't clear it – we say the dose just keeps going round and round…

1-5: Tox Screen Panel Meds, with toxic ranges:

1-5-1: Tylenol (5 – 20 mcg/ml) Patient have a nice bronzed look?

1-5-2: Salicylates (>500mg/l) Ears ringing?

1-5-3: Opiates (usually represented as "present") Breathing? What's Narcan?

1-5-4: Cocaine ("present", or if you're in the service: "Ho!") Apparently it's important to remember that cocaine hangs around in the urine longer than it does in the blood. One reference we looked at said that the drug reaches peak excretion renally about six hours after a dose.

1-5-5: Benzodiazepines ("present") What's flumazenil?

1-5-6: Ethanol (toxic> 300 mg/dl, often reported as % of total blood volume, legal limits often 0.08%): I found a conversion: a level of .08% supposedly equals a level of 80mg/dl, and .3% equals 300mg/dl. Can this be right?

Some toxic ingestions can be handled with dialysis – apparently all the alcohols can be removed this way, although we usually treat **ethanol** overdoses with intubation, and then let them "cook it off".

A short flame: Where is it written that we have to put patients with DT's on benzos to detox them in the ICU? Why in the world don't we just prevent the whole DT thing with an appropriately dosed ethanol drip, then transfer them to detox, and do it the easy way?

1-5-7: Methanol (toxic > 20gm/dl)

Another member of the alcohol family – "wood alcohol", I think they used to call it. Methanol ingestion patients seem to be so desperate for something alcoholic that they'll reach for anything that even resembles it: antifreeze, paint thinner...you'd have to be pretty thirsty. Methanol is converted to a couple of nasty metabolites: formic acid ("Ralphie! I told you not to eat that whole box of chocolate-covered ants!"), and formaldehyde.

Treatment is way cool: giving the patient ethanol will actually displace the methanol in the metabolic pathway – the bad stuff then cooks off slowly and non-toxically. Once in a while we get a glass bottle of – is it 10% ethanol? – up from pharmacy and hang it at some carefully calculated rate that factors in the weight, age, gender, and probably the renal function of the intern ordering it...

1-5-8: Ethylene Glycol: ("Ethylene! You stay out of that glycol! Don't <u>make</u> me get the hose!")

Another dangerous substance found around the house, also appearing in antifreeze, brake fluid, etc. Treatment consists of ethanol, dialysis, and buffer in the form of a bicarb drip. We saw this recently, and it turns out that the lethal dose is – want to guess? 100cc...

A really important point: ethylene glycol is sweet, and your dog or cat will definitely drink it up if it appears in a puddle under your car. I think that there are alternative antifreezes around.

1-5-9: Miscellaneous other things that show up on a tox screen, among many, (usually reported as "present"): **cannabinoids, phencyclidine** ("angel dust"? – I remember a story about a "dusted" patient who pulled his hands right through his handcuffs...), **amphetamines**, **antidepressants** (some of the older ones are very toxic), **oxycodone** (somebody really must've had a lot of time with nothing to do when they figured out about crushing oxycontin and sniffing it. What, did they try everything else in the cabinet before they got to that? Colace? "Hey Ralphie, try one of these!")

1-5-10: A really cool thing:

A completely off-topic but totally neat maneuver popped into mind at the thought of someone sniffing a colace capsule – Jayne taught me this cool thing if a kid (hopefully a kid) shows up with some interesting item inserted in the nose: mom (hopefully mom) puts her mouth over the kid's open mouth, she holds the kid's nostril closed with a finger (hopefully a finger, and not another M&M, or marble, or whatever it is that's plugging the first one), blows with appropriate pressure into the kid's mouth, and with air pressures doing what they do, the item should expel. Ha! Better than calling in the forceps team.

That Jayne – she's a smart one. Thirty years together now, next August.

1-5-11: A scary story.

Wow – this one was really something else. Patient comes in, about 30 years old, with a really unclear recent history. Mild mental retardation, maybe a history of pica as a child – not sure. About 350 lbs. This person was amazing for a single fact: he had no blood pressure. In the middle of trying to figure out what the HECK was the matter with him, we the most incredible struggle trying to measure his blood pressure – it simply was NOT there. On top of this, he had "cryptovascular syndrome" – I made that up – we could NOT access his blood vessels. Someone had managed to get some kind of femoral line in him at some point before he'd gotten to us, and we ran EVERYTHING through that one line until we risked losing it, and rewired it for a triple lumen. That sort of solved one problem – but there we were, running around the unit, getting dopplers, large BP cuffs, running around the bed, cycling noninvasive pressures on his upper arms, forearms, upper legs, lower legs – getting BP readings once out of every three or four cycles, maybe, on tons of pressors, all really low readings... what a scene. And NOBODY could hit an artery for either a blood gas, or to place an arterial line... and I mean, we TRIED! Our resident team guys tried, anesthesia came up and tried, the other anesthesia guy came up and tried, our attending tried, all the while on (straight drips) of levophed at 100mcg/ minute, neo at 1000, dopamine at I forget... finally we got a BP cuff to read on his left forearm, I think it was. Terrible BPs – and a venous blood gas from the femoral line showed a pH of 6.9 something. Yowza!

All this while – NO idea what in the WORLD is causing this hugeous crash, although theories were abounding: meningitis maybe? Not an MI... didn't seem to be septic – no fever, no white count... and then a family member mentioned, finally, that he'd eaten... what? HOW many tubes of toothpaste? Three?

Well... it was quite a night. Surgery finally came up and actually did a cut-down at the bedside to place an arterial line – something I've seen done exactly once before in 20 years – they draped and prepped his wrist, dissected that sucker out, inserted a catheter, sewed it in REAL good...

and the BP was terrible! And finally we got an ABG – and the PH was still 7.03! This is about five or six hours along now…

So we did all the things you'd think of to correct the badness – we ran a bicarb drip, we tried to run CVVH to clear the acidemia – then the stupid catheter kinked, as so often in large patients, and the system went down within an hour… ran HUGE amounts of pressors, ran in ENORMOUS amounts of crystalloid… and I staggered home that morning, at the end of my twelve hours, left a trail of clothes, and face-planted on the bed. Woke up at about 3pm, called Katie to see what had happened…

He was fixed! Hey – don't ask ME what happened! Fixed! Better! He was awake! Moving the extremities! He'd WEANED OFF THE PRESSORS! All this in eight hours! Extubated the next day, left the unit the day after that!

Fluoride poisoning. The attendings were amazed. I was amazed. It was the quickest, MOST amazing recovery from the MOST profound crash that I think I'd ever seen. Pretty sure it was going to be written up for the journals…

1-6 - "Cardiac" labs

The whole point of drawing labs is to get information about what your patient is doing. The first part of cardiac assessment is the patient's rhythm: is he in sinus? Something else? Sinus with ectopy? More ectopy than before? Less? What labs might you think about in this situation? Probably…

Electrolytes first.

1-6-1: Potassium (3.5 – 5.3 meq/l):

Everybody pretty much knows about the importance of K when it comes to issues of cardiac irritability. It turns out that **1-5-2: Magnesium (1.3 – 2.4 meq/l)** counts just as much. (New people, try to remember that the mag thing is still an innovation for us ancient nurses – be patient with us, we'll get it eventually. I still haven't gotten over reaching for lidocaine when my patient has a run of VT. Speaking of which – what should I be reaching for?)

Here's a question – how are you going to give your patient a dose of potassium? Orally? On an empty stomach? What if your patient's been vomiting? (What kind of cardiac event might he be having?) Not orally? How about IV? How dilute does the K have to be – you might have to give 10 meqs per hour through a peripheral vein, in a pretty large volume to keep from burning a hole in the patient's arm. But what if the team doesn't want to give volume – maybe they want to diurese the patient instead? Well, could you mix it with lotion and rub it on his back? How are you going to solve this? (Go back and look at **1-1-2**.)

The effect of repleting electrolytes can be really impressive: lots of ectopy may simply go away.

The other thing to worry about when giving K is the kidneys – these guys usually excrete potassium at a fairly constant rate; if they're failing, they won't. So if your patient's BUN and creatinine have been rising, and his K is 3.2, what should you do?

Magnesium also turns out to be the treatment for "polymorphic VT", which is either the same as, or first cousin to Torsades de pointes. You'll see cardiologists tell the teams to keep a patient's K greater than 4, and their mag up around 3…

Cardiac Enzymes

1-6-3: What are cardiac enzymes?

This is the myocardial infarction thing. The idea is that destroyed myocardium releases specific substances into the blood, which can be measured – nowadays they call these the "serum cardiac markers".

1-6-4: Which cardiac enzymes do we follow on our patients?

For a long time we followed creatinine phosphokinase levels: "CPK"s, and we still send them, but recently we've started sending troponin levels as well, and these are pretty much the standard now.

1-6-5: Can a patient have elevated enzymes without having an MI?

Well, see, that's the thing. It turns out that almost any situation that causes muscular injury – almost anywhere in skeletal muscle or the myocardium – can cause a CPK bump. Apparently not, however, for troponin, which only shows up in myocardial injury.

1-6-6: Can a patient have an MI without having elevated enzymes?

I don't think so. You read about people having MI's without developing q-waves – maybe because the events are physically very small – but I don't believe that a person can sustain a muscular injury to the heart without releasing some amount of enzymes.

1-6-7: What is CPK again?

CPK is released into the blood whenever there is a muscular injury somewhere. Non-cardiac injuries will release CPK: defibrillation, surgery, trauma or seizures – even IM injections. CPK begins to pop up in the period roughly 4 - 8 hours after an event, and starts dropping 48 hours out.

1-6-8: What is the reference range for CPK?

Our lab uses a reference range of 60 - 400 units/ liter. I know that I've seen patients "rule in" with a peak CPK "inside the range" – say, in the 300's – but the thing is that they show up positive for **MB isoenzymes**, which indicate specifically that the CPK release is coming from myocardial tissue. They would presumably be troponin-positive as well.

1-6-9: What are isoenzymes?

It turns out that different muscle tissues produce different sub-species of CPK when injured, which can be measured and expressed as a percentage of the total amount of CPK that's been released.

1-6-10: What is the "MB fraction"?

"MB" refers to the sub-species of CPK isoenzyme that gets released from <u>cardiac</u> muscle after an injury occurs – an MB percentage higher than 3% is a "rule in" for some kind if cardiac injury. MB isn't always diagnostic of an MI specifically, since other situations can cause tissue injury to the heart: cardiac surgery, or defibrillation, or even chest compressions during CPR - you get the idea. You might see a rise in CPK/MB in a patient whose chest had struck the steering wheel, producing a "cardiac contusion"…everyone reading this has a seat belt on, right? I wear mine in the shower, but hey, that's just me.

1-6-11: What are MM and BB?

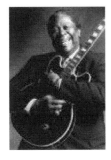

It's been a while since I even saw these used, but I think that MM is the CPK isoenzyme that gets released in skeletal muscle injury, and BB is the one released when brain tissue infarcts. Does that mean that brain tissue is structurally muscular? (Mine isn't. Wish it was.)

1-6-12: Does a higher CPK mean a larger MI?

That's the idea – but you have to make sure that you're looking at the right kind of CPK. If the MB isoenzyme forms more than 3% of the total number, then that points to cardiac tissue as the source of the release. A person who's been knocked off a bicycle by some dope opening his car door might have a result in the thousands, but if the MB "iso" wasn't there, then you'd have to say that the CPK "bump" came from skeletal muscle instead of the heart.

During the Crimean War, Flo and I used to call a small MI a "subendo": sub-endocardial, meaning small, and not all the way through the muscle wall ("transmural"). This kind of event usually went with a CPK peak of something less than a thousand: 400, 500 maybe. I think these are the MIs that nowadays are often called "non q-wave" events, because the muscular injury isn't big enough to generate the dreaded evil q's.

Big MI's on the other hand are pretty unmistakable – you may see CPK peaks of 3 - 4000 or more, with an MB fraction – well, what would it have to be? 3% (or more) of 3000 – um…well, one percent would be 30, right? So 3% would be 90? So if the MB number came back at something like 300, that would be 10% - definitely a cardiac event. Pretty big one. Q-waves for sure.

1-6-13: How many CPKs should be drawn, and how far apart?

We usually send three CPK specs, eight hours apart. If a cardiac patient has some sort of complicating event later on – say a spell of a-fib, or maybe recurrent pain, then we'll probably send another three sets to see if there's been another injury. (A small CPK release is called a "leak", and a really small release is called a "leaklet".)

Remember that CPKs are going to go way up in any situation that produces skeletal muscle injury, but the situation that really makes the numbers get scary is **rhabdomyolysis** – which I think got mentioned somewhere earlier. This is a pretty dangerous scenario that shows up sometimes when someone's been lying on the floor, say, for a couple of days without moving – maybe intoxicated, maybe after a stroke, something like that. We've seen CPKs get up into the range of 100,000. Pretty high.

1-6-14: What is troponin?

It turns out that there's an even more sensitive test for myocardial injury, and her name is troponin. There are three types of troponin: CTnI, CTnC, and CTnT, which is the one we use (we call it "troponin-t").

It turns out that troponin is a really sensitive and accurate indicator of myocardial injury, which makes it preferable to CPK, since you can get knocked off your bike three times a week and not release troponin until the frustration makes you have an MI. Troponin is a definitive indicator for non-q-wave MI; there's no confusion about whether your CPK bump is coming from your broken arm or from the chest pain that you got when that idiot opened his door in front of you for the fourth time this month.

Troponin also stays elevated for something like a week after an MI, so someone who comes in four days after his event - when his wife finally convinces him that he doesn't look so good - will still have diagnostic levels to prove what's going on. Just didn't want to miss the post-game show, y'know.

Nothing's perfect though, and other conditions besides MI can make troponin rise: renal failure can cause the only "false elevation" of troponin that we've heard about. Other causes of troponin release: an episode of CHF, and obviously any myocardial injury besides an MI will do it too: cardiac contusion, defibrillation, myocarditis, ablation (that's where they burn out the WPW thing in the EP lab, etc.), but the important point is that there's no confusion as to the source of the enzyme release. They say that troponin may replace CPK testing entirely sometime soon.

1-6-15: What is the reference range for troponin?

Our range is 0.00-0.09 for "normal". Anything above 0.10 is considered a "rule-in" – here's a quick example: we had a patient whose CPK came back at 184, with an MB of 5.1. If you calculate it out, the MB turns out to be 2.8% of the total (5.1 turns out to be 2.8% of 184. I realize not everyone is as stupid as I am with numbers, but it always helps me to say things several times.) So the MB fraction is a hair under 3% - maybe not an MI? But the troponin at the same time was 0.14 – strictly speaking, a "rule-in". The next set of enzymes showed a CPK of 440, with an MB fraction of 4.4%, and a troponin of 0.19. Helpful. Definitely a little MI.

1-6-16: How often should troponins be drawn, and how far apart?

We send troponins and CPK/MB's on the same schedule – it's the same red-top spec, every 8 hours times 3.

1-6-17: What is "washout"?

This is a "reperfusion" phenomenon that you see when a patient gets clot-busted. Visualization exercise, okay?: everybody see the little clot that's plugging the coronary artery at the narrow spot? (No Ralphie - the <u>heart</u>. The big red thing. No, the one that's <u>moving</u>.) There isn't much gas exchange in the tissue beyond an arterial plug, or exchange of anything for that matter, and CPK will accumulate downstream in the ischemic tissue which is not quite dead yet, but will be soon, if the clot doesn't get busted. If perfusion is suddenly restored, all that CPK gets blown out into the circulation at once – if this occurs within the 6 hour "window", then the affected area of myocardium will hopefully be saved, and the CPK bump will only indicate the transient injury, instead of tissue death. Close one!

What else might you expect during a reperfusion period that might make you a little nervous?

1-6-18: Can cardiac enzymes go up if a patient is ischemic, but not having an MI?

CPK /CKMB may not rise after an ischemic episode, but troponin does in about a third of patients, raising the theory that "micro-infarcts" are occurring. "Angina producing necrosis." Bad prognostic sign, worse than if there's no troponin release.

1-6-19: What is hBnp all about?

This is pretty cool – let's see if I remember this right. It turns out that the ventricles produce a – hormone, is it? A "natriuretic factor"? (wooo…), which helps the ventricles to pump. An inotrope – sort of like an internally produced dobutamine. And that they release this stuff to help themselves pump in times of stress. So – patient comes in, short of breath. You do an EKG, maybe he's had an MI in the past. No new ischemic changes… yeah, he's an old smoker. Well – is it CHF? Or a CHF flare?

Send the BnP. If the ventricles are unhappy, as in a CHF episode, then the BnP will be really high – because the ventricles are stressing, right? And in a COPD flare, they won't… smart!

The ranges we found in one reference were: normal patients, < 100 pg/ml, and patients with LV failure, about 500 pcg/ml. A patient in CHF might have a result in the 30,000's.

1-6-20: What is C-reactive protein all about?

We see this lab get sent now and then. This one looks at inflammation – is it a sytemic indicator of chronic inflammatory things going on? People with higher CRP's: >3.0 mg/ liter, have a higher risk for nasty cardiac events. Lower: <1.0 mg/ liter seems to be better.

1-7: Lipids

A **lipid profile** is made up of a number of tests:

1-7-1: total cholesterol (<200mg/dl)
1-7-2: HDL (30-60mg/dl)
1-7-3: LDL (<190mg/dl)
1-7-4: Triglycerides (<180mg/dl)

We send these as part of the workup on cardiac admissions, and oftentimes our patients get a daily dose of one statin drug or another, but we don't follow them much as a matter of course. One exception: patients on propofol get a <u>lot</u> of lipid from the emulsion that it's made of – sometimes the lipids are removed from their TPN as a result.

We had a patient a while back who had some kind of incredible congenital hyperlipidemia – I forget what the numbers were exactly, but there was a white sediment in his blood spec tubes. Scary.

2- Respiratory Labs:

Obviously the main topic here is blood gases. There's more than you probably ever wanted to know about blood gases in the faq on "Vents and ABG's", so take a look over there for details, but we can take a quick overview:

2-1: ABGs:

2-1-1: pO2 (80 – 100 mm Hg) :

This is the good stuff – this is what you're trying to deliver. A rough rule of thumb that's often helpful if you're trying to figure out how your patient's doing: the pO2 should be something like four or five times the FiO2.

Example: right now, you're breathing room air, which has an FiO2 of 21%, right? And if we stuck you for a blood gas, your pO2 should be something like 80-100, which is roughly four or five times the FiO2 number. So if you intubated me, put me on 100%, and stuck me, my pO2 would be upwards of 400. I hope. The point is, the next time someone tells you how great it is that your patient has a pO2 of 80, and they're on 100% and 10 of PEEP, you'll know that 80 is actually really very low, compared to where they ought to be. Hypoxic. Remember: "oxygenation" means just that: how well the blood is getting oxygen delivered from the alveoli.

2-1-2: pCO2 (35 – 45 mm Hg):

This is the bad stuff, the stuff you're trying to get rid of. "Exhaust gas": comes out of the tailpipe. (So if you use Red Man in your pipe, and you exhale blue smoke, does it mean you need a ring job? As for me, just make me a DNR – I had a cracked block last year anyhow. It's that diabetes, man.) Too much pCO2 and the carbonic acid reaction goes the wrong way – respiratory acidemia results. Get <u>rid</u> of too much and the reaction goes the other way – respiratory alkalosis.

Remember that "ventilation" refers specifically to how well your patient is clearing C02. Different conditions often produce specific effects on blood gases: patients in CHF will usually be hypoxic, but won't have much trouble ventilating. Pneumonia patients are the other way – they may oxygenate fairly well, but they don't ventilate good. Correctly. Properly. Whatever.

Remember that a pCO2 in the sixties can "narcotize" a patient… "Jeeze, he looks narced to me…", and will NOT be breathing much…

2-1-3: pH (7.35 – 7.45):

pH tells you lots of things, and it takes time to learn how to put it in the right context. Just looking at it from the respiratory standpoint, the pH will change as the pC02 does, except in the opposite direction: if pC02 goes up, pH goes down, and vice versa, roughly .08 for every ten points of pcO2 away from 40. So, all other things being equal, a pCO2 of 50 should give you a pH of 7.32, down .08 from the ideal pH of 7.40.

What if the pCO2 was 50, and the pH was still 7.40? What then? What does it mean if a person is a "chronic retainer"?

2-1-4: Bicarb (22-29 mmol/l):

The range for this one is "the age you'd like to be". (Thanks, Laura!) Bicarb is the buffer that floats about in the serum, counterbalancing the carbonic acid. (Something tells me that there's a little more to it than that…). The kidneys do the job of either holding onto bicarb or dumping it, as blood pH conditions change – it takes three or four days to come to a new stable state.

2-2: Venous Blood Gases:
2-2-1: Can I believe what a VBG tells me?

Well – think about this for a second. In a VBG, the oxygen is going to be.. what? High, or low? Low – right – because it's on the "extracted" side – the oxygen has been extracted by the tissues… so that's not going to look good. And the pCO2? High or low? High – yes… because the venous blood is carrying off the CO2 as exhaust gas, right? So that's not going to look good either… and the pH? Hmm… the pCO2 is high… so there's going to be more carbonic acid… so the pH is going to be low… see? – VBG's just don't look nice.

But sometimes they're all you've got to work with. No arterial line? Can't get an ABG, no matter how hard you try to stick the patient? Yeah, you can send a VBG… just remember that the oxygen will be low, the CO2 will be high, the pH will be low… but if the pH on the VBG is still 7.3ish, then you know at least that your patient isn't horribly acidotic… can be useful.

2-2-2: What are central venous sats all about?

This has to do with tissue extraction of oxygen. We follow these when we're looking at early, goal-directed management of septic patients. The number is read off a sensor built into the patient's central line, at the distal port, like the one on a PA line – except this one's a fiberoptic sat sensor, instead of a thermistor. Or a ther-Mrs.

Anyhow - if the number is low – and they want it to be around **70%** - then it means that either the tissues are extracting too much oxygen, being all stressed, or that they're not getting enough delivered in the first place. So – is the patient's crit ok? Might need more carrying capacity. Is the patient all dilated centrally, but clamped down peripherally, making lactate? Tank em up. Is the patient's heart being affected by the sepsis? Happens… throw in the swan, check the output. Low? Think about dobutamine to increase the output… I personally hate that last one, as these patients are already tachycardic, and even saying the word "dobutamine" in the room can put them into rapid AF… have they ever tried milrinone instead? The whole idea seems dumb though…

Radical idea of the week – how about just leaving them on 100% FiO2 for the first day? One day won't kill em…

2-2-3: What's the difference between a central venous sat and a mixed venous sat?

Skip this one if you get dizzy easily…

Someone's dissertation probably hung on this one. Used to be there were hugeous arguments about which central saturation number to believe – which one told us the most about the post-extraction saturation: a spec from the RA/ SVC – that's to say, one from the tip of a cvp line; or one from the tip of the distal port of a PA line, way out in the PA?

Lots of arguments about this… including the fact that the number from a CVP line spec will actually be LOWER than one from the PA, which seems not to make sense… but then they explain that blood from the SVC is more oxygen-extracted than blood from the IVC, because the brain uses up a TON of oxygen… so the blood mixed together from BOTH VC's, reaching the PA, will actually have a slightly HIGHER saturation… jeeze, it makes my head spin.

I ask 'em which one they want, and that's the one I send ☺

2-3: Carboxyhemoglobin (bad effects show up anywhere from 10-30%, serious effects >40%):

This is a scary one. Carbon monoxide just loves hemoglobin so much that it will push oxygen out of the way just to take its place on the Hb molecule – that's to say, it "binds preferentially", and is rather a bear to get rid of. All that CO-saturated hemoglobin (that's the "carboxy" part) is <u>not</u> carrying oxygen around – it would sort of make sense that if 40% of your Hb was saturated with something besides oxygen, then bad things would ensue. Duh. Ever read "Coma"?

Treatment is so cool: serious exposure cases go into the hyperbaric chamber, and are sent "down" to a depth of whatever number of atmospheres, as though they were going down in a diving bell, or being treated for the "bends". Pressurized. ENT has to come in and puncture the patient's eardrums to prevent tympanic rupture. Hyperbaric oxygen is apparently really useful in preventing bad things like neurological sequelae. I hate it when those happen!

Hyperbaric also turns out to be the thing to do when your patient has the "flesh - eating bacteria" – the group A streptococcal infections that are so scary. They're apparently anaerobic, and making a patient incredibly hyper-oxic is just the thing to kill them off. Neat!

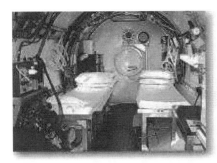

Big one!

2-4: Methemoglobin (goal: <4%):

This is another substance that likes to bind to hemoglobin and that can interfere with oxygen delivery if too much of it accumulates. This one appears when inhaled nitric oxide therapy is used for pulmonary hypertension. (Not <u>nitrous</u> – ha ha! – why are my feet so big? Hmm, that's a big drill…) Too much methemoglobin: bad. I've never seen it happen.

2-5: What is an anion gap (10-14 mEq/l), how do I calculate it, and why is it listed here under "respiratory"?

Acid-base involves everything. After thinking about it, and thinking about what to put in this section, I decided to leave it here under the heading of "respiratory" because the part of acid-base that you're probably going to work with first is the ventilation kind – but remember that the non-respiratory, the metabolic components, are just as important to think about. So maybe this will help you keep them both in mind.

Calculating an anion gap is supposed to help you figure out what's going on with your patient's acid-base balance thing. "Why the hell is he so acidotic?" Or alkalotic. There are "gap" acidosis's, and "non-gap" acidosis's.

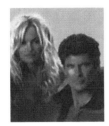

A little-known fact: acid base balance analysis was developed on the beach by the two eminent Bay Area nephrologists Anderson and Hasselhof, in the Anderson-Hasselhof equation.

(Now that IS geek humor…)

After talking about the gap, I'm going to confess that I don't use it myself. Never having learned a lot of the horrible chemistry, etc. that lies behind the ways the physicians analyze these situations, I tend to rely on experience, and I can usually come up with something helpful that way. There are a few main reasons why you're going to see your patient become acidotic or alkalotic, and they'll become very clear to you inside of your first year's time in the unit:

> ### 2-5-1: Acidoses:
>
> - He's <u>gained</u> some acid:
>
>   1- Did his pCO2 go up? (How does that make acid?)
>   2- Is he "shocky"? (How does that make acid? Send a lactate.)
>   3- Has he been running the marathon? Again? Send a lactate.

4- Is he in renal failure? There are a couple of kinds of "renal tubular acidosis".
5- Is he in DKA? (How does that make acid? Send the ketones.)
6- Has he gotten 12 liters of normal saline today? (Can someone explain hyperchloremic acidosis to me? Change this guy to Ringer's Lactate already!)
7- Has he been poisoned? Too much aspirin?

- He's <u>lost</u> some bicarb:

  1- Does he have an ileal loop? They can dump bicarb like mad. Sodium, too.
  2- Profound diarrhea? They, uh… dump bicarb like mad.
  3- Has he been climbing mountains and taking too much Diamox? (Dumps bicarb in the urine. Hey, it could happen! And monkeys could…never mind.)

2-5-2: Alkaloses:

- She's <u>lost</u> some acid:

  1- Has her NG tube been putting out liters and liters a day? (Losing HCL?)
  2- Has she been over-ventilated? (How does that make an alkalosis?)
  3- Has she been diuresed for several days running? (Loop diuretics make the kidneys dump H+ ions as well as potassium. Acid loss, right?)

- She's <u>gained</u> some bicarb:

  1- Has she been getting into the family-sized antacids again? I never go to the warehouse stores any more.

Let's take an example of the thought process: a patient comes in, intubated, history of COPD, maybe having a flare, they put him on a vent at 100% FiO2, rate of 12, tidal volume of 600, 5 of PEEP to hold things open. You send a gas, and here it is:

(pO2 / pCO2 / pH / bicarb):   325 / 40 / 7.56 / 39.

Well – you can turn the oxygen down, that's for sure. PCO2 looks good – right on the ideal number. But what's up with the pH? Wicked alkalotic, as we say in Boston.

Hmm – look at the pCO2 again. That's okay. So this isn't a respiratory thing. So what does it have to be? Got to be a metabolic thing. Look at the bicarb – way high. Definitely a metabolic thing.

Actually, this is a pretty common scenario for COPD people: they walk around with a pCO2 around 50 most of the time anyhow, right? – hence the saying that they belong to the "50/50 club" – meaning their pO2 and pCO2 are both usually around that number.

If you sedated me, say with 0.5mg of morphine (I'm a very sensitive individual…wiping tear away), and made my pCO2 go up to 50, what would my pH normally do? Anybody remember the rule? If the pCO2 changes 10 points, the pH changes .08 – so with a pCO2 of 50, my pH would be… 7.32.

But this guy walks around with a high pCO2 all the time. COPD people never fully exhale, that's on account of they're obstructed, right? Chronically? In the pulmones? They "air trap" – so they never really get rid of their carbon dioxide effectively.

His baseline gas would be something like 50 /50/ 7.40 – how come is that? I mean, why does he have a normal pH?

It's on account of he's compensating – remember compensating? And how does he do that? By holding onto bicarb with his kidneys – look: his bicarb is wicked high. Compensated.

So what happens when he comes in, and you tube him? He's probably been in trouble for a couple of days – his pCO2 has been even higher than usual, and his kidneys are just a-hangin' on to every little bicarb molecule that goes by, and he's doin' okay, keeping his pH fairly normal, but his pCO2 goes up a little more, and a little more, and then bam! Narced. Stops breathing, almost. Gets tubed.

So okay – we tube him, and we ventilate him, and we "blow him down" to a normal pCO2. But by this time he's saved up so much bicarb over the past couple of days that he's got this enormous reserve of it floating around in his blood – so if we blow him down from his pCO2 of about 75 that he's been compensating for all this time, what happens to his pH? <u>Wicked</u> alkalotic.

So – what to do? Well, he'll re-equilibrate in a few days – it takes three or four days for the kidneys to straighten things out again (assuming that they work). Or we could let his pCO2 rise some, which would normalize his pH some. Or we could give him diamox for a day or two, to make him dump out some of that bicarb. But somebody better figure out what pushed him into trouble – pneumonia, COPD flare, CHF, whatever - and treat that at the same time, yo!

2-5-3: Calculating the Gap:

The preceptor had to go look this one up. (Hanging head in shame – the preceptor can't calculate an anion gap?)

Here's a formula: the Anion Gap = (serum Na^+) - (serum chloride + serum bicarb).

In English, this turns out to be the difference between the main serum cation, that being sodium, minus the sum of the main serum anions, chloride and bicarb.

- So: the calculation itself turns out to be easy: take the level of the main cation, sodium - let's say it's 135.

- Now the sum of the two main anions: chloride and bicarb, let's say 100, and 25. Add those up: 125.

- So what's the difference between the sodium and the total of the negatives? 10?

- That's the gap. A normal gap is 8-16. (mEq/liter).

- An example of a "gap" acidosis would be one produced by high lactate – also I think DKA's and some poisonings do it. The gap number gets large – ooo, scary. Then when things get better, the intern will look up from the sheep's entrails – I mean, the computer – and tell you, as if he'd invented the earth: "See, the gap is closed." Now we feel better…

As usual, my explanations will not be the same as those you get from your medical teams – and they probably shouldn't be. Current book-knowledge is exactly what they're supposed to have, and bedside experience is what you and I are supposed to have, and we're supposed to put those together – it often works out very well!

2-5: Alpha-1 antitrypsin

Worth mentioning. This is just really unpleasant. People who don't make enough of this, for genetic reasons, are prone to emphysema, even if they don't smoke. Occurs in something like one in 500 people. These folks apparently get severe lung disease just by reading tobacco billboards…

3- Liver Function Tests

3-1: A story.

A story goes here – just skip this part if you don't want to go off on a sidetrack for a while. I'm not sure how to tell this – if there aren't any numbered questions I get disoriented. It was one of those rare experiences that have made a permanent impression in my memory (and there's not much room in there.) It's lots easier to describe VT – "just the facts, ma'am". (Young people: who said that?) This is harder.

Some years ago – maybe ten?, a gentleman came into the unit with this rare liver thing: "sclerosing cholangitis", which is apparently one of these conditions that can be managed for a while, but which are never cured, and which kill you in the end. The bile ducts become spontaneously inflamed, sometimes they close and have to be stented open. Transplant didn't seem to be an option in his case, and I think that he was in the unit that first time because he had an acute obstructive jaundice that they were trying to treat with stenting procedures.

I have a terrible memory for some things. Maybe that's just a trick my mind plays on me, since I can apparently remember "escape - capture bigeminy" without much trouble, and how arcane is that? Very. House officers will come back as juniors into the unit a year after their intern month – I'll remember the face, usually not the name, and embarrassedly sneak over to the photo list to quickly check – then act like I never forgot it… but I won't forget Charles Mifune (not his name): name, face, case, or family.

I usually ask the same set of simple questions by way of getting to know a new patient – entering a room under the assumption that I may have to do something unpleasant to, or with, someone that I've never met before, I usually will give a nod, and say "Mr. Yakowitz?". You have to be careful to watch how far to extend yourself in this situation – a patient may show you in the first seven seconds that he wants you to stay in his room for the next three hours, and the job being what it is, you have to evaluate time limits right away. Or not. There's a lot of variation.

I was quickly impressed. Mr. Mifune had a surprising natural dignity, which is something you read about – here it was for real. I could never call him Charles – there was something in me that had too much respect for the man, which only grew as I got to know him, to allow for familiarity, no matter how many times I cleaned him up in the bed. But there was no lack of mutual affection either – he liked me, I liked him, maybe because we saw similarities of personality – which means he probably never got a really good look at me, anyhow! He was of Japanese descent, and seemed to embody some qualities that I think of as Japanese, mixed with some American ones: he was reserved, but friendly – there was no social barrier – his whole life had been lived in an American context. He seemed quietly disciplined. Apparently from a poor working background in Hawaii (he used to take his wife on walking dates to an ice-cream stand before they married), he couldn't afford law school, and so became a postal worker until retirement. I think his wife had worked on a pineapple plantation. They'd had something like six children – all of whom seemed to have absorbed his work ethic. I found out later that they had all worked and scholarshipped their way through college – they would gently tease their dad, copying things he'd sternly said to them in the past about homework…and they laughed about the cheap ice-cream dates. I thought they were some of the best dates I'd ever heard of.

The discipline with which he'd raised his family seemed to be of a piece with his personality – who really knows? But it seemed that way. The man carried himself through a really arduous set of tests and procedures with patience, quiet humor, and simple fortitude – and go watch a few ERCP's if you think this stuff is easy, although I hear that they go more smoothly now than they used to.

His wife seemed to share the same kind of personality. She would sit quietly in the room, exchanging comments with her husband while I would draw labs, or start an IV, or hang meds, always present, always very concerned. They seemed to be best friends, used to helping each other. They seemed to be grounded in reality, probably from all that walking, back in Hawaii. She took him home.

Eight years later. We'd moved to a new location – our shiny new ICU, which was nice-looking for sure, but I always thought we did a pretty good job in the old one… and back came Mr. Mifune. The ancient Rolodex that still holds the primary nurse assignments reliably coughed up my name, and I came in to find myself assigned to a patient that I actually remembered. They were very happy to see me - I guessed that they associated me with the time that he'd gotten better. Now things were obviously worse - he looked terrible: jaundiced, thin, big belly, tired. And calm, and sad, and brave. He was back in the unit to see what might be done.

It took a couple of weeks, as I remember it. There was always some family member in the room – usually Mrs. Mifune herself – she hadn't changed: still showing that same sense of restraint, mixed with a totally American sense of humor. And the same feeling of grounding in reality – as if there had never been a TV in their house. They knew what was coming, and they were quite prepared for it, thanks. No hysteria, no screaming, no throwing themselves to the floor, no shouting, or threatening of hospital staff. They were ready.

As jaundice worsens, so does confusion. Bilirubins rise, LFTs rise, ammonia rises, treated with lactulose – we know what that does. Even confused – and I think he was almost unique in this way – Mr. Mifune always remembered who I was. He would gently rouse from his sleepiness and say, a little startled, "Hi Mark!" He never became combative, although he did forget where he was. He would accept our answers to his confused questions, and he would always help turn himself in the bed when he needed cleaning up.

I got to know some more of his family members. One son was angry – not at us, not at the hospital – angry at fate, he was, and he knew it. He would look furious –when I could, I'd bring him a coffee and we'd talk. Mr. Mifune had had relatives and friends who'd been in the 442nd Regimental Combat Team – the Japanese-American unit that lost so many men running uphill into live fire from Monte Cassino in the dead of winter, in 1944. I actually knew about this a little, since my son has a jones for the History Channel, and we like to sit together sometimes on the couch and watch. Did I ever get a grin from the patient's son when he realized that I had heard of that unit!

Charles died, quietly, sleepily, probably very comfortably, and I was there. Mrs. Mifune, crying, hugging me hard, said "You were here at the beginning, and you were here at the end. We were so glad." I had no words. What a privilege. I want to be Mr. Mifune when I grow up.

3-1-1:

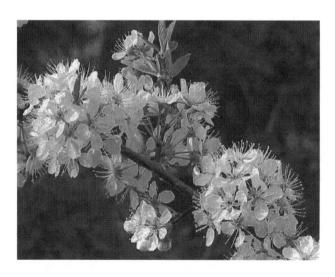

Deep breath. Okay - back to liver function tests. Anybody else need the tissues besides me?

From the point of view of a preceptor, I should say that I don't look at liver function tests as much as I ought to – all I want to know is: are they rising or falling? – since they generally move in a group. ("This way, group!")

(I guess it's clear that humor is my coping mechanism, huh? Better than skydiving, I guess. Cheaper insurance, too.)

The notes here are based on some quick reference checks – anyone with a correction to make, please send it along? It turns out that the ratios of one LFT to another can indicate what your liver-failure patient's underlying problem could be: tissue based maybe, or obstructive. These diagnostic problems don't usually turn out to be something that I worry about when my goal is to keep the patient alive overnight – unlike knowing the difference between rapid a-fib and VT. I find myself checking the PT and PTT much more frequently in liver-failure situations, along with ammonia checks to see if the lactulose is working. Another clue is that the patient wakes up – but that's an assessment detail that I leave to the experts. (grin!)

A couple of the main LFTs:

3-2: Bilirubin, direct (0 – 0.3mg/dl) and indirect (< 1.0 mg/dl):

Let's see if I have this right. Bilirubin is metabolized in the liver – conjugation, they call it. ("I am bilirubin, you are bilirubin, he is bilirubin, they was bilirubin…") Bilirubin has to be conjugated so that it can be eliminated (mostly) in the bile, and (a little) in the urine.

Direct bili is the part that has been conjugated, and the indirect bili is the part that hasn't. The **total (0.3 – 1.9mg/dl)** bilirubin is both of them added together. Basically what I remember is that the normal numbers are very low – anything greater than 1.0 in either one makes me look twice.

An example of how I might use LFTs at the bedside: we had a patient not too long ago, I think mentioned elsewhere in this article, who had taken a really impressive amount of acetaminophen and then waited to come in until she'd absorbed most of it from her gut. This is your basic bad liver situation – you can almost hear the freight train of liver failure bearing down on your patient, who is stuck on the tracks. I think that the LFT specs aren't usually sent more often than qd, but certainly this patient's LFTs are going to be high, and going to get higher quickly – just a matter of time until she starts becoming jaundiced. (Where does the patient become jaundiced first? Yes, Hermione?) Time to call transplant.

Some others:

3-3,4: ALT, AST:

(I think these are the new names for what I used to call SGOT and SGPT). These reflect liver cell damage or death, as opposed to obstructive problems. ALT is apparently the most specific to the liver.

3-5: Alkaline Phosphatase:

("Geez, would ya look at this guy's alk phos rising?") This one seems to be more related to problems in the biliary tree itself.

3-6,7: PT/PTT

For sure the PT and PTT are indicators of liver failure – when the patient is really in trouble, as in maybe thinking pre- transplant, they're often on continuous FFP infusions to supply the clotting factors that the sick liver can't make.

Update: nope, no more continuous FFP drips. Apparently you want to give your patient his FFP's all at once, in a shot. Works more better.

3-8: SPEP: This test separates out four of the proteins made by the liver to see whether there's not enough, or maybe too much of one kind or another: albumin (hold on to that – you need that), and the alpha, beta and gamma globulins.

3-9: Hepatidites (I guess "Hepatitis's" isn't the right word...)

3-9-1: Hepatitis A
3-9-2: Hepatitis B
3-9-3: Hepatitis C

Well... we know about these. Tons of material out there – these guys are pretty unpleasant, virally transmitted hepatic diseases that you really don't want to acquire while working with patients who have them... as always, you should use universal precautions, acting as if ALL patients were carrying some disease that you didn't want to 1- catch yourself and 2- spread around the hospital. Wear the gloves.

4- Hematology

They still call the basic hematology spec the **Complete Blood Count (CBC)** – we'll take the parts one at a time.

4-1: Hematocrit (36 – 46%)

A hematocrit tells you how many red cells are floating around in the serum. The number is reported as a percentage because of the way the test is done – they spin the spec tube in a centrifuge, and the red cells settle to the bottom – if the tube is half-full of red cells, then the "crit" is 50%. If it's a third full of red cells, the crit is 33%. The crit number will definitely go up and down as your patient de- or re-hydrates, and a dry, debilitated person admitted with a normal number may show you that he actually lives really low once he gets "tanked up". Renal failure patients can fool you that way. (Why do renal failure patients run chronically low hematocrits, and how is that treated?)

A crit drop after aggressive hydration is called "dilutional", which is clearly not the same as a "delusional" crit drop, which is where you think the crit has gone down, but it hasn't. That's the kind I have. I think.

The rules for transfusion have really changed over the past few years, and patients are often allowed to run with numbers that would have made us very nervous in the past: low 20's sometimes. It turns out that transfusions are dangerous – well, um - I think we knew that. But the statistics are clear: more patients die if they're transfused than if they're not. This does <u>not</u> mean that you shouldn't get a ton of blood set up for your big GI bleeder – but the lady in room 92 who's just a slow vent-wean may not need to be kept at 30 the whole time she's in the ICU.

4-2: White count (4.5 – 11 thousand/cc): Defenders against evil. There's a number of different kinds, (determining how many there are of each is the **4-2-1: differential**), and there's a basic breakdown of the types in the faq on "Blood and Transfusion": T-cells, B-cells, helper cells, polymorphonucleates, basophils, esosinophils…a few things come up with some regularity in the unit:

- Total number: higher usually means something bad is going on infection-wise. Watching the number rise and fall from day to day isn't always very meaningful – it can vary a lot from day to day without a real change in the patient's status. Watching the trend over several days is helpful. Steroids will make your patient's white count rise.

- "Bandemia": Bands are immature white cells – if their numbers rise, it means that the marrow is cranking them out rapidly, probably in response to a bacterial infection. Developing bandemia is also sometimes called a "left shift" – having to do with the way the cells sort out, I guess. Sounds like when your kid joins the anarchists and starts living in a tree… just like dad did!

- **Eosinophils:** Sometimes you'll see an order for this when the docs are trying to figure out if the patient is having a drug reaction – usually a drug fever or rash.

4-2-2: "It's a bad sign when the white count is higher than the crit." Yup… bad.

4-3: Platelets: (130 – 450 thousand /microliter): Microliter? One millionth of a liter? Pretty small volume for 130 – 450 thousand of anything to swim around in, but I guess they're right – why did I always think that it was per cc? Definitely important – can't clot without these - don't leave home without 'em. We transfuse plates for low counts if patients are actively bleeding or if their count drops below 20K, although that number seems to change at times. Does anybody know - why do platelets come in six-packs?

The problem with giving repeated platelet transfusions is that they don't work very well after the first few – it's an antibody-mediated thing as I recall. I remember giving "HLA-matched" platelets in the past, but we don't seem to do that nowadays. Are they pre-matched now? I have no idea.

4-3-1: Heparin-Induced Thrombocytopenia (positive or negative)

We definitely see patients come up positive for this one now and again. Usually the lab gets sent twice; if a patient's count has dropped drastically over a day or so, we change our line flushes to normal saline and start sending the specs. Stop the sq heparin too, and get out the air boots.

H2 blockers can also really hurt your patient's platelet count, which I understand is why we don't see cimetidine around anymore – we used to give that stuff like water. We use ranitidine now, apparently much better, although still on the platelet-problem list to some degree.

4-4: Coagulation Studies:

4-4-1: Prothrombin Time/ PT (10-14 seconds)

4-4-2: PTT /partial thromboplastin time(normal 20 – 40 seconds, therapeutic 50 – 70 seconds)

4-4-3: INR /International Normalized Ratio (normally 1.0 – therapeutic 2.0 – 3.5)

We still send the "coags" ("co-aggs") the way we used to: the PT and the PTT, but in recent years the INR has become a standard part of the coag report, replacing the PT – newer nurses look at me blankly when I ask what their patient's PT is. In amongst the horrible complexity of the clotting cascade there are two anticoagulation paths that we follow: the PT/INR (coumadin therapy) represents one of them, PTT (heparin therapy) the other.

Sometimes you'll see a patient come in who may have gotten a little confused about his pills at home, with a PT greater than 50, an INR greater than 20. That's pretty anticoagulated. These people often show up with GI bleeding of one kind or another, sometimes with spontaneous bleeding in the head. Ugly.

4-5: D-Dimer (normal <250 micrograms/liter):

D-dimer turns out to be about having clots: it's a material released by the degradation of fibrin, which means that there's a big clot process going on somewhere. Iraq, maybe. D-dimer will pop up if a patient has a DVT, a PE, or in DIC, when supposedly zillions of little micro-clots are being formed. D-dimer is part of the **4-6: DIC screen**, a raft of labs that goes off in two tubes, iced, and includes the coags, a d-dimer, and other measures of clot activity including **4-7: fibrin split products (normal is < 10gm/ml)** – if the FSP is high, then a lot of clotting (and clot breakdown) is going on, as in DIC.

4-8: Fibrinogen (200 – 400mg/dl): Another part of the DIC screen. This is one of the proteins in the clotting cascade – if a patient is in DIC, then fibrinogen gets used up rapidly by the disseminated clotting process – which is to say, its titer goes down. Helpful in making the diagnosis.

4-9: Erythrocyte Sedimentation Rate (0 – 20mm/hour)

I don't see as many orders for these specs as we used to, but they still crop up. This involves measuring how rapidly the red cells in a spec tube settle towards the bottom in the space of an hour. Apparently it isn't diagnostic by itself, but it's used as an indicator for the presence of lots of different kinds of inflammatory processes, MI, or tumor activity. Used in monitoring arthritis, maybe? I've never gone looking up a sed rate on one of my patients and gotten upset on getting the result. If the cells fall faster, the inflammation is worse – as a patient responds to treatment, the cells fall more slowly. Anybody know why?

4-10: Coombs Test – Direct and Indirect:

Direct Coombs testing is an auto-antibody-vs-RBC test. Indirect Coombs tests are used by the blood bank in determining possible reaction to transfusion. Is the one pre-transfusion, and the other for detecting reactions? Pretty obvious I don't know much about these, and while we do send them off, we don't make much use of them at the bedside. Make sure you check blood products properly! (What would you do if you thought your patient was reacting?)

5- ID:

5-1: Cultures: blood, urine, sputum, stool, CSF (Did I miss any?)

We send a lot of cultures – maybe too many, they tell us. We get routine culture reports back in one day, finals in three, and the results include **5-2: sensitivity reports** as to which antibiotics the bug is sensitive to. These are starting to get scary of late – we had a patient recently whose decub wound was colonized by acinetobacter (say that three times quickly) – the report came back something like this:

Vancomycin: RESISTANT   Methicillin: RESISTANT   Metronidazole: RESISTANT
Gentamicin: RESISTANT   Cefuroxime: RESISTANT   Penicillins: ` RESISTANT
Cefazolin: RESISTANT   Amikacin: PARTIALLY RESISTANT
Linezolid: BETTER NOT BE!

You get the idea. Wash your hands.

5-3: A couple of specific tests:

- **5-3-1: TB/AFBs**: we send three sputum specs for **AFB** (Acid-Fast Bacillus). Smear results come back within 24-48 hours, and the culture specs are usually held for something like 8 weeks.

   There is a variation on the TB theme called mycobacterium avium (MAI, or MAC) – this also produces a positive result on AFB smears, and makes people nervous until the result comes back more specifically. MAI colonizes immunodeficient people – you see it in AIDS patients sometimes, I think.

- **5-3-2: Influenza**

   Couple of kinds. Wear a mask within – what is it? Six feet of the patient? Get your shot.

- **5-3-3: H5N1 Avian Flu**

   Haven't seen it. Hope we don't. Could get very ugly. Have some ice cream every day. Hug a puppy.

- **5-3-4: HIV testing/** We send these sometimes. People come in, they have opportunistic infections, it's important to know. We don't give the anti-retroviral drugs much – I'm not sure why. I know we see people with AIDS a whole lot less now than we used to 20-odd years ago.

- **CD4 (T-cell count) (500 – 1500/ml):** trends are the key – lower counts correlate with progression of HIV.
- **5-3-5: Viral Load:** Another part of the HIV test panel: usually reported as high, intermediate or low - depending on the test method used the numbers are variable. Jayne says that with the protease inhibitor cocktail some patients' levels come back "undetectable". Cool.

- **5-3-6: CMV – (presence of antibodies and/or the virus)**

  Opportunistic viral infection. Pregnant nurses? Check up on this one – I think the last guidelines we saw said that universal precautions do make it safe to care for these patients

- **5-3-7: RSV**

  I think this one is detected by viral cultures. RSV itself is not the danger to the pregnant nurses – it's the ribavirin that we treat them with that's really very dangerous to the babies…

- **5-3-8: Herpes cultures**

  We send herpetic cultures sometimes – the lesions show up orally on some patients, and I think they hang around for about a week – less if treated with topical and maybe systemic acyclovir. Once in a while a CSF culture will come back positive, diagnosing herpes encephalitis – not fun.

- **5-3-9: Branch-chain DNA and PCR, "polymerase chain reaction":** These are two methods used to "provide more evidence" when the cultures aren't definitive. I understand that PCR is used to replicate DNA material nowadays to help identify organisms that might otherwise not show up in the dish. Very cool.

- **5-3-10: Kary Mullis:** Another interesting thing about PCR is its inventor: the scientist who won the Nobel Prize for it named Kary Mullis. He's apparently fond of surfing, and thought up the PCR idea while driving on the California highway in his Honda Civic. (With or without his boards?) He won the prize, but his parent company apparently got the rights to PCR, which they sold for some $30 million. Oh well – back to the surf for the next idea.

- **5-3-11: Lyme Disease and Babesia**

  People have heard about lyme disease, but babesia is the same kind of thing, except different. Treated with atovaquone? Lyme can <u>really</u> be a bear…

5-4: CSF: It seems like most of these specs are drawn to rule out one kind of infection or another, so ID isn't a bad place to put them, although there are other reasons for doing LP's as well.

5-4-1 Which kind of infection?: One of the main things that you're trying to figure out here is whether an infection is present at all; and if it is, whether it's viral or bacterial. A clue seems to have to do with how many white cells show up in the CSF, and what kind they are:

Viral infections: mostly lymphocytes, glucose higher than 3.0 mmol/liter. Herpes simplex turns out to cause many cases of viral meningitis, and they use the PCR method to verify it.

Bacterial infections: mostly neutrophils, glucose less than 2.0 mmol/liter - bacteria eat up the csf glucose and, virii don't.

5-4-2 Some normal values for CSF: here's another case where some of the tests should go somewhere else maybe, like chemistry, but they're relevant here. The point is that things overlap for important reasons.

- glucose: 40-85 mg/dl

- opening pressure: 50-180 mm H20

- white cells: not many, i.e. less than 5 per cc – lots of whites may also point to tumor activity.

- red cells: none, unless the LP is traumatic

- color: should be crystal clear – a yellow tint ("xanthochromia", which apparently means "yellow tint") means either red cells have been in the csf, or jaundice, or maybe eating too many carrots. Cloudy csf often points to bacterial meningitis.

- Protein: not much compared to the serum, maybe 35mg/dl. Increased amounts of protein in the csf might mean a breakdown in the blood-brain barrier, pointing to infection, inflammation, or even tumor activity.

- (I don't think I have a blood-brain barrier. What were we talking about? Um - where's my bag of carrots?)

5-5: Opportunistic Infections in the MICU

Seems to me that we should do an article on these infections all to itself. Hmm.

All these guys are either positive or negative by culture… one of the big problems with them is that they're starting to mutate towards the more deadly. It looks like some of the really strict precaution regimens really do work to contain these, but there are so many gaps – I mean, I alcohol my hands every couple of minutes, it seems like, but what about when Ralph the arrogant intern wanders in and out of the room, no gown, no gloves, with his air of importance bearing him in and out – what, does he have a bug barrier of power surrounding him or something? Or the housekeeping guy, who sometimes doesn't change gloves between rooms, but wears the same pair all around the unit? Or the lady who reads the numbers off the tube feed pumps? Or… there are handwashing monitors out there now, and it's probably a good thing, too…

5-5-1: MRSA – lives in the nares? Some impressive percentage of the whole population carries these guys around in the nose…it makes sense that if this bug is starting to be responsible for wound infections, and it's NOT sensitive to Vanco… then we have rather a problem.

5-5-2: VRE

Same idea. This one lives in the gut. Migrates to interesting places – "translocation", they call it, which I think means "migrates to interesting places."

5-5-3: What are survey studies all about?

Got to see who's got these bugs on their way into the MICU, and who's picked them up while staying here. Positive conversion is NOT a happy thing!

5-5-4: C. Difficile

This one is even tougher to kill than we thought – it survives a LONG time out in the environment – encapsulated, is it? Got to do handwashing AND alcohol for this one.

5-5-5: A subject for a study: should ICU nurses be routinely screened to see if they're carriers of opportunistic infections?

"Um… you're going to culture me WHERE now?" It's hard to imagine that we're not all carriers of these bugs by now…

6- Endocrine: We send these often enough to mention them:

6-1: Thyroid studies:

We usually send the "panel": T3, T4, and TSH are the ones that come to mind. Got to have enough TSH coming from the pituitary, otherwise the thyroid won't make the other ones. We give synthroid to patients who need it, usually because they've been diagnosed on the outside and come in with it listed in their history. Recently we had a patient in myxedema coma, which got the resident teams very excited – severe hypothyroid. She got intravenous thyroid treatment, something I don't think I've ever seen before. Cool.

6-2: "Cort-stim" tests:

These are to figure out if your patient's adrenals are working, which turns out to matter in sepsis treatment. Do adrenals shut down in sepsis? Some septic patients who don't respond properly get treated with steroids, which used to be absolute heresy back in the day.

A baseline cortisol level gets sent – why always in the morning? Some circadian thing there. (After working nights for 20 years they'd have a hard time with mine.) Then the patient is given a dose of IV ACTH, also known as co-syntropin – then after an hour the cortisol level is remeasured to see how well the adrenals responded. Sometimes you'll see a seriously hypoadrenal patient wean off pressors after being started on IV hydrocortisone. Impressive.

6-3: Testosterone: ("Yo, I'm a <u>donor</u> for that stuff, man!") Couldn't resist. I don't think I've ever sent one.

6-4: Beta HcG

Once in a while we'll send one of these, often to make sure that, say, some young, unconscious patient isn't pregnant before we give some drug or treatment that might be dangerous to the baby.

7- Immunology:

7-1: A New Discovery - "Anti-RN" Antibodies:

Immune problems in general involve testing for problems in "self-recognition" - a condition which afflicts many nurses. I believe that this may be caused by "Anti-RN Antibodies". I propose a research study: "Healing Our Pain: Exploring Levels of Anti-RN Antibodies in a Hospital Population of Nurses, Physicians, and Assorted Family Members: Do We Immune-Oppress Ourselves?"

Hmm. Maybe the Therapeutic Touch people could help us out here – "Feel the aura healing the antibodies…" Yo, keep your hands off my aura, man!

7-2: ANA:

(No, not that one.) "Anti-nuclear antibodies". These can show up in patients with a number of disease states: lupus, rheumatoid arthritis, scleroderma, and also after certain chemical exposures. The result is reported as a titer: the patient's serum is diluted, and the last dilution that still shows the antibody is the result – i.e. 1:20, or 1:60. Higher would presumably be worse – the antibody is still detectable at higher levels of dilution.

7-3: ANCA:

"Anti-Neutrophilic Cytoplasmic Antibody" – also auto-imune-produced. Titer reults. This tests for a variety of unpleasant rheumatologic conditions: Wegener's granulomatosis, polyarteritis nodosa, glomerulonephritis - rheumatologic things.

7-4: Rheumatoid Factor:

Also a titer–based test that indicates the presence of an antibody, this time for rheumatoid arthritis, positive in 70-80% of cases, usually at > 1:80.

7-5: Scleroderma Antibody:

Apparently not so useful, as it only shows up in 20% of patients with the disease. Phooey. Then again, would I really want to know? I guess so.

7-6: Immunoglobulins:

I wish I knew more about this stuff. Immunoglobulins turn out to be the proteins made by plasma cells in the bone marrow - they attack antigens introduced by specific invaders like bacteria or foreign chemicals. Immunoglobulins get the abbreviation "Ig" (pronounced "eye-gee"), and there are five main kinds: IgG (gamma), IgM (mu), IgA (alpha), IgE (epsilon), and IgD (delta). These guys take various forms, and do a number of different things, but basically their job is to hunt down and help kill off invading micro-organisms.

I know that I've hung IgG in the past, but it seems to have been pretty rare, and I forget what for.

10- Odds and Ends: A few of these that don't seem to fit easily into other categories:

10-1: Tumor Markers

PSA (the prostate one) and CEA (the colorectal one – also marks for others) are the only two that come to mind – I'm sure that there are lots others. Not sent very often, mostly as part of a screening workup when the underlying disease process isn't clear.

10-2: Haptoglobin:

This one's always been a mystery to me, but it doesn't turn out to be too hard – it's an indicator of hemolysis. Turns out that haptoglobin is a protein, made by the liver, that binds to the small fraction of hemoglobin that floats around <u>unbound</u> to any red cells – normally a very small amount, which would only make sense. This normally small amount increases when red cells start to hemolyze, which also makes sense – more hemoglobin breaks loose and floats around.

Next – after binding up free hemoglobin, the haptoglobin-hemoglobin, um, molecule?, is taken up by the liver again, where things get recycled – and the haptoglobin is destroyed. Apparently this stuff isn't made very rapidly, so the level goes down. Low haptoglobin – hemolysis. Can someone tell me: so does this get sent after suspected transfusion reactions?

11- A nice picture.

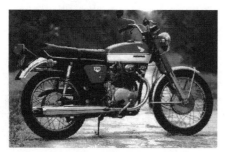

Ain't it pretty? Old. Wahoo!

12- Collecting lab specimens:

12-1: Blood Draws

12-1-1: peripheral sticks

I hear lately that there are nurses on the floors who DON'T know how to stick their patients for bloods. Look guys, this is just not excusable. I don't care where you work – this is just an essential skill for any RN. No excuses – learn, practice, do.

Here's a nice image of peripheral blood drawing with a vacutainer – the needle screws into the thingy, and you swap the tubes one after the other.

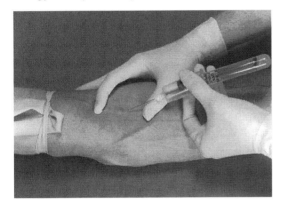

Oh sure, all our patients have veins this good. ☺

http://www.medtrng.net/efmb/handbook1/vacutainer.jpg

12-1-2: Specimens from arterial lines

What if you need to draw labs on your patient every hour? Hyponatremic seizure, maybe, being corrected... how fast? Go back up to the entry on sodium, then back down here... so you'll need a LOT of labs, right? Or DKA – might have to check – what? And how often? Are you going to stick your poor patient that often for all those labs?

You might. Sometimes you can draw labs out of a large bore peripheral IV with a tourniquet above it... but what if you needed frequent arterial gases?

Time for an arterial line: www.icufaqs.org/ArterialLines.doc

12-1-2-1- ABGs: while docs and RRTs do direct sticks, at my hospital we nurses draw these specs from a- lines.. The tricky part is learning which way the stopcocks work:

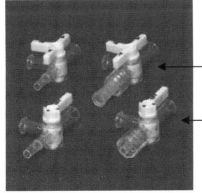

The tricky part is that some stopcocks...

point to where they're open...

...and some point to where they're closed.

http://www.niproindia.com/3waystopcock.htm

You have to learn how to turn the stopcock and draw your specimen from one of the little connectors, usually the one pointing upwards from the line.

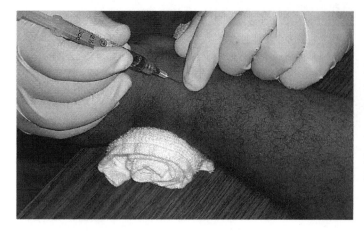

Here's how the docs do it, the respiratory therapists do it, and nurses in some other hospitals do it.

Which blood vessel are they sticking here? And look at the color of the blood in the syringe…

http://www.pcca.net/images/ABG_Picture.jpg

12-1-2-2: Other labs

Other labs are drawn with a vacutainer off the arterial stopcock, just like ABG's are. Remember that you have to waste something like 3cc, because there's a couple of inches of line tubing between the stopcock and the patient, and you don't want to send that to the lab, right?

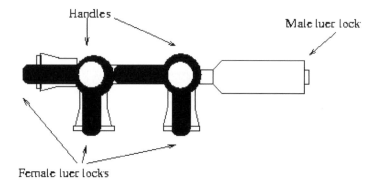

http://www.smtl.co.uk/Datacards/IV/images/manifold-2-tap.gif

12-1-3: specimens from central lines

This is a "manifold" – they go on the ends of the infusion lines that we attach to central line ports. Or sometimes just a single stopcock…. anyhow, you can take a syringe and aspirate your specimen from the central line, screwing the syringe onto one of the female luer connectors.

We usually draw these specs from the "distal port" of the central line.

Important! It's worth remembering however, what's going on along the length of that central line. You'll remember of course, from your careful reading of the FAQ article on central lines, that they have ports emerging at various spots along their length… so let's visualize this for a second. Suppose you have TPN infusing into the proximal port… and you draw a chem 7 from the distal port… which has – wait a second! It has TPN flowing past it! No wonder the glucose came back at 967!

The trick is: stop your TPN, or D10W infusion before you draw these specs. Don't turn the pump off – what if you forget to restart it? Just put it on "hold", then it'll remind you that it wants to be turned back on after you're done.

Would you stop your pressor infusion the same way?

1- **VBGs/ CV sats**

We draw our VBG's / central venous sat specs from the distal port of the CVP catheter. Which one is that, anyhow?

2- **What is a "true" mixed venous specimen?**

I think we talked a bit about this somewhere up above – there's lots of argument about whether you can believe the central venous sat drawn from the distal port of an RA line, or if it has to come from the distal port of a PA line. I let the big guys worry about that, and I just draw the spec from wherever they tell me to.

12-1-4: blood cultures

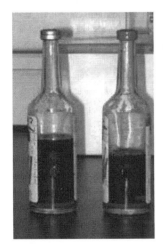

We usually send two sets, two bottles each, from two different peripheral sites. I usually draw these with a butterfly and a vacutainer, swapping the bottles after 5cc each.

http://webcls.utmb.edu/samplecourses/bact/Bact/images/PC001.jpg

A few points:

- Do you want to get your patient's blood cultures BEFORE, or AFTER you start their antibiotics?

- It's NOT a good thing to send "routine" blood cultures – say, when your patient spikes a new temp to 104, from a line that's already in him. The idea is that you're culturing the line, and not the patient. Although if there's nowhere else to draw from, then you'll probably have to…

- It IS ok to send cultures from new lines – they should be the first-ever spec drawn from them, however.

- Which bottle do you spike first?

- We've been told repeatedly that we send too many of these – talk to the team. If your patient spikes every day, and has been "pan-cultured" within 24 hours, you probably shouldn't be repeating the specs yet.

- Blood cultures need to be drawn with special attention to the specimens. Like any other venipuncture site, you have to swab in the circular motion, away from the site, then – and again, there's always argument – we prep the bottle tops with iodine after we pop the caps off. Some places use alcohol. Some places like you to change needles on your blood syringe between bottles, some don't…

12-2: Urines

12-2-1: UA specimens

It think they need 5cc for a UA spec – we send them in clean tubes. Clean specs, not sterile..

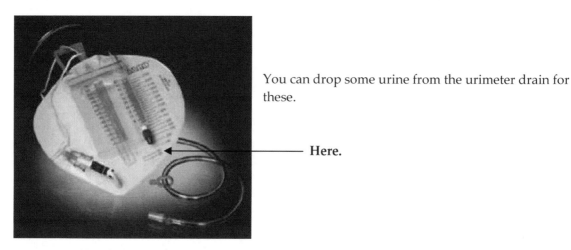

You can drop some urine from the urimeter drain for these.

Here.

http://www.bardmedical.com/urology/metertour2/bag.html

12-2-2: Urine cultures

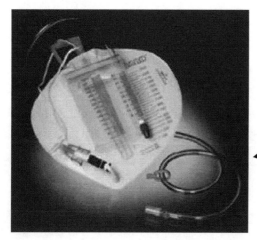

These are very sterile specs. There's a little port on the urine drain tubing for these. You swab the port with whatever prep they tell you to – alcohol, betadine, chlorhexidene – whichever – and then draw your spec. Our adapters are needle-less, but back in the day we needled specs out of these.

The port is here – hard to see in the picture.

12-2-3: 24-hour urine collections

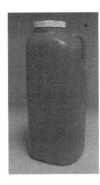

Not sterile.

Big bottle.

Sometimes these guys are iced, sometimes not.

http://www.rush.edu/rml/images/24hrurcon.JPG

12-3: Sputum

This guy hooks up to the inline suction catheter that we use on our vented patients.

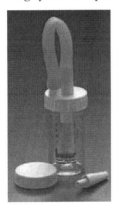

12-4- Stool specimens

Well, gotta do it. Little sterile cup…

12-4-1: stool for O&P

We don't see a whole lot of ova and parasites, but they're absolutely out there. Unpleasant, but a lot of the them are totally curable. Wear shoes crossing streams in Africa.

12-4-2: stool for C.diff

Flagyl. Wash your hands.

12-4-3: stool for occult blood

Otherwise known as the guaiac. Lots of patients have occult blood loss – means "you can't see it just by looking, so you have to use the guiac thing to see if it's there". Is the patient on steroids? Getting "gut prophylaxis'?

Med Tips

Hello all. Here's the latest idea: a list of commonly used drugs, with comments on them by ICU RNs, from novice to experienced. <u>Not</u> a drug reference in any official way – there's certainly lots of those around – but personal experiences and perspectives, some stories. **Take all the material here with many grains of salt,** and always check with your own pharmacy staff and references if you have questions. Which you should. There are lots of meds that are given infrequently, and we're always looking them up when they get ordered, to make sure we're current. Remember Rule # 1 of the MICU: "<u>There are no stupid questions.</u>"

Rule # 2: "Refer to Rule # 1".

What put the idea into my head: a new person was asking "Is it true that tylenol can really make a patient's blood pressure drop?". (It can, but may be a long time before you see it.) Another one: "I <u>hate</u> adenosine – it's ten seconds of pure terror." You get the idea. The meds are organized by system, and broken down in an extremely efficient way, which is to say the way they occurred to us. Please feel free to send in thoughts that you'd like to add!

This one's a little messy – seems unavoidable. Seems like nothing changes so rapidly as meds – new ones coming, old ones going away, regimens changing – it's always in flux. Plus we're adding generic names for the folks in other places... so when the time came to update this – well... it's just a little messy. And the whole point of these articles was to be fun and chatty - so bear with us. ☺

1- CNS Meds:

1-1- Anticonvulsants / Anti-edema

- Dilantin/phenytoin
- fosphenytoin
- Valproate
- Tegretol/carbamazepine
- Phenobarbital
- Mannitol
- Keppra/levetiracetam

1-2- Psychiatric Meds:
- Acute Confusion/Delirium
- Cimetidine (strange story)
- Haldol/haloperidol
- Psychosis
- Risperidone
- Zyprexa/olanzapine
- Clozaril/clozapine
- Seroquel/quetiapine

1-3- Encephalopathy:
- Lactulose
- Thiamine
- "Banana Bags"

1-4- Depression:
- SSRIs: Prozac/fluoxetine, Zoloft/sertraline, Celexa/citalopram, Paxil/paroxetine
- MAOIs: Parnate/tranylcypromine, Nardil/phenelzine
- Tricyclics: Amytriptyline, Imipramine, Desipramine
- Wellbutrin/buproprion
- Lithium
- Dextroamphetamine

1-5- Sedatives/ Pain Meds:

- Propofol
- Opiates: Fentanyl, MS04, Methadone, Dilaudid/hydromorphone
- Narcan
- Benzos: Valium/diazepam, Ativan/lorazepam, Versed/midazolam
- Benzo drips: versed
- Flumazenil

1-6- Withdrawal:

- ETOH, opiates
- Serax/oxazepam, Librium/chlordiazepoxide
- Clonidine

1-7- Paralytics:

A story in which the nurses triumph…

- Nimbex/cisatracurium
- Vecuronium, Pavulon/pancuronium, curare

2- Cardiac Meds:

2-1- Repleting the Elements: K^+, Mag^{+2}, Ca^{+2}, $P04^{+2}$

2-2- Hemodynamics: Controlling the rate:

- Digoxin
- Calcium channel blockers: diltiazem, nifedipine, verapimil
- Beta blockers: propranolol, metoprolol, esmolol, nadolol
- Alpha/ Beta blocker: Labetolol

The volume:
- Diuretics: lasix/furosemide, diuril/chlorothiazide, bumex/bumetanide, edecrine/ethacrynic acid, mannitol, diamox/acetazolamide
- The squeeze:
- Nipride/nitroprusside, nitroglycerine
- Oral antihypertensives

<u>2-3- Antiarrhythmics</u>: (Wasn't that the cardiology group started by Annie Lenox?)

- Amiodarone
- Lidocaine
- Procainamide
- Adenosine

3- Pressors and Vasoactives (drips):

3-1: "Up" meds:

- Neosynephrine/phenylephrine
- Levophed/norephinephrine
- Dopamine
- Vasopressin
- Dobutamine
- Zebras: epinephrine, amrinone, milrinone, isuprel

3-2: "Down" meds:
- nitrates
- nipride
- labetolol
- regitine/phentolamine (in case of local infiltration trouble)

4- Pulmonary Meds:

- Beta agonists: albuterol, ipratroprium
- Mucolytics: mucomyst/acetylcysteine, DNAse
- Theophylline
- Glycopyrrolate

5- Gut Meds:

5-1: Too much acid:

- H2 Blockers: Cimetidine, Ranitidine, Famotidine
- Proton Pump Inhibitors: Prilosec/omeprazole, Nexium/esomeprazole
- Antacids

5-2: Coating the Stomach: carafate

5-3: Moving it Along: colace, senna, mag citrate, go-lytely, enemas, reglan/metoclopramide

5-4: Stop the Bleeding: octreotide, vasopressin/ NTG

5-5: Clearing the Ammonia: Lactulose

6- Endocrine Meds:

- Insulin: drips, sliding scales, regular, NPH, humulin, glargine
- Oral hypoglycemics: glucophage/metformin, glitazones
- Thyroid meds: Synthroid/levothyroxine
- Cort stim tests: cosyntropin
- DDAVP/desmopressin
- Steroids: hydrocortisone, methylprednisolone, pulse steroids, stress steroids

7- Renal Meds:

- renal dopamine
- phosphate binders: calcium acetate
- epogen/epoetin alfa

8- Anti-infectives:

- gram positive infections
- gram negative infections
- fungal infections: amphotericin B, ambisome, fluconazole
- TB meds: rifampin, INH/isoniazid, ethambutol
- Drug resistance: Linezolid/Synercid/quinupristine
- Antivirals: acyclovir, protease inhibitors

9- Antipyretics:

- Tylenol/acetaminophen
- Motrin/ibuprofen
- Aspirin

10- Anticoagulants:

- Heparin
- Coumadin/warfarin

- Low Molecular Weight Heparins: fragmin/dalteparin, lepirudin
- platelet drugs: plavix/clopidogrel, integrilin/eptifibatide, reopro/abciximab, aspirin
- Clot busters: TPA, streptokinase

11- Anti-Anti-coagulants:

- Protamine
- Vitamin K/

12- Miscellaneous Meds and Weird Reactions:

- Cancer chemotherapy in the MICU
- Code drugs
- Malignant hyperthermia and NMS: Dantrolene, bromocriptine
- Mucomyst for preventing renal dye damage
- Glucagon for beta-blocker OD
- THAM/tromethamine
- Reglan – strange extrapyramidal reactions
- Oral meds for low BP: midodrine, pseudoephedrine
- Drug Fevers, Rashes

1- CNS Meds:

Remember, meds are always given in a context: there are things you're trying to accomplish, or prevent, or improve, or get more of, or get rid of. Goals you're trying to reach. Basic goals in neuro-med: preserve what you've got, closely monitor for changes, control seizures, minimize brain swelling. (Neuro is really not my thing – I floated once to a neuro ICU, and the charge nurse says, "So, uh, what do you know about neuro nursing?" I said: "Um, the brain is in the head, don't let it swell up." She said, "You're going to do just fine.")

Preserve What You've Got: to preserve what the patient's got, you have to be able to assess what's going on. This means that you may have to lighten a sedated patient sometimes, which can be problematic in some situations - status asthmaticus requiring paralysis and sedation is a good example. One way to observe neuro function might be to lighten sedation - <u>a little</u> - and see if they start responding vital-sign-wise to changes in position, voices nearby, etc. Rapid lightening may mean using short-acting meds like propofol – for situations requiring barbiturates and the like you'll probably have to check with the neuro folks for advice on how long it may take for your patient to wake up. Frequent pupil checks are good too.

More recently – of course, it's not recent to the newer nurses, but it seems like last week to me – we've started using BIS monitors to follow depth-of-sedation on our paralyzed patients. I understand that the guidelines from On High suggest completely lightening paralyzed or sedated patients once a day – mm. Not sure how practical that really is. BIS monitoring makes for a nice indicator, and we generally believe what they say.

1-1: Anticonvulsants:

Seizures are no fun. (I said I wasn't a neuro nurse, right? Do uncontrolled seizures really damage brain tissue? "Uh oh, he's going to be fried now…")

Dilantin: Dilantin works pretty well – I don't know what the stats are, but lots of seizure situations that I've seen have come under control with a dilantin load followed by regular dosing. Dilantin will definitely drop BP – it has to be given at a rate of 25mg/minute, so loading doses and reloads have to be given on a pump. There also used to be a story that you couldn't give dilantin po if the patient had a stomach full of tube feeds – is that still true? What if it takes four hours for the stomach to empty? Do you shut them off and wait? That long? And what was that old business about the gums growing?

Ok, new ICU nurses: what's the therapeutic range for this drug?

There's a new version of dilantin/ phenytoin, called **fosphenytoin** – apparently it's a lot safer to give intravenously, creates less hypotension.

Valproate: We see this one sometimes, given both po and IV. No big impression one way or the other. They do follow levels on this drug I think, like they do with Dilantin.

Tegretol: Don't see this one used too much lately. Can cause drops in white counts?

Phenobarb: Once in a while people will come in getting phenobarb as a maintenance med for seizure control, but rarely. I'm not even sure if they're using phenobarb comas anymore for status epilepticus – obviously I haven't had a patient like this in quite a while. Somebody check this out?

1-1 also: Drugs for Rising ICP:

Rising intra-cranial pressure is your basic Real Big Bad ICU Thing. Everybody immediately starts thinking about the triad – heart rate down, respiratory rate down, widening pulse pressure, right? Cushing's triad, I think it is. The thing to remember: **mentation goes first**. In other words – the first sign of rising ICP is a change in mentation for the worse. (What do you mean, "How am I supposed to tell with you?") Someone who was oriented becomes disoriented, or progressively unresponsive. **You do not want to wait for the triad to show up before you start treating the patient for rising ICP**. The way I was taught: at the first sign of a problem, get help – and give **mannitol**. It shouldn't hurt, hopefully will help – is that still true? Mannitol always has to be filtered, and the goal is to get the patient's brain "dry": all other things being equal, the serum osm is supposed to get to between 310 and 320 (?)That's pretty dry.

Keppra/levetiracetam – newer anti-seizure med. Not much experience with it, anyone want to contribute?

1-2- Psychiatric Meds:

Lots of psych situations come up in the ICU, and they can take some sorting out, but as I see it at the basic bedside level, you're trying to do two things: keep the patient safe, and try to figure out if something bad is happening. This is often not something that you're going to be able to figure out by yourself, so get help. For really acute situations and questions of competence (what do you mean, "Yours?") there's an Acute Psych Services person on call at all times.

Acute confusion/delirium:

Some situations develop quickly, and you need to have a plan. Sometimes (it seems like less often lately) patients will develop "ICU psychosis" – I remember any number of patients, usually elderly – but not always, who become acutely confused when suddenly taken out of their own environment and stuck in a hospital bed. Managing this can be a tough problem – and sometimes calls for radical measures: intra-aortic balloon patients are famous for getting acutely confused, for example. A ballooned patient <u>can not be allowed to sit up</u>, because the balloon (think of a hot dog at the end of a straightened-out wire hanger) – can be pushed inwards, and poke up through the arch of the aorta.

The result may be that a series of meds get tried on the patient, some of which may work, or not work, or make things worse… the end point however is that sometimes these patients have to be intubated, so that they can be safely sedated. It's always good to have a plan! Of course, a medical intern will look at you like a gunshot buffalo when you suggest that your mildly agitated, ballooned patient may need this at some point… so be ready to climb the chain of command quickly!

• Some patients have weird responses to meds – once in a while you'll see a patient who has a "paradoxical response" to a sedative: in other words, it'll make them more agitated instead of less. Ativan is famous for this, and rarely Versed.

• Another episode I'll never forget: a nice man, who I forget exactly what was wrong with him, who went from oriented to absolutely wild, really screaming crazy, over the period of a couple of hours. Psych came up, took a look, and decided that it was the **cimetidine** he'd been started on. We all looked at each other – this, we'd never heard of. And they were right!

Haldol (haloperidol): Haldol works well sometimes – sometimes very well, sometimes not at all well. The good thing about haldol is that it inhibits respiration the least of all the sedatives we use, which makes it a good choice for patients who are having breathing problems. The last thing you want to do with a patient who's already hypercarbic is to sedate him with something like **Valium**, which will probably double his pC02 and push him over the edge of intubation.

Haldol can also drop a patient's blood pressure, but I think that has more to do with the general effects of sedation, since lots of sedatives will do this. A classic blood pressure scenario involves intubation – you have a patient who's been developing respiratory distress over, say, a week or so. Very dehydrated, hasn't taken in much fluid over that whole time. Comes into the unit in increasing distress – tachycardic, maybe hypertensive, but actually (being so dry), maybe not. Huffing and puffing, agitated, they get a dose of **etomidate** for intubation, or maybe propofol, and boom – blood pressure drops to 60 systolic. And the team is <u>always</u> surprised. Don't you be – make sure that you have good IV access, a running gravity line of normal saline that you can give fluid through, and maybe a dilute mix of **neosynephrine** ready to go on a pump nearby. We use 10mg of neo in 250cc for situations requiring peripheral administration, but only for very short use. Take a look at the "Intubation" FAQ for more on this.

I saw an anesthesiologist give a dose of **ephedrine** in this situation once, and didn't like want happened at all! Heart rate doubled, blood pressure doubled, nothing titratable or controllable about the situation at all! Made me very unhappy, and I don't think the patient liked it either! I like using neosynephrine MUCH better for this situation.

Psychosis

(Just don't say it, okay? What do you mean, "Who are you talking to?") Some people in the unit get treated with antipsychotic meds, usually the ones they were on before they came in. More acute problems obviously take precedence, but I think the idea is to try to keep the treatment going unless it's causing other problems.

Risperidone: I don't know much about this one except that I've seen it work really well a couple of times, for patients who have been severely disoriented and agitated. Sometimes patient will be treated with a variety of meds – say haldol round the clock, maybe along with some antihypertensive to control elevated blood pressure, and maybe a beta blocker to control tachycardia. I seem to remember risperidone working so well that it replaced all of those. You may see this kind of thing sometimes: an agitated patient may be treated with cardiovascular meds, and a more appropriate treatment may not come until psychiatry gets a look at the patient and figures out the problem.

Olanzapine, **clozapine**: these are **zyprexa**, and **clozaril**, respectively. I don't know much about either of them, but I read somewhere that after a patient who'd been in uncontrolled schizophrenia – for many years (maybe 20?, 30?) - was started on one of these, his brother burst into tears, because his brother had finally "come back". If they really work that well, I hope they save some for me….

Something we saw recently about clozaril: we had a patient come in with really high, almost uncontrollable temperatures up to around 106 F, and the team was worried about **neuroleptic malignant syndrome**, because apparently clozaril is on that list somewhere. The fevers actually turned out to be related to her sepsis (pneumonia), and eventually came down, although they treated her anyhow with **bromocriptine** for her possible NMS for the whole ICU admission. Held the clozaril too.

Seroquel – yup, listed as an antipsychotic. A lot of people seem to get this to help them sleep. Works pretty well!

1-3- Encephalopathy

(What do you mean, "You!"? So I like to lie on the couch – so what!?)

Lactulose: The nurse's favorite. Works, though. One thing we've tried that actually turned out to be useful: if a patient has a really sore perianal area, adding lactulose to their tube feed diet a couple of times a day may make their stool liquid enough to be managed with a rectal tube, allowing the skin to heal around it.

Thiamine: Someone explain this one to me: what exactly is Wernicke's thing, and how does thiamine fix it? Something to do with alcoholism. And what is Korsakoff's thing? Rimsky-Korsakoff – he was the russian composer who discovered thiamine?

Banana Bags: 1 amp of mvi, 2 grams of magnesium, 1mg of folate, 100mg of thiamine, in D5 NS (probably), shaken, not stirred. We don't use these, but apparently they're useful in alcohol situations. (Do they keep them behind the bar at Ralph's?)

1-4- Depression

(We're always talking about putting Prozac in the coffee in the nurses' lounge…)

If our patients were the ones you went by - overdoses is what I'm thinking of here - you'd have to say that antidepressants just don't work at all. Of course, that would be like saying that all of us are going to die of ARDS in our 30's. Our patients are sometimes on antidepressants when they come in, and they're usually kept on them while they're with us.

SSRI's: Prozac, Zoloft, Celexa, Paxil – Once in a while we'll get an overdose patient in who's taken all their prozac, or zoloft, or whatever SSRI they're on. These drugs are apparently so non-toxic that they're safe to hand over to horribly depressed, possibly suicidal patients, unlike **tricyclics** and **MAOIs**. (Weren't the MAOIs the native people in Fiji or someplace?) There was an interesting story some years back about Prozac and yawning… try Googling that one…

MAOIs: Let's see if I can remember them without looking – **Parnate** is one, and **Nardil**. Sounds like a couple of the characters in the Lord of the Rings. I guess these are really rare now, hardly used any more. One really critical thing to try to remember is that these patients **MUST NOT GET DEMEROL.** (Is that for all of the MAOIs or only some? – I wouldn't want to get it wrong.) I don't know why exactly – but apparently it produces a potentially **fatal reaction**. Important. Another thing with these drugs is that if the patient makes a mistake and eats something wrong containing tyramine (?)– cheese, or wine of one kind or another, or I think maybe snow pea pods or whatever, they can have a truly severe hypertensive reaction, requiring rapid treatment with **nifedipine** – or maybe something like **nipride**? Never seen it happen. I don't think I've ever given anyone any of these meds.

There's a new version of one of these meds out now in patch form – Emsam, I think it's called.

Tricyclics: We do see tricyclic overdoses sometimes. Unlike the SSRIs, these meds can kill, and I guess pretty quickly – they interfere with cardiac conduction. I don't remember – do these patients ever buy temporary pacing wires? I think they also have to get a **bicarb** drip, something about protecting the kidneys by alkalinizing the urine.

Wellbutrin: I think I've given this a couple of times, but it's not much of an ICU med. I think it's also on the "relatively safe" list.

Lithium: for bipolar disease, right? Famous line: "I don't miss my lows, but I sure do miss my highs." Lithium can definitely be toxic – not sure what the treatments are, but I know that they do draw levels. Come to think of it, it seems as though we ought to develop a "Tox and Poisoning" FAQ. I don't seem to recall giving lithium to patients while in the MICU. My colleague Cathie just leaned over and mentioned that a renal attending told her that chronic lithium use for bipolar disease seems to be associated with eventually developing renal failure. (So should I stop taking it now, or can I still go on for a while? Where's the men's room?)

Dextroamphetamine: Once in a while this one still pops up. I think the idea is that the drug will supply some kind of energizing pop in the morning to patients who can't seem to mobilize themselves. Doesn't seem to do much, and I seem to recall that it effectively stops people from sleeping. Add a sleeping med in the pm, and you wind up with a seriously messed up situation.

1-5- Sedatives / Pain Meds

Propofol: Ah, the "Milk of Amnesia". ICU nurses love propofol. Works well, works quickly, wears off almost as fast as it goes to work. Two main cautions: propofol will drop your patient's blood pressure, sometimes more, sometimes less, so be ready. Second: **propofol will make your patient stop breathing.** So be ready for that too. There's more on all this in the "Sedation and Paralysis" FAQ.

A nice thing about propofol is that it has no effect that I know of on the gut, so your patient can be started on tube feeds without having to worry about opiate ileus problems. Another thing to remember is that it comes as a lipid mix, so your TPN patient may need to have lipids removed from her formula if she stays on the drug for a while.

Opiates: We use a lot of opiates in the unit, sometimes in combination with benzos or propofol. Most people have a pretty good idea of what opiates are all about by the time they get to the unit, but they probably haven't seen them given in the doses that we use for long-term sedation. It's good to keep in mind that their strengths are different: **morphine** is what everything else is compared to – so for example one milligram of **dilaudid** is equivalent to 4 or 6 mg of morphine. I think 50mcg of **fentanyl** equals 2-4 milligrams of morphine – there are equivalency charts around that you can look at.

Fentanyl: Fentanyl is the propofol of the opiates – works quickly, wears off quickly. Used to be, we ran people on morphine drips for the long term, but nowadays we're using fentanyl because apparently it causes less of a histamine release, which is better for patients who have an inflammatory component, like asthmatics. Sometimes we use a lot - we're running a woman now on a fentanyl drip at 2200mcg/ hour, when the usual range is something like 100-300. That high of a dose usually means that they've been on it for a while – at least a couple of weeks. My impression is that people habituate pretty quickly to fentanyl, and may need a higher dose every few days to keep a steady level.

Patients like that will definitely have to be weaned carefully to avoid withdrawal. (You may not avoid withdrawal completely as you wean the med, but you should understand the idea.) The usual method is to try to wean the drip 25% per day – which does <u>not</u> mean 4 days – it means 25% each day of what's running. So the lady on 2200mcg would go down by 25% the first day, to 1650. Second day, you'd go down by 25% of the 1650, or 420-odd, to about 1235. And so on. Even then you may have to pop them back up sometimes.

How would you know if your patient was withdrawing? What could you do to tell?

MSO4: I got my first - ever personal exposure to morphine a couple of months ago, when my rapidly advancing age introduced me to the happy concept of kidney stones. I got a total of nine mg in two doses, and I can't say it made me euphoric, but I sure was happy the when the pain went away. Took a nice nap too. (Apparently I was quite a spectacle. Cried like a baby. My wife points to her uterus and says: "See?")

We use little bits of morphine in the unit for pain management, apart from narcotic drips, because it's easily reversed. A patient with respiratory problems after surgery may only get small doses of morphine on a careful prn basis – there are always lots of things to think about. Ten milligrams of morphine is equivalent to 10mg of morphine…wait a minute…..Doh!

Here's a neat morphine trick: the next time a patient manages to do a Houdini and yanks out everything including ET tube, IVs, and all, and you have no access to try to give something to calm him, try nebulizing five milligrams of morphine through a mask…one of our attendings came up with this on the fly one night, and it worked really well.

A word about PCA pumps in the MICU – "Patient Controlled Analgesia". I'm all for patient-controlled analgesia – I think it's a great idea. Just not in the ICU. A postop patient in the ICU is there for serious problems – blood pressure maybe, breathing more likely. I think the nurse at the bedside should be the one in control of pain management – he needs to be the one giving the doses and watching what happens. Not the patient. Just my opinion.

Methadone: Now and again we have addicted folks in the unit, and they are usually started on methadone right away to prevent withdrawal. (Of course they sometimes come in as Mr. or Ms. Who Knows Who They Are – unresponsive, sometimes no ID, sometimes no clothes…so it can be hard to tell. Tox screens help sort things out.)

Dilaudid: Dilaudid (hydromorphone) is strong stuff. The chart says that 1mg of dilaudid (hydromorphone) is equivalent to 4mg of morphine. We use dilaudid drips occasionally – I'm never really clear on why, since usually we go for agents that wear off more quickly.

A couple more things from the chart: **Demerol** 75mg, and **oxycodone** 30mg are each equivalent to ten of morphine…

Opiate Antagonist: Narcan ("Narcotic Antagonist")

We used narcan last week – we got a patient with respiratory depression, apparently from her patient-controlled-analgesia (she'd had a fractured hip repaired). I guess she got too much. (What did we just say about PCA pumps…?)

I've learned to be careful when giving narcan – if your patient is intubated and lined (or even if they're not), you may want to think about applying restraints before giving the dose. As I understand it, Narcan pushes the opiate molecules off their receptor sites, and if the patient was in pain before, it may be worse afterwards.

In other words, they may levitate, scream, shout, swear, and otherwise demonstrate an alteration in comfort level secondary to an alteration in opiate receptor status mediated by pharmacologic alteration of pain management as evidenced by, uh, screaming. (Got to love nursing diagnosis.) That's to say, they become distressed. So - narcan isn't always a nice thing to do. The hip lady got some, which was before I came on, and I wonder how she felt – would it have been kinder to intubate her and let her "cook off" her opiates to a safe level? Risk? Benefit? Judgment call.

The other thing about narcan is that it doesn't last very long – it doesn't "cure" an opiate overdose. Your patient may have to be intubated for respiratory support until the overdose is metabolized off.

<u>Benzos</u>

Valium (diazepam): seems like we don't use Valium so much these days; it seems like we use **Ativan** (lorazepam) instead. Patients at risk for alcohol withdrawal get put on Ativan doses round the clock, with extra doses prn. Alcohol withdrawal can require really impressive amounts of benzos – back in the Valium days we used to see patients get thirty to forty milligrams IV. Every hour. Or more.

Versed (midazolam): Used mostly for procedures on un-intubated patients, such as those undergoing endoscopy. It seems to work well, and it's very short-acting. I'm supposed to have an upper endoscopy myself at some point, and I'll have a report from the field to add at some point.

Ok, here's my report. So I turned 50 – it happens. Went off for my endoscopy – both ends, such a lovely birthday present. Man, that versed is the greatest! I didn't remember a THING!

Benzo drips – versed drips are the one we use. The other benzos tend to hang around for a long time, which is why we try to use the shorter-acting agents. The idea is to try to shorten ICU stays, rather than lengthen them.

Benzo Antagonist: Flumazenil. This is Narcan for benzodiazepines. Needs to be used carefully, since a patient that takes benzos chronically can be pushed into seizures by this drug. For overdoses, we usually let the patients cook off the drug while they're intubated (since their main lethal effect is that they make people stop breathing). Then once awake, out comes the tube, they get evaluated by Psych, and off they go.

I remember when they were doing the double-blind trials on this drug – apparently the research team was notified whenever a benzo overdose showed up in the ER, so up they came, and there was my intubated patient in the bed, very sleepy, not really rousable, but otherwise stable. The nurse working on the study told me "You know, we never know if we're giving the drug, or just a dose of normal saline." They pushed the dose, the woman's eyes opened wide, she sat straight up in the bed (in her four-point leathers), and almost levitated. The nurse: "I guess that was the drug, huh?" Ya think?!

1-6- Withdrawal

Patients can withdraw from all kinds of substances: alcohol and opiates are the ones we see the most. Lately we've gotten a little better about putting **nicotine** patches on patients who smoke, but I bet it gets missed a lot more than we think.

As we looked at a minute ago, people withdrawing from alcohol usually get treated with benzos – sometimes a whole lot of benzos. It can be scary, and I can remember at least several times being given orders for 30mg of Valium an hour. Or twice an hour. More recently, it turns out that propofol "covers" alcohol withdrawal in pretty much the same way that benzos do. GABA receptors, is it?

So for example, let's think of a scenario: gentleman found "down" in the park, bottles of scotch nearby, vomitus nearby, probable aspiration, intubated at the scene. Comes to the ER, sent to the MICU, nasty looking x-ray (right – you guys who read the X-ray FAQ: any quick and easy clues on a chest film to make you think of aspiration?). The ER nurse gives you report: "He's really been agitated down here – we've given him ten of Ativan over two hours, which is more than I've ever given before, and he's better now, but they had to push a dose of vecuronium to get him through his head and neck CT – he's still got his collar on, and they haven't cleared his C-spines. He's tachy at about 120, sinus, and his pressure is 160 systolic – he only put out about a hundred cc when we put his Foley in…".

This is actually going to be a little bit of a puzzler, because now he's got at least two reasons to be tachycardic. (What are they?) So he comes up from the scanner (thank you, thank you ER, for scanning him <u>before</u> sending him to us), and his vec dose is wearing off, and he's trying to yank out anything out he can reach – his ET tube, his IV's, his Foley, the nurse's fingers, the stretcher rails – at this point the nurse will usually turn to the resident (who hopefully is still in the room), and ask for a propofol order. Our range is 0 – 300mg/hour ("Okay, so I got him on zero of propofol, and he's been really well - sedated with that, so I haven't gone up at all". I mean, why do they write "<u>zero</u> to 300"?) We'll give a small bolus dose of maybe 20 mg to start, and then depending on size and degree of agitation I might start the drip at 100 /hour, see how it worked, and then go up if necessary, or if the patient was absolutely enormous and totally wild, I might start at 300, and work backwards. The nice thing is that you know that not only is their short-term agitation covered, but withdrawal should be too. (Except that it's probably a little early for DT's, unless he'd been lying in the park for about 3 days.)

So the strategy is something like: propofol for the short term, and round-the-clock benzos until it seems clear that an effective "level" has been reached. "Level" is in quotes because we don't actually measure one, the way we might with digoxin or dilantin, but you get the idea – we're trying to figure out what regimen will keep the patient stable so that they can be weaned off the propofol and the vent. Although that can often take a little longer than anticipated…and remember – no vent, no propofol. It's worth repeating: **Propofol will make your patient stop breathing**.

Other drugs used for DT prophylaxis are also benzos, eventually oral, like **serax** and **librium**, although we hardly ever see them used any more – ativan is all the fashion now. It's interesting to see things come, and go, and come back again, and maybe go away again as the years go by, as (presumably) the studies come in showing that one thing works and the other doesn't.

Clonidine – This is an interesting use for a drug – it turns out that clonidine, the antihypertensive also known as catapres, works to block the adrenergic release of endogenous catecholamines during withdrawal episodes. (Whoa! That sounded good! Bet I can't say that again!) Or so it has been explained to me. Anyhow, patients withdrawing from all sorts of things: alcohol, opiates, cocaine, can be started on clonidine, usually in the form of a patch. Neat! Remember that this is <u>not</u> the same as **klonopin** (clonazepam), which is one of the benzos… which reminds me of the time years ago, hunting around in the med closet, we found that vials of **Pavulon** (pancuronium) looked almost exactly the same as vials of something else – **gentamicin** maybe… yikes!

1-7- Paralytics

There's a whole article devoted to "Sedation and Paralysis", so I won't get into all the details here, but there seems to be some basic difficulty that people have in telling the difference between the two. Every now and then I still hear someone say "Okay, so he's sedated with **Nimbex**...". No. No, no, no. Let's recap the basics here:

1. Sedation is sedation.
2. Paralysis is paralysis.
3. They are not the same. As in: **"NOT THE SAME !"**.

Here's a story: patient is being transferred to us from an OSH (Outside Hospital). I'm the charge nurse. Our RN calls their ICU for report:

"Well, we paralyzed him, but he's gotten really tachycardic and hypertensive, so we started him on IV **nitro**, and we've given him a couple of doses of **lopressor**."

At this point our house officers (first-year interns, second-year junior) start looking worried. I can almost read their thought process: "Okay, so the guy's having an MI, maybe he's having an aortic dissection, oh this could be really bad, we better line up the scanner now, maybe we should anticoagulate him, has he gotten his aspirin, what's his troponin, does he have ekg changes, who's the cath fellow on call tonight...". And so on.

I look at my nurse, she looks at me. "What's he sedated with?", we ask, as one.

"Ketamine."

Oh, this is a weird one. I know they use ketamine at the animal hospital where I take my greyhound to get her teeth cleaned every couple of years, and I know that there's some street traffic in it as some sort of hallucinogen, but I've never in my – what is it now? – 23 years in the units, seen ketamine used on people. "Who's managing the patient?" we ask.

"Anesthesia". "Well, is the patient getting enough of the drug?" "I don't know", says the RN on the other end, "I've never given it before."

Uh-oh. This is a patient who's chemically paralyzed but apparently hardly sedated, and he's got to be going bonkers with terror on the inside. We turn to the team, who are still rapidly doing the differential diagnosis thing, and say: "Well, we know why he's so tachycardic." Skeptical looks from the team: "Why?" "He's hardly sedated under his paralysis." We explain about the ketamine. More doubtful looks.

The patient arrives. Report from the paramedics: "He's still paralyzed, really tachycardic and hypertensive, so we kept the nitro going in transit." Apparently the patient got no more sedation on his trip.

In our ICU, starting propofol is pretty much standard practice in situations like these. A patient who is intubated, but who may or may not be adequately sedated, or paralyzed, or both – the immediate goal is to produce safe sedation, and to evaluate the whole picture. Let's say this is a fairly large male patient - we might start him with a 20mg propofol bolus, and start a drip at 100mg/ hour – not an enormous dose. Bingo – heart rate drops from 130's to 74, BP from 230 to 120 systolic. The team looks at us in disbelief, as though we had pulled a moose out of a rabbit-sized hat. The patient rules out for an MI.

This is actually a good illustration of an important point, which is that over the course of some three years, a general medical resident spends three months in the ICU. This means that over the course of one year, a brand-new ICU nurse gets four times as much exposure to ICU patients than the residents do. The result is that some things begin to become very obvious to the nurse, that remain intellectual puzzles for the MDs.

Another quick story about this situation: my wife the CNS (she's a real CNS, the kind that gets into the blood and the poo and the everything else, right there in the bed with her orientees and their patients), goes off to one of these conferences of the Inter-Galactic Association of Critical Care Things and Stuff, having to do with intensive care trends, modalities, interventions, and all like that. Physician is standing up, giving a lecture on vent-weaning strategies. She's a pulmonologist someplace, and says something like: "Now, we did an informal survey in our unit, just keeping numbers for a while, and we found that our staff nurses could correctly predict whether our patients would successfully extubate 86% of the time. Would you believe it?" To which the nurses all responded (on the inside): "Well <u>duh</u>!"

And this actually raises another really important point: ICU nurses develop skills that the physicians don't even know exist. This leads to many of the arguments that nurses have with physicians about management of one situation or another – an attending who takes the time to get to know her nursing staff, who takes the time to get familiar with their expertise, will have an incomparably easier time than one who blows them off when we voice our concerns.

Nimbex: (Cis-atracurium) Back in the days when we used to weave in between the mammoths on the highway to get to work, we used to use **Pavulon** (pancuronium) pushes of 2-4 mg every 2-4 hours to keep our patients paralyzed. Then we started using **curare** drips (the stuff that they shoot monkeys with in the rainforest – what happens when they eat the monkey? They must get very relaxed.) Apparently Nimbex causes less of a histamine release than the older drugs, and so is better for situations like asthma, that have an inflammatory component. Same for the change from morphine to fentanyl drips.

Vecuronium: "Vec" – also hardly used anymore, but once in a while the ER will give a dose – 10mg? to a patient who's severely agitated (**<u>along with sedation!</u>**) for a scan before coming up to us. Wears off in an hour or two. While the OR people do it, I can't say that we ever reverse paralysis nowadays – we just keep the patient sedate and wait for it to wear off.

2- Cardiac Meds:

Well, here's a topic that could (and does) take up whole textbooks. But the goal here is not to create a reference, but just to yak about meds and how well they work or how weird they are, so maybe it won't go on forever. (It'll just feel that way.)

2-1- Repleting the Elements: Very important – but you guys know about this.

K+: You always need to know what your patient's potassium is. If you're diuresing him, plan ahead – do you need to remind the team to order K along with the **lasix**? And by the way, what's the BUN and creatinine? (And why am I asking?) K generally wants to be above 4.0 if the patient is on digoxin...

Mag+2: Mag turns out to be right up there with K+ in terms of keeping the heart happy. If your patient is having ectopy, know both values, and be aggressive in treating them.

Calcium: Lots of argument about replacing calcium, but in practice, we do it. Certainly patients on CVVH need it, because the machine sucks it (along with K+) right out of them, so they usually get replaced continuously. We tend to replace calcium when it's low in our unit.

Phosphorus: We replace P04 with either sodium phos or potassium phos, usually something like 10 or 20 or 30 millimoles. Has to be given slowly – last night I gave the last of a 30 millimole dose, which took up a central line port for the whole shift.

2-2- Hemodynamics: Controlling the Rate

Many of the treatment goals in the MICU have to do with controlling one or the other of these, because too much of either one increases cardiac work, either from the effort of a rapid rhythm or the work of pumping into a really tight arterial system. This is described in typically roundabout fashion as "myocardial oxygen consumption" – which is like measuring a car's horsepower by measuring gasoline consumption. Makes sense I guess...anyhow, the point is that a heart that's hurting doesn't want to beat too quickly, or work too hard at pumping blood into the arterial system. A rate nearer that of NSR is generally better, and a relatively dilated (rather than constricted) arterial bed is easier to pump into. (This last is what "afterload" is all about. "Preload" has to do with the amount of volume arriving in the LV – it's all supposed to get pumped out, right? If not, then things begin to back up – CHF ensues.)

Digoxin: Dig ("Didge") is one of the real oldies – apparently people have been using digitalis leaf to control heart rate for at least a couple of hundred years. I can still just about remember the days before dig levels – the joke was "Load 'em till they start vomiting, then back off." We do it a little better now. Know your patient's BUN and creatinine. Dig is also just about the only oral inotrope around – there used to be a little blue pill in trials called **enoxamone**, which appeared to work very well – at least some of the time. Any new ones coming along?

Calcium Channel Blockers: **Diltiazem, Nifedipine, Verapamil** - these were the original three, and they formed a range of effect: Verapamil slows rate the most, nifedipine drops blood pressure the most, and diltiazem is in the middle somewhere. I know that most places use a lot of dilt drips – for whatever reason, I've only seen it done once or twice.

Beta Blockers: **inderal/propranolol, metoprolol, esmolol, nadolol, etc.**

These are the meds most commonly used for controlling heart rate. A basic concept to grasp is the adrenergic receptor thing – there's lots about this in the "Pressors and Vasoactives" file, but basically there are three receptor groups (this is with a lot of lies thrown in – I understand that there are more, but keeping it simple will help here.) <u>A</u>lpha receptors live in the <u>a</u>rteries. You have **1** heart, so that's where the beta-**1**s live. You have **2** lungs, that's where the beta-**2**s live.

If you <u>agonize</u> a receptor, then it does more of what it's supposed to. If you <u>antagonize</u> it, then it does less of what it's supposed to. So if you give a beta-agonist, like **albuterol**, then the beta-2s in the lungs do their thing, and the bronchi open up. (And the heart rate goes up). Beta <u>agonist</u>.

So then giving the opposite of albuterol, namely a beta-<u>antagonist</u>, or beta-"blocker" (everybody says "aha!" at this point), will <u>block</u> the betas, lowering the heart rate and, if you're unlucky, provoking an asthma attack in your patient. Which is why asthmatics don't get beta-blockers, they get something like verapamil instead.

We use a lot of lopressor and verapamil for rate control in our unit. Once in a while we'll see an **esmolol** drip, but I have to say that I think it doesn't really work very well.

Of course, there's always the heart rate that's too <u>slow</u>, but that's a whole other article…

Labetolol – this is a neat idea: it's both an alpha and a beta blocker. So it produces arterial dilation, and slower heart rate.

The Volume:

Diuretics: Everybody remembers that the three parts of a blood pressure are "pump", "volume", and "arterial squeeze"? Strategies for lowering blood pressure center around picking one of these. The pump component is treated by lowering the heart rate, with one or the other or even a cocktail of the meds we were talking about above.

The volume aspect is what diuretics are all about. There are a couple of kinds – the most commonly used are the **loop diuretics**: **lasix, diuril**, and I think **bumex**, which I understand were invented by the famous medical rock star Don ("Loopy") Henley.

Something like that. I think I'm right when I remember being told that lasix and bumex work on one part of the loop, and that diuril works on another part, and that the combination effect makes the drugs work together more powerfully – "synergistic diuresis" – wasn't that on the flip side of "Hotel California"…?

One recent development in the diuretic world is the idea of giving a big wallop of diuretic to patients who are acutely sliding down the slope into renal failure – the patients who have taken a recent kidney hit because of a prolonged hypotensive episode for example. The theory is that doing this will push the failing kidneys into making good amounts of urine, so that the patient will be able to get rid of fluids, if nothing else. At least that way they won't get into CHF. Obviously this doesn't solve the whole problem though.

Edecrine /ethacrynic acid is a diuretic that can be given to patients with a lasix allergy. Turns out that patients with a sulfa allergy can be allergic to lasix as well…

The two last ones are **mannitol** and **diamox**. Mannitol we use in neuro situations when the worry is increasing ICP – "osmotic" diuresis literally shrinks the brain. (Wouldn't work for me – too small already.) Mannitol easily forms crystals, so it gets filtered.

Diamox is interesting – it causes the kidneys to dump bicarb, so it's useful in alkalosis. Something I heard, which may or may not be true: you go climbing up Mount Everest. The air gets thin, and you start breathing rapidly – producing a respiratory alkalosis, right? Breathing rapidly blows off C02, which leaves you with a carbonic acid deficit, and a relative bicarb excess. (An absolute excess would be if you drank both bottles of Maalox you'd brought along.) Now your fingers and toes start tingling, you get shivery – what to do? Take your diamox pills – you'll dump bicarb, and your ph will come back down. Of course, now you have another problem, right? You come back down the mountain, and your breathing straightens out, and wups! Ack! Where'd your bicarb go! Now you have a new problem!

The Squeeze

The third part of a blood pressure is "arterial squeeze". This is what SVR means: systemic vascular resistance, one of the numbers that comes up when you "shoot numbers" with a PA line. High is tight, low is loose. Another word for this resistance faced by the LV – which determines how hard it has to work to empty itself into the arterial bed – is "afterload". High afterload can be a good thing sometimes, usually in some form of hypovolemic or cardiogenic shock state where getting tight is the only thing keeping your patient's pressure up. But a nicotine addict will walk around in a tight state – which puts lots more work onto his heart. Also bad for anyone with any degree of pump failure – CHF, in other words. Loosening up a tight afterload really helps a failing heart. Flowers and nice dogs work too, maybe through the same mechanism.

Most commonly used in blood pressure situations are **nitrates**, which in the unit usually come in the form of IV nitroglycerine. Nitrates open up the arterial bed – and sure, they do do that - I mean we've all seen patients with angina respond to sublingual nitrate pills. But honestly, IV nitro just doesn't live up to its reputation as an antihypertensive.

For really serious hypertension situations, the drug to use is nipride (nitroprusside). This drug is da bomb. It really is like a bomb, too. This is a really serious, powerful drug, sort of the opposite of norepinephrine. <u>**Nipride must run in a line all by itself.**</u> <u>Anything</u> put to run through a nipride line may kill your patient. (It also isn't compatible with anything.) Don't even <u>think</u> about flushing a heplock with nipride in it – aspirate it instead, then flush with saline. Very serious medicine.

A useful nipride tip: if you use a very concentrated mix, like 250mg in 250cc, then if you decide to doulbe your rate, your rate change may only be a cc or two per hour. This is a bad idea – a much better idea is to use a dilute mix. I like 50mg in 250cc – that way if I want to change the dose, the change in rate will be something like 20 up to 35 cc per hour. The drip is much more titratable that way, and you'll be able to "fine-tune" the drip much more closely.

There are lots of oral antihypertensives: oral nitrates like **isordil**/isosorbide dinitrate, oral **ace inhibitors** like **captopril**, alpha blockers like **prazosin** – (remember about antagonizing the alphas? – makes the arteries dilate.) The thing about oral meds is that they're not particularly <u>titratable</u>, which is something that you really want in the ICU. The nice thing about IV nitro and nipride is that their effects go away really fast – turn the drips off, and their effects are gone within a minute or two. For the same reason, changing the drip rates produces quick responses in the patient. Titratable. It's a lot harder to go down and suck out an oral med that's halfway through the small intestine than it is to turn down the nipride… I have to say that it seems like the best oral BP med is sustained-release nifedipine. Excellent drug, but too powerful in it's regular form.

<u>**Ischemia**</u> We all know about this one, right? Tight coronary artery lesions, not enough **oxygen** is getting to the cardiac muscle tissue, and pain ensues. What to do? Anything that increases oxygen delivery, or that decreases the workload of the heart will help. So: first drug is what? Oxygen!

Next: probably nitrates. Sublingual, IV nitro, etc. Then, or maybe even at the same time, rate control. Ask the patient if he has asthma…

<u>**2-3- Antiarrhythmics**</u>

Obviously dating myself here, but of course the first thing I think of is **lidocaine**. There have been big changes in antiarrhythmic treatments lately though – now **amiodarone** comes first. Great drug – does all sorts of neat things like converting a-fib into sinus rhythm, controls ventricular arrhythmias – in fact, it comes first in the VT/ VF code algorithms now. Two percent of people on amiodarone get nasty fibrotic lung effects.

Very unpleasant. Amiodarone gets loaded, usually 150mg over ten minutes (fast!), then dripped at 1 mg per minute for something like 6 hours, then half a milligram for another 18 hours and then changed to oral.

We really don't see anything like the numbers of VT/ VF codes that we used to back in the Ice Age – the difference is that now we clot-bust most MI patients – it's the MI's that mostly make for the really awful arrhythmic codes.

Lidocaine – yup, once in a while we still use lido. 50 to 100mg load, followed by a drip at 1-2 mg per minute. Lido can make people acutely bonkers, which usually goes away if it's stopped.

Procainamide – second antiarrythmic up until the rise of amiodarone – is it third now? Proc ("Proke") also gets loaded, and then run in mgs per minute. Been a long time since I saw this up and running. Be careful – a proc load can really drop your patient's pressure.

Bretyllium – gone altogether now, I think. I remember being really impressed when they were coding "ET" – before or after he phoned home?, and they called for bretyllium…_that_ was a while ago.

Adenosine – I love and hate adenosine. Very powerful drug, used to break rapid supraventricular rhythms – the problem is, it creates about ten seconds of asystole in both the patient and the nurse giving the drug…

3- Pressors/ Vasoactives

These meds have a FAQ file all to themselves, so that's where to go for the detailed stuff. The idea behind vasoactive drips is that they either raise ("Up" meds), or lower heart rate and/or blood pressure ("Down" meds).

3-1: "Up" Meds

Simple concept – raising blood pressure, which is what the word "pressor" is all about.

This stuff calls for a little memorization. The thing to figure out is: which set of receptors do you want to work on, and why? The answer depends on which of the three parts of the blood pressure is being affected. If it's pump (heart), then it's the beta-1s you want to go after. If it's volume – then you may not want to give a pressor at all if you can avoid it. If it's arterial squeeze (sepsis), then it's the alphas out in the arteries that you want to hit. There's more than you probably ever wanted to know on this subject in the "PA-lines" FAQ, which is where we go into this stuff in more detail. The main point is that "shooting the numbers" with your PA line gives you indices for all three parts: cardiac output/ index tells you about your patient's pump status, the SVR tells you about the arterial squeeze, and the CVP, wedge pressure, and stroke volume tell you about the, uh, volume.

Neosynephrine – (phenylephrine): "Neo" is pure alpha. This is what you want to use in sepsis, when the arteries are dilated. It doesn't have any direct effect on heart rate, but some people worry that it can constrict the coronary arteries too, producing angina, etc. I can't say that I've ever noticed that to happen, although these patients can certainly get angina from the tachycardic reflex to sepsis – "rate-related angina".

Levophed (norepinephrine) – this is sort of a "kitchen sink" pressor – it kicks both alphas and betas, but much more the first than the second. It gets used in sepsis a lot, and it works well, but if you notice that your septic patient is getting even more tachycardic than before, and maybe having some ectopy too, it might be a good idea to change to neo.

Dopamine – dopa is the only pressor that can be started on the floors, so no matter why the patient is having pressure problems, this is the one that they put up. It helps, too, but it's not always the drug you want to go up on – if your septic patient is tachycardic, using a lot of dopamine can only worsen that problem, and sometimes it can provoke VT or VF. Then again, for a patient with an inferior MI (the kind that makes brady-arrhythmias), it might be just the thing. A wire might be better though.

Vasopressin: I just don't understand this drug at all. We use it in two ranges, one for sepsis, one for GI bleeding, in both cases to tighten up arteries. But the dose for GI bleeding is ten times the rate of the dose for sepsis? How come it doesn't produce ten times the blood pressure? We used to use vasopressin together with IV nitroglycerine for GI bleeds before **octreotide** came along – what I do remember is that it causes bradycardia, or some slowing anyhow, often to heart rates in the 50's - that I would never have believed in septic patients who usually run in the 130's for days at a time. But what the heck – it works, I run it.

Dobutamine – This is the pure beta pressor (the only one with a "b" in it.) This is what you want to use when the pump isn't pumping – cardiogenic shock. Two problems with that: first, it "whips" a heart that's already failing – a balloon pump is much better. Second: it very easily causes lots of arrhythmias – something your cardiac patient doesn't need. Make sure their electrolyes are ok.

Rarely used (Zebras): Epi, Isuprel, Amrinone, Milrinone. We'll use these drips sometimes in special situations – like maybe at the end of a code. Epinephrine – very powerful, <u>very</u> arrhythmogenic. Isuprel – "Prel": a powerful beta drug, also causes lots of arrhythmias, can be hard to control. I haven't seen a Prel drip in many moons. (Jayne: "Isuprel is completely gone – nobody even makes it any more.") Amrinone – "the yellow stuff", and it's cousin milrinone – sort of the same as dobutamine, except different – maybe we see these once a year. Anybody know if they're used more in the CCU?

For extravasations: Regitine. This is a good one to know about, even if you never have to use it. A patient who has to get pressors through a peripheral line is at a real risk for injury around the site if the drip infiltrates into the tissue. Regitine is an alpha blocker, and gets injected ("infiltrated") into the tissues around the IV site to relax the vasoconstriction. Never seen it done, but I saw a dopamine infiltration wound once. Ugly.

3-2: "Down" Meds

Nitrates: nitrates are vasodilators – they open up coronary artery flow, and they lower SVR, so the heart gets 1: a better muscular blood supply and 2: less arterial resistance to push against. Nice.

Nipride – the ultimate down med. This is what you want to use if your patient has malignant hypertension, or something very acutely dangerous, like a leaky aortic aneurysm. Very powerful. Be especially careful with this one. The nice thing is that it both works and wears off so quickly, so that you can titrate it very easily – it doesn't take ten minutes for a change to show up.

4- Pulmonary Meds

Beta Agonists: Albuterol, ipratoprium. Simple enough – these are beta agonists, so they make the bronchi open up. Remember that they can make your patient very tachycardic for the same reason.

Mucolytics: mucomyst/acetylcysteine – we used to use this a lot to loosen up secretions, but not in recent years. The in-house CNS (that's as in my house, and my spouse) says it's because it can cause hemorrhagic bronchitis. Sounds like a good reason. Lately we've been giving a couple of doses of mucomyst orally before and after IV dye loads required for contrasted scans – apparently it helps prevent renal failure problems afterwards. How the heck did they figure that one out?

DNAse: Are they still using this? We saw it used for a while some years ago, mostly with CF patients who had very thick, tenacious secretions. I have no idea how well it works.

Theophylline – talk about going in and out of fashion. We used to give this stuff by the barrel, seemed like. Now I see it given once very couple of months, maybe. Those poor COPD patients are shaky enough without being made lots more tachycardic by theo…

Glycopyrrolate – another one we used to use a lot, nebulized, mostly to "dry up" patients with lots of secretions. Also used in place of atropine for bradycardia, I think.

5- Gut Meds

5-1- Too much acid:

H2 Blockers: cimetidine, ranitidine, pepcid. Cimetidine was apparently the wonder of it's day, setting all sorts of world records for drug sales, and it did a lot of good, too.

Then apparently we found out that it often makes platelets go away – we give it rarely now, giving zantac a lot of the time instead. My wife's hospital uses a lot of pepcid (famotidine) – we hardly ever do.

Proton pump inhibitors: prilosec, nexium. ("Mom, I hate my cousin Ralph. Do I have to sit nexium?") Apparently the greatest thing since sliced cimetidine for gastric acid. Sure works well for me…

Antacids – another big change over the years. I remember giving 60cc of **Mylanta 2** every two hours through an NG tube. No more. Do we even stock it now?

5-2- <u>**Coating the stomach: Carafate**</u> (sucralfate)– this is good stuff, but it'll block up an NG tube very easily. I dissolve mine for a while in warm water, and follow it with a warm flush.

5-3- <u>**Moving It Along: Colace, senna, mag citrate, go-lytely, enemas**</u>: You've got to keep it moving, and the sooner you start your patients on this stuff the better. We see lots of opiate ileus, and lots of our patients get **reglan** (metoclopramide) around the clock when they're on fentanyl or morphine drips. Recently somebody got a dose of **neostigmine** for an opiate ileus – I hear it works well for that, but I haven't seen it done myself. And you know that trick they've been trying with narcan through the NG tube for the past twenty years? Doesn't work.

5-4- <u>**Stop the Bleeding: Octreotide**</u>: The word is that octreotide tightens up the arterial flow to the splanchnic-perfused areas, and I guess the studies are clear about its effectiveness. I do know that octreotide has almost completely replaced the previous combination of vasopressin and nitroglycerine that we used to use.

5-5- <u>**Clearing the Ammonia: Lactulose**</u> – it works, but it seems like an awful price to pay for everyone involved. Sometimes patients with varices can't have an NG tube but still need the med – these people get retention enemas through a rectal tube. The trick is not to give too much at once: usually we dilute a dose of lactulose with an equal amount or more of NS, and infuse not more than 200cc or so at a time, letting it stay in place for about 30-45 minutes. Rectal tube balloons have to be deflated every four hours for about half an hour, and the tube itself is supposed to come out of the patient once a shift.

6- Endocrine Meds

Insulin: drips, sliding scales, regular, NPH, humulin, glargine. Lately we've been tearing our hair out (I have less to pull out than most, which may or may not be an advantage) over the decision to put most of our patients on insulin drips to try to keep them in the "tight control" range of 80-120. This means an awful lot of running around with glucometers, a lot of sore patient fingers, a lot of titration between drips and tube feeds, etc., etc. We do a lot of q4-hour checks with sliding scales too. We check patients on insulin drips every two hours, on the idea that regular insulin peaks two hours after a change. **Glargine** insulin, which goes by the trade name of Lantus, is the newest horse out of this particular gate – apparently the dose is given sq once daily, and there are no peaks or drops; just a nice constant delivery. Sign me up!

Oral hypoglycemics glucophage/metformin, glitazones: Lots of patients come in that are managed on the outside with oral meds, but usually they're so stressed during their stay in the unit that they wind up on one of the sliding scale treatments.

Thyroid replacement: Synthroid. We give these when people are on maintenance management.

"Cort stim" tests: the idea here is to check a morning cortisol level (I'm pretty sure the level has to be drawn early in the morning, having something to do with "inner-clock" timing of cortisol secretion). Then a dose of cosyntropin is given, and another cortisol level drawn an hour later. Tells you if your patient's adrenal cortex can respond normally or not. Sometimes septic, hypotensive patients turn out to be "hypo-adrenal", and giving them steroid replacement is supposed to help. Apparently under debate.

DDAVP/desmopressin – this one's interesting. This turns out to be vasopressin, which turns out to be anti-diuretic hormone, ADH. Two uses for this one: first that comes to mind is your hepato-renal patient who's bleeding from here and there, because he's coagulopathic? And uremic? Uremic platelets don't work so well, apparently DDAVP helps them work more better.

The second one is very cool to see, although you may not see it often. Remember any of that pituitary stuff? Hypo-pituitary, all that? We had a young man in awhile back, he'd had some sort of tumor removed, pituitary I guess, and he couldn't make any of his pituitary hormone things any more, had to take them as supplements.

So let's see – two ways ADH can go. You can make too much, which is SIADH, right? You don't pee, much, because you have too much anti-diuretic hormone... ok. Then there's the other way, which is diabetes insipidus – you don't make enough ADH, and you can't hold onto water at all. Right – that's what this fellow did – drank all the time, peed hugely... I mean, scarily – a liter an hour when he'd come in, out of whack. Like a "siphon", which is what "diabetes" means... so he'd get his dose of DDAVP, and it was as though the faucet had been turned off – all of a sudden his urine output would drop to whatever – 40 an hour? "Anti-lasix". Amazing.

Steroids: Couple of flavors of steroids, given for several reasons – hydrocortisone, which is the generic, sort of "weaker" version, and methyprednisolone, which is as I recall about 7 times more powerful as hydrocortisone, which will put your patient's adrenals right to sleep for a while. Some patients in an acute flare of something bad will get started on "stress" steroids – a COPD flare is probably the most common example. They get methylprednisolone, something like 60mg several times a day.

Now and again you'll see someone get "pulse steroids" – this is usually in some really life-threatening situation like a severe lupus flareup, or I want to say BOOP... this is pretty impressive – the dose is a GRAM of methyprednisolone. When you consider the usual dose is 60mg or so… it's a lot!

Steroids will absolutely play havoc with your patient's blood sugars – especially, obviously, if they're diabetic – or even if they're not. Be aware that you may have to work hard with your insulin management while this is going on.

There's been a lot of debate in recent years about giving steroids to people in sepsis. For the longest time this was considered a really bad idea, supposedly because they inhibit immune response – a bad thing when your patient is infected. Then more recently it became the practice to test septic patients for adrenal suppression – which is what cort-stimming is all about – I guess some people's adrenals go to sleep in sepsis. Then the folks with sleepy adrenals got hydrocortisone.

Now the latest rumor is that the evidence is going the other way. Ask around – not sure what the current word is.

7- Renal Meds

Our patients have a lot of kidney trouble, which only makes sense given what's wrong with so many of them. Kidneys are incredibly sensitive to insults ("You stupid kidney!"), and even a hypotensive episode of 20 minutes can put kidneys into ATN. Patients with hypertension often have kidneys that are used to a high perfusion pressure – sepsis or some other kind of hypotensive shock can have a really unpleasant effect. We also see lots of chronic-renal patients who get hemodialysis outside the hospital and who get into trouble for some reason. (Ask me why I take my **glucophage** every six frickin' hours.)

There aren't a whole lot of meds that immediately come to mind when you think "kidney", besides diuretics. Low dose "renal range" **dopamine** sometimes is still used to encourage kidneys when they don't want to go – once in a while it works, too. **Phosphate binders** like **calcium acetate** are used to, uh… bind up excess calcium that can't be excreted by non-functioning kidneys. And we give the new (anything less than ten years old is new to me) **marrow stimulant factors: epogen** for red cells and **neupogen** for whites – I know that epogen replaces endogenous **erythropoietin** ($1.25 for the word "endogenous", please), which is secreted by the kidney – what does neupogen replace?

8- Anti-Infectives

We sure do give a lot of antibiotics in the unit, and it's a good thing too, but I'm pretty sure that we had a patient with a linezolid-resistant bug a while back. (Oh <u>shit</u>…!)

Gram positive/ negative infections: (Why is everyone mad at Gram? What did she ever do to anyone besides make that Christmas fruit bread that everyone hates?) Now I remember why I didn't want to write this part – I am really deficient in understanding antibiotics. Everybody has their thing, and mine is actually balloon pumps. I'm pretty good at blood gases and PA lines too. Daughter number one is doing micro now in nursing school, and she usually quizzes me on things – this time I think it's going to be the other way around.

Ignorance though is no excuse for not knowing the essential points of safety, which in antibiotics usually center around sensitivity reactions, from rashes to anaphylaxis, identifying drugs as the causes of "drug fevers", and knowing which drugs need to be monitored for levels. Vancomycin dosing is level dependent (read: "do your kidneys work?"), and we send peak and trough levels on gentamicin as well. Every drug in the universe has an enormous number of side effects – experience and book time will serve you well when mixed together in fairly large doses. We are always looking things up in our unit, consulting pharmacy, checking calculations with each other. Remember rule # 1: "There are no stupid questions.", to which could be added "Two heads are always better than one."

Fungal infections: Amphotericin B, Ambisome, Fluconazole – Amphotericin B is a toxic drug, and often patients need to be premedicated for it they way you would for a patient sensitive to red cell transfusion: tylenol, benadryl, sometimes steroids. An Ampho-B dose has to go in over something like 6 hours. The liposomal stuff can run a bit faster, and I understand is better tolerated. Fluconazole seems easier in general, but does it cover the same fungal infections? I keep wanting to say "I really should know all this." Which is of course why they publish pharmacy reference books…my wife would look it up on the pharmacy reference that she carries around in her palm pilot at work. The Epocrates reference is a totally cool thing to get if you're at all gadget-head: you download it free – pretty nice of them, huh? into your PC at home, and then the PC sends it into your handheld through the little cradle. Updates itself automatically, too. I wonder if anybody else just gives their stuff away like that on the web…

TB – rifampin, ethambutol, INH, maybe clarithromycin – TB is probably going to earn a FAQ of it's own one of these days – it's a major, serious baddy in the ID universe. Now and then we get a patient who needs to be ruled out, and it becomes a major project: the patient goes into a negative pressure room (it sucks air inwards, to prevent the bug from getting out), and everyone wears N95 masks inside, because it's so easily transmitted. We give the drugs infrequently enough that I always look them up before giving them to make sure I remember what I'm doing. Some years back we had a patient turn positive for something nasty – it was actually Neisseria meningiditis, and all of us who came in contact with him got to take rifampin for two days – makes the urine turn a very pleasant day-glo orange.

Treating drug resistant infections: Linezolid/Synercid - those bugs just don't know when to give up. Of course, we're doing our best to help them mutate, aren't we? This is a battle that is never going to end.

A quick story that goes here: just in case you thought that the superbugs were going to kill us all, and just when you thought that there were no role models left in the world, along comes Dr. Paul Farmer, a physician at one of the big teaching hospitals in Boston.

Dr. Farmer has established a field hospital out in the wilds of Haiti someplace, where he treats the local people who have had the misfortune to be infected with multi-drug resistant TB. Scary one. He's achieved cure rates between 95 and 100% (is this right?) by coming up with innovative treatment plans. So cool.

Antivirals: acyclovir, indinavir, etc. This part of the treatment spectrum is really starting to get going – the development of the whole HIV treatment process was amazing to me, and I think I've read that the antiviral age isn't quite here yet, but soon ought to be. We give these meds as orals / via NGT for patients who are on them on the outside, usually for HIV. I think there's one for CMV as well.

9- Antipyretics

Tylenol – Yes, it's true, Tylenol can drop a patient's blood pressure. Not often, but it happens enough that we old-gome nurses remember it. Nobody's ever had much of an explanation…

Motrin (ibuprofen) – We use ibuprofen now and again for fevers. Good for cramps too, and I sure hope it really works against Alzheimer's the way they say, because, um…what were we talking about? Some article I saw said that ibuprofen actually breaks down amyloid plaques.

Aspirin – Aspirin used to be the best thing for fevers, and I think we used it on my oldest kid when she was small (she's half-way through her first year of nursing school now). Not any more – that whole business about Reye's syndrome and all, but we do still give it to everyone coming in who's suspected of ruling in for MI. Apparently makes an enormous difference.

10- Anticoagulants

Heparin – we see, or at least rule a lot of people out for the heparin-induced thrombocytopenia thing. It's good to think about it if you see your patient's platelet count dropping. We change our patients' flush lines from heparinized saline to NS for this – it seems as though even just saying "heparin" in the patient's room can make this happen if they have this problem.

Coumadin – Most of our patients are pretty acute, so we don't give coumadin/warfarin a lot. On the other hand, we do see patients come in who have taken a bit too much for one reason or another, and it's always worth wondering about if your new admission has a really high INR. Make sure they get vitamin K, and don't brush their teeth for a while.

Low-molecular-weight heparins: Fragmin – this is one of a whole group of new LMW heparins, which are supposed to anticoagulate as well as heparin does, while doing away with a lot of the PTTs, along with most of the worries about HIT. We'll see, I guess.

Platelet drugs: plavix, integrilin, reopro. These are the newer platelet-aggregation inhibitors. Obviously the CCU gets most of the cardiac cath patients, but we still see people from the lab sometimes. I don't know what makes the physicians choose one drip over the other, but they run for a fixed number of hours only, as opposed to heparin running for several days. Plavix is the oral maintenance med in this category – I think there are others, but we rarely give them.

Aspirin: Yup, aspirin.

Clot-busters: TPA, streptokinase – there are some newer ones which the family CNS knows all about, but our patients are hardly ever good candidates for this stuff, since so many of them are coagulopathic already. Once in a blue moon the team will lyse a PE, but as always we'd have to check with pharmacy and our references to run it.

11- Anti-Anticoagulants

Protamine – another med that we give once every year or so. I never have. Remember that it specifically reverses heparin.

Vitamin K – this we give fairly often, at times for those folks we were talking about who get a little too much coumadin. (My wife was doing a community-nursing course years ago, and one of the nurses described an elderly person she had visited at home. She had put all her pills in a candy bowl, and was saying things like "Well, when I'm dizzy I take an extra one of these" – holding up, say, a nifedipine (ack!) – "and when my knees are bothering me I take two of these" – holding up who-knows-what. Good thing she got visited!)

12- Miscellaneous Meds and Weird Reactions

Cancer chemotherapy in the unit

Our hospital requires nurses to go through a certification course to give cancer chemotherapy meds. Now and again we get a patient in who needs them, and the nurses from the oncology floors come down and do it for us. Sometimes we will give a dose of something on the chemo list, but only if it's not at chemo strength – for this we use the special heavy gloves (the coolest purple color), and a special disposal container.

Code Drugs

Atropine, epinephrine, calcium chloride, lido, amio…this is certainly a subject that should take up entire volumes, and does, but here's one thing that immediately comes to mind. Patients will come to the unit after a code sometimes with pupils that appear to be fixed and dilated – atropine will definitely do this. Wears off after some hours. Good thing to remember! Take ACLS. Learn how codes are run. Learn why the meds are given.

Special Situations:

There are some situations that call for specific meds only, and a couple came to mind:

Dantrolene, bromocriptine: Once in a really great while a patient in the OR will develop malignant hyperthermia – a syndrome of very rapid temperature rise, which as I understand it is a reaction to one or the other of the anesthetic agents being given. The fever will go up really fast, and really high – maybe to 108 F. A similar situation is neuroleptic malignant syndrome, where a fever will rise quickly to scary heights, in response to meds like haldol, or zyprexa. I think we had a patient on clozaril who did the same thing. Anyhow, the treatment med to keep in the back of your mind for this situation is dantrolene. Pretty orange color. I think I've seen it given twice, maybe, in the last few years. Supposedly works well – the other med I've seen used for this is bromocriptine.

Mucomyst: lately this old drug has been put to use pre- and post- IV contrast procedures, because there's some evidence that it helps preserve the kidneys from injury. I wonder who noticed that?

Glucagon: for beta-blocker overdose. I've seen this happen once or twice. Another one to keep in the back of your head.

THAM: (Tromethamine) – sort of a "super-bicarb". Powerful stuff, useful for your patient who is horribly acidotic (our patients usually see this drug when they're around 7.0, even with a bicarb drip), and will definitely help your pressors work better as a result. Unfortunately people who get that sick hardly ever get better, so THAM is usually a sign of impending death.

Reglan: This is a strange one: about a year ago we had a patient come in from one of the floors who had developed a sort of "waxy flexibility", which was the term they used to use for catatonic patients who could be put in a position – say, arms above the head – and who would stay that way for hours. The teams finally decided that this poor person was having a very strange extra-pyramidal reaction to reglan. Never heard of it before or since.

Oral meds for low BP: midodrine, pseudoephedrine. Kind of strange, but it's done. I think this is usually in situations when people have some chronic condition that loosens up their arterial tone – muscular dystrophy comes to mind. Pseudoephedrine is the stuff that dries up your nose in cold pills, and midodrine is actually sort of like oral neosynephrine – it's an alpha agonist agent. Used rarely.

NG Tubes for Beginners

We've started seeing new grad nurses in the MICU in recent years, and it's seemed that they might need a hand with some of the basic tools – things that in times past they might've spent time working with on the floors, but which now they have to get a faster grip on, since they've come straight into the higher-acuity area. This is our first is a possible series – topics we have in mind: "The ins out outs of Foley catheters" (sheesh!), "Peripheral IVs for beginners", "Which IV Fluid Should My Patient Be Getting?", "Admitting Your Patient to the Unit"… things like that. Let us know what you think of this one, and as usual, please remember that these articles are not meant to be the final word on <u>anything</u> – always refer to your own policies and procedures, and let us know when you find errors. Thanks!

A couple of cool things: if you're interested, you can follow up on the image and reference links – that's the blue web address lines in this article, simply by clicking on them. If you're reading this article from our website, you'll go directly to the source of the image, or the quote.

The second thing is that the images in these articles can be enlarged. Click the image, grab a corner with the mouse, and drag – bada bing! Big picture! Cool! Helpful with the x-rays.

1- What is a nasogastric tube?
2- What is an orogastric tube?
3- What is a g-tube? PEG tube?
4- What are Salem sumps all about? What's a sump?
5- What is an enteroflex tube? Dobhoff tube?
6- What's a j-tube?
7- Who inserts gastric tubes?
8- How do I insert a gastric tube?
9- How do I assess the placement of the tube? Two really important points.
10- How do I secure these tubes to the patient?
11- How do I check a gastric aspirate with a Salem sump? Another really important point. A quick story. And about Lopez valves…
12- With an enteroflex?
13- With a dobhoff?
14- How much aspirate should I refeed?
15- What can go wrong with a feeding tube?
    - It can go into the wrong place.
    - Coiling
    - Too shallow
    - Too deep
16- While it's in?
17- If it gets pulled out?
18- If it gets plugged?
19- Should these tubes be routinely changed?

1- What is a nasogastric tube?

I think in one of the other articles, we made the point that there are certain professions that require constant examination of all the things you do – I think the example was piloting aircraft. Pilots are forever refining, evaluating, and adjusting their techniques, so that apparently you'll see big arguments break out amongst them about how apparently small things should be done: setting flaps, when to retract gear, whatever it is they're doing, they're always thinking about how it should be done, regardless if it's apparent importance.

This is a good attitude to take into the ICU. There are always things that need thinking about – always things that need to be evaluated – devices or procedures that seem elementary actually aren't... and even the "simplest" device can get you or your patient into serious trouble unless you've taken the time to understand it, and assess it, and use it properly.

Peripheral IVs are a good example – did you check to make sure that the line has a good blood return? Are you sure that your patient is getting the med running through the line? We had a lady recently whose peripheral neo mix infiltrated... yow!

So – NG tubes are another good example of a device that seems totally simple and uncomplicated, but which actually... well, let's see.

Naso-gastric: through the nose, into the stomach.

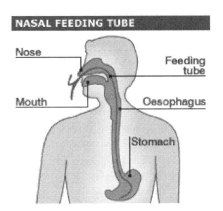

Here it is... "oesophagus"?

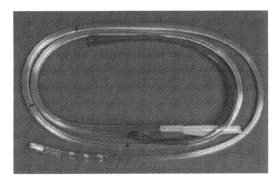

The most common of the nasogastric tubes – the Salem sump. These are large-bore, usually 14 or 18 French, and fairly stiff...

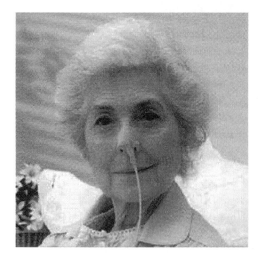

This is the softer variety – the ones we use are called "enteroflex" tubes. There's a longer version that goes the same route, but ends up in the duodenum, past the pylorus – that's the "dobhoff".

"Look, she's smiling!" – "Nah, it's just gas…"

2- What is an orogastric tube?

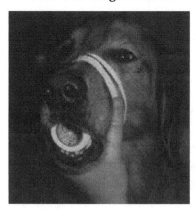

Not too hard – through the mouth, into the stomach.

Guys? I think it's coiled in the mouth…

Nasogastric tubes are painful and uncomfortable, and apparently they cause sinusitis, so our intubated patients get their gastric tubes put in orally.

3- What is a g-tube? PEG tube?

This time it goes through the wall of the stomach, instead of down the oesophagus. "Percutaneous endoscopic gastrotomy" – "PEG tube".

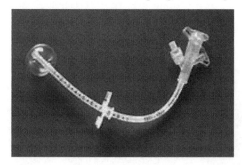

The flat part is sutured to the abdominal wall, and the part with the balloon lives inside the stomach. This one is made of silicone plastic – very nice and soft, doesn't get eaten up by gastric acid, and can stay in place for a long time.

4- What are Salem sumps all about? What is a sump?

This is the clear-and-blue tube a couple of pictures back. These guys are actually two tubes in one – and for a smart reason. Back in the day, nasogastric tubes with a single lumen were the only option – the only ones I saw, anyhow. I think they were just starting to go away when Jayne and I were in school, back in the late 70's. Right around the time of the gold rush. Anyhow – one tube – what's the problem?

The problem is – you hook this thing up to suction, right? Ok – drains the stomach, all fine and good. What happens when the stomach is empty?

Hm – well… stomach's empty, but there's still suction on… well, the tube can either suck up against the stomach wall somewhere – maybe not so good. Or – it can start sucking the air out of the stomach, which is ok up to a point, but when it starts collapsing the stomach… hm – not so good.

Well then, how about this: let's add a second lumen to the tube, so that when the stomach is empty, the second tube will <u>let air come back into the stomach</u>, which won't get sucked all tiny, and which also – hopefully - will prevent the tube from sucking up against the stomach wall. Cool!

That's a "sump". The second lumen – what some people call the "pigtail" – lets air come back into the stomach. Neat!

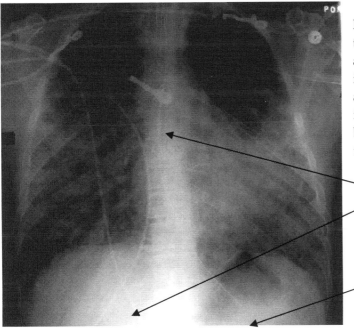

Reading x-rays isn't easy, but there's an NG/OG tube in this one, and you should have some kind of idea of how to find it. I've played around with the contrast of the image to make it a bit easier to find, but you're looking for something that's:

- it's not a chest wire

- it goes down the center of the chest

- and ends somewhere in the stomach….

-

http://www.vh.org

5- What is an enteroflex tube? Dobhoff tube?

These are the softer tubes, like the one Bubbie has in her nose a page or two back. They're much more easily tolerated once they're in, and they're definitely the ones I want. A big problem however is that you **can't reliably empty the patients' stomach** through them. This really matters – if your patients' gut isn't moving things along properly, and he has, say, a liter of fluid in his stomach – he's at an enormous aspiration risk. Yup – even if he's intubated, with the ET tube cuff inflated.

These tubes usually have a sheathed lead weight at the end, which helps them float along into position.

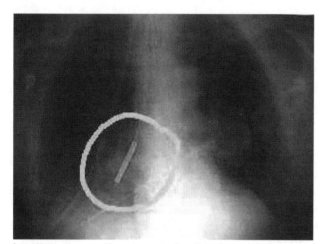

See the weight? Hmm… wait a second… Not a chest electrode… ok. Down the middle of the chest… hm. Ending up in the stomach… uh…

Well guys? Where'd this one go? Think maybe we ought to take it out?

http://www.uam.es/departamentos/medicina/anesnet/journals/ija/vol4n2/feed2.jpg

6- What is a j-tube?

Some patients are at risk for aspirating over and over – it turns out for example, that recurrent GERD – y'know? – acid reflux disease? – can make the lower esophageal sphincter quit working. "Esophageal sphincter incompetence." Not a happy thing – can be a deadly thing. Why?

What to do?

Well – there's a pyloric valve at the bottom of the stomach, right? Hm… if we deliver the tube feeds beyond the pyloric valve… maybe the patient won't aspirate! Woohoo! Time for a Dobhoff tube.

The Dobhoffs are the longer version of the soft feeding tubes, also with a weight at the end.

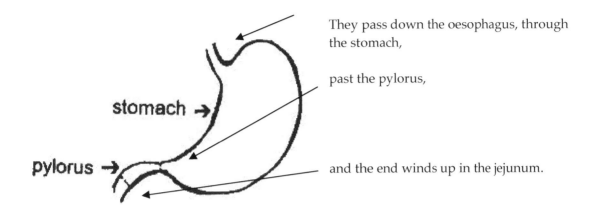

They pass down the oesophagus, through the stomach,

past the pylorus,

and the end winds up in the jejunum.

http://www.wch.ca/images/pyloric.jpg

It's a good idea, anyhow... I'm not too sure how well it works in practice. People secrete stomach fluids all the time – so what you'll see sometimes is an NG tube to suction, and a J-tube for feeding. Complicated. The feeds have to be "elemental", or "predigested", so it's usually something like Vivonex.

7- Who inserts gastric tubes?

At our institution, the nurses put in nasal and oral Salem sumps, along with the smaller feeding tubes **without a stylet**. These decisions, about who gets to do what, are probably made by hospital risk-management committees, working with the insurance companies who provide liability coverage to the hospitals. So don't feel bad if they don't let you place them and make the docs do it.

8- How do I insert a gastric tube?

Carefully! There are lots of descriptions out there on how to do this, and instead of replicating them, we'll just make some comments:

First, as always: make sure the patient consents! Things are a bit simpler when your patient is sedate, because then consent is usually implied, but you still have to be clear that consent for procedures has been given, either by the patient beforehand, or by a proxy. It's worth mentioning that emergency consents for procedures are implied when a patient comes in unconscious, with no family members – every now and then we get an "Unknown White Male", who wakes up and tells us who he is... but the consents still need to be made out and signed by physicians – use the usual forms for blood and procedures.

Next: think about what else is going on with this patient. Does the patient have a history of nosebleeds? Is she anticoagulated? Got platelets? Varices? Just had variceal bands applied? Yup, you have to think of all these things... a patient with recent bands? No way am I inserting that tube – that's why the Great Nursing Supervisor invented GI docs.

Then: you want to make sure you're inserting the tube to a reasonable depth. Measure one way or the other – match the length of the tube from the patient's big toe to her earlobe, subtract pi*R squared, add her shoe size in centimeters times the chi-square regression... hey! Do I get my masters' now? The tube has to go in far enough to drain the pool that should be there in the patient's stomach.

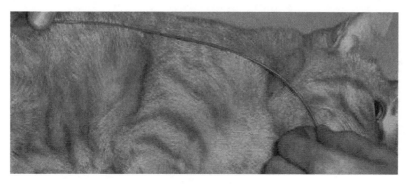 Um... far enough?

Now pick your approach. Nasal? Oral? Does the patient have a history of nosebleeds?

Lots of lubricant. Sometimes I like to wrap the end of the tube around my (gloved) hand for about a minute to help form the curve that will pass through the patients nose.

Pass the tube slowly – and don't force it! You do have to use some forward pressure – experience will teach you how much. Get someone to help you.

Here's a critical trick: as the tube goes in, put the other end of the NG tube to your ear and listen. If the tube is patent, and it ought to be, then if you're approaching the airway, you should hear – what? Breathing? Good guess! Don't advance!

To help the patient swallow the tube, have some crushed ice at hand and give him a little, orally. Or use a saline fish.

Have your gastric suction line at hand. No higher than what – 80mm of negative pressure? Have the little connector gatsy attached – when you get to what seems like reasonable depth, hook up the line, see what comes out. Stomach contents? Good job! Are you sure the tube is deep enough? You can still get gastric contents from the upper part of the stomach...

9- How do I assess the placement of the tube? Two really important points.

Good question. The traditional way of doing this is to attach the hugeous syringe, and quickly push 30cc of air into the tube, while listening over the stomach with a stethoscope. People put the scope bell over the stomach, usually just below the patient's diaphragm, at the midline, and somebody pushes in the air, and people hear a nice woosh, and everybody nods and says: "Perfect!"

Well… it's not always that easy. Sometimes gastric tubes will go to strange places – there are only a couple of places they should be able to go, but very unpleasant and weird things have happened. Want to know?

- "…insertion of a nasogastric (stomach suction) tube through the ethmoid bone of the skull during surgery, causing parts of the patient's brain to be sucked out and causing his death."

http://www.bobtoth.com/anesthesia.html

Whoa. Does that mean that you should push in the air, and listen with the stethoscope on top of the patient's head? Just to make sure? Hmm…   "Well, I was just making sure!"
Yeah, that'll look good.

Similarly:

- "When a fracture of the skull base is suspected, insertion of a nasogastric tube (NGT) should be avoided. The orogastric route is preferred as there have been cases of intracranial NGT placement in the presence of cribriform plate fractures.

http://www.sbiheadlines.com/research/papers/Craniofacial%20and%20Skull%20Base%20Trauma.doc

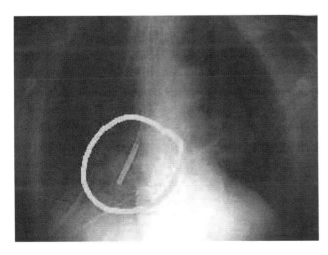

Remember this one? What kind of tube is it? Where'd it go?

The scary part is that you can hear a nice "woosh", even if the tube is in the wrong place…

http://www.uam.es/departamentos/medicina/anesnet/journals/ija/vol4n2/feed2.jpg

So… what do Jayne and Mark say? First off - don't force the tube! Second, assess the patient while you're placing the tube! Third – if you have any questions at all about the placement of the tube – **the standard of care is to get an x-ray.**

If I hear a woosh, (over the stomach!) but I don't get gastric contents, I ask for a film. No exceptions.

A second critically important point: Once the tube is in, and you know it's in the right place: hook it up to suction, and empty the patient's stomach. **I always, always do this**. If that patient has a liter and a half in her stomach, <u>you want it out of there</u>! How much does she need to aspirate to get pneumonia? Or ARDS? Yes, you will find people, as always, who disagree with this… I don't care! ☺

10- How do I secure these tubes to the patient?

For nasogastric tubes, a little benzoin to the skin, and a piece of cloth tape, split, with the splits around the tube (flag the ends so you can get em off later), and the fat end on the patient's nose. Or a tegaderm, which I like better – softer…

For orogastric tubes, almost always for intubated patients, we tape them to the ETT tube, a couple of inches away from the mouth. Cloth tape, flagged.

I am not a fan of using safety pins to pin things to robes/ shirts/ johnnies. What if the patient pulls his shirt off?

11- How do I check a gastric aspirate with a Salem sump? Another really important point. A quick story. And about Lopez valves…

Well – why are you checking the gastric aspirate at all? It's <u>very important</u> – you don't want to let a whole lot of fluid collect in the patient's stomach, so that:

    a- what doesn't happen?

    b- and why might that happen?

    c- and so what else would you want to assess besides the gastric aspirate? And what else?

    d- uh huh, and what if there aren't any?

    e- well, why wouldn't there be any?

    f- and what med do we use all the time that makes this happen?

    g- so what should you do about it?

a- Aspiration. **b-** Because the patient has too much in his stomach! **c-** Bowel sounds. And stooling. **d-** Uh… there might be a problem? **e-** Um…recent surgery? Paralyitc ileus? Gastro-intestinal hypomotility? **f-** Fentanyl **g-** get the patient started on a bowel regimen, possibly including colace, senna, IV reglan, po narcan…

Well anyhow – it's incredibly important to check the aspirate, and to try and prevent aspiration events.

Here's a quick story: I'm the nurse in charge one night, running around, checking the hot spots, helping out, stuff like this. Nurse comes to me, says: "Well, my patient keeps vomiting."

Me: "Um, isn't he intubated?" Meaning, doesn't he also have an OG tube? And if he's vomiting, isn't it hooked up to suction?

Nurse: "Yeah, and I don't know why he keeps vomiting – I mean, I irrigated the OG tube and all…"

We went to take a look. And here we get to the point. <u>OG tubes do not automatically drain a patient's stomach, just because they're apparently at the right depth</u>. Bummer.

Yup, it's true. What a pain. You can hook a Salem sump to low wall suction, and it may very well not work. Mainly, this is because the tip of the tube gets stuck somewhere – maybe it's coiled up in the patient's stomach folds, maybe the tip has coiled up into the antrum, above the pool… or maybe one or both of the lumens is plugged – if the main lumen is plugged, then the drainage is going to try to come out through the pigtail.

Remember the pigtail?

Here's what you want to see: with the Salem sump hooked up to suction, **the stomach will be empty when the pigtail starts whistling.** Make sense? All the fluid inside the stomach comes out- what's left? Air? So now what happens? Air starts coming in through the pigtail – it whistles. Now you **know** – if the tube is in at the right depth – that the patient's stomach is empty.

What if the pigtail won't whistle?

Here's what to do: Irrigate the lumens. Still not draining? Undo the tapes holding the tube in place. Pull the tube back a bit – an inch or so. Or advance it a bit – an inch or so. Draining now? Whoa…. eek! Did you just get a liter out? Good thing!

So – if your pigtail is draining, should you clamp it with a Kelly? Tie it in a knot?

Do this assessment every four hours!

Oh yeah – the other thing. Seen these things?

Lopez valves. We use them to give meds through feeding tubes, so we don't have to disconnect the tube feed setup every time. The thing is – if you decide to drain your patient's stomach by hooking up the suction to the valve here where the red cap goes – well, you can see how tiny the left-side end is, right? Very easily plugged. This means that suction to drain the stomach may not work if it's run through the valve.

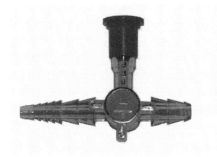

So – if you're worried, take the valve out. Use a regular barrel connector, then hook up the suction.

12- With an enteroflex?

You can't. Or maybe you can, a little – but not reliably. Sometimes you get lucky – but in general, you can't really aspirate through the little feeding tubes, because they're so soft, and their size is so small, that they just collapse when you try to use negative pressure on them.

This came up just last week. Guy had had reconstructive surgery for his oral cancer – partial tongue resection, jaw flap, donor sites, this and that, lube, oil, filter… and then postop… well – why do people get oral cancer? From doing what? And drinking what? And so what are they at risk for when they come into the hospital, and can't get it? Right!

So – he DT'ed. Pulled out his hemovacs – apparently it was ugly. Went back to the OR I think, reintubated, got the hemovacs replaced, straightened out, and then got sent to us for management of the DT's. Started on versed, and fentanyl. Nasal enteroflex tube. Tube feeds…

Well – see? This is a dangerous NG tube situation. Here's a fellow getting all sorts of sedation – I come on, it's day two in the ICU, tube feeds are at 40cc/hour. No bowel sounds, hasn't stooled since coming to the ICU – well, he's on fentanyl. Yeah, he's tolerant to the benzos probably, because why? Right! But is he tolerant of the fentanyl? Nooo, he is not! So what happens to his gut? So… why does it become really important that I know how much is in his stomach?

We explained this to the ENT surgeon when he came in – his response: "Well, is he absorbing the tube feeds?" Us: "We can't tell." Resident: "Why not?" Us: sigh…

I mean – it might've been just fine – no problem at all. But you don't really know for sure – and you really do need to.

13- With a Dobhoff?

Think about this for a second. Where is the end of this tube – that is, where is it supposed to be? Uh huh… and can you expect to aspirate much from there? And through a soft tube, at that?

14- How much aspirate should I refeed?

Well – you can always find a policy for everything – and that's right, you should be able to find some kind of official guidance for your practice. We have a policy that says to refeed all amounts aspirated up to something like 200cc. I don't like it. I think the policy should say: "Refeed all aspirates up to something like 200cc, but only if the patient has active bowel sounds, if they're stooling regularly, and clearly aren't having aspiration events."

(Maybe it does say that... hmm... been a while since I read those. Think it's easy to find them in those enormous folders? A request: please, please, please, **can we have all hospital nursing policies made available on the hospital computer network, in searchable, indexed, printable form?** Please? This should've happened a **long** time ago!)

15- What can go wrong with a feeding tube?

It can go into the wrong place: the tube can coil up into the mouth (if you're placing it through the nose – I've never heard of one going up and coming out of the nose during oral placement – although life is always full of new things!) Or, as above, it can go into the airway, through a bronchial wall, and out into the lung tissue. Or into the head. Bummer.

It can be placed too shallowly. With the tip in the esophagus. Why would this be a problem for someone lying in bed? Why should everyone on bedrest be kept at least 30 degrees head-up at all times?

It can go too far in. Sometimes the end of a Salem sump can make its way into the duodenum, and if you're trying to keep your patient's stomach empty, it's not going to work.

Actually, this can produce unexpected results: a couple of times over the years, I've seen Salems to suction, and the nurse ahead of me will comment on how much drainage the patient is putting out – liters and liters, usually some unusual color, like orangeade... the tube is too far in. Take a look at the film with the team. Where's the tip? Leaving the tube to suction, pull the tube back some... did the drainage suddenly change color? How come?

The soft feeding tubes are inserted with a fairly stiff wire stylet in them, that comes out after the tube placement is confirmed. What could that stylet do?

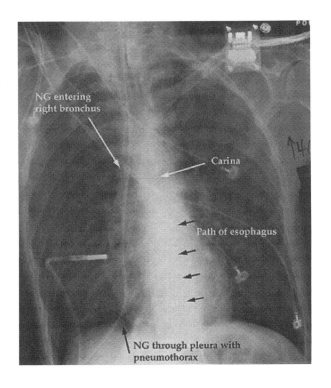

Whoa!

http://www.vh.org

379

16- While it's in?

Stomachs sometimes get erosion injuries from the stiffer tubes, so Salem sumps don't usually stay in much longer than a week.

Oesophaguses also.

What if the tip of the tube gets pulled back up into the esophagus? And your patient is lying flat in bed?

What if the patient has varices?

Question for thought – what if the patient has a trach? Should that patient have a Salem sump in for a long time? What might happen to the tissue between the trach tube and the Salem tube? What is a tracheo-esophageal fistula?

17- If it gets pulled out?

Well – it's not very nice if the tube has to be replaced several times. And as above, what if it gets pulled back only part way? What if the tip got pulled back, say, to the pharynx?

18- If it gets plugged?

Every nurse has her own trick for unplugging a stuck gastric tube. It often has to do with what the tube is plugged with – is it some pill that wasn't crushed up well enough? Some people like ginger ale, some people like hot cranberry juice, some people like hot water – just be sure it's not too hot! Some people like papain, but that's the stuff that you use to dissolve something made of protein, so it probably won't work on a little plug of carafate that's stuck in the tube. Make it a practice to crush up your meds pretty well, and try letting them dissolve some after crushing as well, in some warm water. If you see the plug, try squeezing the tube at the plug with a kelly.

Remember that some meds are NOT meant for NG tubes! Any preparation of sustained release anything is not supposed to be crushed up and squirted through a tube! If some silly doc writes a po order for an SR med without realizing that the patient hasn't swallowed a pill in two weeks… straighten her out!

19- Should these tubes be routinely changed?

In practice we don't usually do this unless the tube is plugged and can't be cleared, or unless we're changing the patient from a Salem to one of the soft tubes. Anybody know how long a soft feeding tube can stay in?

Nutrition

1- How important is nutrition for patients in the MICU?
2- When should I start thinking about nutrition for my patient?
3- What kinds of nutrition are available for MICU patients?
4- How do we figure out what kind of nutrition my patient should or shouldn't get?
5- What kinds of stomach-access devices are there?
    5-1- Salem sumps
    5-2- Enteroflexes and Dobhoffs
    5-3- G-tubes
    5-4- J-tubes (elemental liquid nutrition)

6- How do I make sure that the feeding tube is in the right place, and what can happen if it's not?
7- How do I make sure that the patient is absorbing the nutrition I'm giving?
8- What labs should I watch?
9- What is the big deal with serum albumin?
    9-1- What is a normal albumin?
    9-2- What is oncotic pressure?
    9.3- What does albumin have to do with oncotic pressure?
    9.4- What does "third-spaced" mean?

10- Should my patient be getting IV albumin?
11- What is TPN? What is hyperal?
    11-1- Why does TPN have to run centrally? Can TPN run through a PICC line?
    11-2- Why does TPN have to have a line to itself?
    11-3- Can anything run in the same line with TPN?
    11-4- Why is it white?
    11-5- Why is it sometimes clear and sort of yellowish/greenish?
    11-6- What if my patient is on propofol?
    11.7- Why does the team sometimes seem to wait so long before they start my patient on TPN?
    11.8- Do patients on TPN make stool?
    11.9- What if my patient's TPN doesn't show up on time? What if I contaminate the bag by accident?

12- What are tube feeds all about?

    12-1- What are the different kinds of tube feeds?
      - Jevity, Jevity with fiber, Jevity Plus, Osmolyte, Promote, Promote with fiber, Alitraq, Vivonex, glutamine, Nepro
    12-2- What do I have to know about tube feed pumps?
    12-3- When do I change the pump tubing?
    12-4- How often should I check the aspirate?
    12-5- What if the aspirate is more than 100cc?
    12-6- What happens with tube feeding if my patient is on a fentanyl or morphine drip?

As always, please remember that these articles reflect the experiences and opinions of the authors, without the benefit of academic peer review. When - not if - you find errors, omissions, or things that are just plain wrong, let us know so we can fix them? Thanks!

1- How important is nutrition for patients in the MICU?

Critically important! All sorts of bad things start to happen without nutrition. Surgical wounds don't heal, patients lose muscle mass and strength – and will never wean from a ventilator; patients become edematous and bloated without adequate protein levels in the blood – it seems so obvious! Yet often enough, it gets neglected. Not in your patients, though!

2- When should I start thinking about nutrition for my patient?

At the time of admission. You need to think about nutritional treatment in terms of what's wrong with the patient: will the patient tolerate tube feeds? Will she absorb what you give her? Does she need central TPN? Why? Is she septic, and will the TPN just feed the evil germs? And so on…

3- What kinds of nutrition are available for MICU patients?

We don't see too many dinner trays in the MICU – sometimes we do, but the appearance of a meal tray usually means that the patient is getting ready to leave us. Most of our patients are on some kind of liquid tube feed going in through some kind of tube – and frequently the others are on intravenous TPN.

4- How do we figure out what kind of nutrition my patient should or should not get?

It always depends on the situation, but unless there's some bad thing happening in the gut or abdomen, tube feeds should be started within the first few hours of admission. Someone admitted with one of our common scenarios: say a COPD or asthma flare, or pneumonia, or anything else that might require intubation for more than a day or two should be started right away. If you think your patient may get extubated within a day's time, you might or might not want to feed him enterally - check with the team. (Enterally means using the gut, parenterally means any other way…) Either way, he should probably get some glucose intravenously to keep things like the brain running. Always nice to keep the brain running. What would you do to give nutrition to a patient "flashing" in CHF?

5- What kinds of stomach-access devices are there?

5-1- Salem Sumps

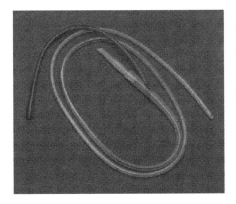

The classic nasogastric tube that we use is this guy, the salem sump.

Actually most of ours are orogastric, because a lot of patients were developing sinusitis when the tubes were put in through the nose. (How would you know? What would you do?) The salem has two lumens – the main one for giving meds and liquids through, and the small blue pigtail.

http://www.buyemp.com/emp_prod/assets/product_images/17b.jpg

Everybody knows what "sumping" means, right? (Do you ever get "sumping for nothing"?) No? Okay – suppose you put a single-lumen NG tube going into the stomach, and you hook it up to low continuous wall suction, because you want to keep your patient's stomach empty. What happens? The tube sucks out the liquid in the stomach, and then begins to suck up the air left behind, and the stomach tries to collapse on itself like an empty balloon. Which it is not built for! What to do? Add a pigtail lumen, which stays open to the air outside the patient. Now what happens is that air whistles back into the stomach to replace the volume that gets sucked out. The stomach stays nice and empty, but retains its normal shape.

The other thing that the pigtail will do is to prevent the tube from sucking itself up onto the stomach wall. Helps prevent trauma.

Nurses at our hospital are allowed to place salem sumps after instruction. Some placement tips:

- Don't force the tube. Duh. You can use gentle steady forward pressure, but if it won't pass fairly easily, stop.

- Lubricate, lubricate, lubricate.

- Put the outward end of the tube near your ear, and try to listen as you pass the tube into the esophagus. If you hear breath sounds, you'll know that you're headed the wrong way.

- Keep your low-wall suction tubing handy as you pass the tube, and if you think you ought to be getting into the stomach, try connecting it to see if you get gastric aspirate. Helps verify position.

- If you think you're in the right place, but you're not getting any gastric aspirate, try the listening-over-the-stomach thing. Still not sure where it is? Are you going to go ahead and use this tube? Nuh-uh! Get an x-ray. Do not allow anybody to push you into giving anything through the tube until you have a clear consensus about where that tube is at!

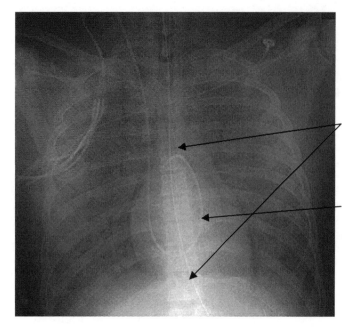

Nice ICU-type x-ray!

Hmm – what's this? Really long, going down the center, all the way down into the, uh… oh!

How about this? Is it in the right place? Really in the right place? I think it might not be in far enough…you could try wedging it to see…

Here's a tangentially relevant story from way back: a nurse wasn't sure where her patient's NG tube was – so she told the house officer, I think an intern at the time, rather full of himself, testing his powers of authority, all like that - and asked for a film. The baby doc insisted that the tube was in the right place, and that the nurse give the dose of oral potassium that he'd ordered. She declined, which produced the inspiring comment: "You seem to have forgotten that I am the doctor."

Well! We were all certainly taken aback, impressed, and intimidated by that, weren't we?

Unfortunately, the physician then elected to give the dose of potassium himself. And was the tube in the patient's stomach? Uh - bad news, baby doc… what's that called? Pneumo-potassitosis?

Here's the important point, which has been emphasized recently in a really well-written article at this website address: http://www.webmm.ahrq.gov/cases.aspx?ic=32 : the best way to tell where your NG tube is, is to get an x-ray. Would you believe that some tubes have made their way into patients' brains? Dropped (or popped) their lungs? (That one's apparently easy with a styletted tube – take a look at the x-ray faq for a neat image of this.) Listening over the stomach may produce all sorts of nice noises when air is injected through the tube, but that does <u>not</u> mean that the tube is where you hope it is. Hooking up the NG tube to suction and getting gastric contents is usually good enough for me, however. Brain contents would presumably be bad…

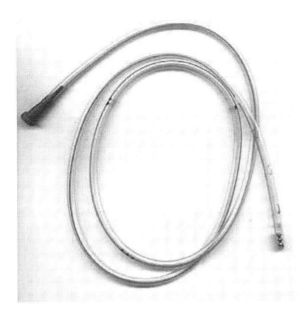

These are the thinner, softer tubes that can stay inserted for very long periods of time - (salem sumps are pretty stiff, and they can injure and erode the esophageal tissue that they rub against.)

Nurses don't insert these tubes in our hospital, but you still need to know the basics – the tube is inserted with a long flexible wire inside it called a stylet. Apparently it's very easy for the tube and stylet to sneak down the trachea and lodge in a bronchus, or maybe pop out into the pleural space (creating a what?) – so the position of these tubes must be checked by x-ray.

http://narang.com/disposable_medical_products/ryles-tube-stomach.html

The difference between enteroflex tubes and Dobhoff tubes is basically in the length: the first ones go as far as the stomach. Dobhoff tubes have a silicone-sheathed lead weight at the lower end, and the idea is that the weight gets carried along by peristalsis past the pylorus into the duodenum, maybe as far as the jejunem? (Oh no - I can't help it, here it comes!: the calendar maker is calling his contractor, checking to see if the months are done: "Well, did ya April 'em? Did ya May 'em? Well then, did jejunem?" Brilliant! Jayne: "You did not put that in the article?!... I married a moron.") The idea is that feeding below the pylorus minimizes the chances that your patient will have gastric reflux – something to prevent when your patient is at risk for aspirating.

There are a couple of things to keep in mind when using these tubes:

- Soft tubes usually collapse if you try to aspirate through them, so you won't be able to check an aspirated residual every few hours. I've found in practice actually that if you aspirate very gently, you can sometimes get these tubes to drain the stomach pretty well, but not always. So don't forget to assess bowel sounds – are things moving along through the gut, or do you think your patient has accumulated a liter of tube feeds in her stomach, just increasing in size every hour and getting ready to try to come up, out, and kill her? What if this patient was wearing a bipap mask? Too awful to think about…

- Feeding below the pylorus means that you're bypassing the digestive abilities of the stomach, which means that you can't give these folks normal tube feeding solutions. We have a couple of "predigested", or "elemental" preparations – I think "Alitraq" (sounds like a town in the Yukon) is one of them, there are probably others.

- Another point about tubes in the jejunem – every blue moon or so I've seen an interesting thing occur because a tube has gone too far along in the gut and gone to suction: patients can drain really impressive amounts when suction is applied below the pylorus – liters and liters a day. Maybe six. Maybe more. Usually this doesn't look like gastric drainage – I seem to remember wondering why this patient seemed to be draining orange kool-aid - and you should get suspicious if the tube looks like it's been inserted too far into the patient. "Geez, doesn't it look like that NG tube should be draining his bladder or something?" I clearly remember the tube getting pulled back while connected to suction, and the drainage abruptly changed color as the tip obviously came up into the stomach, which was where it was supposed to be...

5-3- G-tubes:

G-tubes are a nice thing, I guess. They're certainly part of standard treatment when a patient needs to be trached, at least most of the time, and obviously we use them when they're in place.

But here's the mystery – most of the time I can't get a g-tube to aspirate properly, and no one's ever been able to tell me why. I suppose it's got to do with the position of the tip and all, but why it should be harder to reliably aspirate a g-tube than an NG tube is beyond me. Sometimes it helps to flip the patient over to the other side – maybe the tip of the tube moves and drains better. Except, aren't g-tubes made sort of like foley catheters?

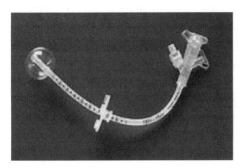

And aren't they sutured in place with the balloon up? Maybe the tubes are so soft that they collapse when you aspirate them? Maybe they don't drain because with the patient on her back, the tip of the catheter is above the collected fluid in the stomach? Not this one...I dunno.

http://www.usendoscopy.com/images/balloon.jpg

Anyhow, do your very best to check gastric aspirates every four hours at least. I checked them every hour last week on a patient who was getting a go-lytely prep...you'd hate to hook up suction and discover that your patient had 900cc in her stomach. Or rather, you'd hate <u>not</u> to find it...

5-4 – J-tubes:

J-tubes are the percutaneous version of soft Dobhoffs. Again, the idea is to feed the patient below the pylorus. Remember that there's no big stomach pouch in there, so aspirates won't really tell you anything. Check anyway. Gently.

6- How do I make sure that the feeding tube is in the right place, and what can happen if it's not?

A little repetition does not hurt. For salem sump tubes do the aspirate thing, or try the listen-over-the-stomach-while-instilling-air thing. X-rays are always better. For soft tubes, get the team to read a placement film, and make sure you've marked the tube so you'll know if it's pulled back – if the tube is still in the nose, but the mark is down by the patient's chest, where is the tip of the tube now? And where are the tube feeds going now? A patient without a gag might absorb several hours of tube feeds into a lung... If you have any question at any time about the position of a feeding tube, don't use it until you're sure of where it is.

By the way, you guys know that patients usually aspirate into the right middle or lower lobes, right? This is because the right mainstem bronchus is roughly a straight shot downwards past the carina, while the left one goes off at an angle, so tube feed being aspirated tends to fall straight downwards...when your patient has suddenly de-tuned, and you're looking at the x-ray with the team, this might be the clue you need. Suctioning tube feeds out of your patient's airway is another – Jayne says you can glucose-test the sputum, but I've never had the courage to do that. This was what methylene-blue coloring was all about.

7- How do I make sure the patient is absorbing the nutrition that I'm giving?

With TPN, as long as the line is in the right vessel and you have a nice blood return, you're probably safe. Certainly the patient on TPN might not be able to handle the sugar load – I think the stuff is based on a D20 solution, isn't it? So insulin treatment might count as an aid to absorption.

Tube feeds are a little trickier. In the old days patients seemed to lose as much, or more volume in liquid stool as we gave them in nutrition. At least we knew if the patient's gut was moving things along! Nowadays the formulations are a lot better, but you still have to assess this carefully. Watch the aspirates. Did they increase when your patient was started on an opiate drip, like fentanyl or morphine? Did the pattern of bowel sounds change? Did they go away altogether? Did the patient get promptly started on a regimen to keep things moving? Is it working?

8- What labs should I watch?

Labs are a big clue to absorption of nutrition. You'll notice that a patient on TPN has all sorts of labs checked, some daily, some weekly, involving all sorts of parameters like electrolyes, glucose, albumin, liver function tests – it's a long list. We spend a lot of time following and repleting electrolytes like potassium, phosphorus, magnesium, calcium...make absolutely sure that you know the rules for giving these. Potassium is a good example. We have a strict hospital policy: no more than 20 meq of IV potassium goes into a patient in one hour. If the route is central, the dose is mixed in at least 50cc, and must be run on a pump. No exceptions! Rapid infusion of potassium is extremely hazardous to your patient's health!

And follow up! Did you give a dose of a critical electrolyte? Measure it after the dose is done. (You might want to wait an hour. You might not.)

9- What is the big deal with serum albumin?

Albumin turns out to be really important, and it's something you might not think about right away, but you should learn to worry about it early on. I'll explain this - as usual - as I understand it, so everyone who knows better should come right along and straighten me out!

9-1- What's a normal albumin?

Normal albumin should be 3.5 – 5 grams per deciliter. Albumin levels drop really fast in a patient who's not getting fed, so we try to start everyone on some kind of nutrition within the first day of admission.

9-2- What is oncotic pressure?

This is not something that we normally think of as a pressure, which is to say something pushing on something else. This is actually a sort of negative pressure, which is holding the water component in the blood serum. If the oncotic pressure is high, then water happily stays in the blood vessels, along with the serum. If the pressure is low, then the water starts to leak out of the vessel walls, into the "third space".

9-3 – What does albumin have to do with oncotic pressure?

Albumin turns out to be the component of serum that "holds" water. Simply put, if the albumin level drops, then the water doesn't want to stay in the serum any more. This can be absolutely critical…

9-4- What does "third-spaced" mean?

Normally you think of bodily fluid as being mostly in two places: either pumping around in the blood, or sitting inside the cells. Two "spaces", that would be. If the oncotic pressure in the vessels drops, the water component in the serum starts to leak into a third space – which is to say, into the tissue, between the cells. This shows up as edema, and this is why assessment of edema, both in the extremities and centrally, is really important. Does your patient have edema of the feet and legs because he has right-sided heart failure? Is he developing total body edema because he's been starved for ten days, his albumin is almost in negative numbers, and he's still getting only normal saline or D5W as hydration?

A patient who is severely third-spaced can get into all sorts of trouble, and clearly one of them is dehydration, which sounds stupid at first. But think – this patient is continuously losing water volume into his tissues, everywhere. He may be total-body positive, say, 3 liters over 24 hours, but his CVP may be 2. His urine output may be 10cc per hour. If an inexperienced team member sees the positive number and reacts with an "automatic" order for lasix (Jayne calls this "reflexive diuresis", which I think is hilarious) are you going to give that dose? Remember: are they treating the patient, or the numbers? See where you can wind up with nutrition?

My wife points out that there's another place that your patient may have problems with third-space fluid: the brain. I am no neuro nurse at all, so I'll quote her: "50% of signs and symptoms around a stroke are from cerebral edema. If the patient isn't getting any nutrition and their albumin gets low, fluid is going to leak into the brain, making the intracranial swelling worse."

10- Should my patient be getting IV albumin?

This is a big debate. Medical folks will shake their heads, and tell you that "meta-analyses of the available literature studies indicate a higher probability of adverse sequelae resulting from administration of parenteral serologic derivatives." Which means, I think, that it's a bad idea because it tends to cause problems. I mean, this is Boston, right?

Surgeons, especially the burn teams, seem to go the other way: "Yeah, hang it every hour. Make it two an hour. Then call me this afternoon. Make it a couple of days."

The nurses, meantime, look one way, and then the other, and wind up saying "okay" to all of them…my own point is that if the patient were started on appropriate nutrition right after they were admitted, the albumin problem might not be rearing it's ugly head. Do your best, but remember, as with many aspects of your patients' care, this may come directly under your supervision. Make sure it happens!

11- What is TPN? What is "hyperal"?

TPN stands for total parenteral nutrition, while "hyperal" is short for "hyperalimentation", which is the same thing. TPN is all about great big bags of very complicated IV solutions which are very expensive, and which contain all sorts of interesting things like amino acids, lipids, vitamins, electrolytes – it really is very impressive stuff, and we old guys have seen it evolve over the years to include more and more components. It can change composition as the patient's course changes, too – for example more or less insulin can be added to the mix if the patient isn't tolerating the dextrose load, or lipids can be added, or removed.

11-1- Why does TPN have to be run centrally? Can TPN run through a PICC line?

As I understand it, small peripheral veins are just not able to take the irritation produced by this stuff, which is very hypertonic. TPN can run through a PICC line, but you'd hate to tie up the patient's only central access that way if they needed anything else. This is why all inserted PICC lines should have double lumens.

11-2- Why does TPN have to have a line to itself?

This has always been the policy on our service. I understand that elsewhere in the hospital it isn't true – that meds and drips of one kind or another are routinely given through running TPN – but where I work this is absolute heresy. If a TPN line is ever used for anything else, it can't be used for TPN again. If your TPN bag were to become unusable for some reason, you can run D20 at the same rate through the line (get an order for this), and then use the line for TPN when it becomes available again, but I think this is the only exception to the rule.

11-3- Can anything run in the same line with TPN?

No. You may find yourself in a tough position if your patient is critical – should you stop their TPN because you need the line? You can only make this kind of decision on the spot, but make sure the team is aware ahead of time of what you're planning to do. There are definitely situations when you are going to have to do this – your patient is getting into trouble big-time, and you need all the lines for pressors, maybe for sedatives, maybe for paralyzing agents, maybe for all them. Do your best to check for compatibilities – DC'ing TPN is a big step. But do it if you have to.

11-4- Why is it white?

It's white because in recent years the lipid component has been directly added to the mix.

11-5- Why is it sometimes clear and sort of yellowish-greenish?

Years ago, early TPN mixes were just amino acids in a D20 base, with vitamins added (anybody remember "Freamine"?) – if a patient doesn't need lipids for some reason, the orders get changed, and the mixture stays clear.

11-6- What if my patient is on propofol?

Excellent question – who thought of that one? Propofol is lipid-based. A patient getting 20 or 30cc an hour of this drug, around the clock, may get so much of a lipid load that way that they don't need any added to their TPN. This may change if their sedation orders do, so keep track! I understand that you may also have to stop a propofol infusion if your patient has pancreatitis and can't handle much in the way of lipid administration.

11-7- Why does the team sometimes seem to wait so long before they start my patient on TPN?

At first glance, it would seem like a simple step to take, but actually starting a patient on TPN involves a couple of decisions that might take some time to make. One of the biggest worries is that our patients, often seriously infected and maybe even septic, might get worse with the addition of TPN, which is apparently the best culture medium ever invented. This situation can be made even trickier if steroids are involved – a patient with a COPD flare getting steroids, who might develop a pneumonia sepsis, might hover for a while in what they call a "metastable" state. Add TPN, and the infection might use it as fuel to just go wild – and maybe the next addition to treatment would be pressors. Not to mention the insulin drip she'd need…

11-8- Do patients on TPN make stool?

Yes.

11-9- What if my patient's TPN doesn't show up on time? What if I contaminate the bag by accident?

Our standard maneuver in this situation is to hang a bag of D20 at the same rate that the TPN had been going at – make sure the team is aware of what's going on, and get an order for the new fluid. You can speak to pharmacy about getting another bag.

Last thing about TPN – it always has to be filtered. We have special filters for TPN only, which come from pharmacy.

12- What are tube feeds all about?

This is another thing that most folks are very familiar with by the time they get to the MICU. We use all sorts of formulations.

12-1- What are the different types of tube feeds?

Here's what it says on the Ross Products/ Abbott Labs website (thank you Ross/Abbott):

- Jevity: Isotonic liquid nutrition with fiber.
- Jevity Plus: 1.2 Cal/ml high nitrogen liquid with fiber blend
- Promote: high protein liquid nutrition
- Promote with fiber: that would be, uh, promote with fiber…
- Osmolite: low residue, isotonic, high nitrogen liquid
- Promod: whey-based protein supplement that can be added to liquids
- Alitraq: this is the "elemental" stuff that we use to feed patients with jejunostomy feeding tubes. Vivonex is the same thing, except different.
- Glutamine: "to nourish the gastrointestinal tract". There's actually an interesting theory that says that giving just a little bit of tube feeds to "line the gut" will prevent the "translocation" of bacteria out of the gut, and into the abdomen. Does that mean: "They move from one place to another."?
- Nepro: "specifically designed to meet the unique dietary needs of people on dialysis"

I think that's most of them. They seem to work quite well.

12-2- What do I have to know about tube feed pumps?

These pumps take a little bit of getting used to, just like any new gadget does. They're simple enough to set up – spike the liquid bottle, install the tubing in the pump, which actually, for once, is really a simple and easy thing to do. Set a rate, set a volume, turn it on, and off it goes. The pumps are very sensitive to occlusions, and will sometimes become unhappy if the supply bottle isn't hung up high enough above them for gravity to help the flow.

12-3- When do I change the pump tubing?

Every 24 hours.

12-4- How often should I check the aspirate?

At least every four hours. Be sure that you assess your patient to see if she's absorbing her tube feeds. This means checking aspirates, assessing bowel sounds, noting the frequency and character of stool, blood sugar tolerance, all that good stuff.

12-5- What if the aspirate is more than 100cc?

If my patient's aspirate is less than 100cc I'll usually refeed it. If I'm getting more than two large syringefuls of aspirate, I'll usually hook up the NG tube to low suction to see how much more is in there, because I wouldn't refeed an aspirate that large anyhow. I've found aspirates as large as 800cc in my day…

Tube feeds usually start at 10cc per hour, and are increased by 10cc roughly every four hours until the goal rate is reached, or until big aspirates become a problem. If the aspirates are consistently larger than 100cc, but the patient is stooling regularly, I'd keep them going.

Never hesitate to assess aspirates more frequently if you think you need to – I think earlier on I mentioned checking them hourly when running a go-lytely prep at 300cc per hour. That was an interesting situation, actually – the patient was a very agitated and confused gentleman who had a lower GI bleed – he was to be prepped overnight for a colonoscopy in the morning. Given the fact that he was receiving intra-arterial pitressin through a femoral arterial catheter, and the fact that he was really severely agitated, requiring four-point restraint, I asked the team if it might not make sense to consult anesthesia about intubating him so that he could be safely sedated. I also liked the idea of having my confused patient's airway protected by an inflated endotracheal tube cuff while I gave him the better part of 3 liters of NG fluids overnight…and the team agreed. Nice piece of critical-care management, I thought…

12-6- What happens with tube feedings if my patient is on a fentanyl or morphine drip?

12-6-1- What is the narcan thing? What is a bowel regimen?

Opiate drips are really hard on tube feeds, since they put the gut to sleep so quickly. It can be very hard to continue with tube feeds at all in this situation – the aspirates rise quickly, the bowel sounds fade away, and nutrition problems start to arise.
A couple of things that are used:

- Reglan (metoclopramide) sometimes works well, sometimes not so well, in keeping the gut moving.

- Narcan (naloxone) is sometimes given along with the tube feeds to try to get the gut to wake up by itself, apart from the rest of the patient. I've seen this tried for many years now – I've never known it to work very well. The dose nowadays is 1.2mg po, tid.

- Bowel regimens are sometimes useful, more so if the patient can avoid long-term opiates. We use a combination of liquid senna, colace, and bisacodyl on most of our patients routinely.

- At one point there was a brief flurry of adding erythromycin to the bowel regimens as an aid to motility, but this seems to have faded for now…didn't seem to do much.

- If your patient ends up with a persistent "opiate ileus", you may be forced into advocating for TPN. Try to make sure that you always save a port on any inserted central line, to keep available for the possibility of TPN.

12-7- Why did some patients used to have blue tube feeds? (That English is?)

They don't any more – methylene blue turned out to be pretty toxic for some patients – I think there were a couple of deaths. The idea behind it wasn't a bad one though, so I've left the description in the article.

A critical part of the tube feed concept is the idea that "things in the gut need to be moving forward along the gut." Forward is good, backwards is bad. Usually backwards is only from the stomach, which is because things are not moving along below it. As a result, some of our patients come to us with recurrent aspiration pneumonias. This can happen for a number of reasons: maybe they've got an ileus for one reason or another – opiates maybe, or being post-op, or maybe bad perfusion. I understand that GERD happens because the stomach acid makes the esophageal valve stop working – apparently treatment with omeprazole, or whatever, lets the valve heal up and start working again.

Whatever the reason, this of course is why you're checking aspirates and listening to bowel sounds. Adding methylene blue to the tube feeds will help you figure out if your patient is aspirating them – if you suction the ET tube and get blue sputum – doh!

What to do? It depends – does the patient have bowel sounds? Are things moving along forward? Has she stooled lately? Maybe metoclopramide would help move things along. Maybe the patient should be fed below the pylorus one way or another – either a dobhoff, or a percutaneous j-tube.

Methylene blue will also have cute effects on the patient's urine color, sometimes also their stool. Sometimes when we're checking blood products, we get an FFP that we'd swear had methylene blue in it…

12-8- Should I stop the tube feeds before my patient is extubated?

Yes, absolutely stop the tube feeds if they're thinking about extubating your patient. We used to stop them at midnight if the patient was going to be extubated in the morning, but nowadays the word is that the stomach empties itself in four hours – so we use that to figure out the time to stop the feeds. Always, always try to make sure that your patient's stomach is nice and empty before extubation – or before intubation! Hook the NG tube to suction even if the tube feeds have been off for days!

12-9- What if he's going to the OR?

NPO after midnight is the rule. Does he need some glucose started up to replace the tube feeds overnight?

13-   How do we use insulin drips in the MICU?

It turns out that everything works better, patients with all kinds of illnesses do better, sepsis clears better, wounds heal better…if their blood sugars are kept under tight control. Really significant, this, apparently makes an enormous difference. Makes for a lot of work, too.

Here's how we do it: say your patient has a glucose of 250. First you need to think about what she's getting for nutrition – has she just been started on TPN? Tube feeds? Is she getting D10W for some reason? Do we know that she's diabetic anyway? The point being – is what she's getting going to stop because of the high sugar, or is the team going to leave it running and treat the glucose with insulin? It would be sort of a mistake to stop the nutrition and hang an insulin drip…

What else could raise glucose? Is he on steroids? "Stress" steroids? Maybe "pulse steroids" – which means giving a gram (I can never get over that – it seems so enormous) of methylprednisolone for some inflammatory process, usually having to do with the lung.

Anyhow, let's say that the patient has type 2 diabetes maybe, and she's been started on TPN, and you've been covering her every four hours with insulin by sliding scale, her fingertips are getting into really tough shape, and her glucose is still 220. Time for an insulin drip. Typically the team will order a bolus – 10 units IV maybe, maybe less, and then a drip at, say, 4 units an hour. Your job now is to check sugars every two hours. Actually, in the setting of DKA we have to check a complete set of lytes, what some people call a "Chem-7" every two hours.

The idea here is that the regular insulin in the drip peaks at two hours – so a change that you make in the drip should reflect accurately in the blood sugar two hours later. The usual range is up to about 10 per hour. Since these are often the folks on TPN, more insulin is added to their daily mix if their requirements increase. As the patient's blood sugar comes down, the drip is decreased so as to keep them from getting too low. Sometimes the team will order a dose of NPH insulin at the same time as the drip starts, and as that peaks you'll certainly be turning the drip down as well. Be really careful about this – remember that with blood sugars, too high is bad, but too low is worse!

PA Lines

Hi all: here's another Frequently Asked Question file. As usual, please remember that this is <u>not</u> meant to be any kind of final reference – it's supposed to be a collection of answers that a preceptor might give to a newer ICU nurse, based on experience, rather than "official" information. <u>Please</u> find as many errors as you can (probably lots), and get back to me, and we'll update the file. Thanks!

<u>PA Line Basics</u>

1- What is a PA line?
2- Why are they sometimes called Swan-Ganz lines?
3- What are PA lines used for?
4- How are they inserted, and who inserts them?
5- What's the difference between the introducer and the PA line?
6- What is a "cordis"?
7- What is the little syringe for?
8- What about the little balloon at the end – what's that for?
9- Why do PA lines have multiple lumens?
10- What's the difference between the colors : yellow, blue, white, purple?
11- Why do they call them "ports"?
12- What are the little black lines that show up along the length of the catheter?

<u>Setting Up</u>

13- How do I set up for a PA line insertion?
14- Why do we use a double-transducer setup?
15- How do I set up the monitor?
16- How do I set up the printer?
17- Where do I level the transducer?

<u>Insertion</u>

18- Who puts in the PA-line?
19- Why do they call it "floating" a Swan?
20- What is a "wedge pressure"?
21- What are all those waveforms that I need to know?
22- When do I turn the printer on?
23- What does a normal CVP trace look like, and what are normal CVP numbers?
24- What does a normal RV waveform look like?
25- Why does everyone look nervous when the catheter tip is passing through the RV?
26- What does a normal PA trace look like?
27- Wedge trace?

28- What does "stuck in wedge" mean?
29- What do they mean when they talk about "right-sided" or "left-sided" pressures?
30- Why does the patient need a stat chest x-ray after the swan goes in?
31- Can I use the PA line before the film is read?
32- How do I make sure the line doesn't get pulled out?
33- What is the clear wrinkly sheath thing for?
34- What is the aluminum clippy thing with the sponge for?
35- Why is it important to put on an "air-occlusive" dressing?

Reading the numbers

36- Okay, the PA line is in, and the x-ray is read. How do I interpret the numbers?
37- How should I wedge the line?
38- What is "overwedged"?
39- What if I lose the syringe – can I use another one?
40- What should I do with the syringe when I'm not using it?
41- How often should I wedge the line?
42- How do I read the CVP?
43- How do I do a cardiac output?
44- Why do we delete the previous ones?
45- How many should I do?
46- What if the numbers make no sense?
47- What is the difference between cardiac output and cardiac index?
48- What is the BSA?
49- What is SVR?
50- What is SV?
51- What are the classic patterns of numbers for different situations, like sepsis, or cardiogenic shock?

Using the ports

52- Which port should I use for what?
53- Can I infuse things through the distal PA port?
54- What goes through the CVP port?
55- Can I use the PA line for TPN?
56- Can I do blood draws from the PA line?
57- What is a Fick output, and how do I do one?

Bad things that can happen

58- What do I have to worry about when the line is going in?
59- How can I tell if those things are happening?
60- What do I do if the line is stuck in wedge?
61- What if the line pulls back to the RV?
62- What if the line gets pulled all the way out?

63- Why do they pull the line "back to CVP"?

64- What should I do with the ports and the transducers if the line is pulled back to CVP?

65- What if the balloon ruptures?

66- How do I know if that has happened?

Taking the line out

67- How do we know when the PA line needs to come out?

68- Who takes it out?

69- How do I get certified to take out PA lines?

70- What should I look for on the x-ray before I pull a swan?

71- Should I culture the tip?

72- Now that the line is out, can air get into the patient through the black diaphragm thing in the introducer?

73- What is an obturator?

74- Can I put in an obturator?

PA-Line Basics

1- What is a PA Line?

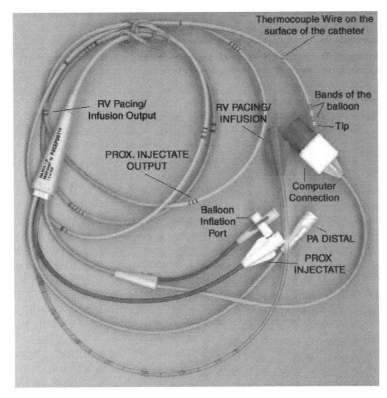

Scary-looking object. This one is a just a little more complex than the ones we use, as it has an extra port for a pacing wire…

A PA-line is a long multilumen catheter (a catheter with several tubes in it, instead of just one), that is inserted through one of the large veins, and threaded through the right side of the heart, up into the **p**ulmonary artery.

http://illuminations.nctm.org/imath/912/cardiac/student/images/catheterbig.jpg

2- Why are they sometimes called Swan-Ganz lines?

PA lines were invented by Drs. Jeremy Swan and William Ganz at Cedars-Sinai, in California. They were first used in the early and middle 1970's.

3- What are PA lines used for?

You need three things to make a blood pressure: you need something to pump with, some volume for the pump to pump with, and some resistance in the vessels that the volume is being pumped through – they have to be at least moderately tight, constricted, contracted, since if they're all floppy and loose, then the pressure in them will never rise to the point that you need if you're going to perfuse your end-organs. Or any other organs.

Pump, volume and squeeze. Snap, crackle, and…I forget what the third one was.

If you're faced with a patient who can't make a blood pressure, and it just isn't really clear why – then what you need to do is to try to "quantify" each of these.

This is what the PA line is for: "when you shoot the numbers", you're generating information that tells you exactly what's happening with all three items: cardiac output (pump), CVP and wedge pressures (volume), and systemic vascular resistance (squeeze).

The thing to understand is that as there are three parts of a blood pressure, there are only three main types of hypotension ("shock states") that you're going to see in the ICU, and each of them originates in one of the three. The "numbers" organize themselves into patterns that will become very familiar to you: here's a quick look.

Before the quick look, some normal ranges: your cardiac output is probably something like 4-6 liters/minute, your wedge pressure is probably around 10 to 12 mm Hg, CVP 8 to 10, and your SVR is probably somewhere around 1000, plus or minus some.

- "**Pump**" problems? "Cardiogenic" shock? The cardiac output will be low, because the pump ain't pumping. Blood pressure drops. The body says to itself: "What to do? Got to keep the blood pressure up somehow!", and starts to tighten up the arterial bed. What number tells how tight the arterial system is? – SVR.

  So – in **cardiogenic** shock, the cardiac output goes down, the SVR goes up – the pattern is usually plain as day. "Ooh, look! The output is only 2.2, and the SVR is 2400!" What does the wedge pressure do? (Remember, the LV is pumping poorly, and <u>can't empty</u> itself…)

- "**Volume**" problems? "Hypovolemic" shock? Lost a lot of blood? Running too many marathons? Cardiac output will probably be low, since there isn't enough volume to pump with. CVP and wedge pressures? Low, right? – again, not enough volume. SVR? Same as cardiogenic: the arteries clamp down, trying to maintain pressure.

  Hypovolemic shock: cardiac output low, central pressures low, SVR high.

-   **"Squeeze"** problem? Any idea what makes this happen? Anybody say, "sepsis"? All that bacteremic endotoxin makes the arteries dilate – blood pressure drops. What to do? Now the body uses the mirror reflex of what it did in the cardiogenic setting: instead of clamping down the arteries, which it can't do, because that's where the problem is – now the heart picks up the slack, pumping both faster and harder: heart rate goes up, and cardiac output does too.

Septic shock: cardiac output high, central pressures low, SVR low.

Give it time. Don't try too hard to memorize all this – instead, get some mileage under your belt. Work with the PA lines, shoot lots of numbers, think things over, then come back in six months, read the article again, and explain to me how much of it I got wrong…

4- How are they inserted, and who inserts them?

PA lines are usually inserted in our unit by the pulmonary fellow, who may supervise the residents and interns, letting them do it. They are threaded through an introducer, which is put in first, usually in one of the internal jugular veins, or in one of the subclavians. The introducer can be placed by the team before the pulmonary fellow gets to the unit to place the swan itself.

5- What's the difference between the introducer and the PA line?

The introducer is a single-lumen large-bore central line that can be placed by the resident team in one of the big neck veins – usually internal jugular or subclavian- which acts as a guide for the swan when it is going into the patient. The introducer is about 4 inches long, and is about half the diameter of a soda straw – it's shaped like an L, with one end going into the vein, and the other end coming off at a right angle, also about 4 inches long. This second end is sometimes called the "side arm". At the point where the two parts of the L connect is a hub, which holds a black diaphragm. The diaphragm is perforated by the swan as it goes into the patient, and it makes a tight air seal around the swan to prevent air from getting into the bloodstream between the introducer and the swan within it. It's important to remember that if the swan comes out, as long as the introducer is still in place, that diaphragm is **not** airtight any more, and needs to be covered with tegaderm, lest the patient suck air inwards through the opening. This would produce an air embolus in the venous circulation, which would move towards the lungs, and produce similar effects to a big PE.

6- What is a "cordis"?

The cordis is the introducer. Somehow, in the jargon, the name of the company that makes a lot of this equipment got attached to just one part of it. The side arm of the introducer is made nowadays of very large bore, clear tubing, and is very useful for rapid fluid boluses, or blood, or the like. We often use it with multiple stopcocks to give a number of infusions together – usually a combination of "background" IV fluid, pressors, etc.

Confusing-looking picture, at first. This would be a "left IJ" insertion.

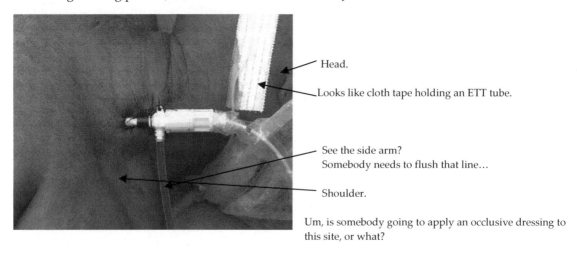

Head.

Looks like cloth tape holding an ETT tube.

See the side arm?
Somebody needs to flush that line...

Shoulder.

Um, is somebody going to apply an occlusive dressing to this site, or what?

http://www.med.umich.edu/anes/tcpub/glossary/graphics/anesthesia_glossary-36.jpg

Don't forget that if you change the background rate of a combination infusion, you also change the rate of the pressors. Be very careful!

7-   What is the little syringe for?

The little syringe is for inflating the balloon at the end of the catheter.

8- What about the little balloon at the end – what's that for?

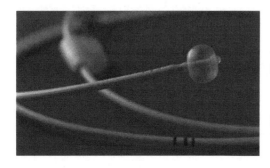

The team will check that the balloon inflates properly, before the line goes into the patient.

http://www6.ocn.ne.jp/~taisho2/katarogu/a/a_wedge.htm

The balloon does a couple of things. First – during insertion, the balloon is inflated in the vena cava – usually superior, since most of our insertions are from the neck. The inflated balloon guides the tip of the catheter along as it is pushed by blood flow through the chambers of the heart, until it "wedges" in place in one of the pulmonary arteries. This is why they call it "flow-directed" catheter placement. The second is the wedge function.

9- Why do PA lines have multiple lumens?

The first thing to visualize here is that each of the lumens has an opening somewhere along the length of the catheter, and the first thing to remember is that the terms "proximal" and "distal" here are **reversed** from their usual meanings – which is to say, they usually mean "closer" or "farther away" from the center of the **patient**.

This time – just to make sure you were paying attention – they mean "closer" or "farther away" from the **point where the line enters the patient.** So the "distal port" – the yellow one - is the one at the tippy end, out where the balloon is. The proximal port - the blue one - is the one closest to the insertion point - but which actually opens up in the right atrium – so it's also often called the RA port. Some swans have extra infusion ports that open up near the blue port in the RA – in our unit these are the white and purple ports. The manufacturer calls these Variable Infusion Ports – or VIP ports (snazzy!) - so these are called VIP swans. All of our swans are VIP swans. The RA ports, by the way, are where you should push meds in a code – never through the distal port if you can avoid it – to get the best drug/blood mixing.

The second thing to remember is what these lumens are really for, which is pressure monitoring. The distal port is hooked to a pressure transducer, which translates the varying pressures it senses into waves that you can see on a monitor, and shows the pressures in the PA, along with the wedge pressure when the balloon is inflated. The proximal port shows the pressure in the RA.

10- What's the difference between the colors: yellow, blue, white, purple?

The colors in themselves don't mean anything except to help you remember where the ports open up. All the swans I've seen from different makers use the same color code. It's important not to mix these up!

11- Why do they call them "ports"?

I'm not sure. "Portal of entry", maybe?

12- What are the little black lines that show up along the length of the catheter?

The black lines measure the length of the catheter, starting from the tip, so that you know how far the swan has gone into the patient.

Setting Up

13- How do I set up for a PA line insertion?

You need to know a number of things to get properly set up for a swan insertion:

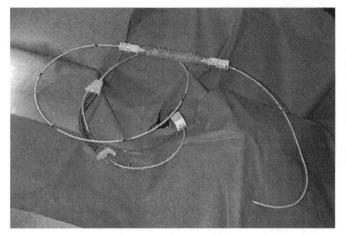

Here's the PA line all nicely set up for insertion on some sterile drapes. You're going to want to have your transducer setup ready, and the doc will pass the distal port connection to you to screw onto the stopcock at the end of your transducer line.

See the curve in the line? Why do you think they make them that way?

http://www.med.umich.edu/anes/tcpub/glossary/anesthesia_glossary-21.htm

- How long do you have until the team will be ready to go?

- Where will they insert the catheter into the patient? That's to say, where in the patient will the team be inserting the catheter, rather than "in the clean utility room", or "in the nurse manager's office"…

- Is the patient going to be able to tolerate the procedure? For example, can he lie flat, or is he hypoxic, and short of breath, and would he need to be intubated first? Or hypotensive – do you have stable access for pressors before the swan goes in? Or very agitated? Oftentimes the doctors are so focused on the insertion procedure that they forget about everything else – so these considerations become **your** responsibility! Your goal is to produce a situation in which this very invasive maneuver can be done under stable, safe conditions. **Always** let your resource nurse know what's going on so that she can help you out.

- Try to make sure that the patient's cardiac electrolytes are okay before the swan goes in; having a normal K+ and Mg+ can make all the difference in preventing VT when the swan passes through the right ventricle. Let the team know what the values are ahead of time!

14- Why do we use a double-transducer setup?

We use a double transducer because it lets us monitor the traces (waveforms) from the PA port and the CVP port at the same time. I usually connect only the distal port cable during insertion so I don't get confused as to which is which – you only want to see the distal trace during insertion anyway.

15- How do I set up the monitor?

What we do is: go into "monitor setup", then "parameters", and turn off all the waveforms except one of the EKG leads and the distal port of the swan. Don't turn the parameters off – just the waveforms – since you still want to monitor things like BP and O2 sat during the procedure – you just don't want their traces cluttering up your screen. Then set the swan trace to "full grid", which will blow it up big on the screen, and which will put scale numbers on the side so that numbers can be easily read from the different chambers in the heart as the swan goes in.

16- How do I set up the printer?

Go into "monitor setup", then "graph setup", and you can highlight the traces that you want printed – usually only the EKG and distal port traces. You can also change printer locations from the standard little printer on the outside counter to one of the laser printers by hitting the "printer" option and choosing the laser. Don't forget to switch back!

17- Where do I level the transducer?

Level the transducer where you level them all: mid-axillary line, roughly at the 4th intercostal space. Mark the patient's chest with a felt-tip pen to make sure that everyone is levelling at the same point – this may make the difference between hydrating your patient and giving her diuretics!

Insertion

18- Who puts in the PA line?

The swan is put in by the pulmonary fellow, or by the resident team under her direct supervision. She **must** be present in the room for the line placement.

19- Why do they call it "floating" a swan?

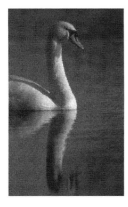

The balloon at the tip of the catheter gets "floated" along by blood flow through the chambers of the heart until it reaches the right position.

20- What is a "wedge pressure"?

Here's how PA lines work, physically:

Let's take a second to remember how invasive lines work: monitor, transducer, stiff tubing filled with saline, then the monitoring catheter itself.

Remember that all these lines are "looking at "something, with their transducers acting as their "eyes" . An arterial line transducer "sees" the pressure in the patient's radial artery (if that's where it's connected to) through the column of heparinized saline in the stiff pressure tubing.

PA lines work the same way: there's an open lumen between the transducer and the tip of the PA line, filled with saline, right? The column of fluid sends the pressure waves back to the transducer. As the line is floated into place, the tip of the PA line passes through the several structures in turn: first the right atrium (CVP), then the right ventricle, then pressures in the pulmonary arteries, and finally the "wedge" pressure.

Now let's talk about the balloon. All these pressures are what the transducer sees as the line goes in, with the little balloon at the tip **inflated**, to let the blood flow push the tip along. As the line makes it's way into the pulmonary artery of its choice, it moves smoothly along until its inflated sides **wedge** up against the sides of the vessel that it's in. Now what does the transducer see?

Well – now it doesn't see what's all around it any more. Now the transducer is only looking **forward**, through the lungs, into the left side of the heart. Only looking forward…sometimes I wish I could do that.

Here's a question: how does the PA transducer look all the way through the lungs to see the left side of the heart? Aren't they sort of in the way? Answer: I have absolutely no idea, and I've always wondered! One of our our correspondents explained that the answer is "magic", which sounds right to me.

So - looking forward, the catheter looks down into the LV, producing the **"wedge pressure"**.The wedge number reflects the pressure in the left ventricle at its fullest – at the end of diastole – so the wedge number is also sometimes called "LVEDP": "left ventricular end-diastolic pressure". If the pressure is high, then the idea is that the LV is having trouble emptying itself, maybe from ischemia, maybe from low EF, maybe from overhydration, maybe from cardiogenic shock. Too low, and the patient is probably dry.

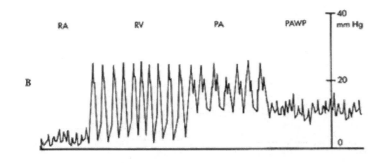

Here's what the PA line transducer "sees" as the line floats into place…

www.rocket.pwp.blueyonder.co.uk/

See how the trace changes as the balloon floats along, finally into wedge? I would read the wedge in this diagram at about 14 or 15 – does that make sense?

21- What are all those waveforms that I need to know?

The waveforms in the diagram above reflect the pressures in the different places that the tip of the catheter travels through – first the vena cava/RA (usually nearly the same wave and pressure number), then the RV, then PA, then wedge. You need to learn what these look like – study up! There are only a few, and they're all quite different and clear.

22- When do I turn the printer on?

Turn the printer on and start "graphing" as soon as the doc gets the tip of the catheter into the vena cava – you want to start your graph with the CVP tracing, and finish up with the wedge.

23- What does a normal CVP trace look like, and what are normal CVP numbers?

The CVP trace has a narrow amplitude – meaning, it goes up and down, but not much, on the screen. Normal CVP numbers might be anywhere from 4-8, depending (always depending!).

24- What does a normal RV waveform look like?

Normal RV traces are much different – you should be able to notice the change from RA immediately. RV pressure waves have a very wide amplitude – they go way down, then way up, from a very low number – single digits – in diastole, to a pretty high number – 20-30, (depending!) in systole. Looks like slow VT. See that on the diagram above?

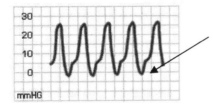 See how the diastolic presure goes <u>way</u> down, almost to zero?

http://classes.kumc.edu/son/nurs420/unit4/hemomon.html

25- Why does everyone look nervous when the tip of the catheter is passing through the RV?

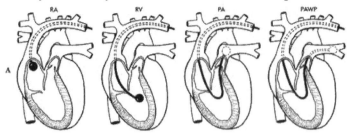

www.rocket.pwp.blueyonder.co.uk/

The tip of the catheter can tickle the inside of the RV and produce runs of VT – you've probably seen this during CVP line placement when the guide wire goes in. Your position during the swan placement is in the room looking at the monitor the whole time, because the doctors may or may not be able to see the runs. Usually by continuing to advance the catheter steadily, the balloon will guide the tip up into the PA and out of dangerous territory. If not, and the runs are prolonged, the team needs to rapidly back the line out and try again. As mentioned above, you want to try and make sure that the patient's K+ and Mg+ are okay before the swan goes in.

26- What does a normal PA trace look like?

Normal PA traces have a smaller amplitude than RV waves – they don't go so far up and down. As the catheter tip passes from RV into PA, the diastolic pressure will come up – you'll see the lowest part of the wave rise upwards, and the systolic will come down – the highest part of the wave will get lower – and you should see a distinct dicrotic notch. Normal numbers might be 30's over 10's. Depending

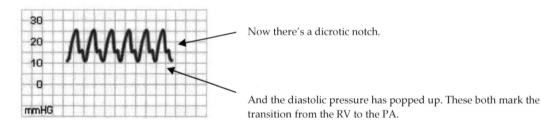

Now there's a dicrotic notch.

And the diastolic pressure has popped up. These both mark the transition from the RV to the PA.

http://classes.kumc.edu/son/nurs420/unit4/hemomon.html

27- Wedge trace?

Again - as in going from RV to PA - the transition from PA to wedge trace should be very clear – the trace will suddenly drop, and compress, and look much like the CVP trace did. Normal might be around 10 to 12.

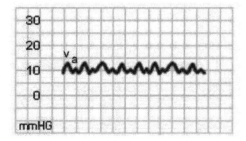

Suddenly the tracing really loses amplitude ("gets a lot smaller, going up and down.") "Yo, Ralphie, you, uh, just lost a lotta amplitude, know what I'm sayin'?"

So – what's this person's wedge pressure?

http://classes.kumc.edu/son/nurs420/unit4/hemomon.html

28- What does "stuck in wedge" mean?

"Stuck in wedge" means just that: you walk into a room, you look up at the monitor, and where you should see a PA wave coming from the distal port of the swan, you see a wedge trace. Even with the balloon down. The line has migrated inwards for some reason – sometimes they stretch out a little as they warm up inside the patient. It will definitely have to be pulled back – notify the team immediately, as this can produce tissue death in the lung.

29- What do they mean when they talk about "right-sided" or "left-sided" pressures?

"Right – sided" means the RA and RV – "left-sided": well – you know! A little better explanation might say that the "right side" is talking about the whole venous circulation, which leads to the RA and RV; the "left side" is everything leading back to (or from) to LA and LV, which is the "what" circulation? (Only one thing it can be.)

30- Why does the patient need a stat chest x-ray after the swan goes in?

Even though the pressure waves may tell a clear tale, you need to be visually sure that the line is in the right place. It might be too far into the patient, for example – you wouldn't know without a film.

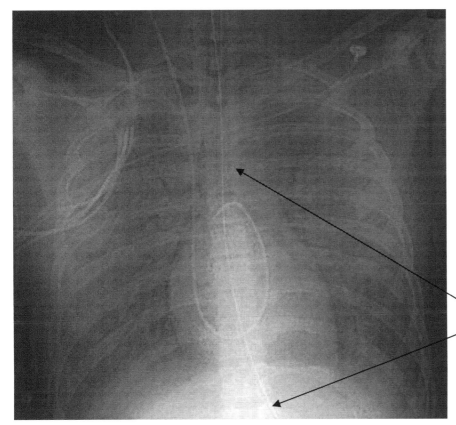

Here's a really nice image of a PA line in good position.

Remember: if you're looking at these images online, or on your own computer, you can easily make these pictures bigger and easier to look at: click the image, then click and hold on a corner, then move the mouse away from the picture. Then let go. So cool! You can leave it that way, or hit the back arrow in Word to make it go back…

ICU nurses: what's this, marked by the arrows? (Easy one…)

http://www.vasilev.com/medinter/files/images/rbm011.jpg

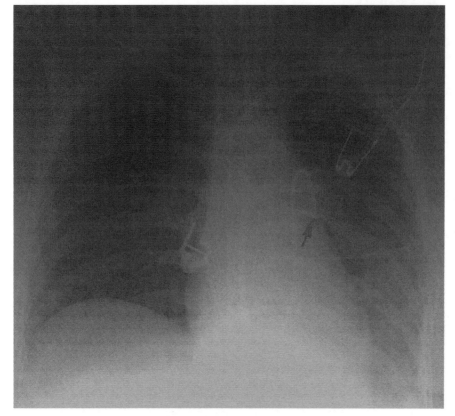

Sometimes they go into a different pulmonary artery. They still work, but it looks strange. This one is a little hard to see – try grabbing the image and making it bigger...

http://www.med.virginia.edu/med-ed/rad/chest/line_q1a.htm

31- Can I use the PA line before the x-ray is read?

No. Hospital policy. Unless it's a code. Use the <u>blue port</u> to push meds – it supposedly gives the best mixing with blood going into the RV.

32- How do I make sure the line doesn't get pulled out?

First, apply an occlusive dressing in the regulation manner. Then what I do is to coil up the outer part of the catheter in large loops, and flag it to the patient's shoulder (not the johnny!) with a big tegaderm. The johnny may get yanked off the patient for some reason, but her arm won't!

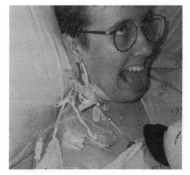

Flagged to the shoulder...another happy PA-line recipient!

http://www.happybeagle.com/shelby-hospital/neck-detail.jpg

33- What is the clear wrinkly tube thing for?

The clear wrinkly thing is called the "sheath" – it keeps part of the swan line sterile so that it can be advanced further into the patient if need be. Policy is: this can only be done for the first 24 hours after the line goes in.

34- What is the aluminum clippy thing with the sponge for?

The clippy thing is supposed to get clamped around the end of the clear sheath further away from the patient. Mostly it gets chucked out – I like to put a tegaderm around that end of the sheath anyway,because I worry about air getting pulled inwards through there. I may worry too much, but that's what happens when you get old in the ICU.

35- Why is it important to put on an "air-occlusive" dressing?

The goal here is to prevent air from entering the patient at the insertion site. Central venous pressures can actually go negative (read: they make a suction) when the patient inspires forcefully – this could suck a whole bunch of air into them – bad!

Reading the Numbers

36- Okay, the PA line is in, and the x-ray is read. How do I interpret the numbers?

The first set of numbers that you see – the way we set it up, they'll be yellow – are the PA numbers, systolic and diastolic. These reflect the"ambient" or "all around and in every direction" pressures inside the lungs. If these numbers are low, chances are the patient is dry.

High, and the patient may be overhydrated. Very high – maybe pulmonary hypertension. There are lots of interpretations that can be made – just try to get used to getting accurate numbers in the beginning. Learn to quickly level and zero the line, set up the monitor properly, get used to the procedure itself – you can learn to argue with the docs later!

37- How should I wedge the line?

Carefully - wedge the line very gently with the syringe. Only insert enough air to produce a wedge tracing, and no more, since you'll only be forcing the balloon to inflate harder against the walls of the PA. Ideally it should take about a cc of air to do this – less, and the catheter may be too far in. More, and it may not be in far enough. The PA walls narrow quickly as you go farther into the lung, and it's easy to over-inflate, which can injure the arterial walls. Inflate only long enough to read the wave.

38- What is "overwedged"?

"Overwedged" refers to how the wedge trace looks often if the balloon overinflates against the walls of the PA. The trace begins to rise upward, becoming less wavelike and more linelike – you'll see this sometimes. Deflate the balloon and talk to the team about the line position – if this is happening with only a little bit of air, say half a cc, the line may be too far in.

39- What if I lose the syringe – can I use another one?

You can, but remember that the original syringe is made so that you can only push in about 1.5 cc and no more – it's got a stop built into the plastic of the barrel. If you switch syringes for some reason, be **extremely** careful of how much air you are using to inflate the balloon.

40- What should I do with the syringe when I'm not using it?

Some people let the balloon deflate and then lock the hub- there's a little locking hub that they use to keep the balloon inflated while feeding the catheter along into the patient - leaving the air in the syringe.

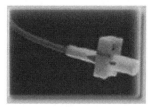
I don't like this myself – what if the hub were to unlock for some stupid unforeseeable reason – then if the patient rolled over on the syringe, the balloon might get inflated, and stay that way. I like to take the syringe off the open hub, which guarantees that the balloon is down, and then reattach the syringe empty. That way the air can't get accidentally pushed into the balloon.

So: is this hub open or closed to the balloon? Are you going to leave it this way?

http://www.irisoft-medi.ru/Products/sg_monitor.htm

41- How often should I wedge the line?

There are times when I wedge the line every hour. Patients who are "moving", or "doing something" (I love technical language) – in other words, actively working their way through some change in their hemodynamic state – will often show important changes from hour to hour. In the case of an ischemic/anginal episode for example, the wedge number might double in the space of ten minutes – and go back down as you treat the patient over the next hour or so. Or maybe not. It depends. Learning how to use a swan as a tool is something that comes with training and experience. In a stable situation I would wedge the swan every couple of hours. Depending.

42- How do I read the CVP?

Read the CVP (and the wedge) by using the cursor built into the monitor. Remember to read at end-expiration. Try this: if your patient isn't tubed, and is alert (seems rare in our ICU, doesn't it?), you can try asking him to hold his breath, just for a couple of seconds, at the end of expiration – a funny feeling if you try it. "Breathe all the way out normally, but then just wait a couple of seconds before taking a breath."

This lets the waveform settle out smoothly without any respiratory variation at all. Get bedside help with this if you have a question, and remember: even the senior staff are always asking each other to check their readings. Humility is a virtue. Two heads are always better than one. ("Why does she always look at me as if I had two heads?")

43- How do I do a cardiac output?

The idea here is that you are using two of the ports on the swan- one in the RA, and the distal one, which is further "downstream". There is a little temperature sensor built into the tip of the swan where the balloon is, and it measures the ambient blood temperature around it continuously. If you inject NS at a cooler, measured temperature into the RA, then the temperature of the blood flowing by the sensor will change, because the blood passing by has been diluted some by the cooler water that has been injected. Suppose you are sitting by the bank of a stream, and your feet are in the nice warm summertime water. Suddenly about a hundred feet upstream someone dumps in say, 20 gallons of ice water. You'd notice! Same way with the swan. The time it takes for the cold injectate to pass the sensor is measured by the computer in the monitor, and it comes up with a cardiac output number, measured in liters of blood pumped per minute. You should shoot at least three times, with a firm steady pressure on the syringe. The monitor will average the numbers for you. This is called doing cardiac output by "thermodilution" – there's another way, called the Fick output, which we'll look at a couple of questions further along.

44- Why do we delete the previous outputs?

We delete the previous numbers because we don't want them averaged into the ones that we're shooting now – if the patient's condition has changed, then the new numbers will be mixed up with the old ones, and won't be specific for the situation the patient is in now.

45- How many should I do?

I always shoot at least three.

46- What if the numbers make no sense?

Lots of things in life are like that… sometimes you get weird readings – very high, or low – in that case I do five, throw out the highest and lowest ones, and average the three that are left. You have to consider that sometimes the equipment doesn't work properly – check with a co-worker, or try talking with biomedical engineering. Let the team know if you're not getting meaningful numbers!

47- What is the difference between cardiac output and cardiac index?

Cardiac index is a "size-adjusted" form of cardiac output.. A measured CO of 4 liters/minute in a 100lb woman is not going to mean the same thing as that same number measured in a 300 lb man. Or vice versa. The cardiac index includes a correction for how big the person is, so the number stays meaningful from one person to the next. Like running mikes/kg/minute using pressors, instead of running straight drips – it takes the size of the patient into account. Normal is 2.5 – 4.5 liters/m² of BSA.

48- What is the BSA?

Body Surface Area is the number entered into the equation to derive cardiac index from cardiac output – it's the number that tells the computer how big the patient is. To get the number you need the patient's height and weight, and then either the computer in the monitor will calculate the number for you, or you can futz around with nomogram diagrams and have all kinds of geeky fun.

49- What is SVR?

Remember "Pump, Volume, and (Arterial) Squeeze": the three parts of a blood pressure? Cardiac output/index was "pump", right? This one is "squeeze". Systemic Vascular Resistance is the number that tells you how tight the arterial system is. (This is also the definition of **afterload**.) High is tight, low is loose. Normal is around 1000 (rounding off to make things easy) - a septic low might be 300, a cardiogenic high might be 2000.

50- What is SV?

This one, along with CVP and PCW is "volume". Stroke volume – how much blood in cc's is pumped with each systolic contraction. Easy – divide the cardiac output (liters pumped in one minute) by the heart rate. Low is empty, high is full. Low can also mean that the pump isn't pumping well...Normal is 60-90cc/beat.

51- What are the classic patterns of numbers for different situations, like sepsis, or cardiogenic shock?

We talked about these way earlier on, and I want to take another look at them again here. These should become absolutely crystal-clear in your mind. Remember the three parts of a blood pressure? The way to think about it is: where's the problem?

Sepsis:

In sepsis, the problem stems from the fact that the arterial system is being poisoned, and dilated, by bacterial endotoxins – so the arteries loosen up (unsqueeze), and the SVR goes down, along with blood pressure. The only reflex that the body has available to compensate – to try to keep up the blood pressure- is by using the heart, which pumps both harder and faster. So cardiac output goes up, and heart rate goes up.

So in sepsis: **SVR down, CO (and CI) and heart rate up, and SV usually goes up**. This last part doesn't seem to make sense though, because now that the arteries are dilated, the circulating volume that used to fill them up quite nicely, thank you, isn't enough any more. So wedge and CVP usually both go down, and you'd think that the SV would, too.

An example: **CO/ CI/ SVR/ PCW/ CVP** might look like: 12.4/ 3.6/ 325/ 6/ 4 – where the corresponding normals might look like: 4.5/ 2.1/ 1045/12/ 8. Why <u>does</u> the SV go up?

Cardiogenic shock:

In cardiogenic shock, the mechanism works in almost precisely the opposite way. Again: where's the problem? This time, it's not the arterial system – this time it's the <u>pump</u> that isn't pumping. So this time it's the cardiac output that goes down. So – what reflex can the body use to fix the low blood pressure that results? Tighten up the arteries! Just the reverse of sepsis. So in this case, SVR goes way up. An example using the same order of numbers as above might be: 2.0/ 1.1/ 2050/ 22/ 12. This time the output and index are down, and the SVR is way up – again, the body is doing this because it's the only thing it knows to do in this situation. The wedge pressure is very high, indicating that the LV is having a hard time emptying itself. Again, in cardiogenic shock: **CO/CI down, SVR up**.

Bear in mind that things can always fool you to some degree. Run your numbers past another co-worker, and the team, and get lots of practice thinking about how the numbers reflect different shock states.

Puzzler:

Or maybe not even shock states: here's a puzzler we saw a week or so ago. A patient comes to the unit postop after a nephrectomy, with a history significant mainly for having an EF of about 15-20% - low, in other words. He had a cardiac output of 3, index about 1.8, SVR 2000. The man had been treated intra-operatively with <u>only red cells</u> for volume, because the surgeons thought he was going to lose a lot of blood during surgery. So he comes to the unit with his swan in place, and he's tachycardic to the 120's, his blood pressure is around 85 systolic, his wedge is around 16, and his CVP was about 10. What exactly is going on here?

Well, his pressure is low, that's for sure. He's tachycardic, as though he might be septic. But he's not hot, nor does he seem dilated arterially, as his SVR is 2000. And he seems maybe fluid overloaded, because his wedge is so high. So... hmm - a mixed-up picture.

Actually, the key here is the history of low EF. This patient's LV doesn't pump very well, even at baseline. An LV with low pumping ability doesn't contract effectively – the walls move in and out only a little with each contraction - and it needs to be kept nice and full to empty itself as a result. (This is called "needing a high filling pressure.") A clue might be how much urine the man made during the case – probably hardly any. The doctors didn't want to throw a lot of IV fluid at the man with a low EF, because they didn't want him getting into CHF – which was smart. So they only gave him red cells. But they maybe they forgot something – after belly surgery, patients wind up effusing <u>lots</u> of fluid into the abdomen. Liters and liters. But he didn't have enough water component in his blood to do that <u>and</u> keep his blood pressure up.

This man is "dry". (Did you notice that we'd left out one of the shock states? This is actually a "trick question" puzzler – the third shock state that we see in the MICU besides sepsis and cardiogenic is, rarely, hypovolemia.) He's tachycardic for the same reason that a septic person is tachycardic – there isn't enough circulating volume in the arteries to pump around – except that it's not because he's dilated, it's because he's dry. The anesthesiologist maybe should have hydrated the patient somewhat, intraoperatively. The high wedge pressure is a false clue – the man probably walks around with a wedge pressure of 18-20, and needs it, because his heart contracts poorly. And so the medical team, maybe inexperienced with postop major belly case management, looked at the lowish cardiac output, high wedge, and high SVR, and decided, quite logically, that the man was probably having a big heart attack (he'd had them before), and was in cardiogenic shock. Although he didn't have EKG changes. The other clue here is the tachycardia (and maybe somebody should've asked how much urine the patient made during the case.) Usually people have a reason to be tachy – they're hot, or agitated, or dry. Or possibly ischemic, which fits in with the heart attack theory. But experienced eyes might've noticed that with his history, and not much urine output, and the belly surgery, and the weird cardiac numbers – "dry" is not uncommon, postop, especially as patients warm up after being in the cold OR for hours- they dilate, and their BP falls until they are rehydrated.

So things are not always straightforward, and it takes time to learn how to apply the information. Always ask around for opinions on what you think is going on, and study up!

Using the ports

52- Which port should I use for what?

- Yellow port: use this one for monitoring the PA pressures and wedge – that's what it's there for.

- Blue port: use for monitoring CVP, for giving intermittent meds like antibiotics, and for IV push meds like Lasix. **Do not use this port for vasoactive infusions!** Someone might come along and hang a med for you, or someone might do a cardiac output through the line. The blue port is also the one to use for pushing drugs in a code, the thought being that it allows for the best mixing with central venous blood.

- White and purple ports – use these for continuous infusions of fluid, meds, whatever you need. It's always a good idea to save one for TPN – flag it!

53- Can I infuse things through the distal PA port?

No. This is a strict policy. Unless it's a code, and there's absolutely nowhere else.

54- What goes through the CVP port?

As above – intermittent and push meds only.

55- Can I use the PA line for TPN?

Yes – we use the purple or white "VIP" ports for this.

56- Can I do blood draws from the PA line?

Yes. Draw off the blue CVP port, and discard the first 5cc. You might want to stop a TPN infusion if it was running through the white port, since it would contaminate your chems: you might get back a K+ of 10, or glucose of 1200! Confusing.

57- What is a Fick output, and how do I do one?

Such an unfortunate name. This is another way of doing a cardiac output, which you might use if you have a reason not to believe your thermodilution output numbers. What you do is to draw two blood gas specs at the same time: one from the arterial line, and the other from the distal port of the PA. <u>This is the only time you ever draw off the distal PA port.</u> Mark the specs clearly : the first one is "arterial", and "mixed venous" for the one from the PA port. Remember to write "add calculated O2 sat" on both slips, and send them off together. When the results come back, you can use a formula in the clinical references section of the unit's computers to figure out the cardiac output: at the clinical references screen, enter Fick in the search box. Click on the blue link that comes up, and you'll see a screen where you can enter the sat numbers, along with a recent hemoglobin– then hit the button and out comes a cardiac output. You might do this if the patient has TR – tricuspid regurgitation – because then the normally smooth flow of blood from RA, to RV, to PA is confused by the valve problems.

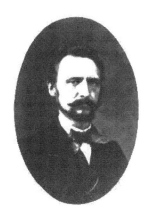

Adolph Fick: 1829-1901. Unfortunate name. Sadly, as it turns out, it does mean what you think it does, over there in Germany…hmm. I wonder if he did research on… nah.

http://www.corrosion-doctors.org/Biographies/FickBio.htm

Bad Things That Can Happen

58 and 59- What do I have to worry about when the line is going in? How can I tell if those things are happening?

- During the introducer insertion, the doctors could line up the carotid artery instead of the jugular vein – this will probably be obvious unless the patient is extremely hypoxic (dark blood) or hypotensive (not pulsatile). One way to check would be to hook up your transducer: even if the patient is hypotensive, the pressure in one of the great veins isn't going to be 60 systolic…the only thing to do is to pull the line, and start over after appropriately compressing the site. You might draw a blood gas if you needed one…Know your patient's coags and platelet count (and make sure the team knows) ahead of time!

- Any procedure associating the neck or chest with a long finder needle can cause a pneumothorax. This may not be immediately obvious, but should show up on the x-ray that you get after the line is in. Treatment would probably involve a chest tube. If the patient became unstable, what might be done before that could happen?

- The patient might have short (or long!) runs of VT as the PA tip passes through the RV. Try to make sure that electrolytes are normalized before the line goes in.

- Advancing the line too far can perforate the pulmonary artery. I've only ever seen this happen once in 21 ICU years. It's frightening – the patient immediately begins to cough up large amounts of bright red blood. Probably the thing to do would be to get the person intubated, keep her airway clear of clots, and then have a thoracic or pulmonary person use a flexible bronchoscope to insert a fogarty balloon into the affected lobe through the trachea, inflated, and left in place. Then a trip to angio might be in order, to try to plug the leak from inside the vessel.

60- What do I do if the line is stuck in wedge?

The line needs to be pulled back. The team needs to do this promptly, because the patient is at risk for perforation or tissue infarct. Interns usually do not do this procedure. Juniors can do this, but with great caution, and probably ought to have a senior around.

61- What if the line inadvertently pulls back to the RV?

Flagged it to the patient's shirt, did ya? Told ya! If the line does slip back to RV, you'll need to know what the difference is in the waveform. **You are responsible for knowing where your patient's PA catheter is positioned.** It will either need to be re-advanced into the PA, or pulled back to the CVP position. The line can only be advanced if it's been in less than 24 hours, and the clear sheath must be in place. Monitor carefully for VT! **This is a critical situation**. Again, a junior/senior procedure.

Actually this happened recently – it was UGLY! I mean, it's not always quite so ugly, but this time, wow! Some people make a pressure with VT, and others don't… this person made NO blood pressure with the runs of VT that the PA line created, tickling her RV.

What you can do: inflate the balloon. It may float back into the PA…but won't wedge. **Not** a permanent fix.

62- What if the line gets pulled all the way out?

If the line is all the way out, (and the introducer is still in place), cover the insertion diaphragm with tegaderm to prevent a possible air embolus. Assess the patient. Notify the team immediately. Has the patient lost a pressor infusion through one of the ports? Swap to the introducer. Stay with the patient until the team has a chance to assess with you.

63- Why do they pull the line "back to CVP"?

Sometimes the swan gets inadvertently pulled back to RV after the 24 hour repositioning limit has gone by. The line then has to be removed. If you need a port for infusion, the line can be left with the distal port in the RA – in this case you would change the transducer setup, because the RA ports would not be usable any more – they'd probably be outside the skin – cap them and flag them "Do not use". The only port left working now is the distal one – so the yellow port now becomes your CVP, and you're working with one transducer instead of two. This line should be taken out. If necessary, a triple-lumen can be inserted in it's place, but it may not work well if it's own ports open up within the introducer.

64- What should I do with the ports and the transducers if the line is pulled back to CVP?

As above: cap them, and flag them appropriately. Disconnect the old CVP transducer, since the distal port is now at the CVP.

65- What if the balloon ruptures?

That would be a bad thing. Not only would you then be left with an unusable swan, but the patient would be at risk for an air embolus entering through the inflation line.

66- How do I know if that has happened?

Blood would show up in the syringe. Cap and flag the inflation port, and notify the team immediately. If the patient still needs a swan, a new one may have to get floated in.

Taking the Line Out

67- How do we know when the PA line needs to come out?

Pulling a swan is always a judgment call. If the patient has stabilized and doesn't need the numbers any more – they may still need the access for meds. Can the site be rewired for a quad port central line? (Why don't they just go ahead and make a 12-lumen central line already?)

The last time I looked, the rule was that all central lines were supposed to come out within seven days of being put in. Obviously this doesn't always happen, but that's the guideline. Sometimes patients are sick enough that another swan has to replace the one that's being pulled. If a central line has to come out because of a temperature spike, think carefully with the team about whether the same site can be rewired for a new line, or whether the patient needs a new stick altogether. Also, remember that it is your responsibility to maintain access for critical meds like pressors. You may have to remind the team of this before they enthusiastically remove your only central access! If no other access is possible, then the line may just have to stay in for the time being.

68- Who takes it out?

Usually a house officer will remove a swan. Nurses can be certified to do swan removals, but you need to do three under supervision, which can be hard to come by.

69- How do I get certified to take out PA lines?

Speak to the CNS, and you can start collecting the experience that you need – you need to document the process as it goes along.

70- What should I look for on the x-ray before I pull a swan?

You want to make sure that the line isn't kinked or knotted – yes, it does happen! There may be other things to think about, since I haven't done this myself, so be sure to follow up carefully with the CNS.

71- Should I culture the tip?

I would definitely culture the tip of any central line that I remove from any patient.

Here's a comment from a correspondent on this, "DocVoc":

Nice site. Have a question/clarification on culturing PA lines. I think it depends upon the setting. For example, in a medical intensive care unit, or even a surgical intensive care unit, and when the line has been in for say, > that 24-48 hours, it may well be good practice and policy to have it cultured. However, say in an Open Heart Setting, where the patient has had that sucker in only in surgery and the immediate post-op period--say 16-24 hours or so: no, the PA line would not necessarily need to be cultured. Of course there are individual particulars that need to be considered even in that situation. A successful, straight-forward OHS patient who has stabilized, and may even have CT's d/c'd etc, and is well on his way out of the OH unit, may not need to incur the expense of this test. Of course, again it may depend on the individual particulars.

72- Now that the line is out, can air get into the patient through the black diaphragm thing in the introducer?

Yes! This is something that people forget about. You should immediately cover the opening of the diaphragm with something air-occlusive (tegaderm is perfect).

73 - What is an obturator?

An obturator is a plastic piece that is fed into the place through the diaphragm where the swan used to be. It's the same length as the introducer, and the top of it screws onto the introducer hub where the clear sheath would. It's designed by the manufacturer to seal up the hub diaphragm and prevent air from entering the patient.

74- Can I put in an obturator?

The last time I went over this with our previous CNS, the answer was yes. As always, re-check to make sure this is correct. A tegaderm should serve well to seal the opening if this can't be done.

Pacemakers

1- What is a pacemaker?

2- What does "intrinsic" mean?

3- How exactly do pacemakers work on the heart?

4- What are the parts of a pacemaker?

5- Are there different kinds of pacemakers?

6- What is the advantage of two wires over one?

7- How are pacemakers inserted?

8- What do they mean by transvenous, transcutaneous, and transthoracic?

9- How does the generator box work?

10- How long do the implanted batteries last?

11- How much electricity does the pacemaker use to actually pace the heart?

12- In English, please?

13- What is "capture threshold?"

14- Why do paced beats generated by a ventricular wire look like PVCs?

15- What does "asynchronous" mean, and what does "demand" mean?

16- What do those letters: VVI, DDD, etc. stand for?

17- What is "failure to capture?"

18- What is "failure to sense"?

19- How can an implanted pacemaker be reprogrammed?

20- What is the magnet thing?

21- What are some reasons for placing a permanent pacemaker?

22- What is an AICD?

23- Can AICD's also function as pacemakers?

24- What problems do AICD's have?

25- How do you stop an AICD from shocking the patient incorrectly?

26- Can you shock a patient with a pacemaker?

27- What is external cardiac pacing?

28- Who was Zoll, anyhow?

29- What else do I need to know about running the external pacemaker?

30- How do I know if capture has been achieved?

31- What's the tricky part?

32- Does external pacing hurt?

33- How long can a person stay on the external pacemaker?

34- How does the Zoll go into demand mode?

35- Any other Zoll tricks?

36- Can you do CPR with the external pacer in place?

37- How effective is the Zoll?

Pacemakers

1. What is a pacemaker?

A pacemaker is an electronic device that provides an electrical signal to make the heart beat when it's own, built-in pacemakers fail. The anatomical, built-in pacemakers provide what's called the "intrinsic" rhythm, and they can be disrupted by various conditions – ischemia for example, or by an MI.

2. What does "intrinsic" mean?

Intrinsic means "built in". In this situation, it means: "coming from the patient's own built-in, natural pacemakers" : the SA or AV nodes; or sometimes from lower down in the ventricles.

3. How exactly do pacemakers work on the heart?

The pacemaker essentially does two things : it <u>senses</u> the patient's own rhythm using a "sensing circuit", and it <u>sends</u> out electrical signals using an "output circuit". If the patient's intrinsic rhythm becomes too slow or goes away completely, the electronic pacemaker senses that, and starts sending out signals along the wires leading from the control box to the heart muscle. The signals, if they're "capturing" properly, provide a regular electrical stimulus, making the heart contract at a rate fast enough to maintain the patient's blood pressure.

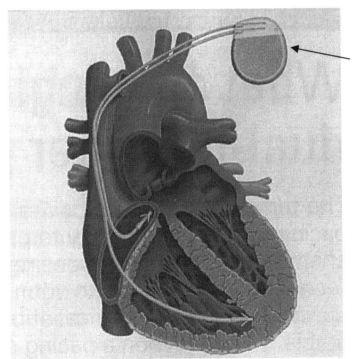

Here's the "box", implanted.

How many pacing wires?

http://www.borleyrectory.com/myessays/pacemaker.htm

4. What are the parts of a pacemaker?

The pacemaker box itself is called the "pulse generator" – the generator is connected to either one or two wires, which carry the electrical signals to the heart muscle. Permanent pacing generators are implanted in the chest under the skin – nowadays they're very small – and the wires leading to the heart are threaded through the subclavian vein.

5. Are there different kinds of pacemakers?

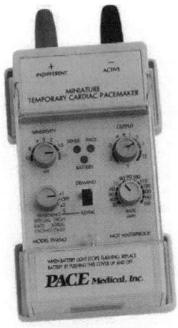

Pacemakers can be either temporary or permanent. The temporary pacemakers that we see in the MICU are made up of a control box and one single output wire leading to the inner wall of the RV (thus called a ventricular wire, or "V-wire"), and provide simple rate control by pacing the ventricles. Permanent pacemakers come in several flavors, but the main difference between them is that some have only one wire leading to the RV, and some have two – one to the right atrium (RA), and another one to the RV. A pacing system that paces both the RA and the RV is called an "atrioventricular" pacer, and paces both right heart chambers in sequence. The signal affects the left-side chambers and stimulates them to contract as well. The signal from the wire generates a visual signal on the EKG that looks like, and is called a "spike".

Here's an example of a temporary, external, single-wire pacing box. The wire has two pole connections, so one pair of connectors: single wire box.

http://www.pacemedicalinc.com/4543.htm

Here's a nice example of single-wire pacing, with spikes coming at a rate in the 70's. The reason we can tell that there's only one wire going is simply that there's only one spike. Two-wire systems generate two spikes.

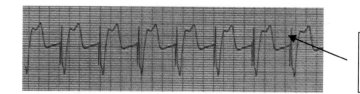

These spikes go both up and down in front of the QRS's, which you see sometimes – a "normal variant".

How many spikes this time?

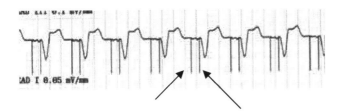

Everybody see the two spikes? The arrows aren't perfect – but clearly there are two pacing functions going on here: the first spike is generating atrial kick, and the second is kicking the ventricles: two spikes, two wires.

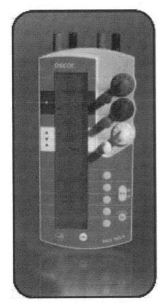

Two sets of connectors: two wires. So what kind of box is this?

http://www.oscor.com/default.asp?owc/temp%20pacing.asp~main

6. What is the advantage of two wires over one?

If you pace the ventricle alone, the patient doesn't get the "atrial kick" – the push of the atria into the ventricles. This can actually add 20-25% to the cardiac output, and improve the blood pressure accordingly. A nice example of this was a patient we saw recently who had a temporary V-wire in place. When she was paced at a rate of 70, she only got a blood pressure of about 85, systolic. But when the pacer rate was turned down, her intrinsic rate took over at about a rate of 60 – sinus rhythm, which meant that she started getting her atrial kick again – and her blood pressure rose, even with the slower rate, to about 105. Also a nice example of how the fastest rate will capture: first the wire, then the intrinsic one.

6.   How are pacemakers inserted?

A temporary pacing wire is threaded through an introducer placed in a central line site, usually the right internal jugular or subclavian. (The right IJ is the straightest shot down into the RV, which is where you want your temporary wire to go.) Nowadays we rarely use transvenous wire insertion at the bedside – we apply the transcutaneous pacer, or "Zoll" instead. Once in a great while a transthoracic wire placement is attempted, usually at the end of a code when nothing else is working…

7. **What do they mean by transvenous, transcutaneous, and transthoracic?**

Transvenous means that the pacing wire is threaded down the jugular vein through an introducer (the same as a PA line introducer). The introducer is put in first, like any central neck IV line, and the wire is passed through it, like a PA line is, until it makes contact with the inner wall of the RV. Then the wire is attached to a generator box, and the heart is paced using the wire. We hardly ever do this at the bedside anymore, since the coming of the Zoll external pacer.

Transcutaneous pacing means using external pacing pads connected to a device like the Zoll machine, or one of the defibrillators that has external pacing ability.

Transthoracic pacing means using wires inserted either during cardiac surgery – small wires that sit on the outer wall of the heart – "epicardial" wires, that lead out of the chest, to a control box - or doing a maneuver that involves pushing a pacing wire into the RV up through the chest wall, subxiphoid, during a code. I've only ever seen this tried once and it didn't work. According to a web source that we looked at, the procedure isn't very popular, can create a whole slew of nasty complications, and usually isn't any use anyhow.

8. **How does the generator box work?**

The generator box consists of a small computerized chip controller that's run by a battery. The box senses and paces through the same set of wires that lead to the endocardium.

9. **How long does the battery last?**

As I understand it, implantable pacers use lithium batteries that last anywhere from 6 to 10 years. The battery in a temporary pacing box is a regular hardware-store type 9-volt battery.

10. **How much electricity does the pacemaker use to actually pace the heart?**

The output of the pacemaker is measured in two ways: "signal amplitude", and "pulse width".

11. **In English, please?**

Signal amplitude means "how much juice the box puts out through the wire with every pulse". This is measured in milliamperes, and is called MA – there's a twisty dial to control the MA on the front of the temporary pacer box. Pulse width means "how long each pulse lasts". The electrical pulse has to be strong enough, and last long enough, to capture the myocardium.

12. What is "capture threshold"?

Capture threshold is the minimum amount of electricity that the box has to emit to pace the heart – as above, it's measured in milliamps, and the twisty knob is turned up until the heart is paced 100% - then turned down again until the minimum is determined.

13. Why do paced beats generated by a ventricular wire look like PVCs?

The reason that PVCs look "wide and bizarre" is because they originate down at the bottom of the heart, at the opposite end from where they usually come - the path of depolarization is backwards as a result. Think of the normal lead II signal, going from northwest to southeast: Oregon to Florida. A paced signal is going backwards, upwards ("retrograde") - the reverse of the normal QRS waveform. Since the v-wire generates a rhythm by emitting electricity from a wire whose tip is embedded in the wall of the RV, the deflection follows the same path as a PVC – so it looks like one.

Here's the two-wire pacing strip again: one wire is in the right atrium, and the other's in the right ventricle. With two wires, the ventricular path is still backwards, just as with one – makes sense, right?

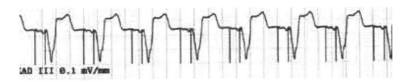

14. What does "asynchronous" mean, and what does "demand" mean?

A temporary control box can bet set to run - just run - at a fixed rate, ignoring any signals that the patient's heart may be making (asynchronous); or it can be set to pace only if the intrinsic heart rate gets too slow ("pacing on demand"). Needless to say, you would use the first way of pacing only if the patient's heart rate was either much too slow, as may happen if the patient wipes out some of her conduction system by infarct, or if the rhythm just isn't there, as in asystole, maybe for the same reason. There's a second twisty dial that controls how sensitive the box will be to the patient – for full control, you would turn it all the way until the control knob's arrow pointer was all the way towards the word "asynchronous". Insensitive. Take the pacing generator out of the emergency pacing tackle box a few times, and get familiar with it.

Here's the strip we looked at on page 3. This is fixed-rate pacing. Not necessarily asynchronous, but this is what it would look like:

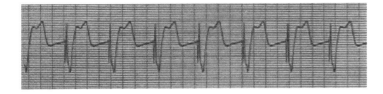

This same dial can also be turned in the other direction, away from "asynchronous" – this increases the sensitivity of the box, so that it will start sensing the patient's own rate. If you want the box to start pacing the patient only when the intrinsic rate gets too slow – "on demand", then you adjust the sensitivity of the box so that it can see the patient's rhythm. This will "inhibit" the box from firing when it sees intrinsic beats. The cardiology people are usually responsible for these settings, but the idea is pretty simple: it's better if the patient's own rhythm controls the heart, especially if all you have is a V-wire (no atrial kick with only a v-wire, remember) – but if it slows down below a certain point, the box will wake up and take over. The intrinsic rhythm stops or slows, and the interval is long enough for the pacer to turn on.

Remember that the wire has to generate a rate that's fast enough to make an adequate blood pressure. If the demand rate is set so that the box only kicks in at a rate of 60, that may not be enough, especially if you're only working with the one wire.

15. What do those letters: VVI, DDD, etc., stand for?

We really only see two kinds of pacemakers in the MICU – single v-wire pacing (usually temporary wires placed for bradycardias and the like), and permanently implanted A-V pacers. Single v-wire systems are called VVI pacers, and the A-V pacers are called DDD.

The first letter stands for the chamber that is paced, the second letter is for the chamber that is sensed, and the third letter stands for the response the pacer makes to a sensed intrinsic beat. So a VVI-mode pacer paces the RV, senses the RV, and is Inhibited from firing if it senses an intrinsic beat. DDD pacers pace both chambers (D stands for "dual"), they sense both chambers, and each of the two wires is inhibited by an intrinsic beat.

This can produce a very cool result: a patient may generate her own P-waves, but fail to conduct them – maybe she has a fritzed-out AV node. The A-wire will be inhibited by the patient's P's, but the v-wire will sense, and follow them. So the patient will be in a "sinus rhythm, with v-pacing", and will be able to increase and decrease heart rate in a normal way in response to exercise, and the like. Excellent!

16. What is "failure to capture"?

Here the idea is that the pacing box sends an impulse to the heart at the right time, but the heart doesn't respond. The box is sensing that the intrinsic heart rate is too slow, but the output signal isn't making the myocardium respond. You see this on a rhythm strip when there are clear pacing spikes coming from the box – at the right time after either an intrinsic beat or a paced one – but they're not followed by a QRS response. There can be all sorts of reasons for this: broken wires, pacemaker box failure, acidosis, alkalosis, bad connection to an external pacing box, battery failure, the moon in Virgo… this can be serious if the patient is depending on the pacemaker to maintain a blood pressure. Various maneuvers can be made with the pacer control box to re-establish proper capture – the quickest one is usually to turn up the MA output. Call the team. While you're waiting, have atropine at the bedside, and the Zoll nearby in case "bad" capture goes to "no" capture!

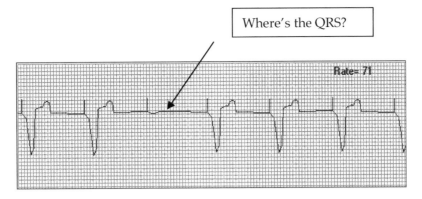

The point to remember: the pacer spikes are coming at the **right** time relative to the patients rate, or lack of a rate – but they're not capturing.

17. **What is "failure to sense"?**

Remember, the pacemaker has both a sensing circuit and an output, or pacing circuit. The pacer has to sense whether or not the patient is generating a rhythm, so it will know when to pace and when not to. In this case the pacemaker will generate spikes that do capture, but the spikes come at the wrong time, and the box is clearly unable to see what the patient's heart is doing. Clearly a bad thing – it can result in the infamous R-on-T situation, producing VT or VF.

The thing to keep in mind: the pacer spikes will be coming at the **wrong** time. This may just be an improper sensitivity setting on the box.

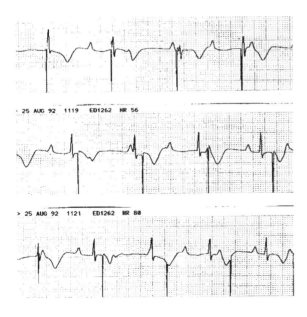

Here we are failing to sense. (Usually a guy thing…) The spikes are certainly regular, but are they coming at the right time, relative to the patient? No – the box isn't seeing the patient's rhythm, and it's firing off blindly. (Three doctors go duck hunting…)

www. monroecc..edu/depts/pstc/paracar5.htm

427

18. How can an implanted pacemaker be reprogrammed?

There's a machine that the physician uses to communicate with an implanted pacemaker.

19. What is the magnet thing?

You've probably seen the physicians do this mysterious maneuver with a ring-shaped magnet that gets placed on the patients' chest over the pacemaker. The idea here is that there is a switch inside the pacemaker with a ferrous reed, which is pulled from one position to the other by the magnet. This is involved in figuring out how much longer the pacers' battery has to live, and also changes the pacemaker into fully asynchronous mode for testing purposes.

20. What are some reasons for placing a permanent pacemaker?

There are lots of things that an unhappy heart can come up with that will indicate the need for a pacemaker: sick-sinus and tachy-brady syndromes will do it, certainly recurrent bradycardias that drop the BP will do it, heart blocks (especially which one?) – you get the idea. If the heart isn't generating a rate for whatever reason, pacing will probably be needed.

21. What is an AICD?

AICD stands for Automatic, Implantable, Cardioverter-Defibrillator. This is a variation on the idea of a pacemaker – the device has a sensing circuit and an output circuit, but instead of acting as a pacer, it spends it's time waiting for the onset of some nasty tachyarrhythmia, like VT, or SVT – which it then tries to shock the patient out of. Apparently they will also sometimes try to override-pace a patient out of a rapid rhythm.

22. Can AICDs also function as pacers?

Apparently the newest generation of AICDs can do both.

23. What problems do AICDs have?

Clearly you wouldn't want to be defibrillated at the wrong time. I have no idea how common a problem this is – I have heard of it happening, and of patients having to come in and have the box reprogrammed, or shut off. Similarly to pacemakers, AICDs can fail to sense, or to capture...

24. How do you stop an AICD from shocking the patient incorrectly?

Apparently the ring magnet will shut off the cardioverter, but will allow the pacer function to keep going if necessary. We need to check into this...

25. Can you shock a patient with a pacemaker?

The last time this came up in the MICU, we called the CCU, and they told us that it's generally safe to shock a patient with an implanted pacemaker.

26. What is external pacing?

Transcutaneous pacing is the use of the Zoll machine, or its equivalent. External pacing capability is built into the defibrillators that we use in the unit. Large sticky pads are applied to the patient's chest and back (it's important to check the placement diagram on the pad package), and connected to the Zoll output cable. The cable delivers electricity to the pads, hopefully capturing and pacing a heart that's too slow.

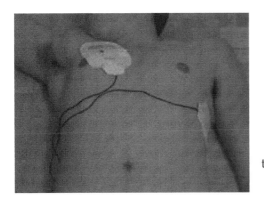

There's been an important change in the way the pads are applied:

Here's the way we **used** to do it. These pads are in the same position used for cardioversion, defibrillation, those things…

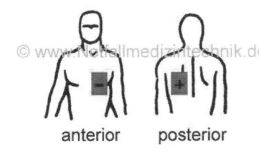

anterior   posterior

Here's the way we do it now. The idea is sort of to "sandwich" the heart between the pads. Apparently works much more better.

This really is important: take the time to go over this stuff before you need to do in emergently. Grab the resource nurse, or a senior staff person, or another newbie, and take a good look at how the parts of the equipment fit together, how they work, where replacments are kept…

27. Who was Zoll, anyhow?

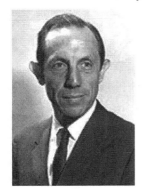

Dr. Zoll was apparently the medical researcher who did the original research and development of transcutaneous pacing, and who patented the machine in the early 1980's.

http://zoll-aed.com/dr-zoll.jpg

28. What else do I need to know about running the external pacer?

Our machine has only three controls that you have to worry about: one changes the box from monitor mode to pacing mode, and the other two are the pacer control knobs.

The basics are really not hard. Remember that the external pacing box should be able to <u>see</u> the patient, as well as pace the patient, so there is a <u>sensing cable</u> that attaches to three chest electrodes. You can pace the patient without this, so in an emergency just get the pads on and go - but having the ability to sense is better.

The pacing electrodes are the big white sticky things – one goes on the front of the chest, one goes on the patient's back – again, check the positioning diagram on the package that they come in. These connect to the cable that lets the box <u>pace</u> the patient: an <u>output cable</u> coming from the box.

29. How do I know if capture has been achieved?

This is a bit tricky, but obviously important. If there's time, make sure that the Zoll's sensing cable is attached to the patient – 3 electrodes in a standard lead II pattern, because it helps if the machine can see the patient's heart rate.

Now the knobs - start with both knob controls: rate, and power (MA) output - set at zero. Turn the heart rate knob up to a rate that you'd like to pace the patient at – this is pretty simple: if the patient's rate is 20, pick something like 60 - 80 beats per minute. Now start turning up the power output knob – it sometimes takes a lot of power to capture – something like 100 to 150 MA.

30. What's the tricky part?

Here's the tricky part. If you look at the patient's monitor for evidence of capture, you may be fooled. The electrical activity of the external pacer shows up clearly on the monitor as large funny-looking-beats, and they will occur at whatever rate of bpm that you chose. The appearance of these beats does <u>not</u> mean that the patient's heart has been captured! You need to actually have some way to tell that the heart is being paced - and generating blood pressure - at the rate you're trying to pace them at. So if the patient has an a-line, try looking at the waveform heart rate counter to match your desired rate, or the pulse oximeter heart rate counter – or feel the patient's pulse, which may be hard to do if they're hypotensive. See if the patient's blood pressure is responding. Don't assume that the electrical activity of the pacer means that the heart is being paced!

31. Does external pacing hurt?

Yes, depending on how much juice they get, but also depending on how big the external pacing pad is. It seems that the larger electrode size does away with most of the pain involved. I hope so - it doesn't look very comfortable…

32. How long can a person stay on the external pacemaker?

Probably not too long. In my experience, an hour or two if the patient really needs a wire. The whole point of the device is to provide temporary pacing in a critical situation until the patient can get a wire inserted in the cath lab. This has almost completely replaced the placement of transvenous pacing wires in code situations, although sometimes it's still tried. The external pacer may stay on in "demand mode" in a patient who doesn't need a wire, but whose rate only rarely goes too low – maybe while waiting for a digoxin level to come down. (Look up "digi-bind"). This is a cardiology judgment call.

33. How does the Zoll go into demand mode?

Once you've determined that the MA is set high enough to capture 100% (all the time, reliably), try turning down the rate knob to let the patient's own heart rate take over (assuming they have a rate at all!) – if they do, and if that generates an adequate blood pressure, the Zoll's rate can be left at a number low enough not to interfere with the patient's intrinsic rate unless it drops too far – at which point the Zoll will kick in on "demand". The Zoll will also run "blind", that is, without the sensing cable attached: if you're in a real hurry, say, in an asystolic code, you can just slap on the pads, pick a rate, turn the MA up to max, and go. Establish capture first, and try to find the capture threshold later…

34. Any other Zoll tricks?

A useful one is: if you have time, benzoin the skin under the <u>outer</u> part of the pacing pads – not on the gel part – because people tend to sweat the pads off. Dangerous. A quick additional point about this: if you should come across sticky defibrillation pads, which are used for patients that require repeated shocks, <u>don't</u> benzoin them on – it can cause arcing!

35. Can you do CPR with the external pacer in place?

The literature I've read says yes – but that you should turn the pacing box off. (Duh.)

36. How effective is the Zoll?

Apparently pretty effective - the survival rates are reported as ranging from 50-100%. The secret: get it up and running promptly. Did your patient just need a dose of atropine? Put the pads on, right now, and get the cables and box hooked up, ready to run. Any time wasted, any time the patient spends hypotensive or becoming even moderately acidotic increases the chance that the device won't work. And get a call in to the cath lab at the same time…

Peripheral IV's for Beginners

This article: the work, the thought, and especially the humor that went into it, is dedicated to the memory of our good friend; hilarious, smart, and loving colleague, Robin Holloway...

Here's the next in our series for new grads coming into the MICU – this seemed like a pretty useful topic. As we gain experience with putting these articles together, we're using more embedded links, like this one (try it): http://www.aic.cuhk.edu.hk/web8/Very%20BASIC%20venous%20cannulation.htm - remember that if you're looking at our articles online, you can click on any of the blue links to open your browser and go to the page that the link came from.

We're also including some questions for the newbie nurse to ponder, maybe with the help of the preceptor...

Hardware

1- What is an intravenous?
   a. The bag
   b. The tubing
       1. the spike
       2. the drip chamber: maxi and mini
       3. roller clamps
       4. pump tubing
       5. buretrols and solusets
       6. blood tubing
   c. The ports
   d. What are needle-less connectors all about?
   e. The connection to the catheter – what are Luer connectors?
   f. The dressing
   g. Filters
2- What is a heparin lock?
3- What does the gauge number mean?
4- How do I know if my patient needs an IV or a hep-lock?
5- Who inserts IV's?
6- Where should they go?
7- How do I choose a catheter size? What do they look like?
8- How are IV's inserted?
9- How do I know if my patient's IV is working properly?

Problems

10- How long can peripheral IV's stay in?

432

11- What does "infiltration" mean? An ugly picture that you do need to see...
12- What is phlebitis?
13- What is thrombophlebitis?
14- What is phlebothrombosis?

Pumps

15- What are infusion pumps all about?
16- What does "KVO" mean?
17- What is a flush line?
18- What is the "primary rate"?
19- "Secondary rate"?
20- How do I figure out where to plug things in to the connectors?
    a.   Above the pump?
    b.   Below the pump?

Treatments

21- Volume infusions.
22- Blood products.
23- Types of IV fluids.
24- What is a rapid bolus? **Something incredibly important!**
25- How much of a bolus should my patient get?
26- What kind of IV fluid should I use for a bolus?
27- Intermittent meds
28- Continuous med infusions.
29- Multiple infusions.
    a.   Compatibility
    b.   Incompatibility
30- What is a med bolus?
31- How do I give a med bolus?
32- What is an IV push med?
33- How do I give IV push meds?

Peripheral IV's for Beginners

Hardware

1-   What is an intravenous?

Most people have some kind of idea what IV's are about before they get to the MICU, but for new grads, a review of the basics is probably in order, since it's pretty hard to imagine something more important to patient care. Let's have a look:

a.   The bag

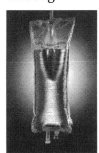

433

Yup, that's the bag. Looks like normal saline. Ok new grads, what's "normal" about normal saline? What does "isotonic" mean? What other commonly used IV fluid is isotonic?

This stuff that's "clear as crystal" is commonly referred to as "crystalloid".

Sterile! The entire IV setup has to be EXTREMELY sterile: the bag, the tubing, the connectors, the catheter, the dressing...

Why?

b. The tubing

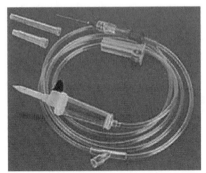

The whole fluid path from the spike to the needle is sterile.

1. The spike

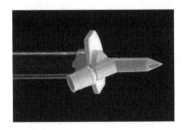

This one's vented – you use this kind with bottle mixes; it lets air get into the bottle, so the fluid can come out, while with bag mixes, the bag just collapses closed.

2. The drip chamber

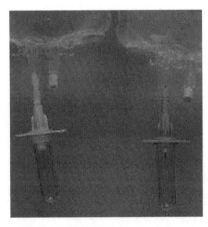

A little hard to see, but the one on the left is "maxi" drip, or ten drops per cc, and the one on the right is "mini" - 60 drops per cc. We never regulate constant infusions by eye anymore – most everything goes on an infusion pump nowadays.

But for a rapid IV volume bolus of something (**not** meds) – normal saline, Ringer's lactate, whatever, we still use gravity. Which one of these are you going to reach for? In other words, which one is going to run more rapidly?

3. Roller clamps

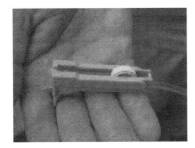

We only use gravity tubing in two situations nowadays: for rapid IV bolus infusions, and for blood. For boluses, the roller clamp has two positions: "all the way open", and "closed". For blood – mm… depends. For acute bleeds? – all the way open. Otherwise we titrate by eye to infuse the blood over an hour or two.

http://www.crvetcenter.com/ivflui9.jpg

4. Pump tubing

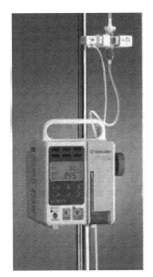

They're all different. The only thing to do is to learn the system where you're at. One important thing that's developed recently: **ALL the sets have to self-clamp if they come out of the pump.**

Why?

http://www.terumo.co.th/Medical.htm

5. Buretrols and Solusets

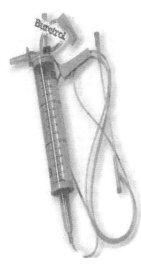

Interchangable names for the same thing, so far as I know. I still use these once in a while for premixed meds – Flagyl/metronidazole comes to mind. The problem is that single doses of intravenous meds really need to be given over predictable periods of time – an hour is usually good for most doses of antibiotics. Vancomycin I usually give over two. The problem is that anything with a roller clamp is never going to be as precise in timed delivery as a pump, so these are rapidly vanishing.

http://www.accd.edu/sac/nursing/math/peds10.html

6. Blood tubing

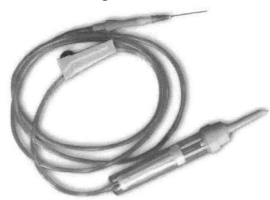

The drip chamber is a bit different for this one – there's a filter built in to catch debris and the like, anything larger than a red cell...

Open sharp! (Might be a blunt, actually...)

b. The ports

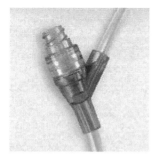

This is where things get plugged into the line. Are you running, say, normal saline at 53.7 cc's per hour? And you want to plug in the patient's dose of IV colace? This is where you go...

Wait a second
... IV what?

c. What are needle-less connectors all about?

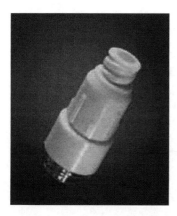

It's been a long time since we used needled connectors, but it's worth mentioning, I guess. Needles, or "sharps", as we call them, are generally considered a Bad Thing. This doesn't mean we don't use them all the time for various things – we draw up meds with them, we give subcutaneous and intramuscular injections with them... but poking yourself with one – whether it's been in contact with a patient or not – is pretty much a Bad Thing. People were getting hepatitis from patients, I think there were a few cases of HIV... so the word went out: the fewer needles, the better.
And lo - non-needle connection systems were created. And they were pretty good...

d. The connection to the catheter – what are Luer connectors?

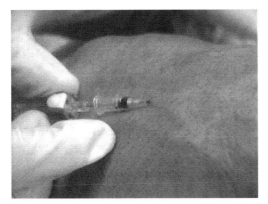

Not a bad picture of the end of the catheter. The tubing actually screws onto the yellow end there – except sometimes it's blue, or green, or pink, or whatever, usually depending on the catheter size. But the screw technology is pretty uniform, all under the name of Luer connectors. That guy Luer – what a genius!

What the heck part of the patient is that, anyhow?

http://www.silverlon.com/images/iv_catheter/iv_catheter_patient1.jpg

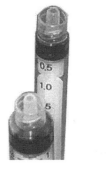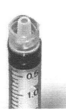

These syringes have female luer connections at the ends.

The catheter hub of the IV, the hubs of injection needles, the connector hubs at the ends of IV tubing – they all use **the same size and type of connector**, which was probably what developing the Luer standard was all about.

http://img.alibaba.com/photo/50347934/Luer_Lock_Syringe.jpg

e. The dressing

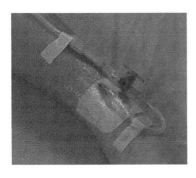

We like to be able to see the site (why?), so we put a clear tegaderm over it…

Change the dressing if it gets loose, or dirty.

http://www.puntex.es/busqueda/descripciones/3M/imagenes/tegaderm.jpg

f. Filters

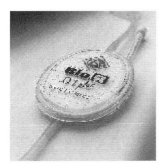

Some infusions need filtering – this is an inline **blood filter** that a company makes, I guess for people who don't use the filtered IV tube sets that we do. (You mean there are OTHER hospitals in the world?)

Patients with PFO's need **air filters** attached to ALL their IV lines.

Why?

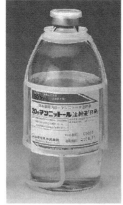

Mannitol needs to be filtered. Crystals! There's a special little filter thingy that goes on the end of the infusion line.

Well – they SAID it was mannitol…

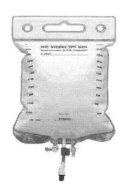

TPN is always filtered – check with the pharmacy to make sure which filters to use for which.

2- What is a heparin lock?

Trick question! A peripheral IV that's been capped and flushed with saline is still called a "hep-lock" nowadays, but we flush very few lines with heparin any more – dialysis catheters come to mind, and even they get flushed with ACD these days. More and more patients are being found sensitive to heparin – someone in the group tell us what HIT is, please?

3- What does the gauge number mean?

I think I have this right – this is a pretty antiquated measurement system, based on the number of tubes that will lie, next to each other, in the space of an inch. Inch? Wow – that IS old… so an 18 gauge catheter? – 18 of them will lie in the space of 2.54 centimeters. 20 gauge? Um… I give up! But it explains why <u>higher</u> numbers means <u>smaller</u> catheters, right?

4- How do I know if my patient needs an IV, or a hep-lock?

I don't think any patient sick enough to be in the MICU should have less than two IV's – whatever they're getting, they probably really need! What are you going to do when the only line they have suddenly infiltrates, and they've got nothing?

5- Who inserts IVs?

We do. I happen to think that the more you can do for your patient, the better, as long as you're staying in constant practice, and these skills are practiced all the time in the MICU. Different institutions have different rules: some places only let IV nurses place peripheral lines, some places let all nurses do it – go with what your local rules say. We do have an IV team, and they really are amazing - they can get lines in rocks, seems like.

6- Where should they go?

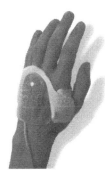

In practice, we stick to the arms for peripherals. Only very rarely will a patient get an IV in a foot – it's risky for dislodging DVTs…

Hands are good…

http://www.asaging.org/awards/awards02/images/ivhouse.jpg

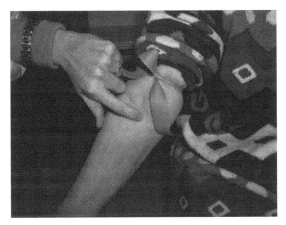

I like antecubital veins. I know that people will sometimes try to avoid them for one reason or another – the patient might need them if they get really sick!

What's wrong with **that** statement… ?

http://www.eyetec.net/group5/images/inject2.jpg

7- How do I choose a catheter size? What do they look like?

What are you going to be running through the line? It's pretty hard to run blood through a tiny little 22-gauge IV. An 18 is good for giving blood – once in a while a patient with really excellent veins will come up from the ER or the OR with a couple of 14's in place. (14's are BIG IV's…)

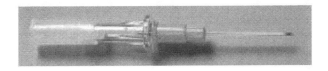

This is what I would call a 20 gauge straight angiocath… this is the one that we use for arterial lines, too. See the stylet in place, sticking out beyond the tip of the catheter?

http://www.rimed.com.br/img_produto/3562.jpg

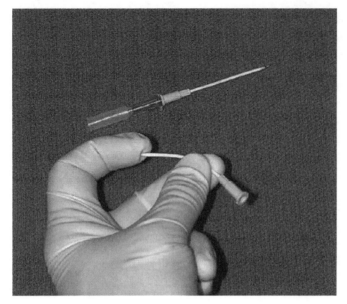

On top, the stylet in place – after insertion, the stylet comes out, leaving the soft, bendable catheter in the vessel.

Hm – gray hub – that a 14? Wooo…

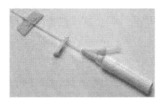

Then there's the butterflies – we use these a lot. What the heck size is a yellow one? 24? Pediatric, probably.

For continuous infusions of crystalloid, intermittent meds, most situations, we use 20's and 18's.

8- How are IV's inserted?

Here's a link to look at:

There's no lack of insertion guides, classes, certification programs, trainings… you just need to find the one near where you are, and learn what they have to teach you. That said, there's a couple things we can mention here…

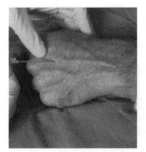

This is pretty good technique. Nice and flat relative to the hand (not coming in straight down). Nice veins! You know you're starting to get into it when you admire strangers' veins at the bank…

Learning to find un-obvious veins is tricky – it comes with practice, so get as much as you can.

9- How do I know if my patient's IV is working properly?

Well… there are certain basics: for one, the catheter is supposed to be <u>in the vein</u>. How can you tell if the catheter <u>is</u> in the vein?

Couple of tricks:

- if you're running the patient's IV fluids through a gravity line, open the roller clamp, unhook the bag from the hook, or the pole, or whatever else it's hanging from, and lower it down below the level of the bed. What should you see backing up in the line?

- Another way to do the same thing without unhooking things: crimp the IV tubing with your fingers. Now with the other hand, squeeze the tubing below the crimp, and release. Get a blood return?

- Third trick – sometimes you just can't get a blood return. This doesn't mean the IV's no good, but it can be hard to tell. Try this: hang your gravity bag up so you can see the drops falling in the drip chamber. Now compress that patient's arm a couple of inches up above where the IV catheter should end. Did the dripping stop? What does that mean? What if it didn't?

Problems

10- How long can peripheral IV's stay in?

Where we work, they're supposed to stay in no longer than three days. If a peripheral site looks ok, and you're stuck for other access, you might not want to pull it even if it's older than it should be. Talk to the team about your patient's access needs.

11- What does "infiltration" mean? An ugly picture that you do need to see…

Sometimes the tip of the catheter pokes its way out of the vein into the surrounding tissue, and what's going through the catheter goes into the tissue spaces instead of the vein where it was supposed to be. If the fluid is something isotonic, like normal saline or D5W, then this is usually not a big deal, and once you recognize the problem and stop the infusion, the fluid is rapidly absorbed by the tissues and the swelling goes away.

What if the fluid has potassium in it? Vancomycin? Dopamine?

The trick of course is to recognize what's happening – which is why checking your peripheral infusion sites is one of the first things you do in your assessment survey.

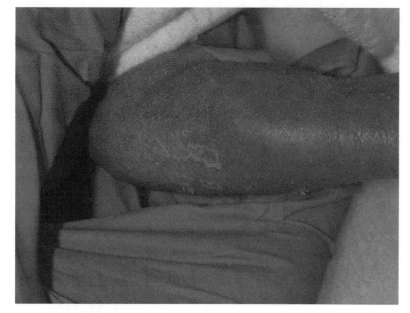

That's a pretty good one. Might've been something with K+ in it...

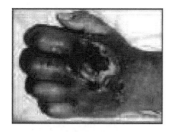

Sorry about this one, but you do need to know – this might've been peripheral dopamine. If a vasoconstrictive drug gets into the tissues... this is why we use central lines for pressor drips.

12- What is phlebitis?

"Inflamed vein.", right? The vein is becoming sore, and unhappy. If you see a red streak tracking upstream from an intravenous site, this is probably your problem. Your patient's problem!

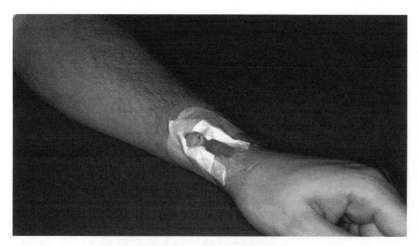

I left this image big, because the phlebitis is hard to see otherwise. Can you see the reddening, heading upwards from the stick site? This IV needs to come out. Soon!

But! What if this is your patient's only IV?

It still needs to come out. Get a new one in as soon as you can, then get this one the heck out.

Can't get another one? Call the IV team. Call the medical team – has the patient run out of veins?

What could you do?

13- What is thrombophlebitis?

This is phlebitis, caused by a clot in the vessel. This is rather worse, and can obstruct flow back from the affected limb.

14- What is phlebothrombosis?

This is the obstruction of a vessel with a clot, but without the inflammation. Ok, who's the wise guy with the big words?

Pumps

15- What are infusion pumps all about?

We use these all the time, and they've almost completely replaced gravity drips for everything.

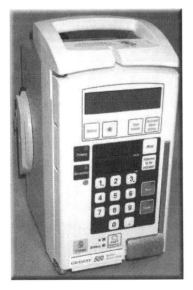

This happens to be the kind we use – we hate them every time we get new ones – then we get used to them... then after a few years we get to hate some newer ones. They'll try to tell you that change is good, but...

Of course, the fluid is pumped towards the patient through whatever kind of tubing comes with the particular pump your institution bought. All of them need part of the tubing to sit inside the pump – this one has three little ball chambers in a row that sit in little openings, and is held in place with little prongs. You learn to use 'em...

If the little pump chambers aren't full, the pump will holler at you – this is technically known in our unit as "having air in the balls".

http://www.qmc.nhs.uk/Divisions/Diagnostics/MESU/images/Graseby%20500%20Infusion%20Pump.jpg

These big pumps are for volume infusions: D5NS with 20 of KCL at 100/hour – stuff like that. We also use them to give antibiotics – most antibiotics like to be given over an hour, and the pumps pretty much guarantee properly timed delivery. I give Vancomycin over two hours – why?

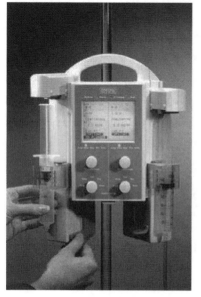

Then there's these guys – syringe pumps? We've used these for a lot of our pressors in recent years, and while we've gotten used to them, there's are a couple of reasons not to like them, which I'm going to try to explain:

A syringe mix of almost anything is – by definition – extremely concentrated. That's fine – lots of patients can't handle a lot of IV fluid – renal failure patients, CHF patients – like that.

But think about it – you may be delivering your drug at one cc per hour. Is that enough to keep the blood vessel open?

Also – if you're using a pressor – how quickly will your patient "see" a change in rate from one to two cc's per hour?

Now hold that thought for a minute while we go on.

http://www.devicelink.com/mpmn/97/05/9705_18b.jpg

16- What does "KVO" mean?

The pump will also holler at you if the line is blocked – is the IV tubing kinked? It's worth remembering that it does take a certain amount of flow to **"keep the vein open"**, so that the blood vessel doesn't clot itself off – lots of opinions about this, as usual, but you really need to keep something running through the line at a rate of at least 10cc per hour to keep things infusing smoothly. This is why we always use flush lines for slow infusions, and for any drug being delivered by syringe pump.

17- What is a flush line?

It's a simple idea – suppose you've got a patient on an insulin drip, and the insulin is mixed one-to-one. One unit of insulin in one cc of diluent – right? If you run that drip by itself, is that enough volume to keep the vein open? Probably not. So - rig a normal saline line with a stopcock manifold at the end, and plug in the insulin at the manifold connector, like this one:

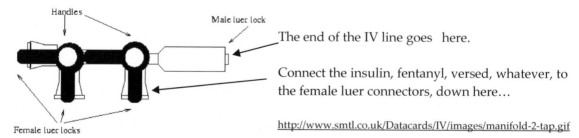

The end of the IV line goes here.

Connect the insulin, fentanyl, versed, whatever, to the female luer connectors, down here…

http://www.smtl.co.uk/Datacards/IV/images/manifold-2-tap.gif

But - why use this fancy stopcock business? Why not just plug the insulin into one of the line ports on the main IV tubing? The "Y" connectors?

Well – you could do that. People do do that. But – suppose you were doing your q2 hour glucose check, and your patient's blood sugar was 52… ok – you stop the insulin. What's the problem?

The problem is that the whole length of IV line from the port downwards – from where the drip was connected – **is still full of the insulin solution**, been driven into the patient by the flush line. Are you going to want to take the whole line down? Nah… just disconnect it from the stopcock, all the way close to the patient. No problem!

18- What is the "primary rate"?

You can set the infusion pumps to deliver fluid at a fixed rate – right? D5NS at 100 hour? And the pump will run until the bag goes dry, or until it reaches the end of the volume you've told it to give – say, 900 of the liter bag you hung. That's your primary rate.

19- "Secondary rate"?

Suppose you want to give a rapid dose of something being pumped – the one that comes to mind is propofol. Say your patient is doing fine on 10 cc of propofol per hour, but now you have to suction him, and you know from experience that he bites his ET tube closed when you do. Bad. What to do? Give him a little squirt of sedative? Probably a good idea. (a "bolus") How we do this?

Our pumps have a secondary rate setup: this means, "Ok pump, what I want you to do is to give the stuff you're pumping at a **different rate, but only for a while**, and then **go back to what you were doing before**". So – in this case – I would set the secondary rate at something fast – say, 500cc per hour, and set the volume for 2cc. This would zip in 20mg of propofol as a bolus dose – the pump would then go back to the regular delivery rate. The patient would relax, the suctioning would go smoothly, no biting, all would be well. Nice trick.

Bear in mind that small – gauge IV's don't like really rapid infusions – 22's and the like will not work well if you set a pump at a really rapid rate – so I usually set my secondary rates at 555 cc/hour or something, instead of 999.

20- How do I figure out where to plug things in to the connectors?\

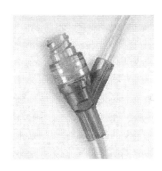

These guys.

a. Above the pump?

Someone wrote in to ask this one – and since there are no dumb questions – we'll answer it here: **are** there any connectors above the pump?

b. Below the pump?

Has to be – they only put the connectors below the pump on the tubing. But would a newbie nurse know that? Well – she ought to. But who know what they're learning in nursing schools now? Alteration in cosmological reality of the human spirit, potential versus actual? I don't care! But they should be teaching them how to run infusion pumps!

Treatments

21- Volume infusions.

We mentioned these before – this is your simple, plain-vanilla volume-over-time infusion of something really simple: normal saline at 80cc per hour. D5W with 20 of K at 100 hour. Stuff like that.

22- Blood products.

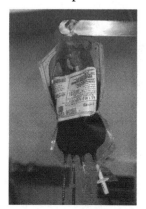

Mostly, we still give blood by gravity – hang it up with a filtered tubing set, open the roller clamp, and time it so it runs in over an hour or two.

http://www.castenholz.org/ptguide/Blood.JPG

23- Types of IV fluids.

These take a bit of learning about, but one thing to understand is the idea of tonicity – some fluids are equal to blood in concentration, some are more, and some are less. Hypertonic: more concentrated. Hypotonic: less. Iso – the same.

The point is that solutes in the body – in the blood and in the cells, are going to respond to whatever IV fluid you give your patient.

Most of the time, your patient who needs hydration is going to want some kind of isotonic IV fluid – something like normal saline – D5W. Maybe with a little KCL…

Thinking about how different IV fluids act on your patient is something that comes with time. It's more complex than it seems, so work with them for a while and see what situations call for what kinds of fluids – then study up some more.

24- What is a rapid bolus?

Sometimes you want to give a whole lot of volume, really quickly. Gravity is still the best way – the pumps will go up to about a liter per hour, but if you really want to give volume at high speed, hang your liter of saline way up on the pole, open the clamp and watch it fly in. You'll need the right kind of access – an 18 gauge in a large vein will do just fine. Central lines are even better – a cordis is the piece of hardware you want in this situation. Take a look at the FAQ on "Central Lines" for lots more on that topic.

Lately with the advent of "guided sepsis therapy", the volume resusciation has gotten a LOT more aggressive: we see the docs running something like 6 to 8 liters of fluid into a septic patient in the first couple of hours… wow!

A word about giving these rapid boluses – sometimes you'll see people do this by squeezing the IV solutions, with one of the white pressure bags that we use to keep A-lines pumped up. This is ok, but it needs to be done the right way:

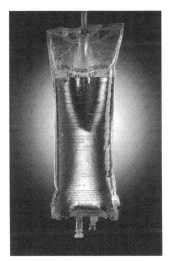

Something incredibly important!

Look at this bag. Hasn't been spiked yet – hmmm… what's that, inside the bag, up at the top?

Ok – now, suppose you put this bag under pressure, to push the IV fluid into the patient?

What happens when the fluid runs out?

What is an air embolism?

How could you avoid one?

http://www.uthscsa.edu/mw/photogallery/Media/biomed/images/IV_BAG.jpg

Simple: before giving a bolus this way – spike the bag upside down. Squeeze the bag with the line clamp open to get all the air out of the bag. Then hang it up, and off you go!

Don't forget this!

25- How much of a bolus should my patient get?

Well – what are you trying to do? Raise her blood pressure? Is she really dry? Or is she oversedated? My point is that your treatment decisions always depend on the context – lots of patients become hypotensive to one degree or another when they're sedated – to you give them a lot of fluid? Or "touch" them with a bit of neo?

You'll gain experience in figuring out whether your patient is "wet", or "dry" – partly it's about the CVP, or the wedge – partly it's about how much pee they make, partly it's about whether or not they're septic and having leaky capillaries, partly it's about how well nourished they are comng in, and what their serum albumin is (why?)… it's about a whole lotsa stuff! Your job as a newbie in the unit is to absorb, osmose, and learn – gain experience – and let it all soak in. Just be aware, at the beginning, that there's more to it than just adding up the Ins and the Outs…

A puzzler for the newbie nurse and her preceptor: your patient has, say, ARDS. He's on the vent, on 100% oxygen, a rate of 26/minute, and 15 of PEEP. His CVP is 10. Why's he only making 10cc of urine an hour?

26- What kind of IV fluid should I use for a bolus?

We usually use normal saline for "volume resuscitation". This works well for a while, but after many liters, patients can develop a hyperchloremic acidosis – it can be pretty severe, too. At this point we usually switch to Ringer's Lactate.

27- Intermittent meds

Yup – as we looked at earlier: most doses of intermittent meds do NOT want to be infused too rapidly – most antibiotics like to go in over an hour. I clearly remember reading an article about an antibiotic error on an otherwise healthy young person: some med, a dose of antibiotic, was pushed, rather than dripped into her – she coded, and died a couple of days later. Anaphylaxis? Hard to know – most people survive anaphylactic events in the hospital – and this was a preop dose, given in the OR! Anyhow – as always – check with your local authorities and references. Slower is better. To a point.

28- Continuous med infusions.

Yup, we run em all the time. Heparin bag mixes, propofol drips, all sorts of continuous bag mix drips that have to be run at fixed doses, every hour. We ancient nurses were sitting around telling stories last weekend: we remember dropping whatever number of cc's it was into a burette EVERY HOUR – usually of heparin – and infusing a controlled volume that way, before infusion pumps became common.

29- Multiple infusions.

Lots of old sayings about "bad signs": "it's never good when a patient's white count is higher than her hematocrit". That's true. Another one is that it's never good when the patient is surrounded by a forest of pumps – more than six – not a very good sign.

It makes for a lot of things to think about, doesn't it? Not least of which is the fact that a lot of these meds may not like each other, may actually form precipitates or crystals in the IV tubing if you try to make them run together.

    a.   Compatibility

An important concept, and one that you have to make sure you check. Will these meds run together in the line, or will they create smoke and flame, or whatever? Not that I've ever seen that, but I have seen lines go crystallized along their length. This is certainly not good for the patient. It almost always means the loss of the catheter as well, which can be pretty tough to deal with in a grossly edematous patient on a zillion drips.

    b.   Incompatibility

What we were saying. We use an online compatibility reference. Make sure – every time.

30- What is a med bolus?

Didn't we talk about propofol up above, a while back? You can use the infusion pumps to give bolus doses over time: heparin comes to mind, propofol... make sure you understand how to set up the pump to do this.

31- What is an IV push med?

Now you're getting into serious territory. The old saying is quite true: once you push a med into a patient, you ain't getting it back! Although how you'd get other meds back isn't quite clear... you really need to remember to take the time, every time, to do all those right things: right drug, right dose, right patient, all that – every... single... time. You just do! And you need to refresh your memory on how fast these drugs can be given – also every single time. Heparin for example: I think it's supposed to be pushed at no more than 1000 units per minute. Digoxin doses are supposed to be given over a couple of minutes. These rules don't exist because some mean unpleasant person decided they wanted to tell other people what to do all day – these rules exist because giving these meds too fast can hurt your patient!

Take the time to think about how fast your patient is going to see this drug. It's hilarious sometimes to see some intern grab an IV line, grab a med, push the drug into a port eight feet away from the patient without clamping the line above the port, stand back, and be amazed when magical things DON'T happen... why is it that doctors develop this idea that they can turn to a nurse and say: "Make such and such happen immediately, nurse!" . This same idea applies to things like IV meds – they'll decide they need to give it – shove it into the line, probably most of it goes back up towards the bag – then stand back with the line not running, and wonder why their treatment hasn't produced a miracle cure.

Then they'll turn to you, and in this patronizing way tell you how much they have to learn from you...

Then they come back in a year and they REALLY want to know what you think...

32- How do I give IV push meds?

Well – there's a way, and you need to know. First, the IV has to be working, right? Not sort of, not maybe, not kind of, not iffy – it's either working, or it ain't. If it ain't – don't use it. If a rotten IV is the only one your patient has, do all the tricks to try to see if there's a blood return. If there isn't, try to impress on the doctor's head the fact that you have no reliable IV access – they hate this kind of thing – reality intruding, as it interrupts their intellectual process. However, it's not your fault if the patient has no veins.

I clearly remember an anesthesiologist who insisted on using the IV that some patient had, which was clearly infiltrated, until I practically tied him up in a corner while I put in a new line. Interrupted his discussion – very annoyed. Sorry, dude.

Let's use the instance of intubation to talk about pushing IV meds – it's something you'll see often enough, and it's a good example of how it needs to be done properly.

Now – what you're going to be giving here are the push meds for the anesthesiologist. Etomidate, maybe – maybe some propofol. Maybe some succinylcholine – I hate that stuff.

What you want to do is to rig a gravity flush line, with maxi drip tubing. Got that? Liter bag of saline, with a drip chamber halfway full, that you can visibly see dripping. All set?

Now – got a good vein? Nice blood return? All hooked up? Get the gravity line running. Now pick a port close to the patient. Plug in the drug syringe. Use an alcohol swab.

Ok? Now – crimp the IV tubing above the injection port with your other hand. This prevents what you're pushing from going backwards, up the IV, towards the bag, instead of towards the patient. If you do it wrong, you'll know right away, because the drip chamber will fill up...

Now push – slowly. Give the etomidate over at least thirty seconds. Propofol the same – ask the anesthesia person how fast, if you're not sure. (No comment…)

Now let go of the crimp in the tubing – let the gravity flow flush the med into the patient.

And there you are! So cool!

Pressors and Vasoactives

Hi all – here's a new update of our first-ever article. As usual, please remember that these articles do not mean to be the final opinion on anything! They are only meant to reflect our own experience and knowledge, which is – scary – getting up to about 50 years combined. **Always check with your own references and authorities!** And when you find mistakes, let us know? Thanks!

1- What is a pressor?
2- What is shock?
3- Are there different kinds of shock?
4- What are the three parts of a blood pressure?
5- What does "pump" mean?
6- What is "inotropy"?
7- What about "volume"?
8- What's "crystalloid"?
9- What is "squeeze"?
10- How does this relate to shock?

   10-1- PA Lines
   10-2- **Something that will make you look really smart!**

11- Which shock state reflects a "pump" problem?
12- What is "ejection fraction"?
13- Which shock state reflects volume?
14- Which shock state reflects arterial squeeze?
15- What measurements do we use at the bedside for treating shock states?
16- How do pressors fit into the treatment of shock states?
17- How do pressors work on receptors?

   17-1 Agonizing receptors

The Quiz!

1- What is a pressor?

"Blood pressure medicines" come in a couple of varieties: there are some that make blood pressure go up, and there are those that make it go down. The word "pressor" is usually used to mean the first kind. Another word that describes these drugs (both kinds) is "vasoactives", which is to say: affecting blood pressure, or heart rate, or both. The major use for pressors is in the treatment of one kind of shock or another.

2- What is shock?

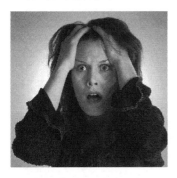

n. (noun)

1. "Something that jars the mind or emotions as if with a violent unexpected blow."

http://www.thefreedictionary.com/shock

2. The realization that you <u>are</u> working in the MICU…

Shock is usually described as a state in which the body's tissues aren't getting enough blood flow for one reason or another. The peripheral tissues – way away from the major vessels, and supplied by smaller vessels whose perfusion suffers when blood pressure drops – lose much of the blood supply that they depend on for oxygen and nutrient delivery. So they switch gears at the cellular level: they change from <u>aerobic</u> respiration, in which they use delivered oxygen to make energy, to <u>anaerobic</u> respiration, which works, but poorly. The byproduct, or "engine emission" of aerobic respiration is carbon dioxide, which we get rid of by breathing. But the emission from anaerobic respiration is unfortunately lactic acid, and since the blood vessels are not carrying wastes away effectively – being underperfused – the lactic acid builds up, creating a metabolic acidosis. The acidosis makes blood pressure even harder to maintain, since most pressors like adrenaline (epinephrine) and norepinephrine (levophed) depend on the blood pH – if the pH is too low, they won't work very well.

3- Are there different kinds of shock?

Yes – three main ones, but to understand them, we need to talk about how exactly a blood pressure is maintained. It turns out that there are three major components of a blood pressure.

4- What are the three components of a blood pressure?

We think of them as: **"pump"**, **"volume"**, and **"squeeze"**. Of course, it's lots more complicated than that, and as always, most of the information in all of these articles is written "with a lot of lies thrown in" – there are shelves of textbooks that have been written on each subject that we try to cover in a few pages. But the point is: how can you organize the ideas in your head to figure things out at the bedside? Quick-and-dirty is what will help most...

Keep in mind as we go along that **each of these components needs to be measured**, and that many of the tools we use in the unit are designed to do just that.

5- What is "pump"?

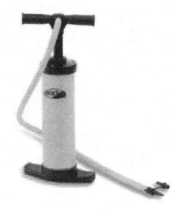

Pump is the heart. Anything interfering with inotropy, heart rate, or cardiac output, be it an MI, an arrhythmia, ischemia – is a pump problem.

How might you measure your patient's ability to pump? Numerically, I mean?

http://www.klangundkleid.ch/img/moebel/sofina/08510_double-stroke-hand-pump.jpg

6- What is "inotropy"?

Inotropy means: "how hard the left ventricle is working to pump, to empty itself".

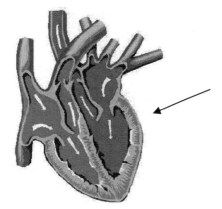

That's this one. Why do we worry about the left ventricle so much, in relation to blood pressure? I mean, we worry about   the RV too – but for sort of different reasons. Take a look at the article on PE's for more about this. (www.icufaqs.org/PulmonaryEmbolism.doc)

Hmm – think we could measure this?

http://www.everyschool.org/u/wcms/tanaka/Heart.jpg

7- What about "volume"?

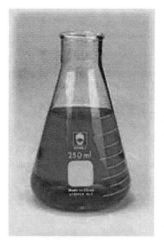

Easy enough: the circulating volume in the blood vessels. You have to include the relative volumes of red cells and plasma to this idea though – there may be plenty of red cells, but if a patient's plasma volume is low – which is to say she's dehydrated, hypovolemic, but not from bleeding – you wouldn't give that person blood, would you? Or the other way around – you wouldn't give just crystalloid to a person with a low crit from bleeding, would you?

8- No. What's crystalloid?

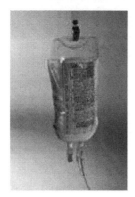

Any "clear-as-crystal" IV fluid is "crystalloid" – it's a word used for a kind of IV volume replacement - as opposed to "colloid", meaning anything protein-based such as albumin of one kind or another, or plasma – but as I understand it, not red cells. Anyhow, right – you would correct volume loss with what the person needed, based on what they needed: red cells, or the '"water" component of the circulating volume.

How might you measure your patient's volume status?

http://www.fluvaccine.com/Stat/images/itemslarge/2U4.jpg

9- What is "squeeze"?

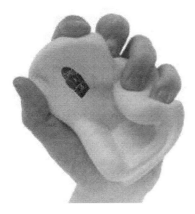

"Squeeze" has actually been used around ICUs for long time to mean two different things – some people use it to describe how tight the arterial bed is - which is to say how tight, or constricted the entire system of arterial vessels is. Other people use "squeeze" to mean inotropy. I use it the first way, because it helps me think about what's happening to the patient – it's a useful concept when you're faced with a hypotensive situation that you're trying to sort out.

We need to measure this too…

http://www.mikkis.co.uk/admin/images/Stressball-Home.jpg

10- How does this relate to shock?

The three components of a blood pressure actually reflect the three kinds of shock that you're likely to see in intensive care. The trick in treating each of these correctly comes from our ability to measure each of the components precisely. Any idea how we might do that?

10-1- The tool you need in this situation is a **PA line** – a pulmonary artery catheter, also knows as a Swan-Ganz line, or just a "Swan".

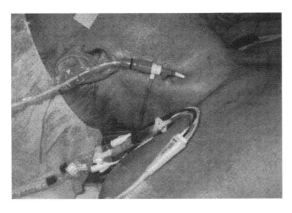

That's the yellow thing, going into the blue thing, there at the patient's ear, sort of? Which is connected to the white thing, going into his neck?

PA lines tell you everything you want to know:

-   how well the **pump** is pumping (**cardiac output, cardiac index**)

-   how full the right side of the heart is (**CVP**), and how full the left side is (**wedge pressure**) – that's the **volume**…

-   and how well your patient's arteries can **squeeze** : that's the **SVR** – the "systemic vascular resistance"…

PA lines are serious juju – they're invasive, they're tricky to place, they need very serious care and feeding – in fact, they've got a whole enormous FAQ all to themselves, and they need one! But understanding how pump, volume and squeeze all go together is important to understanding how pressors work. Go take a look! (www.icufaqs.org/PALinesApril04.doc)

10-2- Something that will make you look really smart.

An alternative – if your patient has no PA, but does have a central line and a radial a-line, you can call the in-house IABP tech to come and do a "green dye" cardiac output. They hook up a little color-measuring thing to the arterial line, and they inject some form of dye - (probably green!) - through the distal port of the CVP. Then they measure how long it takes for the dye to show up at the a-line, multiplied by this, divided by that, aligned with the coefficient of Hammerschmidt, over the square of the patient's shoe size… and out come the numbers. Cool!

11- Which shock state reflects a "pump" problem?

The kind of shock that reflects "pump failure" is **"cardiogenic"** shock, which is to say: "originating in the heart". Simple idea: the blood pressure is low because the pump isn't pumping. This is usually because of a sizable MI, but people with end-stage heart disease of one kind or another, such as cardiomyopathy ("heart-muscle-disease"), or people who have had multiple MI's - leaving them with a very low ejection fraction - can live on the edge of cardiogenic shock much of the time.

12- What is ejection fraction?

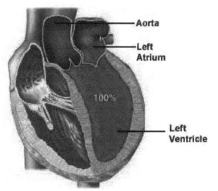

"EF" is the amount of blood ejected from the left ventricle into the arterial circulation with every systolic contraction, expressed as per cent. Normal is something like 50-70%. Impressively low is usually said to be less than 30%, and "cardiac cripples" who can't get up from the chair without shortness of breath sometimes run in the low teens.

Here's the LV at the end of diastole – all full, ready to go.

http://www.heart1.com/images/content/ejection1.jpg

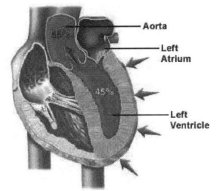

Here's the LV at the end of <u>systole</u> – the LV is contracted. 45% of the blood in the LV is left, so 55% has been ejected into the aorta.

See? That's "pump". So what happens if the pump can't pump?

http://www.heart1.com/images/content/ejection2.jpg

13- Which shock state reflects volume?

"Hypovolemic" shock reflects low volume – and again, the fix depends on which component of circulating volume the patient has lost. You probably wouldn't give red cells to a patient with heat stroke, whose crit might be up around 60%. And you would try not to give crystalloid to a person with a big blood loss. Would you give this patient a pressor?

14- Which shock state reflects arterial squeeze?

"Septic" shock reflects "squeeze". (Cardiogenic shock affects squeeze too, but we get into that in the FAQ articles on PA lines and balloon pumping (www.icufaqs.org/IABPFAQ.doc) – take a look at those for more than you ever wanted to know on the subject!)

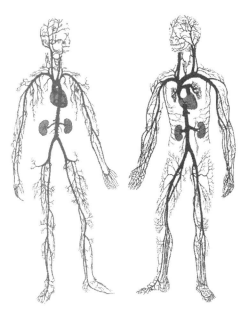

It turns out that the arteries are contractile – they can be made to open up ("dilate"), or tighten up ("constrict"). The whole system of arterial vessels is sometimes called the "arterial bed" – and it helps to think of the whole bed, the whole system, loosening or tightening up in response to various states.

In septic shock, the germs floating about in the systemic circulation produce a set of unpleasant chemicals called endotoxins. These specifically affect the arterial vessels , loosening them up, causing the blood pressure to drop. An analogy would be a garden hose turned on full – if you squeeze the hose, the pressure rises, and the water squirts across the yard. If you release the squeeze, the water pressure drops, and the water runs all over your shoes. Similarly, if the arterial system as a whole tightens up, the patient's blood pressure rises, and if the system loosens up, the pressure falls – which is the cause of hypotension in septic shock.

http://www.eurobloodsubstitutes.com/images/heartCircul_arteries.gif

So the trick in diagnosing hypotension is to figure out: which of the three components is the problem? There's lots more on this subject in the PA-line FAQ.

15- What measurements do we use at the bedside in the ICU for treating shock states?

Well, we start with blood pressure, but you probably knew that part. Use the tools at hand. A blood pressure cuff is a good start. A seriously hypotensive patient, on pressor drips, really ought to have an arterial line. www.Icufaqs.org/ArterialLines.doc

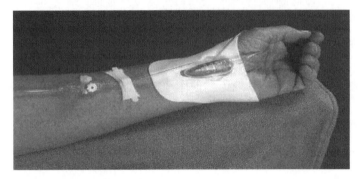

The same catheter as an IV, usually a 20 gauge angiocath, inch and a quarter, in the radial artery, hooked up to a transducer.

http://www.zefon.com/medical/aline.htm

A "labile" blood pressure – an unstable one – needs constant monitoring, because... well, because it's unstable! The need for pressor titration (dialling the dose up or down) is ongoing – you want to wean these drips down whenever you can, while still keeping the blood pressure in the range your patient needs. An actively septic patient, or a cardiogenic one, can require pressor titration every few minutes! You didn't think you were going to get to sit down in the ICU, did you? (grin!) If you don't have an a-line – use the non-invasive BP cuff, and set it to cycle frequently. How frequently? What if the patient is coagulopathic? What is coagulopathic? What if she has a low platelet count? What is a low platelet count – less than what?

Then there are the central line numbers: CVP, wedge pressure, and the ones we get from "shooting numbers": cardiac output/ index (CO/CI), stroke volume (SV), and systemic vascular resistance (SVR). Each of these measurements corresponds to one or the other of the three parts of the blood pressure, and each kind of shock has a characteristic "appearance" that is often immediately obvious once you shoot your first set of numbers after a PA line goes in.

16- How do pressors fit into the treatment of shock states?

The choice of pressor depends on the nature of the problem. To explain this, a quick review of adrenergic receptors will help. There are three adrenergic receptor sets that we worry about in the ICU: the **a**lpha receptors which are located in the **a**rteries, and the two kinds of beta receptors: beta-1's (you have one heart, that's where they are), and beta-2's, (you have two lungs, that's where those are.)

17- How do pressors work on receptors?

This is really helpful to understand:

17-1- To **agonize** set of receptors means to **stimulate** them, to make them "do their thing". If you agonize the <u>a</u>lpha receptors in the <u>a</u>rteries (a little repetition never hurts), then the arteries **tighten up.**

17-2- To **block**, or **antagonize** those receptors means to "stop them from doing their thing." If you antagonize the alphas, then the arteries **loosen up**. (This is how some antihypertensives work: doxazosin/ Cardura, terazosin/ Hytrin, prazosin/ Minipress. Hydralazine too, maybe?)

17-3- You might remember that the **number** we use to measure how tight or loose the arterial system is as a whole is the **SVR** – the "systemic vascular resistance" - the normal range is something like 800-1100. The thing to remember is: **higher is tighter, lower is looser**. So to take the example of sepsis, the basic problem producing the hypotensive, acidotic state is that the arterial system has been made to dilate by the action of bacterial poisons floating about in the bloodstream. Low SVR. To counter that dilation, we use (usually) a pure alpha-agonist pressor: **neosynephrine** (phenylephrine). "Neo" agonizes the alphas, and makes the arteries tighten up again. So the SVR, which might be as low as 200-300, should rise as the arteries constrict. In sepsis, the pump isn't the problem, it's the "squeeze" that's not right.

The volume component becomes a problem too in sepsis, since as the arteries dilate, the volume in them is suddenly not enough to keep them filled up – so the CVP and wedge pressure are low. People describe this by saying "the tank is dry" – the "tank" being the capacity of the arterial system, which has just been increased dramatically by dilation. The heart tries to compensate for the loss of arterial "squeeze" and volume by pumping both harder and faster, so the classic appearance of the numbers is: high cardiac output and index, low SVR, and high heart rate.

The strategy against sepsis is simple:

- fill the tank: hydrate the patient to increase her circulating volume,

- squeeze the tank: apply an alpha pressor to tighten up her arteries.

- kill the bugs: find the source, and give her the appropriate antibiotics.

Nowadays there's been a big move to act more aggressively when sepsis rears it's ugly head, and there are a number of rules for treating it in the early stages, based on a whole lot of review work done by some eminent docs led by R. Phillip Dellinger. In my ICU, these translate into a set of specific steps that elaborate on the three rules I made up myself (grin!), and involve <u>rapid</u> hydration – something like 8-10 liters over the first six hours (whoa!); measurement of CVP and central venous oxygen saturation with specs drawn from the distal central catheter port, careful application of pressors to achieve MAP goals and preserve organ perfusion, tight control of blood sugar levels – stuff like that. Good stuff!

Levophed is often used interchangeably with neo, but has broader effects on both sets of receptors, which sometimes produces problems: for example, a patient in sepsis will already be reflexively tachycardic. Sometimes levo can aggravate the tachycardia , sometimes disastrously, producing unpleasant things like rapid AF, or even nasty ventricular arrhythmias – think of using neo in this situation.

18- How do you treat other shock states?

The other two states that we see are hypovolemic and cardiogenic shock. Hypovolemia is treated by "fluid resuscitation" with the appropriate component of volume that the patient needs: red cells (along with stopping the blood loss), or crystalloid for dehydration. In hypovolemia, you see a similar picture to sepsis in that the heart rate rises to compensate for loss of circulating volume, and the central pressures: CVP and wedge will be low, but the SVR will actually <u>rise</u> very high – maybe up towards 2000, because the arteries will tighten up to try to maintain blood pressure. These folks make lactic acid out in the peripheral tissues not because their arteries are too loose, but because they're too tight, and the little arterioles can't get their supply – they're shut out of the circulation, out there at the toes and fingers and the like. These people have cold, sometimes dusky hands and feet.

19- Do you use pressors to treat hypovolemic shock?

Not if you can avoid it. If blood pressure doesn't recover with the right kind of fluid treatment, then something else is probably going on. If you apply an alpha-agonist pressor to an "empty tank", you'll tighten the arterial system to the point where the patient may lose their fingers or toes to necrosis. If you apply a beta-agonist pressor to increase the heart rate – well, their heart rate is already up, isn't it? A patient with this kind of "reflex" tachycardia can be pushed from sinus tach into something like rapid AF or even VT by using a beta agonist pressor – this is why levophed sometimes doesn't work in septic situations the way you want it to. Lately there's been a move to **dobutamine** (pure beta agonist) in septic situations, and while it may make scientific sense, it seems like a dicey move to me, for the same reasons, so be careful.

Dopamine has similar effects – it's "chronotropic" – that is, it raises heart rate, even at low doses, and because it's often the only pressor available for peripheral use, it is used in situations where it probably shouldn't be – although in a code, or near-code, you do what you have to do to save a life. If there's no option but to run a vasoconstrictive pressor through a peripheral vein while the team is getting, say, a femoral line placed – well, that's what you have to do. Change over quickly – the patient could lose an arm if the drug infiltrates!

An important point:

- **Regitine/phentolamine**. This is worth knowing about – if your patient manages to develop an infiltration of a pressor, probably through a peripheral vein, what's going to happen to the tissues at the site? Why?

  Regitine is the drug for this situation: it's an alpha-blocker. What the docs will do is draw it up in a syringe, and with a subcutaneous injection needle, they'll infiltrate this stuff into the tissues around the IV site, hopefully reversing the alpha effect of the pressor. Apparently it works – I've only seen it done once or twice, but you might save someone's arm this way…

Another important point, and a specific caution about central lines should go here. A femoral central line placed emergently for giving pressors is a good thing – it's the right thing to do – but **you** need to make sure that it's in the right place. You're using the line, it's your responsibility.

Once the patient gets to you, wherever that line is: **transduce it**. You'll immediately get lots of arguments about whether or not the number is "real", and all this, but that's not the point. You're trying to make sure that you're not sending pressors <u>downstream</u>, towards the leg, right? What would happen in that case? What if the line wasn't in a vessel at all – maybe in the peritoneal cavity? What then?

So – transduce the line. If it's arterial – you'll know! If it's venous, you'll know that too. Who cares if the number is correct – as long as there's a CVP waveform of some kind, and the mean pressure is about, say, 12, and not 60 – you're probably ok. So – what does a CVP waveform look like?

Phenylephrine (neo) can be given peripherally in a dilute mix of 10mg in 250cc, but should only be used temporarily while the patient is waiting to have a central line inserted. Try to use a big vein. We got a patient last week with a "peripheral" mix of levophed running: 4mg/ 250cc bag… I dunno about that one. They tried to tell me it was allowed – I have to ask about that.

20- What about cardiogenic shock?

Cardiogenic shock is produced by "pump failure" – usually from a big MI. In this case, the set of adrenergic receptors to work on are the beta-1s, and the pressor to apply in this situation is **dobutamine** – a "pure" beta pressor. (Assuming you want to use a pressor at all. You don't want to "whip" an already failing left ventricle if you don't need to – you use an intra-aortic balloon pump – but that's another FAQ.)

You have 1 heart – that's where the beta-1s are. The "numbers" for cardiac output, central pressures and the SVR form a pattern that is just as "classic" and recognizable to the experienced ICU person as the ones for sepsis: in this case, cardiac output is <u>low</u> (because the problem is with the "pump"), and the wedge pressure will probably be high, since the left ventricle can't empty itself, and the pressure backs up.

(If the pressure continues to back up, the rising pressures will reflect back to the lungs, forcing "water" out of the capillaries into the alveolar spaces – "congestive heart failure" – this is why cardiogenic patients are almost always intubated.)

The SVR will be <u>high</u> - as in hypovolemia, the only reflex the body has available to try to keep up the blood pressure is by tightening the arterial bed. (You'll notice that this is the "mirror" reflex of the one the body uses in sepsis – tachycardia/ increased inotropy. There are only the two reflexes the body has available to use in these situations. Well – that's a big lie. But you get the idea.)

Agonizing the beta-1s increases both heart rate and inotropy, which increases cardiac output and, hopefully, blood pressure. Be careful! Beta-1s can often be stimulated by beta -agonist drugs used for other reasons: the classic one is **albuterol** – supposedly only a beta-2 agonist. Beta-<u>2</u> receptors are in the lungs (you have <u>two</u> lungs): when you agonize them, the bronchi dilate. But these drugs aren't all that specific: albuterol can kick the heart rate up as well as opening up bronchi. Increased heart rate in cardiogenic shock = badness.

The opposite case is also true: giving a beta <u>antagonist</u>, or beta -"blocker", like **Inderal**, can have a bad effect on the beta receptors in the lungs – producing broncho-constriction (asthma attack!). **Lopressor** is supposedly "beta-1 specific", and hopefully leaves the lungs alone. Just something to think about. Might want to switch to verapamil.

21- What other pressors are there?

We talked a little about dopamine above. Dopamine effects come in three flavors, related to the dosage being given: low, medium, and high. At low doses, say 150-300 mcg/minute, dopamine is thought to affect "dopaminergic" receptors, which in turn is supposed to increase blood supply to the kidneys : this is what they mean by "renal-dose-dopa". Does it work? People argue about this one all time in very learned fashion, but it seems to work enough of the time that we still do it occasionally.

At middle ranges: 300-600 mcg/minute – dopamine has beta effects – it increases heart rate and inotropy. There's lots of overlap in these ranges, and many is the patient started on "renal dose" dopamine whose heart rate pops up to 150 – time to shut it off! Again, this is probably <u>not</u> the pressor to use in a septic situation, because the heart rate is already too high, right? So applying a beta-agonist pressor may push the septic patient with sinus tach at 150, into rapid a-fib at 200, or even VT. At high ranges: 600-1000 mcg/ minute using the ancient method of the "straight-drip" technique (as opposed to the mcg/ kg/ minute technique that everybody else in the universe uses), dopamine finally has some alpha effect. But do you want to push a tachycardic patient all the way through the beta range, to finally get to the alpha range to get their blood pressure up? Negative! Use neo.

Another couple of pressors, more rarely used: **epinephrine**, which is a "kitchen-sink, kick-everything" pressor, hardly used except in codes and as a last-ditch in hypotension that's not responding to anything; **isoproterenol** – (Isuprel, or just "Prel") – a very powerful beta-agonist, <u>really</u> rarely used, only as a bridge to try to keep heart rate up in situations where atropine doesn't work – the drill used to be: A-I-P for symptomatic bradycardia: atropine, isuprel, pacing wire. Nowadays we use the Zoll pads.

22- What basic considerations do I need to keep in mind about using these drugs?

A few words about using vasoactives in general: try to think about how the drug is being delivered to the patient: is anything (besides you) speeding up or slowing down the flow? Sometimes big changes in blood pressures can mean that somebody gave, say, an antibiotic through a line carrying levophed. **Big mistake**. This would initially cause a dramatic rise in BP, followed by many inches of IV tubing carrying no pressor at all (and if the flush is running at 5cchr, it may take two hours for the pressor to fill the line back to the patient!)

22-1- Setting up the drips:

Precise, consistent delivery is your goal. Here's what to do:

Hang a bag of normal saline, with tubing, **on an infusion pump**, (not a gravity line!), set at a **fixed rate**. This is your **flush line**. Choose a rate that is going to deliver the vasoactive fairly quickly – not 10cc/ hour! You can turn it down later, but if your patient's blood pressure is squat, you want to deliver the pressor fairly quickly. This does **not** meaning bolusing the patient with pressor – it means getting the **column** of the drug delivered to the patient quickly.

Now the question is – where to plug the pressor into the flush.

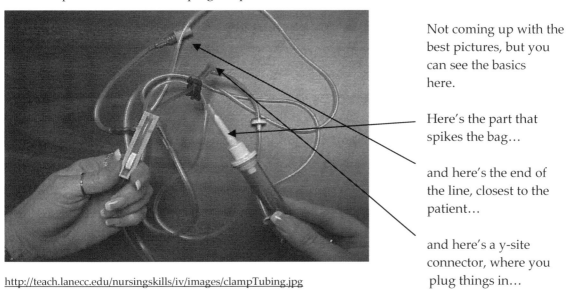

Not coming up with the best pictures, but you can see the basics here.

Here's the part that spikes the bag…

and here's the end of the line, closest to the patient…

and here's a y-site connector, where you plug things in…

http://teach.lanecc.edu/nursingskills/iv/images/clampTubing.jpg

So the question is – where do you want to plug in your pressor? And why does it matter?

Well – the whole point is that you want your patient to see this drug pretty soon! If you're using the little syringe pressor mixes, they run at rates of what – a cc? Per hour? Vasopressin runs at 2.4 cc per hour. If your flush line is running at 10cc/ hour, and the tube holds, say 30cc, and you plug the vasopressin into a y-connector halfway up the line… it might be hours before the patient sees the drug!

You don't want to hook up the syringe directly to the infusion port either – a drip running at 2.4 cc/ hour isn't enough to keep the lumen from clotting off – that's what the flush is for.

So okay – you don't want to use the y-connector… what to do?

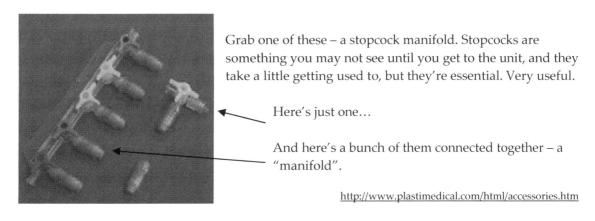

Grab one of these – a stopcock manifold. Stopcocks are something you may not see until you get to the unit, and they take a little getting used to, but they're essential. Very useful.

Here's just one…

And here's a bunch of them connected together – a "manifold".

http://www.plastimedical.com/html/accessories.htm

Screw the manifold onto the end of the flush line tubing, and the other end onto the infusion port of the patient's central line. Now screw the luer connector of the pressor into one of the manifold connections. This is easier to do than it is to describe…

Now your pressor is connected as close as possible to the patient, and being "driven" by the flush line. This means your patient will see the drug soon.
I try to use flush lines running at a fixed 100cc/hr when possible – this means that the pressor is never going to take very long to reach the patient down the line. Whenever possible, run (compatible!) vasoactives at constant rates, **and with a line all to themselves**. Try not to change the rate of a flush attached to a pressor line rapidly – move in small increments, and try to be patient.

Never (really never!) bolus patients with pressor during hypotensive episodes. These are the big gorillas of the drug world, and you can kill your patient with them! Make sure the drug is actually reaching the patient at a controlled rate, and make small changes. Be patient! Anticipate big changes when increasing pressor rates, and be ready to dial down rapidly when you first see the change you're looking for.

Also – **don't** get into the habit of turning the flush rate way up briefly if your patient goes hypotensive. Turn it up a little! It can be very hard to be patient, with the team breathing down your neck… remember that if you do give a bit of fluid through that line, that **you've washed all the pressor out of it**, and you're going to have to wait all over again for it to work, which means the patient will get hypotensive again…

22-2- Drug Rates:

Let's talk briefly about rates. In almost every hospital in the universe, vasoactive drugs are delivered based on the patient's weight, measured in kilos, over time. So the dosage is measured in micrograms per kilo, per minute. This standardizes the dosage number from one patient to the next, no matter how big or small they are, which makes thinking about it relatively easy. An example is dopamine: low medium and high range effects are supposed to roughly correlate with sections of the range, from 1 to 10 mcg/kg/minute. Maybe up to 12.

We do it a bit differently – we run "straight drips", which just means setting the pump to deliver, say, 200 mikes of dopamine/minute. It's easy, and in practice, you're titrating the drug for effect, right? So it doesn't really matter what dose technique you use, **as long as you stay in the ranges in your policies. Check them frequently!**

Here's a quick example of how it doesn't matter: lady came in, bad heart, low EF, PA line, the docs want to try one drug, then another, to see if they can tweak her cardiac output. Actually, she was lying there in the bed on 2 liters of oxygen, quite comfy, good blood pressure, mentating, but she'd recently developed acute renal failure, and the docs are all a twitter to technologize her and optimize her, and this, and that… the older nurses are looking at each other: "She looks fine! Why don't they just leave her alone?"

So anyhow, they float in a PA line. Poor lady. Now we start shooting numbers, and they ask me to start dobutamine – I think they were hoping for a little inotropy, a little afterload effect if possible, a little this, a little that… so the intern calculates her weight, which is pretty impressive, and then calculates the straight drip rate, and turns to me, and says: "Ok, so go ahead and start her on 300 mikes per minute."

No way, man. I am an old, beat-up, battle-weary ICU nurse, and I've seen many and many a bad thing happen over the years… even low doses of dobutamine can produce an impressive tachycardia – not a good thing for a hurting heart. So I mention this in a friendly way, and, what with the grey hair and all, I convince him that I'm going to start at 100mcg instead. He has this look: "Ok, I'll indulge the old nurse. Poor old guy."

An hour later the lady's heart rate has gone from 74 to 118. She's not getting sweaty or having chest pain… yet… I go and grab intern boy. We change to a different drug.

See the point? Sure, she was way below the calculated dose range expected for her size. But: **responses to these drugs are extremely variable**. She hadn't read the intern's textbook.

23- Are there other vasoactives I need to know about?

We haven't talked much about the other kind of vasoactives: the ones that make blood pressure go down instead of up. These come in a couple of flavors:

- Receptor **antagonists**: The opposite of an adrenergic pressor. I don't think there's a pure alpha antagonist blocker drip that I can think of, although remember regitine? The alpha blocker? Only used for infiltrations…

  You will see **labetolol** – this is a cool idea: it's **both** an alpha and a beta blocker – so it loosens a tight arterial bed when your patient is hypertensive, and slows his heart rate as well. Nice!

  Otherwise, you'll see beta-blocker drips sometimes for heart rate control: propranolol sometimes, sometimes esmolol – stinky drug, works poorly. (Did I really say that?), and sometimes calcium-channel blocker drips: diltiazem mostly I think. Works much better than esmolol, as far as I can tell.

- A drug sort of in a class of it's own which does about fourteen nice things at once for the heart is **Amiodarone**. Neat drug – it has complex effects, including beta blockade, and the ability to sometimes chemically convert people out of a-fib. Or v-fib! Very cool!

- **Nitroglycerine** (TNG) is used for controlling anginal symptoms and for acute blood pressure control (it doesn't seem to work very effectively for this in most people) – it works by dilating both arteries and veins, decreasing SVR (afterload) and preload, by increasing the venous capacity. Less volume arrives at the LV because the venous tank is bigger, and it's easier to pump it out, because the arterial tank is bigger - looser.

- **Nipride** (nitroprusside) is the third antihypertensive that we use. This is the Big Gorilla in the antihypertensive zoo. **Be extremely cautious with this drug** – it is very powerful. (Some people call a nipride bag wrapped in foil the "silver bullet".) It must **always** have a separate, dedicated IV lumen all to itself, and **nothing must ever be run through that line** – it **will** bottom out your patient's pressure.

The bad thing about nipride is that it works so rapidly – you have to move very carefully when titrating up on the dose.

The good thing though about nipride is also that it works so rapidly – it has a very short half-life, and within seconds after you stop the infusion, its effects (should!) go away. Nipride can produce a really poisonous cyanide metabolite called thiocyanate – usually this gets measured at least daily while a patient is on this drug. Worse in renal failure.

24- How do we use vasopressin?

Vasopressin, which is also ADH? Anti-diuretic hormone?, is used in several situations in the MICU, but mostly, lately, for sepsis. The confusing thing is that the ranges are very different.

- For GI bleeding, the range is <u>0.1 to 0.4</u> units/minute. Nowadays we've mostly gone to octreotide for this situation, but it's worth mentioning.

- For use as a pressor in sepsis, the dose is <u>0.04</u> units/ minute. Sometimes we wean it to 0.02, but mostly we just shut it off when the patient's pressure recovers.

The theory as I understand it (not very well), is that in sepsis the body gets into a vasopressin-deficient state, which contributes to the systemic arterial vasodilation. I have to say that I've really been surprised at how effective this stuff is – actually the really impressive part for me was how SVR recovers with this drug. It's a weird but true fact that applying "regular" pressors to a septic patient with a PA line... well, the BP comes up, for sure, but the SVR often stays low – really low, in the 300's, maybe. I have no clue why – you'd think it would rise as the pressure did. Not until vasopressin came along did the numbers actually start to reflect what you'd expect.

The other significant thing about vasopressin is that you'll see your patient's heart rate drop, sometimes down from say, the 130s, to around 60 or 70. It may take a day or longer for the heart-rate effect to show up, but blood pressure usually responds within an hour or so in my experience. This can make your team nervous – we've seen some patients on vasopressing get into bradycardias in the 40's, with serial EKGs, troponins, much head-scratching... remind the team that it may be the drip. They'll look at you as though you're mad, until the attending comes in and agrees with you. Then they'll look at you as though you're magic, which is just as bad...

Vasopressin has also showed up in code situations, which was new to me – at the last code I went to, I found myself pushing a vasopressin dose, which made me a little nervous...

We also give a drug called DDAVP/ desmopressin, which is a synthetic version of ADH, sometimes for uremic bleeding, and sometimes – rarely – for people who don't make their own ADH. "Diabetes insipidus". Remember that "diabetes" means "siphon" – water goes in, and comes out almost at the same speed! We had a young man a year ago who was pan-hypo-pituitary, after a brain tumor was removed. Didn't make any ADH. So if he missed his DDAVP pill (used to be nasal spray, now I guess there's a pill), it was like Niagara Falls in his room until we could get it into him! So it's good to know that there's an endocrine aspect to hemodynamic management too, although you don't see it too often.

25- Why don't we use the Trendelenburg position for hypotension any more?

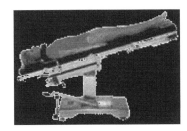

Ok – which one is this?

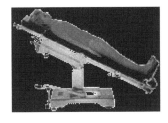

And this?
http://www.denyers.com.au/versatility.html

This one was hard for an old nurse to get used to – after doing it for something like 20 years, another piece of "basic knowledge" gets chucked out… they say that putting patient in T-berg makes blood flow north in the patient, increasing the intravascular pressure on the carotid bodies, making them think that things are better than they are. Remember that these are the guys who live in the aortic arch, looking downwards toward the heart. If the amount of volume coming out of the LV suddenly drops, they get on the line to the adrenals saying: "Yo! Secrete some epi!" So if you put the patient in Trendelenburg, they see this as more "volume" (which it isn't, really), and it just defeats your whole purpose. Plus it makes it hard for the patient to breathe. Jayne says that the best thing to do is to: "Lie 'em flat, and put their feet up on two pillows, which will improve the blood pressure some because it improves the venous return." Sounds good to me. But I have yet to see a patient lose blood pressure in T-berg…

What I have seen is reflex bradycardia when patients are inadvertently bolused with some powerful pressor. Typically someone gets impatient with waiting for a pressor change to take effect, and dials up too rapidly. The patient will suddenly respond with a blood pressure that may rise from, say, 70 up to 240 systolic – this does indeed produce a reflexive bradycardia, which is the carotid bodies doing the <u>other</u> thing, yelling "Whoa!" down the phone line.

<u>Don't</u> give this patient atropine! Just dial them right back down again, or even shut off the pressor/flush flow altogether for a short time, then **carefully** re-titrate. You have to be a little patient with pressor changes… be alert to this situation in the ICU. A patient with a sudden drop in heart rate, and a sudden spike in blood pressure… on the bedpan? Or did someone get hasty with the Levophed?

26- Here's a little chart thing for those who like them:

Condition	CVP/PCW	CO/CI	SVR	SV	Pressor to Use?	Receptor to Treat
Normals:	8-10/ 10-12	4-6/ 2-3	1000	80+/-	Coffee!	Caffeine!
Sepsis:	↓ ↓	↑ ↑	↓	↑	Neo, Levo, Vaso	Alphas
Cardiogenic:	+/- ↑	↓ ↓	↑	↓	Dobutamine?	Beta-1s → IABP?
Hypovolemia:	↓ ↓	↓ ↓	↑	↓	Fluid or blood only?	

The Quiz!:

Ready for the quiz? No answer key! Any and all of the answer choices may be relevant! Discuss, compare and contrast!

1- Pressors are:

   a- drugs that press on things
   b- pills that raise blood pressure
   c- pills that lower blood pressure
   d- very precisely titrated intravenous drips, which work on specifically targeted adrenergic receptors, and which are carefully chosen depending on the situation of the patient
   e- I give up!

2- Vasoactives are:

   a- drugs that act on vaso things
   b- different kinds of Vaso-line
   c- the name for pretty much any kind of drug infusion that affects heart rate, peripheral arterial or venous constriction, dilatation, and therefore blood pressure, along with the size of the pupils
   d- I lied about the pupils

3- Shock is:

   a- how you feel when you come to work in the MICU
   b- when your patient has low blood pressure
   c- when she has high blood pressure?
   d- Low blood pressure, for any of three main reasons, causing peripheral lactic acidosis, and a lawnmower
   e- B and d, except for the lawnmower

4- The three parts of a blood pressure are:

    a- pump, crackle, and pop
    b- snap, squeeze, and Dopey
    c- squeeze, pump, and volume
    d- Huey, Looey, and Sneezey

5- Cardiogenic shock results from:

    a- pulmonary failure
    b- a big MI
    c- a low EF
    d- a high EF?
    e- B and C

6- Volume is measured with:

    a- a CVP line
    b- an arterial line
    c- a foley catheter
    d- a blood pressure cuff
    e- feeling the inside of your patient's mouth for moisture
    f- all of the above

7- Pressors are for:

    a- all shock states
    b- some shock states
    c- Only states where they're allowed by law
    d- Certain shock states, depending on what the cause is

8- How many adrenergic receptors do we mainly think about?

    a- One
    b- Two
    c- Three
    d- Eighteen

9- Pump is measured, numerically, using:

    a- cardiac output
    b- cardiac index
    c- pulmonary output
    d- pulmonary index

10- Squeeze is measured with:

    a- a girdle
    b- a PA line

c- a green dye output
d- SVR
e- PVR

11- To agonize a receptor means:

a- To really hurt!
b- Just to make it a bit nervous
c- To – generally – increase the "tone" and activity of the organ that it's attached to

12- To antagonize a receptor is to:

a- make it angry
b- to – generally – decrease the activity of the organ it's attached to

13- The pure alpha pressor that we use is:

a- levophed
b- nipride
c- phenylephrine
d- dopamine
e- colace

14- The pure beta pressor that we use is:

a- dopamine
b- dobutamine
c- milrinone
d- amrinone
e- saxamophone

15- Vasopressin is:

a- run at a rate of 0.4 units per minute
b- run at a rate of 0.04 units per minute
c- run at a rate of 4.04 units per minute
d- run at a rate of 44 units per minute

16- An infiltrated peripheral pressor:

a- is no big deal, nothing to worry about
b- might be a big deal, but nothing to worry about
c- **an incredibly big deal, that you really have to worry about, that you should do your utmost to prevent, that could cause the loss of the patients' limb, and which should be immediately reported to the physicians, assessed, and possibly treated with a regitine infiltration**
d- what's an infiltration?

True or False:

17- **All central lines, regardless of where they are placed**, should be transduced as soon as possible, to make sure they're in the right vessel.

18- All central lines should be transduced as soon as possible, to make sure they're in the left vessel.

19- I can run my pressor drips through a gravity flush line.

20- I can run bag mixes of pressors on a gravity line.

21- I can run Nipride on a gravity line. (Shudder…)

PE's

As usual, please remember that these articles are not meant to be the final word on anything – instead, they're supposed to represent the kind of information passed on by a preceptor to a new ICU nurse. When (not if) you find mistakes, let us know, and we'll fix them right away. In the meantime, make sure to check with your own references at all times!

We decided to have some fun with images this time around – if this makes the file a little tricky to handle, let us know, and we'll take them out.

1- What is an embolus?
2- What is an embolism?
3- What is a pulmonary embolism?
4- What are the bad things that result physiology-wise from a PE?
5- What are the two relevant concepts of badness (COBs) involved in problems with the lungs?
6- What is the confusing thing about the two COBs?
7- So then which one is the problem that happens after a PE?
8- What other bad things happen to people with PEs?
9- What is a DVT?
10- Why do people get DVTs?
11- Is it really true that you can get DVTs and PEs if you sit too long on the plane?
12- What does smoking have to do with it?
13- What does taking birth control pills have to do with it?
14- What if the patient has a cast on?

Preventing PEs

15- Can DVTs be prevented?
16- What are air boots all about?
17- What about compression stockings?
18- What is SQ heparin all about?
19- Should my patient get sq heparin if she also has air boots on?
20- Should my patient get air boots if she is already getting sq heparin?
21- Can sq heparin be bad?
22- Can air boots be bad?
23- Can putting someone on a heparin drip be bad?
24- Can a patient develop a DVT anywhere besides a leg?
25- Can air boots prevent DVTs that happen, say, in my patient's arm?
26- Does it have to be two air boots?
27- What about those little air boots that just squeeze the feet?

Detecting DVTs

28- How do I know if my patient has a DVT?
29- What is Homan's sign?
30- What is a venogram?
31- What are LENIs?
32- Should my patient have LENIs before getting air boots applied?
33- What does d-dimer have to do with it?
34- How do I know if my patient has a PE?
35- Can you see a PE on a chest x-ray?
36- What is a VQ scan?
37- What is a pulmonary angiogram?

Kinds of PEs

38- Are there different kinds of PEs?
39- What is a saddle embolus?
40- Are there different kinds of emboluses?

Treating PEs

41- How are PEs treated?
42- How long does a patient have to stay on heparin for a PE to dissolve?
43- What does TPA have to do with it?
44- How is a big PE or a saddle embolus treated?
45- What is clot lysis all about?
46- What does coumadin have to do with it?
47- What are IVC filters all about?

Other Kinds of Embolisms

48- What is an air embolus?
49- What does a patient with an air embolus look like?
50- An incredibly important point involving rapid IV boluses.
51- What should I do if I think my patient has just pulled in an air embolus?
52- What is a fat embolus?
53- What is an amniotic fluid embolus?

Embolisms

1- What is an embolus?

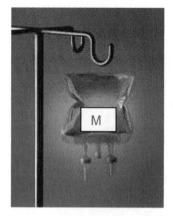

Um, it looks like your patient is about to get an Mbolus!

2- What is an embolism?

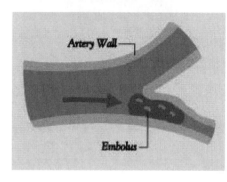

You just don't want to have things floating along in the bloodstream that aren't supposed to be there. Just not a nice thing – clots are the one you always think of, but anything that hangs together and moves along will do it: a big air bubble maybe, or a hunk of fat, or maybe a big blob of amniotic fluid, moving along the vessel... anything capable of holding its shape and plugging up the vessel, whether on the right side or the left. Meaning, on the venous side, or the... what?

http://www.stanford.edu/group/neurology/stroke/images/embolic.jpeg

3- What is a pulmonary embolism?

Clots, usually, and most often from the big veins in the upper legs. These guys break loose, float downstream through the venous system and end up making their way through the right side of the heart to - where?

Apparently nasty PE events coming from the calves are much less frequent. Emboli can also develop in the arms, and around central line catheters.

Question for the group: suppose your patient came in with a black big toe from an embolus. Where would that one have come from?

4- What are the bad things that result physiology- wise from a PE?

Couple of things:

- There's a loss of blood flow through part of the lung. Blood stops flowing through whatever part of the lung is normally perfused by the vessel that gets plugged by the embolus. This can produce a pulmonary infarct. If the PE is big enough, blood flow through the lungs will be obstructed so much that relatively little will make it through to the left side of the heart, producing what amounts to hypovolemic hypotension.

- There's a loss of some gas-exchange in the affected part of the lung, because the little capillaries in the alveoli aren't being perfused. The air goes in and out just fine, but the capillaries aren't working.

- So the air going in and out doesn't match up with the blood flow that's supposed to be there to meet it.

- So let's see: air going in and out - let's call that …oh, pick something at random. How about "ventilation"? And perfusion - hmm. Let's call that "perfusion". Do they match? No, they do not. A ventilation/perfusion - "V/Q" mismatch.

5- What are the two relevant concepts of badness (COBs) involved in problems with the lungs?

Okay: the two concepts of badness:

- **COB #1 - Shunt:** The **bronchi** are plugged up. Pneumonia (sputum), CHF (water), that kind of thing. What happens: blood goes past them, but doesn't exchange gas. That's "shunt". The percentage of blood that doesn't get to exchange gas is the "shunt fraction". Maybe a whole lung lobe is plugged up - left lower lobe pneumonia, maybe? Then a whole lot of blood goes by alveoli with no gas in them. Big shunt.

- **COB #2 - Dead space:** the **blood vessels** are plugged up. That's PE. This time the air goes in and out without obstruction, but there's no blood going by them, so all that alveolar space isn't being used. It's "dead" – "dead space". ("Mr. Scott, head for the … no, I can't say it.")

6- What's the confusing thing about the two COBs?

The confusing thing is that while the problem happens on <u>one</u> side: either the bronchial, or the vascular, the bad effect is described by what's happening on the <u>other</u> side. So – if you have a PE on the vascular side, you wind up with a big hunk of dead space on the bronchial side. And if you have a big pneumonia on the bronchial side, you wind up with a big shunt on the vascular side. Confusing.

7- So then which one is the problem that happens after a PE?

Increased dead space. Air goes in and out, but the blood isn't going through the alveolar capillaries in that part of the lung.

8- What other bad things happen to people with PEs?

Think about this for a second. Remember "preload"? (Half the audience screams and runs for the door. Ha! Locked!)

Preload is the volume arriving in one of the ventricles. The amount of blood. Got to have the right amount of preload - not enough, and the BP drops; hypovolemia. Too much preload and the ventricle starts to get overloaded, and things start to back up - if this happens on the left side, you get CHF. (What if it happens on the right side? How come my shoes feel so tight?)

Preload has to come <u>from</u> somewhere. For the right side of the heart, the volume comes from the venous system, right? Everything drains into the vena cavae, then into the RA, then the RV, and then - where?

What about the left side? Where does the preload come from? Who said "lungs"? Very good.

So - if a big PE comes along and blocks off, say, a whole lung, what happens to the blood supply to the left side of the heart? So what happens to the blood pressure? And what do you think the PA pressures might look like?

Would you give this patient a lot of IV fluid to support her blood pressure? Or a pressor?

Oh, and yeah - how do you think all this might affect the patient's breathing?

Oh, and yeah #2: the patient could infarct that part of the lung too – but apparently that doesn't happen all of the time.

9- What is a DVT?

"Deep Vein Thrombosis" : a big clot that forms in one of the big veins in one of the extremities.

10- Why do people get DVTs?

Remember all that stuff about "the hazards of immobility"? This is one of 'em. Think about it – were you evolved to sit in front of the tube with a bag of Doritos? No! – you're supposed to be foraging for roots and tubers and all, and chasing down the occasional antelope. So get going!

11- Is it really true that you can get DVTs and PEs if you sit too long on the plane?

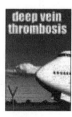

Apparently quite true and factual: the famous story is that Richard Nixon developed both while flying around doing the diplomatic thing. Couldn't have happened to a nicer guy. And what about those 18 minutes, huh? That whole thing about the secretary reaching around the desk like that was just total BS! And you know what else!? He offered a million dollars….okay! Okay. I know – it was a long time ago… He <u>was</u> a crook! And what the hell were we doing in the 'Nam anyway, dammit?

A year or so ago, one of the senior residents was trying to figure out if he should dose himself with Fragmin before flying to Thailand. I'd just get up and walk around the plane...

12- What does smoking have to do with it?

Definitely increases the risk of forming DVTs. I bet Nixon smoked...

13- What does taking birth control pills have to do with it?

Combined with smoking – <u>really</u> increases the risk of producing thrombi. I saw a young woman in the surgical ICU once, years ago, who'd infarcted her entire bowel. Hmm. Would that embolus have come from a DVT? Hmm. You think Nixon took...?...nah.

14- What if the patient has a cast on?

Definitely a problem – a little prophylaxis is obviously the way to go, since detecting a DVT in a casted extremity is going to be difficult. Ortho nurses: should I take an aspirin every day if I get casted for a broken leg? Broken arm?

Preventing PEs

15- Can DVTs be prevented?

This is really the key to the whole thing. So many people develop DVTs, and so many DVTs and PEs never get caught because they're so "silent", that really the only thing to do is to use preventive measures in almost every admission who's undergone surgery, or who is stuck in bed for other reasons for more than a day or two.

Then again, it turns out that less than half of patients who look like they're having a PE, actually do have a PE. But you'd hate to be wrong!

16- What are air boots all about?

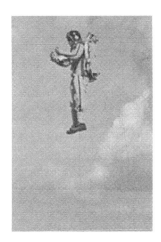

(What do you mean, "Not those!" - I like those!)

Air boots apparently work really well – so well that there's a separate little category that you'll see on physician's admitting notes: "Prophylaxis" – by which they mean: "Routine prevention of awful things."

Like PEs – air boots or subq heparin bid are routine, along with something to prevent gastric stress: carafate maybe, or some kind of acid-production blocking med. Actually I think they're getting away from heparin now, as fragmin apparently works better, doesn't provoke the HIT thing, only needs to be given once a day, and can

477

even substitute for systemic heparin treatment. Cool. I don't know enough about fragmin and all those LMW heparins.

The air boot concept is easy: squeeze the calves every now and then, keep the blood moving through the veins, prevent it from standing in one place ("venous stasis"), and prevent the formation of DVTs. Somebody seems to be making a <u>lot</u> of dough on this one. Actually I think it was an entrepreneurial spinoff from some people at MIT…

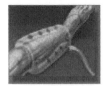 Hard to find a picture of those things we all work with. We did find an article on the website of one of the major health insurance companies, indicating that they required these for patients immoblized after surgery, trauma, etc. Now you <u>know</u> they work!

A weird thing is that some studies are apparently showing that even one air boot is effective in preventing DVTs – even a single air boot applied to one arm. Doesn't seem to make sense on the face of it.

17- What about compression stockings?

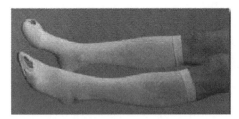 Cute!. Wish those were my legs! Wait - those are my legs!

Apparently these guys just don't do the job very well by themselves, although you can get real fancy ones custom-made that will help a lot. Are they called Jobst stockings? Somebody actually sat down and figured out that proper stockings increase the velocity of venous return by some enormous amount. I remember that at one point you weren't a really cool SICU nurse until you'd had your own pair custom-made…

18- What is SQ heparin all about?

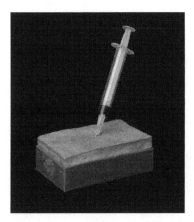 Right – 5000 units subq, q 12 hours, apparently reduces the chances of DVT by 50%. Whoa – looks like a lot of heparin there, mate! Maybe time to change to fragmin, anyhow.

19- Should my patient get sq heparin if she also has air boots on?

I've had house officers tell me that patients need one or the other, but not both. The trick is to make the right choice.

20- Should my patient get air boots if she is already getting sq heparin?

See question 19.

21- Can sq heparin be bad?

Sure – the HIT thing can apparently be provoked just by going into the patients' room and saying the word "heparin". Seriously – you'll see platelet counts drop drastically even in response just to the subq stuff, or the small amount that gets infused through the central line flushes. Put these patients on a no-heparin diet.

22- Can air boots be bad?

Absolutely yes – if the patient has a pre-existing DVT, and you slap on the boots, and compress those legs, and dislodge those clots... yowza!

I put the question to one of the senior residents a week or so ago: "Hey Ermintrude, listen, do you just go ahead and slap airboots on patients routinely when you don't think they have pre-existing DVTs?"

Answer: "Yah – if vee don't sink zey've got any pre-eggzisting DVT, vee joost shlap 'em on." Dutch, she was, I think...

What if the patient never got the boots put on in the first place after admission – what if the nurse forgot, or never got to it, or the team never ordered them, and you came on a couple of days later and said: "Uh, hey - shouldn't this guy have air boots on or something?" Would you go ahead and put them on?

23 – Can putting someone on a heparin drip be bad?

Absolutely yes. Doing almost anything to, or for a patient involves the possibility that something bad might happen – a "negative outcome". Your patient has CAD, and is started on a baby aspirin every day, and comes in with a GI bleed. Common? – no. Possible? - sure! And will you see things like that? Absolutely. And the docs sweat that one all the time: "If I put this patient on heparin, what are the chances that she'll spontaneously bleed into her head?" Low. Has it ever happened? Sure. Can you predict it? You can try – this stuff gets refined all the time. Stay current, y'all.

24- Can a patient develop a DVT anywhere besides a leg?

Arms for sure – I think that the doppler studies can see them, and I know that we've heparinized, or argatroban-ized patients for them. Anticoagulated them.

25- Can air boots prevent DVTs that happen, say, in my patient's arm?

That seems to be what the studies are saying – so I guess so.

26- Does it have to be two air boots?

I know I've seen people with only one boot on – was that because they had a DVT in the other leg, and the idea was to prevent more from forming? Wouldn't they have been heparinized for that DVT?

27- What about those little air boots that just squeeze the feet?

Yeah – did you see those at the NTI too? Was it hot in Texas, I tell you what? That Riverwalk thing was pretty nice, but that whole business about the free dinner with a lecture didn't work out so well. Which classes did you… what? Oh! Sorry! Yeah, we saw these little gadgets at the National Teaching Institute in San Antonio (I got this totally corny Alamo belt buckle, I wear it everywhere), which only compressed the feet, and the company rep claimed that the studies showed that they worked as well as the long boots do. Sounded good, looked a little funny. Anybody seen these in use?

Jayne says that these are used on really large patients, because their calves are too large for the standard boots.

Detecting DVTs

28- How do I know if my patient has a DVT?

This is a very tricky business. Not only do lots of other things act like DVT: leg cramps, strains, sprains, all that stuff, but many DVTs and their subsequent PEs don't ever get diagnosed at all. There are studies that show that only something like a third of patients that you might think have a DVT, actually have a DVT. This needs to be carefully looked at, because you don't want to be anticoagulating people who don't need it, but you don't want to not treat someone who needs it.

29- What is Homan's sign?

Homan's sign is the thing where you gently pull the patient's foot north towards her head, and ask if she's having pain in her calf. Apparently not really useful.

30- What is a venogram?

This is a dye study that is considered the "gold standard" for DVT testing. Nowadays however they try do Lower Extremity Non-invasive Testing, which is an ultrasound procedure. Apparently quite accurate. Always good to try and avoid exposure to contrast dye. Why?

31- What are LENIs?

"Lower Extremity Non-Invasives" – a kind of ultrasound testing that tries to look for DVTs – apparently a pretty effective and accurate test, although there are sometimes problems seeing the deeper veins.

32- Should my patient have LENIs before getting air boots applied?

I can remember when this was the rule – nowadays if there's no reason to think that the patient has an active DVT, the usual plan is to just put them on a bedrest patient routinely.

33- What does d-dimer have to do with it?

Jayne says that d-dimer goes up whenever there's a clotting process going on somewhere in the body. So yes, d-dimer will go up if a patient has a DVT or a PE, and you will see the spec sent when they're doing the workup, but the d-dimer can also go up if the patient has recently had surgery, or maybe has a tumor process going on. It's not much of a specific signal by itself, but when added to the workup it helps narrow things down.

Detecting PEs

34- How do I know if my patient has a PE?

Even though the whole picture can be really hard to sort out, some things usually don't look right.

- The patient may have chest pain without ischemic EKG changes. (Jayne: "You'd look for the EKG changes that go with right heart strain." Well, see? - now that's a CNS for you, right there.

Smarty. <u>My</u> smarty.) It makes sense though – if the right side of the heart is trying to pump through a partially obstructed lung, it's going to be working harder than it normally would. Actually, only about 20% of PE patients show right-heart-strain EKG changes. (I looked up that last one – you have to look things up when you're talking to Jayne..)

- The patient will probably be short of breath. Makes sense.

- And tachypneic. And tachycardic.

- Even the most expert practitioner can be completely fooled one way or the other.

35- Can you see a PE on a chest x-ray?

Apparently hardly ever.

36- What is a VQ scan?

This is one of those radiation-tagged-perfusion-nuclear-imaging jobs. The results are either "high" or "low" probability – in the case of a patient who is likely to having a PE, even a completely silent one, a suspicious VQ study has to be followed up with some other kind of confirming scan. Lately a lot of our patients have been going for a spiral CT with contrast to rule PE in or out.

37- What is a pulmonary angiogram?

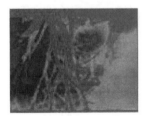

Wow, man - far out! "PLEASE DO NOT TAKE ANY OF THE BROWN ACID!" (I will personally send a nice present to anyone who can tell me who said that, and where.)

This is apparently the gold standard diagnostic test at the current time. Go in there, inject some dye, light up the vasculature, do lots of fluoroscopy, and see if there are places where perfusion just isn't happening. Nice to avoid dye studies if possible – bad for the kidneys. Keep the mucomyst thing in mind whenever you hear the "dye" word. 1200mg po qid now, I think. Also the bicarb thing.

<u>**Kinds of PEs**</u>

38- Are there different kinds of PEs?

Apart from where they're coming from, apparently it has mostly to do with how big they are, and how much lung they plug up. Bigger would be worse, I would guess.

39- What is a "saddle embolus"?

(Mr. Ed – you want to handle this one?) This is the PE equivalent of an antero-lateral MI – the widower-maker. The (very large) clot goes and lodges itself at the bifurcation of the pulmonary artery. Ack! That's sort of the root of the pulmonary circulation, right there. These people are going to be in serious need of some serious treatment, seriously soon. Sometimes the surgeons will actually go in after a clot like this: "embolectomy". A while back somebody told me about a clot that a surgeon pulled out of some patient's PA that was "the size of a carrot". I hope he got better! The patient, too!

40- Are there other kinds of emboluses?

Remember – anything that can hang together and move along the lumen of a vessel can be an embolus: clots for sure – what else? There are air emboli, fat emboli, amniotic fluid emboli…
I seem to recall that bullets can do weird things if they get into blood vessels, although they don't usually come under the category. Lead embolus, maybe? More on these below.

Treating PEs

41- How are PEs treated?

Clot lysis and anticoagulation are the main things. (And maybe handgun control?) Heparin followed eventually by coumadin is apparently the way to go with anticoagulation, because it prevents the formation of additional clots – apparently where you have one clot, you have the high likelihood of making more – maybe many more. So anticoagulating the patient can save her life by preventing more clots from forming and being thrown into the lungs.

Obviously the patient may have to be treated for hypoxia, right? You're an ICU nurse now. What should we do?

42- How long does a patient have to stay on heparin for a PE to dissolve?

Trick question – heparin doesn't dissolve a clot. You eat up the clot yourself: you phagocytize it, or whatever. Chomp, chomp, little white cells! Apparently it can take a while to eat up a PE. One source we looked at said that existing clots can go away within a very variable period of time, ranging from a week to several months.

43- What does TPA have to do with it?

Potentially lifesaving, potentially deadly. This one really takes some careful consideration, and I can't remember seeing it used in MICU patients more than a couple of times. I guess sometimes it's safer to intubate a person, heparinize her, and wait for the PE to get eaten up than it would be to give a fibrinolytic. Imagine if the person had a history of hemorrhagic stroke? Or recent surgery? Horrible to even think about…

On the other hand, Jayne tells a story about a code she saw – big, nasty, chest-pumping, defibrillating, intubated code - nothing was working, just wailing away, and up pops the emergentologist, who says: "Give TPA – it might be a PE." And it worked! And the patient went home!

44- How is a big PE or a saddle embolus treated?

Well, see, there you are: faced with your decision tree, right there.

45- What is clot lysis all about?

As above: this stuff – not heparin – is what's going to dissolve that nasty PE. Apparently TPA and streptokinase work equally well, and the results in the initial studies were so impressive that sometimes the studies were stopped – almost everybody getting lysed was getting better, and everybody else was doing badly. The thing is, the stuff is so dangerous that they usually save it for patients who are having serious blood pressure trouble…why?

Another neat thing about lysis is that it not only dissolves the clot that's made it to the lung, but the other ones hiding in the leg veins just waiting to break loose and make more trouble…

We recently had a patient come in after a transatlantic flight, during which he apparently never moved a muscle, who went down in front of the stewardesses at the end of the flight. Hypoxic, hypotensive: he'd developed several huge PEs. Looked terrible – got lysed. Got better! Extubated the next day – his wife was crying, he was crying ("I thought I was dead!"), we were practically all crying…big save!

Here's a comprehensive reference article that was written by an ER doc at Jayne's hospital: http://www.remotemedicine.org/Paths/chestpain.pdf - an excellent and thorough resource.

46- What does coumadin have to do with it?

If you've got the kind of body that's going to produce a DVT/PE once, then the chances are that you're going to do it again. I'm not sure what the study numbers are exactly, but I know that given a certain age, history, body habitus, etc., some people are going to go home on coumadin for life.

47- What are IVC filters all about?

Here's an example of one of the filters that are sometimes placed   in the IVC to trap thrombi before they can get to the lungs – this is a Greenfield filter, and that's either a clot or a red chili pepper that it's caught there.

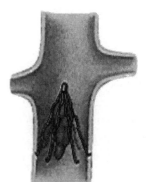

Other Kinds of Embolisms

48- What is an air embolus?

A big bubble of air injected into the circulation will travel along the vessels as a blob, and you can effectively plug off pulmonary circulation with big bubbles just as well as you can with clots. In the ICU you want to worry about this happening in connection with central lines, and a couple of main points should be made:

- remember that at times the pressure inside the chest can go <u>negative</u>. If you have an uncapped port on a central line, **it will suck air into the patient**.
- If you've removed the PA line from one of the introducers with the little black membrane, then you need to remember that the membrane isn't airtight anymore, and unless you cover it with a tegaderm or insert an obturator, **it will suck air into the patient.**

- If you remove a central line and forget to slap an air-occlusive dressing over the site, it may remain patent and **suck air into the patient**.

Just don't let this happen.

49- What does a patient with an air embolus look like?

Usually awful – like someone with a big PE. Blue, short of breath, chest pain – and what's that horrible sucking sound?

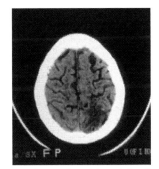

That's if it goes to the lungs. Everybody see that nasty thing down there on the lower right? According to the U of Iowa's website, this is an image of somebody who managed to send an air embolus to his/her head. Left-sided-circulation embolus. Scuba diver maybe? Don't hold your breath on the way back up! Pwing!

http://www.uiowa.edu/~c064s01/nr320%20copy.jpg

Apparently the big risk for air embolism is during surgery – and it's pretty dangerous: something like 50cc can displace most of the blood on the right side of the heart, and 300c can be lethal.

50- An incredibly important point: rapid IV boluses.

This raises a point that does come up fairly frequently in the MICU. Giving a rapid fluid bolus from a liter bag of saline involves putting the IV solution into one of the while compression bags that we use for arterial and central lines. Hold a liter bag of NS up to the light – how much air is in that bag? <u>If you don't vent that air, the compression bag will pump it right into your patient</u>. Don't let this happen. Spike the bag upside down and squeeze the air out through the tubing. Every time.

51- What should I do if I think my patient has just pulled in an air embolus?

A little tricky – let's see if I can remember this right. What you want to do is try to trap the air in the RV in such a way that it won't get pumped out towards the lungs, so you're supposed to:

- Get the person into trendelenburg position with the right side up, which will trap the air in the right atrium (ventricle?) and prevent it from getting into the circulation.

- Apply oxygen.

- Get the team. The maneuver is to try and aspirate the air from the RA (RV?) through a CVP line until no more can be removed.

52- What is a fat embolus?

I've never seen one, but I understand they happen sometimes after long bone fractures.

53- What is an amniotic fluid embolus?

These are really rare - something like once in 20-30,000 deliveries, and I don't think we've ever seen one come into the MICU. Deadly, however. The idea is that amniotic fluid gets injected into the systemic venous circulation, and from there makes its way to the lungs. I don't think I've ever seen one, but once in a great while we do get an obstetrical patient into the MICU.

Reading 12- Lead EKGs

I'm not sure if updating these articles is such a good idea - they just get bigger and bigger, and we throw more and more stuff in, and they just get monstrous and probably scary for the new kids. It's fun to a point – but we're trying to convey the basics here, or at least what passes for the basics as we understand them. Well… let us know what you think. Too big? Too much? Or too full of mistakes? (grin!). The whole thing already prints out like the telephone book…

1- What is an EKG?
2- What is a 12-lead EKG?
3- When you do an EKG, what are you looking for?
4- What do EKG lead groups have to do with cardiac anatomy?
 4-1: Inferior
 4-2: Lateral
 4-3: Anterior
 4-4: Septal
5- What is the difference between coronary ischemia and a myocardial infarction?
 5-1: A brief rant.
6- What does ischemia look like on a 12-lead?
 6-1- What do I do if my patient is having ischemia? What is "flashing"?
7- What are the stages of an MI, and what to they look like on a 12-lead EKG?
 7-1- Acute Injury: ST elevations.
 7-2- Necrosis: Q-waves.
 7-3- Resolution: persistent Q-waves or flipped T's.
 7-4- What do I do if my patient is having an MI?
8- What is reciprocity?
 8-1- What is a right-ventricular MI, and why is it going in the section on reciprocity?
 8-2- How are RVMIs managed?
9- Going through the evolving EKGs of an MI.
 9-1- Stage 1- the acute infarct.
 9-2- Stage 2- necrosis.
 9-3- Stage 3- resolution
10- Another one.
11- What are intervals all about?
 11-1- PR interval
 11-2- QRS interval
 11-3- QT interval
12- What does a 12-lead EKG look like if a patient's potassium is too high? Too low?

A couple of words about confidence: EKG interpretation often gets classified a nurse's mind as one of those things that he should just stay away from. I really think that this is just plain wrong. I think that any nurse who is smart enough to make it into an ICU in the first place is certainly smart enough to learn the basics of EKG interpretation: what the stages of an MI look like. What big ischemia and its resolution look like. And where in the heart it's happening.

This does <u>not</u> mean that you are supposed to be able to tell the difference between a "neo-Stalinist pre-excitation syndrome", and "variant Lown-Ganong-Beethoven-versus-Hootie-and-the-Blowfish, Type 2". This is why the Great Nurse Manager in her wisdom created cardiologists, and am I ever glad she did, because I don't want to stay up nights studying all that stuff.

But - now trust me on this - the basics are not that hard. And they really are an essential skill.

So let's do it!

What is an EKG?

Everybody remember that the heart works electrically? SA node, AV node, all that? The signal travelling along its normal pathway goes from roughly northwest to roughly south, uh…southeast?

This shows the electrode placement for lead II, the "reference lead", which follows the normal conduction pathway – unlike the other leads, which look at conduction from all sorts of other directions.

Northwest: negative electrode goes here

(the ground electrode goes here…)

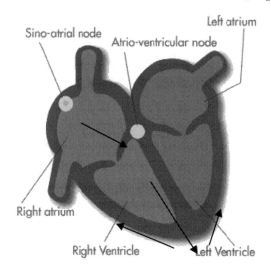

Southeast: Positive electrode here

www.arrhythmia.org/ general/whatis/

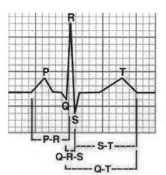

As the impulse goes along in lead II, it makes - or it ought to make – the normal conduction complex that we all learned, like so:

And everybody remembers what the different parts of the complex are: the PR interval represents the signal going through the atria, so it makes a small-sized wave? And the QRS represents the signal going through the what? So it makes a what-sized wave? And the T-wave represents the re-setting of what?

Right - no problems so far.

However, when bad things happen, things start to look a little different.

It might look like this:

(What is this? What's it called, I mean?)

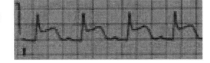

Or this:

(This?)

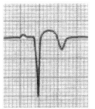

Or this:

(Doesn't look right, does it?)

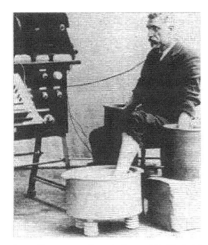

First we need to look a little more at what a 12-lead EKG really does.

What is a 12-lead EKG?

"Willem Einthoven! Are you <u>sure</u> there isn't going to be any lightning tonight?"

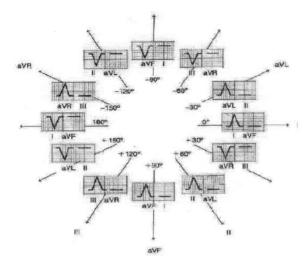

Even though the electical signal travels through the heart in only one direction, it can be looked at from any other direction that you want: upwards, from the feet. Downwards, from the head. Side to side, front to back - that's what this diagram is telling us: it's a matter of moving the monitor wires around, and looking from different vantage points. So, they use 12!

http://www.medspain.com/curso_ekg/ekg5c.jpg

3- When you do an EKG, what are you looking for?

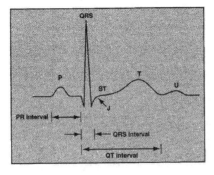

- **Rhythm:** you're trying to figure out what rhythm the patient is in. Rhythms and arrhythmias have their own FAQ, so take a look over there for more on this subject.

- **MI:** you're looking for changes in the normal complex - like this one on the left - that indicate one phase or another of an MI. ST elevations? Q-waves? This is where you look.

http://www.clevelandclinicmeded.com/medical_info/pharmacy/novdec2002/Normal-EKG.gif

- **Ischemia:** you're looking for changes in the normal complex that indicate the presence, or resolution of ischemia: ST depressions, or flipped T-waves...

- **Intervals:** you're trying to figure out if the intervals are normal. Too long, too short? We'll get into some of it.

- **Changes associated with electrolyte problems:** There are also a couple of waveform changes associated with electrolyte disturbances that you should get a look at – we'll take a look at a couple of them as well...

4- What do EKG lead groups have to do with cardiac anatomy?

Twelve lead directions apparently cover the whole heart pretty well. The important part for us as ICU nurses is to understand that there are only a few "territories" of the heart: inferior, lateral, anterior, and so on, and that each of them is reflected in a group of the twelve leads.

"Localizing" bad things on the EKG means using the 12-lead to figure out where in the heart the problem is taking place. To do this, you have to do a little – but really not a whole lot – of memorization:

- you need to learn which groups of EKG leads reflect which parts of the heart.

- you need to learn what the stages of an MI look like on an EKG.

- you need to learn what ischemia looks like on an EKG.

All of this really adds up to less than your average Spanish quiz. Um…unless you were taking French…

The twelve-lead EKG looks at the heart from, uh, twelve! different directions, at the same time. Some areas (also called "territories") of the heart that you might hear about in report, or in patient histories:

- **anterior**
- **lateral**, (or sometimes both of those, as in **antero-lateral**),
- **inferior**, and maybe we'll look at the **infero-posterior** territory, but I think I'm going to leave it out on purpose, as interpreting it gets very confusing to beginners. Remember however to check up on it later.
- **septal**

Each of the big areas is perfused by its own respective artery – there are only three main ones:

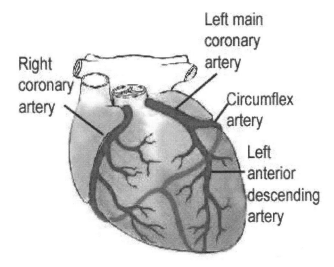

http://www.clevelandclinic.org/heartcenter/pub/guide/disease/cad/cad_arteries.htm

- The **right coronary artery (RCA)** perfuses, uh…the right side of the heart! See how the right side is actually on the **bottom** of the heart? **Inferior** territory: right ventricle.

491

The left side is twice as hard: two arteries! The big vessel there, the "**left main**", divides into two:

- the **left anterior descending (LAD):anterior** LV territory.

- the **circumflex (LCX): lateral** LV territory.

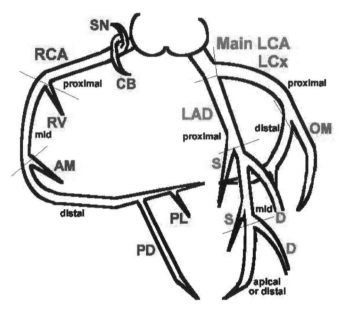

Here's the same system of arteries, except schematic this time.

If you look at this for a minute, it starts to sort itself out: there are really only three main arteries in the system: RCA, LAD and LCX.

You need to see how the left main divides, where it says "Main LCA": a plug there will produce ischemia or infarct in two places downstream. See that? Both the LAD and the LCX are threatened – at the same time - by a problem in the left main artery. **Antero-lateral.** Bad.

The same kind of thing can happen on the right side: a single occlusion can threaten the inferior territory (RCA), and the posterior one (PDA, or just PD in this diagram: "Posterior descending artery", which perfuses the back of the heart. **Infero-posterior.** Also bad.

http://soback.kornet21.net/~heartist/coronary/cag-ori.gif

There are obviously more arteries, and they're important too, but these three (or four) are the main ones. Knowing how they show up on a 12-lead will cover about 98% of the crucial territories that you'll have to worry about at 4am when your patient is having chest pain. (You might be having chest pain too – last week a floor nurse who sent us her very sick patient went into an SVT…)

The key concept: **as each artery perfuses a specific part of the heart, so each part of the heart has a group of leads on the EKG that reflects its activity.**

The different groups of EKG leads only reflect what's happening in their own part of the heart (most of the time – as usual, this is "with a lot of lies thrown in".)

4-1: Inferior Territory/ Right Coronary Artery: Leads II, III, AVF

The heart lies sort of on its side in the chest, with the RV downwards, inferiorly. This territory is perfused by the **right coronary artery**. It's worth mentioning that the inferior part of the heart is innervated partly by the same structures that innervate the stomach – the wall of the one organ lying near the other – and I understand that this is why people with inferior ischemia or infarct often have nausea or vomiting, or sometimes hiccups in place of anginal pain. (They call that an "anginal equivalent" – instead of having chest pain, they do something else.) An infarct here is an

inferior MI: an "IMI". Likewise, we say that a person with ischemia in the RCA is having "inferior ischemia", which does <u>not</u> mean that it's less important than any other kind!

Try to invent some useful memory device to help you remember the lead groups until they become more familiar. Remember "On Old Olympic Towering Tops…", and all that? I understand that the really useful ones are usually dirty – anybody heard what the angry ER doc said to the abusive patient: "AMF, YOYO!"? Hey – I'm not telling what it means - but I understand that surgeons usually know that one…

4-2: Anterior Territory/ Left Anterior Descending: V2, V3, V4

The next time you do a 12-lead, look at where you're putting the sticky precordial chest electrodes – they look at the front: the anterior part of the heart, really the septal and anterior parts of the left ventricle, which are (mostly) perfused by the **left anterior descending artery**.

See how it makes sense that V1 and V2 would be right over the cardiac **septum**?

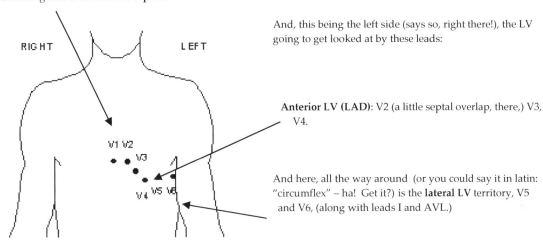

And, this being the left side (says so, right there!), the LV going to get looked at by these leads:

Anterior LV (LAD): V2 (a little septal overlap, there,) V3, V4.

And here, all the way around (or you could say it in latin: "circumflex" – ha! Get it?) is the **lateral LV** territory, V5 and V6, (along with leads I and AVL.)

<u>Any</u> EKG changes representing ischemia or MI should make you worry, but as they show up in different territories, they should make you worry about different things: these left-sided arteries supply the Big Pump, the LV – think about what interrupting it's blood supply might do. Brrr! Infarcting LAD territory produces an **anterior MI**.

4-3: Lateral Territory: I, AVL, V5, V6

Look at where you stick V5 and V6 – all the way around the left side of the chest. Along with I and AVL, they reflect the lateral part of the left ventricle - also Big Pump territory. This part of the heart is perfused by the **circumflex artery**. So an infarct here produces what kind of MI?

If you were still awake several paragraphs up, you'll recall that the **left main artery** divides into the LAD and the LCX, which between them perfuse most of the left ventricle. So if your patient infarcted <u>there</u>…the widowmaker. See that? Take another look at that diagram of the arteries – see how the left main supplies the two Big Pump arteries?

So: a **left main artery** occlusion will threaten both areas of the LV at the same time, and will produce an **antero-lateral MI**, with characteristic EKG changes in V2-4, as well as I,L, and/or V5-6. In a minute we'll start looking at some 12-leads – one of them is for exactly this situation: both territories are being threatened.

Make sense? Any MI is a bad thing, but injury to the Big Pump is a very bad thing, and is responsible for cardiogenic shock. There's lots more on cardiogenic shock and its treatment in the "PA-line" and "intra-aortic balloon pump" FAQs.

4-4: Septal Territory : V1, V2 (V2 overlaps sometimes: both septal and anterior areas)

These leads are right in the center of the chest, and look at the septum between the ventricles. As I recall, the septum is perfused partly by the RCA, and partly by the LAD. A **septal MI** would show in V1 and V2.

(I hear the CCU nurses yelling: "Hey! What about posterior reciprocity in the septal leads!?" Listen: don't confuse the kids. This stuff is hard enough. We'll work on reciprocity towards the end of the article, okay? Maybe.)

Starts to make sense when you look at it, doesn't it? Give it time…

5- What is the difference between coronary ischemia, and a myocardial infarction?

It's surprising to me that people get mixed up about this. What do they teach the kids in nursing school, anyhow?

A brief rant needs to go here. (After 25 years, it appears on your license renewal: "permitted to rant.")

A while back, we had a nursing student working with us as a tech – she was in her fifth year (<u>fifth</u> year out of a five-year BSN program!) – and she was hoping to work with us after school – new grad in the unit, that kind of thing. So by way of gentle encouragement, I pointed to the monitor where as I recall the patient was in something only moderately complicated - like, say, normal sinus rhythm, and I said: "So, Louella, what's this rhythm that this patient is in here?"

Poor Louella, looking very sad, shook her head: "I don't know."

"Louella dear", says I, not a little appalled, taken aback – I mean, five years is longer than med school, right? – "Louella, what exactly are they teaching you in that nursing school of yours?".

"Um, a lot of theory?"

Ladies and gentlemen, here is a jewel. A student who looks the old, beat-up, battle-ax ICU nurse in the eye and says: "I don't know." A jewel! – because she understands the following essential point of ICU practice:

There are two - count 'em - two correct answers to any question:

1- The correct answer.
2- "I don't know."

The second of these answers is equal in value to the first. It reflects honesty, the willingness to find out the answer, and the courage to admit ignorance when you feel that everyone else around you is so obviously smarter than you are. Our daughter #1, a brand-new RN, comes home every day holding her head: "Oh Goddess, (nurses pray to the Goddess of our profession, whose nickname is "Flo"), there's so much I don't know!"

Here is the beginning of wisdom. Any honest ICU nurse with experience will tell you, still holding her head: "The more you know, the more you realize you don't know!" Truer words were never spoken...
Oh, and something else – don't let all that "theory" get in the way when you need to know how to do CPR, or when to hold your patient's digoxin, or why to argue that your patient is too unstable to go for their third MRI in three days, or why they might be on the wrong pressor, or why they need to stay in the ICU instead of being pushed out too soon, or...

Sigh.

Okay. Onwards. Where were we?

Ischemia vs. infarct:

It really is very simple: the difference between a blood vessel that's still open – even a little – and one that isn't open at all.

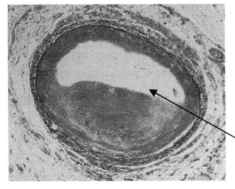

Here's the lumen (the "tube") of a coronary artery, which has been reduced to about half it's normal width by the development of a big ugly red plaque thing, in the lower part of the picture. Usually the plaques occur in one spot along the lumen or another, rather than all the way along the length of the artery, and so the plaque is called a "lesion" – which is said to be more or less "tight". Tighter being more severe, probably producing more symptoms, and more dangerous...

Still open.

http://www.medscape.com/viewarticle/460224_7

The tight lesion reduces the flow of blood to whichever territory happens to be affected. So while enough blood might get through when this person was at rest, that might not be true if the patient got up and started carrying groceries upstairs from the garage. The heart starts working harder, calls for more blood, can't get it, and responds with pain (and EKG changes.)

This is **ischemia**. (CCU nurses: what kind of ischemia is this? Why is this "better" than the other kind, and what's the other kind called?) The lumen of the artery isn't completely plugged, but there's a mismatch that develops between the demand of the cardiac muscle, and the ability of the artery to supply the oxygenated blood that it wants – not enough gets through.

How about this one?

Uh-oh. Looks like there was a little bit of opening left, where the arrow is pointing, but it's gone now. This vessel isn't just narrowed, it's **plugged**. So now the muscle tissue beyond it isn't just getting less blood, it's getting **no blood at all**, and unless something is done pretty quick, that muscle tissue is going to die. This is **infarction**. (Up here in New England we call this an "infahction", as in: "Yah, he took a wicked infahction, but not a shock.")

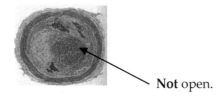

Not open.

http://www.healthandage.com/html/res/aging_of_you/content/13.htm

Okay ICU nurses, what's probably plugging up that last little bit of vessel lumen, and what should this patient be receiving by way of treatment?

6- What does ischemia look like on a 12-lead?

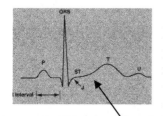

Remember the normal complex? Lead II – nice normal complex. Here's the thing: ischemia and the stages of an MI are different processes, yes? So – they produce different kinds of changes in the normal complex of an EKG. The normal complex goes through a whole series of evolutions as it's heart goes through an MI (look down a bit to see a quick chart of that.) But in ischemia, what you get is usually **ST depression**, below the isoelectric line:

Not depressed.

Way depressed.

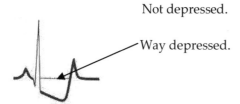

Depressed.

496

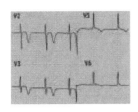 Or you could see
flipped T-waves:

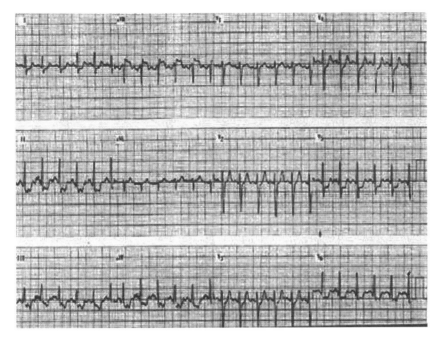

Here's a pretty nice example of an ischemic EKG: so, what do we see?

ST depressions? Very good! Where?

II, yup – what goes with II? III, yup, depressions there too… and AVF. Nice! So this is ischemia, where in the heart? Which territory? Which artery?

Did I fool you? No? There's ischemia in two other territories as well, isn't there?

Ponder this one for a second: what do you think is meant by "rate-related ischemia"?

http://www.le.ac.uk/pathology/teach/CA/Cases/ecg_ischaemia.jpg

So: even before this patient goes off to the cath lab, which arteries do you think are going to show problems?

6-1- What do I do if my patient is having ischemia? What is "flashing"?

Your patient is short of breath with ischemia? (Which means which vessel/s are being ischemic? Producing what EKG changes, in which leads?) This is what is really meant by "flashing" – a point which is often confused with other acute shortness-of-breath scenarios. If the **left** coronary arteries (there, I gave it away) suddenly become ischemic, then the blood supply to the papillary muscles, and the chordae tendonae – remember them? – may drop off. So the chordae may stop working. So what's the problem?

The problem is that the chordae are what make the valve leaflets work – so if they don't work, then the valve goes flooey, and starts not to valve anymore. (You must not say "flooey" however – very low-class. You must say: "incompetent", which comes from the original Latin, meaning, I believe, "flooey".) Leaky. "Regurgitant": with each systolic contraction, some of the blood is pumped backwards instead of forwards. If it happens on the left side, "mitral incompetence", then blood being pumped backwards goes – where? Increasing the pressure in the what? Causing what to leak into the alveoli, filling them up? Very quickly?

Just like drowning. "Ischemic mitral regurgitation." Sounds awful, and it is…

CCU nurses: how does this show up on a wedge pressure? How do you measure it?

Well – what to do? Everybody knows at least some of this by the time they get into the MICU: your patient is having chest pain, flashing maybe – what <u>do</u> you do?

One way to remember the moves to make is to think: "**L,M,N,O,P**":

> - Your patient is getting "wet" – give some **L**asix. (Actually, lasix isn't really what she needs, is it? Although it's quite right to give – what she really needs is something to make that coronary artery dilate – what could you give that would make that happen?) If you're really quick on the draw, sometimes you can head off intubation in someone who's flashing – sometimes no matter how quick you are, you can't.

> - She's probably having chest pain – give her some **M**orphine.

> - What do you give everybody with cardiac ischemia? Under the tongue? **N**itrates – IV nitroglycerine in the ICU. (That's probably what the patient wants instead of lasix, right? But give the lasix too…)

> - What does her heart tissue need more of? Administer some **O**xygen. What if she's a COPDer?

> - **P**osition her properly: sit her way up, high Fowler's position, and put pillows under her arms to ease her work of breathing.

Now you want to see if her ischemia responds – this can be tricky if she doesn't have classical, substernal chest pain – maybe her anginal equivalent is nausea, or shortness of breath. People with diabetic neuropathy who can't feel their feet may not feel anginal pain either… But true cardiac ischemia should produce some kind of characteristic change in the EKG - you're going to look for the ischemic changes to **reverse** – for the ST depressions to come back up, for the flipped T-waves to pop back up, in the same lead groups where they appeared at the beginning.

These maneuvers don't repair the underlying problem though, right? – which is why people get cathed, and angioplastied, or stented, or bypassed.

But what if all that stuff doesn't work? What if you do all that good stuff: L, M, N, O, P – and the patient is still ischemic? Now what? Maybe a trip to the cath lab? Maybe. It might, though, be time for the CCU nurse's favorite toy…

Begins with "I", ends with "P"…?

CCU nurses: What is "pseudo-normalization", and what's it got to do with ischemia?

(Is pseudo-normalization what really weird people do, but only on Halloween?)

(I actually thought that one was pretty good, myself!)

7- What are the stages of an MI, and what do they look like on a 12-lead EKG?

This time the problem is different: the muscle tissue beyond that little plug is not just inadequately supplied – it's **not** supplied. Going to die. I hate it when that happens!

The underlying process took a surpisingly long time to clarify, but finally in the 1980's they figured out that little clots were the culprits in causing MIs, suddenly occluding what was left of a tight arterial lumen already almost blocked by plaque. The 'tight lesions' are the places along the lumen of the coronary artery where the cholesterol plaques have nearly – but not completely – closed the lumen to blood flow. As I understand it the theory says that platelets, loving as they do to stick to rough places, tend to form clots that plug what small opening is left – which is what lies behind the whole concept of 'clot-busting'.

Apparently there's a whole inflammatory aspect to the process of infarction as well, involving the plaques rupturing, which doesn't sound healthy at all. Also there's a story around that bacteria from the mouth may be involved in plaque formation, and that flossing can help prevent it. Just something else grandma was right about.

There are several phases that an MI "evolves" through, and each phase has its own clear EKG characteristics.

Before we go through each bit in detail, here's a quick look at the whole process.

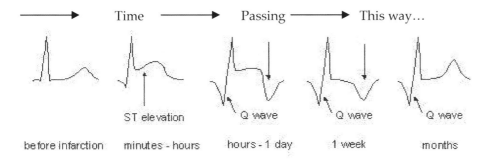

http://heartkorea.com/ecg_guide/ecg_04_2.htm

7-1- First Stage: Acute Injury (ST Elevations):

Let's make sure that we know what we're looking at here, exactly:

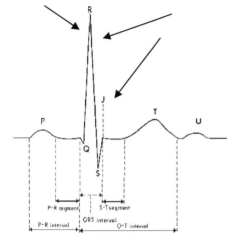

Take a look at the QRS complex, in the middle of the diagram. You need to know exactly which wave is which. Again, it's not too hard:

The arrow on the left is pointing at the R-wave, which **rises** up from the **isoelectric line**, which is this one...

... here. The flat part.

The upper right-hand arrow is pointing to the S-wave, which **slides** back down.

www.bilgi.umedia.org.tr/ yayin/tejm/ekg.htm

The lower right-hand arrow is pointing to the ST segment – the same part that became depressed back in question **6**.

So - now that there's a clot occluding the lumen, the process of infarction begins. It turns out that there are three clear stages in the progression of the MI – the first is the period of the 'acute injury'. This stage lasts some hours - I remember being taught that it's roughly six - and represents the period of time between the acute blockage of the lumen, and the start of tissue death in the part of the heart that is distal to that plug. On an EKG, this stage of infarct will show as **ST elevation** in all the leads that reflect whichever part of the heart is being affected.

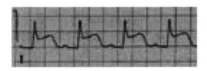

See how the S-wave doesn't go all the way back down, and is holding the T-wave up with it? S-T elevation. Early-stage, acute injury MI. Bad.

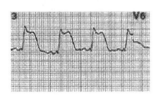

These are really elevated! "Tombstones"...

Very important: This six-ish hour period is the time when you want to try and get your TPA up and running – if you wait any longer, it may be too late to salvage the muscle tissue.

Just as important: what if the patient had had a CVA six months ago?

500

7- 2- Second Stage: Necrosis (Q-waves):

Up.

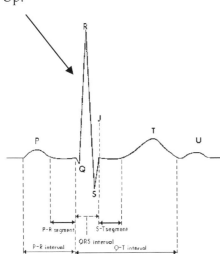

Here's the normal complex again. Take a look at the QRS complex. Is there really a Q-wave here? Until they get to the ICU, lots of nurses never even see a Q-wave, and so don't really know where they should be?

Sort of, kind of, maybe, that little tiny wave there at the end of the PR interval – see it? That little thing, says "Q"? Not much of a wave...a "non-pathologic" q-wave.

The idea is that normally, ignoring that wee little Q, the first move that a QRS complex makes after the PR interval is to go – which way? Who said "Up!"? Yes, correct. Up is right. See that? Up, after the PR?

Big q-waves represent the progression of the MI from the stage of acute injury to the stage of necrosis. Brrr! They show up as the QRS moving **downwards first**, after the PR interval.

Take a look at this normal 12-lead. In every lead except AVR – we'll leave AVR out of this, since it doesn't fall in any of the lead groups, and in fact I don't really know what it's for – in every lead, after the PR inteval, the QRS goes up. Can you see that, all those movements up?

All those arrows: upward QRS's.   What about this one?

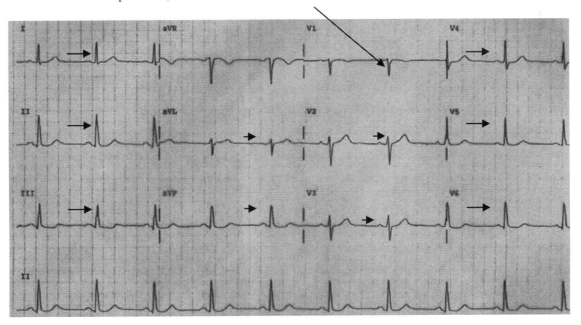

http://www-personal.umich.edu/~danielbc/2004/study/normal%20EKG.jpg

What about V1? Looks like a big q-wave: a **downward** movement after the PR. But see – is it the only one there is? V1 goes with which other lead? (V2.) Is there a q-wave there as well? (No.)

This is important: if you're going to see some kind of change in a 12-lead EKG, you should clearly see it in all the leads of a group, or it may not really mean anything – artifact maybe, or iffy lead placement. My own EKG has a consistent q-wave in lead III – but not in II or AVF. My little pet q-wave – it just lives there…

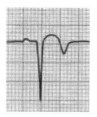

Here's another one. See the PR interval? What does this QRS do – go up first, or down first? Down is correct. This is definitely a "pathologic" q-wave: greater than a third of the total size of the QRS. This one is the whole size of the QRS!

The appearance of q-waves means that the patient has missed the time "window" for clot lysis – which makes sense, considering that the artery has now been plugged for more than four to six hours. Not much tissue can survive without blood that long. You figure – cardiac tissue must be really tough stuff – how long does it take before irreversible brain damage occurs in an untreated, hypotensive arrythmia? Six <u>minutes</u>? Mine's probably even less…

Here's an interesting strip, below.

See the ST elevations, <u>and</u> the Q's, all at the same time? This person is <u>evolving</u> from the first stage to the second – moving from the stage of acute injury to the stage of necrosis. The ST segments will come back down to the baseline (the "isoelectric" line) as the Q's develop.

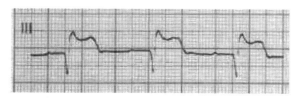

ST elevations, sliding back downwards as the Q waves grow…

7-3- Third Stage: Resolution (Persistent Q's, or flipped T's):

The resolution stage represents the development of scar tissue in the infarcted area, which happens roughly two weeks after the necrotic stage of the MI. The affected part of the heart will still show EKG changes, possibly forever – either what are called 'persistent Q-waves', or flipped T-waves. Unless he's having ischemia again!

A lot of the interpretation depends on context. If an elderly gentleman – say, myself (!), came in with a broken ankle, and you saw Q's, or flipped T's the routine EKG that you do on every older person, you'd cleverly ask me: "Uh, Nurse Markie, did you have an IMI in the past at some time?" You would probably say that the Q's or T's represented an old MI, rather than one I was in the middle of.

Unless I was having chest pain…

Here's another look at the whole process. Any clearer now?

Before the MI **1st Stage** **Necrosis** **Resolution: the Q's remain, and maybe**

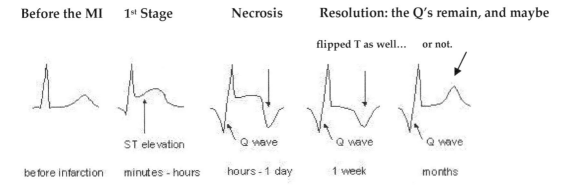

Let's say it again: remember that these evolutionary changes will stay in the same group of leads the whole time, reflecting the events in the part of the heart that they represent.

7-4- What do I do if my patient is having an MI?

In two paragraphs? Did you leave your copy of Braunwald at home?

Well – timing is everything. Is the patient in stage 1? – time to think about the cath lab, or TPA, unless there's some really good reason not to give it. Which there may be…

If your patient does get TPA, look for the ST elevations to come back down to baseline without the development of q-waves.

Stage 2? Too late – the patient is going to have to "take her hit". Watch out for the usual stuff: ectopy, changes in rhythm, blood pressure, all that.

Remember that different kinds of MIs present in different ways: for example, inferior MIs often affect the conduction system: they may "brady down", buy atropine or external pacing pads (ow!), or a temporary pacing wire – neat stuff like that. They may get the hiccups, or nausea and vomiting instead of having chest pain, as the inferior cardiac nerves also innervate the top of the stomach, so I'm told.

Anterior, lateral, antero-lateral MIs – Big Pump Mis: they can get into all sorts of nasty trouble: cardiogenic shock, maybe. Big "flash" events, for another. Make sure that the specs for cardiac markers get sent every – what is it now, still every eight hours? Troponin, maybe still CK and MB isoenzymes – and I think they still have us do EKGs with every set. Take a look! Watch for evolution, all that good stuff!

8- What is "electrical reciprocity"?

"You mean there's more?" (sigh)…there's always more! Why do you think they write those enormous books and all?

This is a fairly important concept, and it does have to go into this article, but in the swirl of ST elevations, depressions, mountains, valleys, rivers, plagues of frogs…you might want to put this bit off until later. It's a lot to soak up at once.

I hate reciprocity – it's very confusing. Describing reciprocity is like describing how you can look at something through binoculars: if you look one way, the image is right side up – but if you flip the binoculars and look through the wrong end, the image is upside down, even though you're still looking at the same thing. Some EKG lead groups act this way – they "mirror each other" electrically, so that ST elevations in one group will show up as ST depressions in the other. Not ischemia – "mirroring". You may need to reflect on that for a while…

There are only two main areas of the heart that do this: the inferior and lateral ones; the septal and posterior ones. A set of inferior ST elevations in II, III and AVF can produce lateral ST depressions in I, AVL, V5 and V6. You'd think that this would mean lateral ischemia, but no – it's a reflection, bouncing electrically across the heart from the inferior injury, showing up in reverse.

Yup, it's confusing. The trick is to remember that when assessing EKG changes, **ST elevations always come first** – ahead of anything else on an EKG. If there are ST elevations **anywhere** on an EKG, you should wonder if any ST depressions on the same EKG might be reciprocral, instead of ischemic. See if they fit: inferior-lateral? If there are no ST elevations, go with ischemia as your interpretation.

Inferior MI, lateral reciprocity.

Here's a pretty good example: see the inferior ST elevations? So that's going to be the primary process.

Now - see the ST depressions in I, and AVL? Lateral leads? That's not ischemia – it's the "mirrored reflection"of the inferior MI. Question for the cardiologist – why isn't there reciprocity in V5 and V6?

There's more here, though.

See the ST depressions in V1 and V2? Read on, we'll talk about posterior reciprocity, and why it makes sense that it would show up in this situation. But ST depressions show in V3 and V4 – too many changes for me. Call cards!

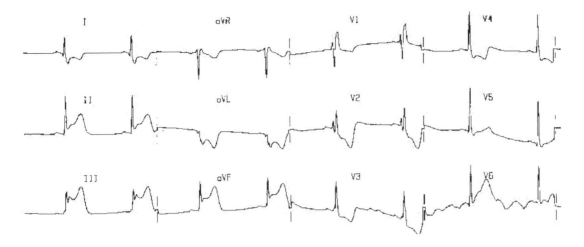

Lateral MI, inferior reciprocity.

See the ST elevations, this time in I and AVL? They're subtle, but they're there. Again, for some reason the entire lead groups isn't represented, but enough of it is, and in the right way, to be convincing – the primary process is a lateral MI.

So let's get reciprocal: what's happening in the inferior leads? Not ischemia.

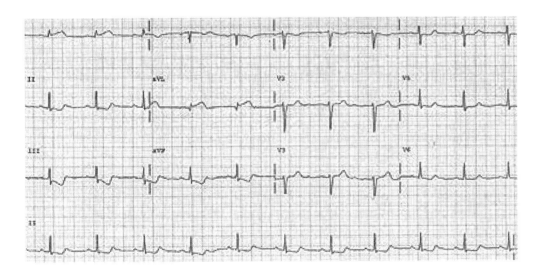

Posterior reciprocity is even more terrifying and complicated. If you don't like horror movies, don't read this part – it's just too awful.

The septal leads (they look at the **front** of the heart) will reflect a posterior event (which is in the **back**) in the same way that the inferior/lateral ones do, but it's even more ridiculously tricky, since reading the posterior leads is made sort of difficult by the fact that…well… there aren't any posterior leads! (At least not on a normal 12-lead.) Sheesh!

See - on a 12-lead - the way you look at the **back** of the heart, is by looking at the leads that look at the **front** of the heart, only **backwards**. And upside down. Don't hurt your neck. Remember the binoculars? If you reverse them, then the image is upside down and backwards?

So: here are a couple of sets of septal leads: V1 and V2.

ST depressions!

Now – here are the same groups of leads, flipped and reversed:

ST elevations!

See the ST elevations? This is what you would see if you put real posterior leads on the patient. Posterior MI – in fact, you'll see MDs do just this with an EKG – they'll flip it over and hold it up to the light, looking for just this effect.

Sometimes the clue is: is the patient having an inferior MI? Remember that the RCA perfuses both the inferior and posterior areas – is there ST elevation in II, III and AVF? And ST depression in V1 and V2? Those septal leads may be giving you a "mirror" of an infarct process, rather than showing ischemia – an infero-posterior MI.

Uh-oh - Jayne's here: "Did you tell them about the posterior leads?"

The Preceptor: "What posterior leads?"
J: "You're telling me that you don't know how to do posterior leads?"
The P: "There **are** posterior leads?"
J: "Of course there are posterior leads, you… listen. Dopey. You take three more electrode stickers, and you stick 'em on the patient's chest, going around towards the right, continuing the right-sided chest leads. You told 'em about the right sided chest leads, didn't you?"

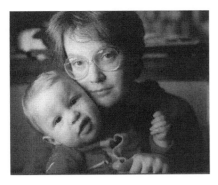

The P: "Well, um no…"
J: "Well then tell them, you enormous goof!"
About…1986?

Just like an old married couple… cute baby, huh? We were all a lot cuter back then… he's taller than I am now, and doing all that great 18-year-old stuff…dreadlocks, last summer. I thought about them myself for a minute, until somebody reminded me about the bald spot…I mean, I can't see it, can I? And there's still some hair in the front… so on the principle of anterior reciprocity, does this mean that I can pretend that the bald spot isn't there if I want to?

Daughter #1 weighs in: "<u>No</u>, you can <u>not</u> have dreadlocks with a bald spot. That's almost as bad as an old hippie with a bald spot and a ponytail. Eww!"

Well. You should've seen my hair when I was 17 – down the middle of my back, flew in the wind when I would cycle around Central Park in the summer of '72…nope, no helmets back then. "Moondance" on the radio. Had Dwayne Allman died? Janis and Jimi were gone…ten years after that, daughter #1 was born. And now she's a nurse. And now I'm "The Man". Sigh…but my son and I found a 1972 Honda, little motorcycle, fixed it up…but I don't take it faster than 30!

What does this have to do with the heart? Everything!

8-1: What is a right-ventricular MI, and why is it going in the section about reciprocity?

Well – it's going here because I was going to leave it out… let's see if I can remember this. Posterior events go along with inferior ones, because the back of the heart is perfused by the **posterior descending artery (PDA)**, which branches off of the **right coronary artery (RCA)**.

This is the same kind of process as a left main infarct: two areas can be affected at once. Both the inferior and posterior territories will by affected by a single plug in the RCA, producing an **infero-posterior MI**.

A plug here...

produces an inferior infarct here...

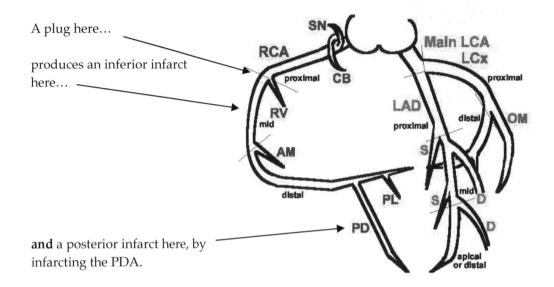

and a posterior infarct here, by infarcting the PDA.

Now go back and look at the EKG on page 17. Infero-posterior, you think? Plus some anterior ischemia? Eww!

Infarcting all this territory can produce yet another kind of MI, the **"right ventricular" MI/ RVMI**. Jayne says that up to 50% of all inferior MIs affect enough RV territory to "stun" them into "hypokinetic inactivity" – meaning "they don't move much, and don't pump much." To see this on an EKG, you need to do a 12-lead with the chest leads applied backwards – going around towards the right, instead of towards the left. "Ralph - do a right-sided EKG, will you?"

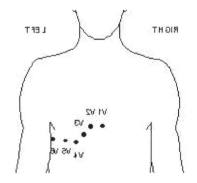

Something's not right – it looks familiar, though...

I couldn't find an image of right sided leads...but this is the basic idea. The placement is the same as usual, except going in the other direction.

Jayne says that to do **true posterior leads**, here's what you do: take all the chest lead wires off.

Now stick on three more chest electrodes along the same line of V5 and V6, along the fifth intercostal space, using the same   spacing that you used for the chest leads, ending up under the scapula: V7, V8, and V9.

Now start reattaching the wires: put the V1 lead wire on the V4 electrode. See? The V2 lead goes on the V5 electrode. And so on around the chest. Now when you do your 12-lead, you'll get a clear picture of what the entire RV is doing: inferiorly and posteriorly.

8-2- How are RVMIs managed?

RVMIs are a different kind of beast entirely from the left-sided kind. By definition, a left-sided MI involves the Big Pump – and your patient is going to get into fluid-management problems, CHF, that sort of thing, right? High wedge pressures, because the LV can't empty itself? Lasix, fluid restriction, hypoxia…

In a right-ventricular MI, the idea is that the ventricle becomes hypokinetic ("It doesn't move much.") – just sort of sits there, stunned, instead of sending blood along to the lungs. So what?

So: if the blood doesn't get pumped along to the lungs, then how is it going to get through those lungs and over to the other side, so that it can get pumped out into the arteries, which is after all how you make a blood pressure? The LV needs a steady supply to work with – instead of being suddenly injured and overloaded, it suddenly doesn't have enough volume coming in. "Preload".

These people get lots of volume, to flood that sluggish RV and keep the blood moving along to the lungs – just the opposite of a left-system MI. Lots and lots of fluid – liters and liters. Ten in a day, maybe. Maybe more. Give them normal saline – isotonic; stays in the vasculature…

Well. I did warn you about the posterior stuff…look, I know, it's hard. And maybe I lied a little about how hard it really was. Maybe a lot. But aren't you learning all kinds of cool stuff? Soak up what you can, then forget about it for a year – then come back and read this again, and see if more of it clicks.

9- Going through the evolving EKGs of an MI.

Okay – ready to look at EKGs all the way through an MI, all three stages? Let's go.

9-1- Acute Injury - Stage 1

Look at the ST elevations in leads II, III and AVF in this first EKG – pretty impressive. They're not quite high enough to be called "tombstones", but they're impressive.

Important question: what kind of MI is this? Which territory is being affected? Anterior? Inferior? Lateral? Septal? Yukon?

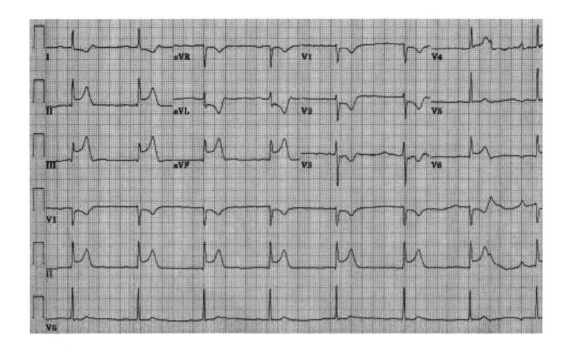

Take another look at those ST elevations. Has the patient "Q'd out" yet? Is it too late for clot lysis, you think, or is there still time?

I think we also see some reciprocity: see the ST depressions in I and AVL? That would be lateral territory, which is reciprocal to, or reflective of what area? Inferior – correct. So what kind of MI is this? See that? The reciprocity doesn't show in the whole lateral lead group though, does it? Happens that way sometimes – but certainly there's a nasty primary process going on in II, III and AVF.

How about the septal leads?

Which coronary artery is being affected? What about the PDA?

What kinds of specific bad things do these people do? What might you specifically want to have on hand? (Take a look at **7-4** again.)

9-2- Stage 2 - Necrosis:

How about now? Not the same patient - same kind of MI though, same territory. But now things are looking a little different down there in II, III and AVF. See how the Q-waves are starting to show up?

Not just starting! This person is in the process of "Q-ing out" inferiorly. "Can we lyse this guy?" "No – look, he's q-ing out."

Are there other interesting changes to find on this EKG? What territories do they represent?

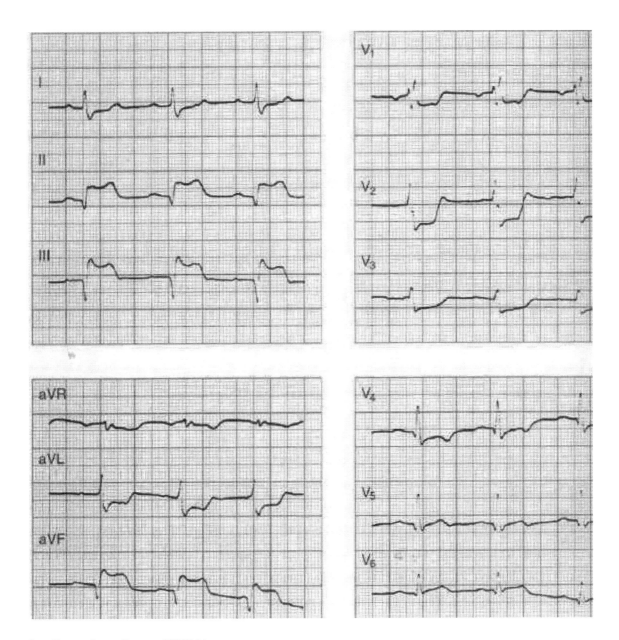

I think there's some interesting reciprocity happening here: remember, ST elevations always come first in interpretation. "So: if the ST elevations are inferior, and inferior is reciprocal to lateral, then...oh, my head hurts!"

No – keep going, you were doing great! The inferior territory "reflects" the lateral one. So the ST elevations in the one show up as ST depressions in the other. Sure enough: I is a little depressed, AVL is definitely depressed, but once again I think V5 and V6 are sitting this one out.

How about the ST depressions in V1 and V2? Could be septal ischemia...hmm -I think this is even yet another inferior-posterior MI. This person's primary process is an IMI, right? Remember the diagram: the RCA perfuses the back of the heart...I think those ST depressions are "mirrored" – they're "reflecting" an ST elevation process going on, way in back there.

And what's going on with V3 and V4? Uh – would somebody please call the cardiologist?

9-3- Stage 3 - Resolution

Well, clearly these aren't all from the same patient. For one thing, the rhythm is different – what rhythm is this? In this "post-MI" EKG, try to find the "persistent" Q-waves in II, III, and AVF.

But the idea is pretty well conveyed, I think, isn't it? Evolution of an inferior MI from the acute stage, to necrosis, to resolution?

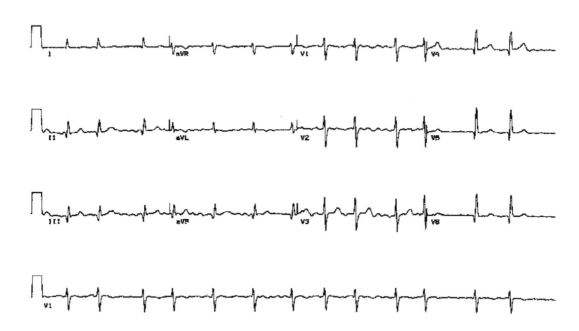

Do you see Q's anywhere else here? Are they large enough to worry you?

Whew! Reading EKGs takes it out of you, doesn't it? Can we go out for mimosas now?

10- Another one.

Ready to try another one? You sure? You want a sublingual nitro? Me first, I'm the old one...

What's going on this time? Whoa – all kinds of neat badness!

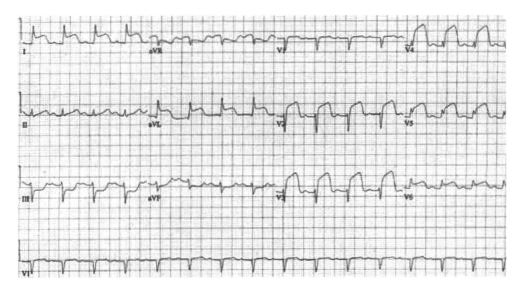

Okay - let's be systematic:

Lead I shows ST elevation, so there's an acute MI going on. Lead I goes with AVL, V5 and V6: ST elevations throughout the lateral territory. Oooh: a circumflex infarct, right?

After starting with lead I, go on to lead II: anything there? Small QRS…how about the rest of the group: III and AVF? ST depressions in III for sure, maybe just a little in AVF. Hmm – lateral ST elevation, inferior ST depression…

Wait a sec – didn't we say a while back that ST elevations always come first in interpretation? So ST elevations laterally…and infarct is always interpreted as the main process…ha! Inferior reciprocity!

Onwards. Where were we? We did lateral, we did inferior, what's left? The chest leads – ok, start with V1. Yow, a q-wave! And it gets worse from there – V2, V3, V4 – big anterior ST elevations that are already starting to form q's…another infarct area!

So there are two areas with ST elevations: the lateral group, and the anterior group. That would mean infarct in the circumflex and the LAD…wait a minute…uh-oh – this guy is infarcting a left main lesion!

Excellent!

11- What are intervals all about?

Remember these? People memorize these, spit them out on quizzes, but sometimes they don't get the real idea. What is an interval, actually?

It's a length of time -how long it takes for something to go from one place to another.

So – what is it that's doing the going? What's moving?

It's the signal – the signal actually <u>moves</u> along the conduction pathways. It would probably look something like an ocean wave – if you were standing somewhere along the pathway, and slowed everything down so that you could watch carefully, you'd probably see the wave coming along at you as it moved along the path. Or you could surf that wave and watch as you passed by the cardiac anatomy.

This first arrow on the left shows the signal as it generates the p-wave – the p-r interval.

The second arrow shows the movement of the signal through the ventricles: the QRS. Which one moves faster?

Who remembers what the T-wave is?

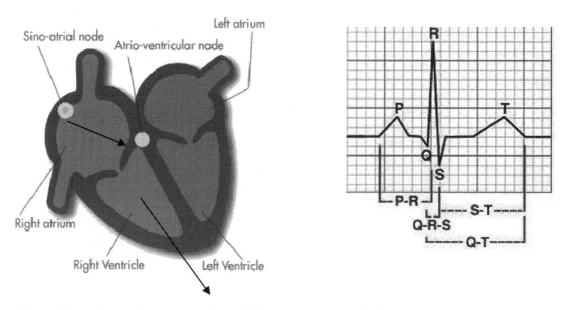

Intervals can be too long, or too short. Makes sense. Let's take them one at a a time:

-PR interval: Too long? Greater than .20 seconds? First degree heart block?

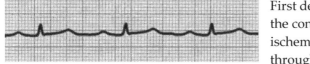

First degree heart block, right? Probably because the conduction system has taken some kind of hit: ischemia, or an infarct, the signal isn't travelling through the atrial tissue at the normal speed.

Too short? What's your patient's heart rate? In the 40's? Why am I asking?

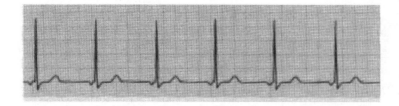

That is short. The rate's not that slow…still, this is probably coming from the AV node. Junctional tachycardia: a faster-than-normal junctional rhythm, with the p-waves going backwards along their normal pathway through the atria. Take a look at the FAQ on arrhythmias for more info on that kind of thing…

- QRS interval:

Now that I think of it, I don't think I've ever heard anyone complain about a QRS interval being **too short**. Other things, maybe…

Jayne points out that QRS's are very short in SVTs…

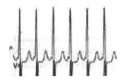

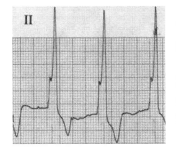

This is more what you tend to see. **Too long**: greater than .12 seconds…probably one of the bundle branches is blocked.

I think the bundle-branch-blocks are going to have to get an article of their own one of these days – mostly because I don't know how to tell the one from the other, myself…

- QT interval:

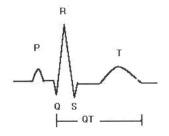

This is the one that a lot of people get worried about in the ICU, usually because it's getting longer than it ought to be. Remember that the QRS is the time it takes for the signal to depolarize the ventricles? And the t-wave is the time it takes for the conduction system to reset? So: the QT interval is the time it takes to do both of those.

Apparently it can be **too short**:

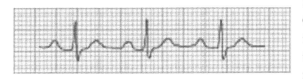

Looks okay to me – the website said this "short QT interval strip" was supposed to indicate that someone's calcium was too high. I think they got this one wrong – long PR interval, maybe?

Too long is what they don't like to see:

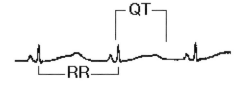

Looks long to me. Dangerous. The heart is taking too long to re-polarize – nasty arrhythmias such as Torsades can result. **Haldol is famous for** (occasionally) **provoking this.**

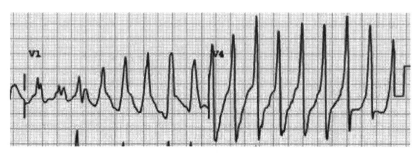

Yup – that's it! If you hang around the ICU long enough, giving haldol now and then, you will definitely come across this one…grab the magnesium.

I seem to remember that this is also why cisapride and – what was that antihistamine that everybody used to take? - Seldane – were both taken off the market.

I'm pretty sure that we used to measure the QT intervals when we were loading patients with oral quinidine – but now as I come to think of it, I hardly remember doing that in recent years. Nor do I remember much else, unfortunately…

Here's the thing: the QT gets shorter as the heart rate speeds up, and longer as it slows down. So what you really need to know is: is the QT interval too long - at all? Regardless of the heart rate - fast <u>or</u> slow? So the thing to do is to calculate the QT interval with the heart rate factored in, and indeed, this is called calculating the "corrected QT interval" – the "QTc".

Happily, our monitoring equipment will actually do this for you – the thing to try to remember is that average of 380 – 400 milliseconds. Longer than 440 milliseconds is too long.

Take a look at the strips on the slide from the website link that appears below. If you got out your calipers and measured the intervals, you'd see that the QT interval is longer at the slower rate, shorter at the faster one. But the ratio of lengths probably stays the same, regardless of the rate. Too long is too long. Dangerous.

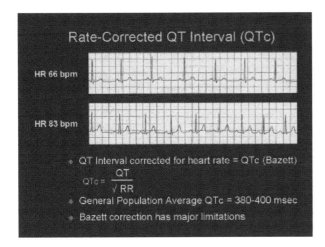

12- What does a 12-lead EKG look like if a patient's potassium is too high? Too low?

Potassium is the main electrolyte that we see causing EKG disturbances in the MICU.

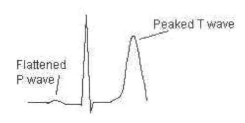

Hyperkalemia. A really high potassium – say, greater than 6.0 – is an unhappy and dangerous thing. You'll certainly be treating that – but the development of the peaked t-waves is what really sets off concern, probably indicating the development of myocardial toxicity.

How would you anticipate treating this?

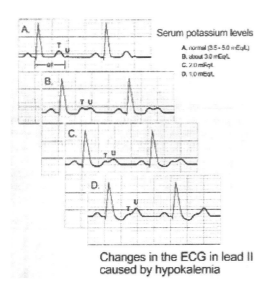

Changes in the ECG in lead II
caused by hypokalemia

This chart is a little hard to read – this is going the other way: **hypokalemia**, getting worse from the top strip downwards. See how the U-wave develops? What's this patient's creatinine, and why do we care?

Cardiologist goes into a bar, sees a cute EP fellow sitting alone: "Hey, nice waves U've got..."

(Hey! No hitting the preceptor!)

Reading EKGs, II – a scary situation, and a big save.

The usual disclaimer goes here: this article is <u>not</u> meant to be an authoritative reference in any way – instead, it's supposed to reflect the thinking and experience of a couple of rather "over-experienced" ICU nurses. <u>Please</u> check with your own local references and authorities on any questions about our content – and let us know what you think!

Special thanks go out on this one to our latest guest editor, daughter #1, Nurse Ruth, RN, who provided criticism, questions, comments, and patience with the project in general!

Here's a really nice example of applied EKG-reading. This was a totally scary, unexpected, out-of-the-blue situation, which we thought would go well as an example of what ICUs are all about.

The scenario was terrifying to start with, although pretty straightforward; young woman comes in through the ER with an acute meningitis: the bad one, turned out to be neisseria meningitidis, which kills at a mile unless treated absolutely as soon as possible. So: young person, not a college student as sometimes happens, but who works in a popular coffee shop. She picks up the big bad bug, which maybe had colonized some customer of hers without causing the disease, and rapidly gets sick: complains of a headache to her roommate at about 5pm, and is found by the roommate, incontinent of stool, at about 10 that night.

A side story: the roommate is a student from somewhere – Bolivia? They're good friends – she literally picks up the sick girl and washes her down in the shower, and then with the help of another friend who also was here from somewhere on foreign exchange - Bulgaria? - the two of them, with about 100 words of English between them, one of which <u>isn't</u> 911, carry her down five flights of stairs, flag down a cab, get in with her with the $25 that they have in the world, and manage to say "hospital" to the driver, who brings them to us. One of the friends apparently carried the girl into the ER in his arms…

In the ER, she's pretty unresponsive, seizes, gets intubated, gets CT scanned, then LP'd. (Somebody in the group tell us: why does the scan need to be done first?) – then started on antibiotics. Comes up to us – an ugly scene. Apparently acute DIC likes to accompany this disease entity: she had little areas of purpura growing in spots all over her; she's gone on a couple of pressors, bacteremia, sepsis…she's very sick.

Couple of days go by. She's still intubated, weaning off her pressors, still on propofol, since every time they lighten her she starts to become uncontrollably agitated, pulling at equipment, lines, not responding to voice…this is actually really good news, because at least she's moving everything. Now the plan is to get keep her safe, finish her antibiotic regimen, and then try to wean her from the vent as – hopefully – her head clears up.

I come in, take report, and notice something odd on the monitor…

Ok new ICU nurses – something's wrong with this picture. What is it?

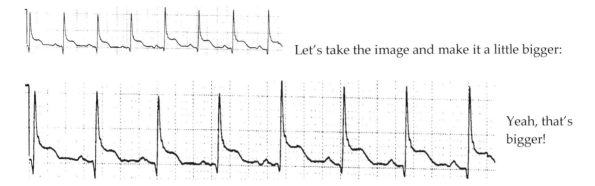 Let's take the image and make it a little bigger:

Yeah, that's bigger!

Anybody see the thing that shouldn't be? Are these normal looking complexes?

This is where a lot of people get a little lost: they've learned some arrhythmias, but for some reason never get a grasp of some of the other, really basic observations that you really have to know about when you start working in the ICUs…yes, there are p-waves. Yup, every p-wave is followed by a QRS complex…but this is not an arrhythmia problem; something else here is very wrong. Scary wrong – so wrong that the appropriate response from you should be something like: "Holy s&*t!"

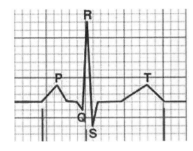

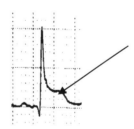

Here's a normal one complex… added…

And here's the problem one, with helpful arrow

See it now? What's the arrow pointing at – which segment? And what's up with that segment? Elevated? Depressed? Cone-headed? So who remembers what ST elevation means?

Holy s&*t!

This is alarming – here is something that is really not supposed to be: ST elevations on the monitor, from a 22-year old kid with meningitis? Say <u>what</u>!?

So – what do you do at this point?

Who said call the physicians? Sounds right to me…

Something to remember – if you're opening this article as a word document, you can click on any of the ekg pictures, then grab a corner and drag them bigger, to see the details more closely…you can then just drag it back, or leave it, and close the document without saving changes – then everything will go back to the original size.

Here's the first of a series of 12-lead ekgs – the times that they were done didn't scan in all of them, but they're in sequence :

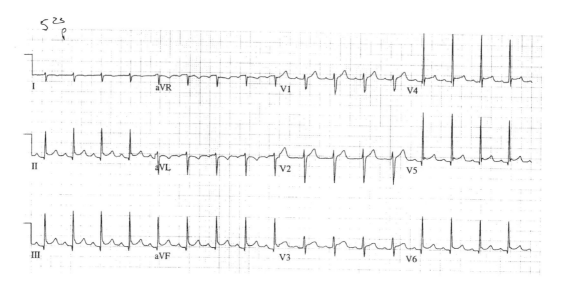

Since it's first in line, lets start with lead 1: don't see much going on. Small complex, maybe – not sure what to make of that. Along with lead one in the lateral group goes AVL, and V5 and V6. (Which coronary artery are we looking at here?) AVL is inverted, with a flipped T-wave, but the other leads look ok, so since the whole group isn't showing a problem, I'd tend not to get very worried just yet. See the non-pathologic q's, however? Little baby q's? Hmm…

Finished with the lateral group – next comes lead 2, along with 3 and AVF. A little suspicious – is there a little ST elevation in the whole group?

What's left: antero-septal leads: V1-2-3-4: v4 might be thinking about something, just a little…

On the monitor, the ST elevations are getting worse – next ekg:

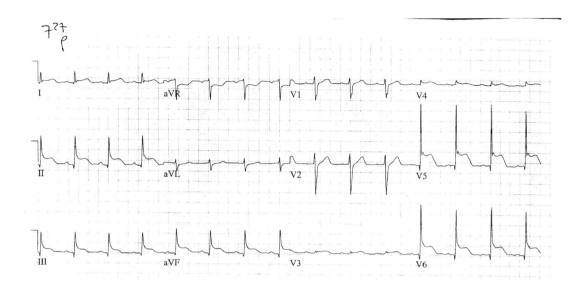

Ack! Worse! See it now? This is bad. ST elevations in...who said two areas of the heart? WTF?

I'm starting to get really unhappy now. The junior resident calls "cards" – the cardiology resident on call for the house, whose response was: "Holy s&*t!" He's on his way down.

Next ekg: even more worse. Everybody sees this, right? ST elevations in two lead groups: lateral/circumflex, and inferior/RCA, right?

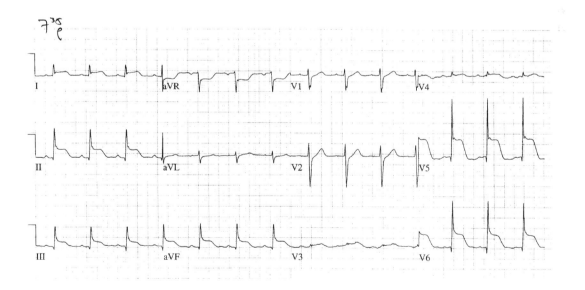

Next EKG, 20 minutes later...you've heard of "tombstones" on an ekg? Those there are them, right there...this s&*t is really evolving rapidly... the cards guy is here.

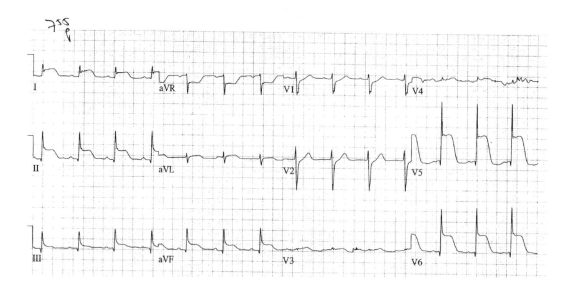

Let's try to anticipate him here – what <u>could</u> be happening? How could the kid be infarcting two areas of her heart at once? Something is blocking flow through two of the main coronary arteries…

There are two main possibilities that occur to my ancient mind:

> 1: - she could have thrown little microemboli to her coronary arteries, which is possible, since she's DIC-ing; two main cores out of three, or

> 2: - she could be having some totally bizarre vasospastic thing going on, and a couple of her coronary arteries have tightened up so tight that they're occluding themselves closed.

The only reason I think of that is that I saw it happen once – years ago. A woman in her 40's, I think, came in, and had an enormous MI – they cathed her, and she had clean coronary arteries…they put it down to severe vasospasm, and I think somebody called it "syndrome X"…

The cards guy arrives, with an echo machine: if the two coronary arteries are seriously and completely plugged, then the echo will probably show that the two areas of the heart they supply won't be moving very much, and the kid may have to go emergently to the cath lab, maybe for stents…

…but they <u>are</u> moving! So the vessels <u>aren't</u> plugged.

Sure enough, the cards guy thinks this is a vasospastic response to something, possibly the propofol that the kid is on.

This has all us old ICU nurses scratching our heads…I mean, we use a <u>lot</u> of propofol! Never seen this! The plan: stop the propofol, (der!), apply some…some what?

Come on now, new ICU nurses, let's apply the process here. You're learning about all those cool intravenous ICU drip meds – some of them <u>tighten</u> up arteries, right? You want to use those here? Nooo, you don't. You want the other kind, right? One of the ones that <u>loosens</u> arteries up. And which one loosens up the tight coronary arteries? Nitroglycerine? Perfect choice! Loosen up those arteries!

All of the arteries?

Wait a minute – isn't she on pressors? Bacteremic, septic, all that?

Uh - yeah…so?

So that means that we're gonna be giving her one drip to make her arteries tighten up – that's the pressor, and at the same time we're gonna give her another drip to make her arteries loosen up? That sense makes?

Hope so! The idea is that the nitro is going to specifically loosen up the coronary arteries – does it work with that much specificity? Who the heck knows? We need to try something though, because we've got a four-hour window here before this acute myocardial injury turns to necrosis…and long before then we're going to have to decide whether or not to take this kid to the cath lab and start drilling, or stenting, or…yeesh!

We sneak on a <u>little</u> nitroglycerine – straight drip, 100mcg/minute, just to see if the kid is going to bottom out her pressure in response to it or not…then we crank, and get it up rapidly to 500mcg, sort of arbitrarily – this is the middle of our usual dose range, which sort of ensures that you're both giving a hefty dose, and that you still have room to give lots more if you want to…

Next ekg, about 15 minutes after cranking up the nitro: what's happening? You're looking at the same areas, right? – inferior and lateral. Is anything changing? This ekg is a little noisy, patient moving around, maybe…

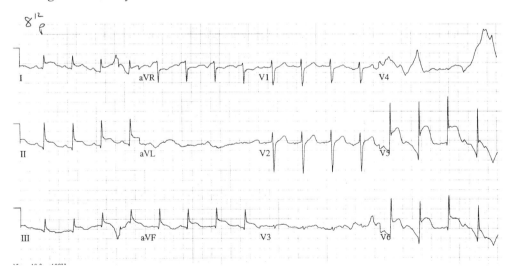

What do we think? Anything happening?

Well – how would you know? What is it exactly that you're hoping is going to happen? Let's visualize: two of the coronaries are so tightly spazzed that nothing – hardly – is getting through them. Along comes the nitro – what's supposed to happen? So what's supposed to happen on the EKG?

Thirty minutes - how about now?

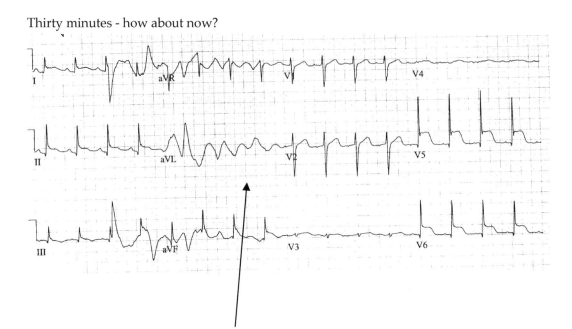

Why are we <u>not</u> worried about what this might be?

And now? About 45 minutes.

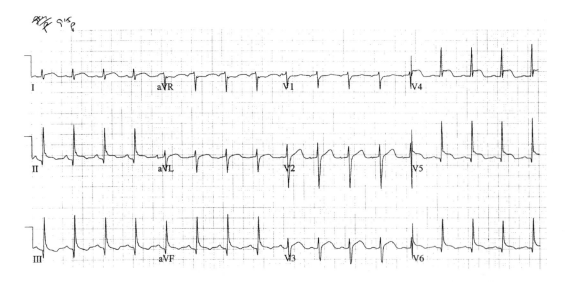

Here's the last in the series, about 3 hours along…whew!

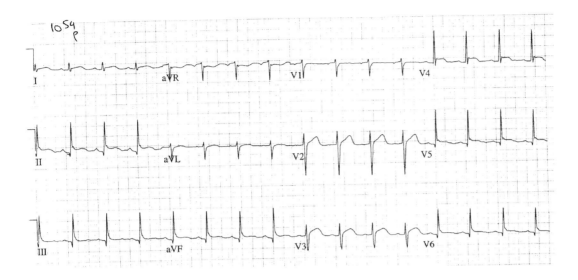

Big save! Never happened again- the kid went on a low-propofol diet, which made things a little complicated for the neurologists and their wakeup regiment – we wound up using fentanyl, then changing to versed, which alllowed us to keep her safely sedate, and to lighten her when needed - but nothing works or wears off as quickly as propofol, which makes it ideal for quick neuro checks like that. She weaned off the nitro within the day – weaned off the pressors, weaned off the sedation, the vent, got extubated, was totally nuts and confused (but increasingly verbal, moving all fours, all that good stuff), said a lot of really interesting things, went to the floor, and last we heard, went home! Fabulous! Intensive care!

X-rays

It's just my opinion, but I think that ICU nurses should have some basic (really basic) idea of how to look at x-rays of some of their "tools of the trade": ET tubes, central lines, PA lines, maybe a couple of others. Obviously you aren't going to be trying to compete with physicians in reading them, but still I think it's useful to be able to look at a stat film and say "Gee, it looks like that ET tube is in the right main stem." Or "Wow, no wonder the PA line is stuck in wedge, look how far in it is!" Things like that. So I went out on the web and surfed around, and I found some film images that may be helpful.

As usual: please remember that this material is not meant to be an official reference of any kind – it's supposed to reflect the experience and knowledge of a preceptor as it is passed on to a new RN orientee. Also please let me know when you find errors or omissions – we'll put them in right away.

A word about the x-ray images: film images can be impenetrably hard to read, even if you have, as radiologists are said to have: x-ray vision. (Ha!) A lot of these images are clearer on the computer screen, I guess because the resolution is lots higher than what's produced by most printers. Mine, anyhow. Try a laser printer, or try looking at the pictures on your monitor and adjusting the contrast - sometimes it helps.

1- What is an x-ray?
2- What are some common x-ray procedures that my patients may have in the MICU?
3- Who takes x-rays?
4- Who reads them?
5- What is a stat film? How stat should stat be?
6- Can I stay in the room if my patient is being x-rayed?
7- What are those clip things that the x-ray techs wear?
8- It seems like my patient has been x-rayed twelve times today – is that safe?
9- Who was Roentgen?
10- Is it true that Marie Curie glowed in the dark?
11- What about Pierre?
12- What is a CAT scan? What is a spiral CAT scan? How long to CT scans take?
13- What is a CTA?
14- What's the difference between a CT scan and an MRI?
15- What is an MRA?
16- Why do some tests use contrast?
17- What's the connection between IV contrast and renal failure?
18- What is this I hear about mucomyst? Bicarb?
19- Do we give contrast in the MICU?
20- What kind of IV access does my patient have to have to get IV contrast?
21- What about Gastrografin?
22- What is the problem with Glucophage (metformin)?

1- What is an x-ray?

Here's what I know – I mean, I could look up all sorts of information, but this is supposed to be what your preceptor knows, right? Is your preceptor a medical physicist? No! But can your preceptor work an intra-aortic balloon pump, a CVVH machine, and a Zoll pacing box (how about one at a time, okay?) Hopefully!

So: x-rays are a kind of dangerous but useful ionizing radiation. They produce images on silver-coated film that lives in the x-ray plates that we're forever putting behind one part of our patients or another.

The dangers in exposure to x-rays are two: how much power they use to shoot, and how close you are to the shot. "The exposure varies inversely with the square of the distance from the source." Meaning: that your risk of exposure drops a <u>whole lot</u> when you get away from where the machine is pointing at. So stand way back. I usually stand behind the tech shooting the film (grin!).

2- What are some common x-ray procedures that my patients may have in the MICU?

Our patients get "imaged" a lot. Most of our images are portables, shot in the bed, although all too often patients will have to travel to the radiology suites for CT or MRI studies. Some common situations:

"Plain films":

- After intubation.
- After the insertion of any central line in the neck or chest, or after repositioning a line.
- After the insertion of a chest tube.
- After the insertion of a soft nasogastric tube – in fact, I hear that nowadays there's a push on to get a film after the insertion of Salem sump tubes as well, which to me doesn't seem to make sense if you're getting gastric materials from it, although it might just be in the distal esophagus...
- Whenever your patient looks like they're in worsening respiratory distress.
- To help evaluate "before" and "after" treatment of pulmonary edema.
- Daily to evaluate changes in, say, pneumonia, or any other developing disease process.
- Rarely, we'll have bone-fracture films to shoot, but usually fractures in our patients are stabilized in the most basic way by orthopedics, and then left to be resolved once the more life-threatening problems are settled.

CT scans and MRI's: (starting from the top and working south, and only listing the ones that come readily to mind)

- Head: Any kind of acute neuro event, or symptoms of a neuro event, will often buy your patient a head CT. In CVAs, the critical question is: is it embolic, or hemorrhagic?

- Neck and spine: usually a traumatic neck injury can be "cleared for c-spines" with plain films, but now and again you'll see a CT or MRI for these. Encephalitis and meningitis also show up nicely on CT's, I understand.

- Chest: lots of reasons for chest scans – traumatic injuries, bleeds, tumors, fluid collections...

- Abdomen: also lots of reasons – specific organ disease, fluid or air collections, retroperitoneal bleeds (we see our share of these – lots of our patients get "hardware-ized" in one fem or the other).

- Pelvis: Also for looking at retroperitoneal bleeds, I believe – in the MICU anyhow. SICU patients might have an unstable pelvis after a car crash.

3- Who takes x-rays?

X-ray techs shoot all our films. There are specialty techs who run the CT scanners and the MRI machines. I believe that there is a single tech who does all the portable CT scans. Don't forget though, that on trips to the scanners you are the person in charge of the patient clinically. If you think there's a problem, or the chance of a problem – speak up! The techs are used to this, and are more than willing to help you get the patient through the scan safely. There's a detailed "trip to the scanner" section in the "New in the ICU" FAQ.

4- Who reads them?

Our house officers do quick reads on stat films, but if they have any questions about what they're looking at, there's always a radiologist available in the house to help them out. All the films are reviewed on radiology rounds within 24 hours.

5- What is a stat film? How stat should stat be?

This can vary a lot, depending on how busy the techs are. Stat in my mind really ought to be within 30 minutes at the most. Sometimes it just takes longer…

6- Can I stay in the room with the patient if my patient is getting x-rayed?

I find that I rarely need to – the only time I can think of is if the patient is having lateral decubitus films shot (side-lying – they're usually looking to see if a collection of fluid moves downwards with gravity and "layers out"). It can be hard to keep a patient in this position when they're hooked up to lots of hardware – check with the tech - you may find yourself wearing lead and holding the patient up.

By all means, use appropriate measures to safely, briefly sedate your patient if she needs it for the x-ray. If you're taking your patient off the floor for CT or an MRI, check with the team – if your patient can't be accurately scanned because of agitation, there's no point in making the trek if you can't safely give them sedation to help them hold still.

7- What are those clip things that x-ray techs wear? Should we wear them?

The techs all wear film dosimeters – gadgets that measured their cumulative exposure to radiation over some given period of time. As for nurses wearing them – I need to ask around about this. (Update – the techs said no.)

8- It seems like my patient has been x-rayed twelve times today – is that safe?

It's obviously a question of priorities: will the patient benefit more from having the x-ray studies, or from not having them? Looking around on the web I found an interesting way of looking at the problem: you compare the amount of radiation from the x-ray study with the amount of normal "background" radiation the patient might receive just by lying still in bed, bombarded by cosmic rays, and radon from the rumpus room in the basement. They call this the "Background Equivalent Radiation Time" – or BERT. Here are some of the numbers:

- Dental x-ray: 1 weeks' worth of normal background radiation.

- Chest film: 10 days.
- Upper GI series: 1.5 years (uh-oh…)
- Lower GI series: 2 years
- I understand myself that KUBs use a lot more radiation than chest films do – I always stood way back when we were having our kids…

The website giving this information went on to say that "no studies of radiation to humans have demonstrated an increase in cancer at the doses used in diagnostic radiology…". I'm obviously not trying to do a comprehensive review here – but as far as I went, the information was reassuring. Your milage may vary…

9- Who was Roentgen?

Worth mentioning – he discovered that these strange rays generated by his vacuum tube could pass through certain materials, make interesting images on silver-coated photographic plate. Not knowing what the rays were or where they came from, he called them "X" - like the unknown quantity in an algebra formula.

Here he is:

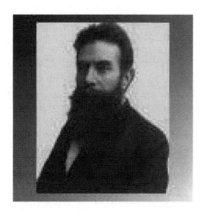 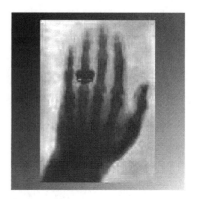

The second picture is of Mrs. Roentgen – part of her, anyway – maybe the first or second x-ray ever taken.

10- Is it true that Marie Curie glowed in the dark?

Neat rumor, huh? My daughter did a report on Marie in high school, and says that to this day they still can't handle her diaries – they're too radioactive.

11- What about Pierre?

I have no idea, but my daughter says there's an old joke:

Pierre: (going to bed at night) Marie, turn the lights out.
Marie: They <u>are</u> out, dear.

12- What is a CAT scan? What is a spiral CAT scan? How long do scans take?

Nurses have a pretty good idea of what CT scans are – they produce a series of "cuts", images across the body working upwards or downwards through the body section in question.

Spiral CTs are a newer kind of scan – the scanning tube rotates continuously as the patient moves along through the scanner – the result is better imaging with lower radiation exposure. Most scans nowadays take less than half an hour – it's transporting your possibly unstable patient to the scanner and back that makes for all the stress. There's a full description of how you might plan and carry out a trip to the scanner in the "New In the ICU" FAQ.

13- What is a CTA?

CTA stands for CT Angiography – the idea is to do a spiral CT scan while IV contrast is injected. CTA can apparently require a lot of contrast – 100-150 ml. This may be a bad thing for your patient's kidneys…CTA seems to be the scan of choice when evaluating PE's and vascular aneurysms of one kind or another.

14- What's the difference between a CT scan and an MRI?

MRI stands for Magnetic Resonance Imaging – it uses radio-frequency waves instead of ionizing radiation to generate an image. The machine involves the use of <u>very powerful</u> magnets – they will pull <u>anything</u> made of ferrous material (iron/steel) right off of you into the machine, and you will not be able to get it out until the techs shut the magnets down – this usually makes them very unhappy. There was a famous story from somewhere about a code cart getting whipped entirely up off the floor…

Likewise, taking a patient with implanted objects can be <u>very dangerous</u> – how about pacemakers? Hip replacements? Cerebral aneurysm clips? <u>Think about this every time you take a patient to the MRI suite</u> – check with the team, and check with the scanner techs to make sure the scan is safe.

MRI scans take much longer than CTs – get orders for appropriate sedation (I find a little propofol in my coffee is very helpful – ow! Oh, you meant the <u>patient</u>!) before you go. Here are a couple of nice images to show the difference in quality:

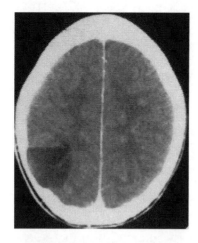

This is a CAT scan of - what? And what's that thing over there on the left? At least it's not pushing everything over to the other side...

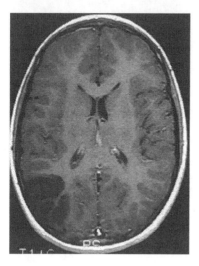

Look a little clearer? Same patient. This is an MRI with gadolinium contrast. The difference is that this is a much more expensive study. I know which one I want my brain surgeon looking at...

15- What is an MRA?

MRA is "Magnetic Resonance Angiography" – which is to say, MRI looking at blood vessel flow, probably using contrast. MRI studies use a contrast material called "gadolinium" - you'll hear the techs say things like: "With or without gado?" Gadolinium turns out to be an element – here's what I could find out about it: "Gadolinium, chelated to a carrier molecule, is an intravenously injected MR contrast agent which ...normally stays in blood vessels...it has the effect of making vessels, vascular tissues, and areas of blood leakage appear brighter." (Thanks Ray Hsu, Washington U. School of Medicine!) So this is what you'll probably see them give when you're looking for a bleed somewhere... "Gadolinium is excreted through the kidneys, with a half –life of 1.25 – 1.6 hours." Gado has the reputation of being very low on the allergic reaction list.

16- Why do some CT tests use contrast?

They help light up the structures that you're trying to see. In CT scanning, the contrast dye is iodine-based – which is why patients with allergies to shellfish aren't supposed to get them. These dyes definitely have dangers associated with them: obviously, some people are going to have severe allergic reactions. The other problem, and we see this one more often than we'd like to, is the fact that a dye load can really, seriously hurt a patient's kidney function, especially if they've got some degree of renal failure already. Here are some of the main points:

- IV contrast dye can cause reaction that is about the same anaphylaxis, and is treated the same way. If a patient reacts it has nothing to do with previous exposure to the dye.

- Reactions occur in less than 5% of the patients who get IV contrast dye. There's an alternative "low-molecular weight" dye that lowers the risk of reaction to less than 1%.

- Hives is what most people show as a reaction to contrast.

- The risk of a fatal reaction is something less than 1 in 100,000.

- Pretreatment helps. Antihistamines and corticosteroids, as well as using "non-ionic, low molecular weight" contrast dyes means lower rates of anaphylactoid reactions. The reaction may not be related to previous exposure, but people who have reacted before may react again – the rate is 17-60%. Asthmatics and people with multiple allergies are at greater risk for reaction.

- Severe reactions are very rare… 1 in 6250 exams using LMW contrast.

17- What is the connection between iodine-based contrast and renal failure?

Here I'm going to summarize one of a really neat series of clinical pearls from the US Army Pharmacy website, edited by Major Dave Andersen. This one was comprehensive yet succinct, and extremely clear. Thanks, Major Andersen.

A 62-year old patient with diabetic nephropathy is booked for a CT scan with contrast. All labs are normal except for a glucose of 135, and a creatinine of 2.4. (Uh-oh…I've been in too many of these situations myself. Can you spell CVVH?) The radiologist is concerned about giving contrast to a patient with a creatinine over 2.0. Is there anything that can prevent or minimize further kidney damage?

Acute renal failure from IV contrast – this they define as a rise in creatinine of more than 0.5 within 48 hours after the dose – ranges from 9-40% in diabetics with mild-to-moderate renal insufficiency, to 50-90% in diabetics with severe chronic renal insufficiency. (Ack! I take my glucophage, don't I? And the doc says my feet tingle because I stand up all night…)

Some summary points:

- Lots of things have been tried.: Ca^{+2} channel blockers, mannitol, lasix, dopamine, others, with little or no success. "Mannitol and furosemide actually worsened renal function more than saline alone."

- The problem is that CT scans of many areas are basically worthless without contrast. (How about going straight to MRI instead? Or is there no advantage?)

- Non-ionic, LMW contrast may cause less kidney damage.

- IV hydration before and after a contrast dose is shown to limit kidney damage. Normal or half-normal saline at a rate of 1ml/kg/hour for 12 hours before, and 12 hours after the contrast seems to be effective.

18- What is this I hear about mucomyst? Bicarb?

A recent study showed that a 600mg dose of Mucomyst (acetylcysteine) on the day before and the day after the contrast dose significantly lowered the incidence of contrast-induced acute renal failure. Anybody know how this works?

Additionally, we've started hydrating patients pre- and post- dye studies with normal saline and sodium bicarb infusions. It looks like the combination of the two saves the most kidneys.

19- Do we give contrast in the MICU?

We give oral contrast in the form of gastrografin. The CT orders have built-in dosing orders to tell you what to do – usually it's something like 7.5cc of gastrografin orally (ack!) or through an NG tube, repeated several times. Check with the team if you're worried about your patient's kidneys. There are template orders and advisories about renal failure built into the CT scan forms to help guide decisions about prophylaxis for contrast injuries.

20- What kind of IV access does my patient have to have to get IV contrast?

We take patients with all sorts of IV access to the scanners, but for some reason the techs down there want the patient to have a plain, garden-variety heplock in one arm or the other. Anybody know why they don't use a central line? Make sure the IV is patent, and in a sizable vein – that contrast gets injected pretty fast…

21- What about Gastrografin?

Appaarently this stuff is very safe to use. It is iodine based.

22- What is the problem with Glucophage (metformin)?

(I took a personal interest in this one…) Glucophage has the rare but unhappy ability of provoking a severe lactic acidosis, especially in renal failure situations. If the IV contrast dose were to push a patient from, maybe, CRI to ARF, then the presence of glucophage in that situation would be a bad thing. It appears that the routine is to hold glucophage for a day before the exam, and for two days afterwards… good to know.

a- Normal Chest Film with Markers

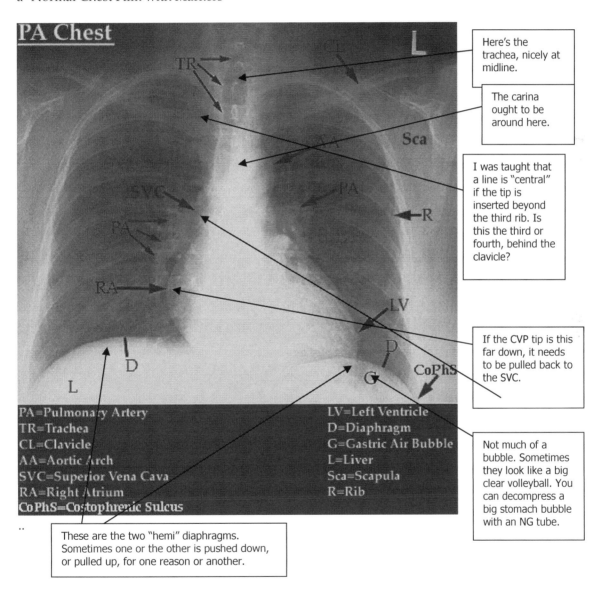

PA Chest

L

TR

Sca

R

SVC

PA

PA

RA

LV

D

D

L

G

CoPhS

Here's the trachea, nicely at midline.

The carina ought to be around here.

I was taught that a line is "central" if the tip is inserted beyond the third rib. Is this the third or fourth, behind the clavicle?

If the CVP tip is this far down, it needs to be pulled back to the SVC.

Not much of a bubble. Sometimes they look like a big clear volleyball. You can decompress a big stomach bubble with an NG tube.

PA=Pulmonary Artery
TR=Trachea
CL=Clavicle
AA=Aortic Arch
SVC=Superior Vena Cava
RA=Right Atrium
CoPhS=Costophrenic Sulcus

LV=Left Ventricle
D=Diaphragm
G=Gastric Air Bubble
L=Liver
Sca=Scapula
R=Rib

These are the two "hemi" diaphragms. Sometimes one or the other is pushed down, or pulled up, for one reason or another.

b- Chest film with a really clear trachea and carina.

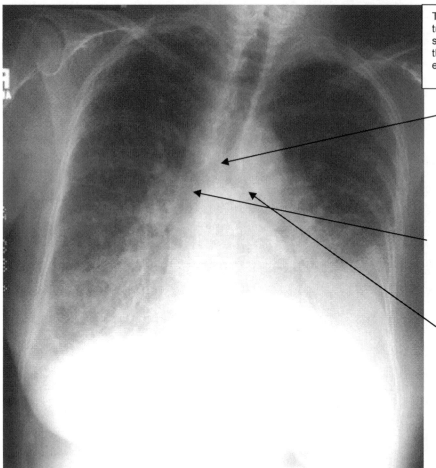

This film shows the trachea, carina, and main stems very clearly – they're not always so easy to see.

Here's the carina. An ET tube that's too far in may poke the carina – this may be why your patient is hacking and choking all the time. Check the film!

The right main stem is where patients often aspirate to - it's more in a straight vertical line downwards than the left one. ET tubes that are advanced too far also usually wind up here.

This is a pretty unpleasant looking x-ray. Compare these fluffy looking lung bases to the nice clear ones in the first picture – probably pneumonia. See how the left hemidiaphragm has been pulled upwards? That's a pneumonia thing.

c- Chest film with ETT and NGT

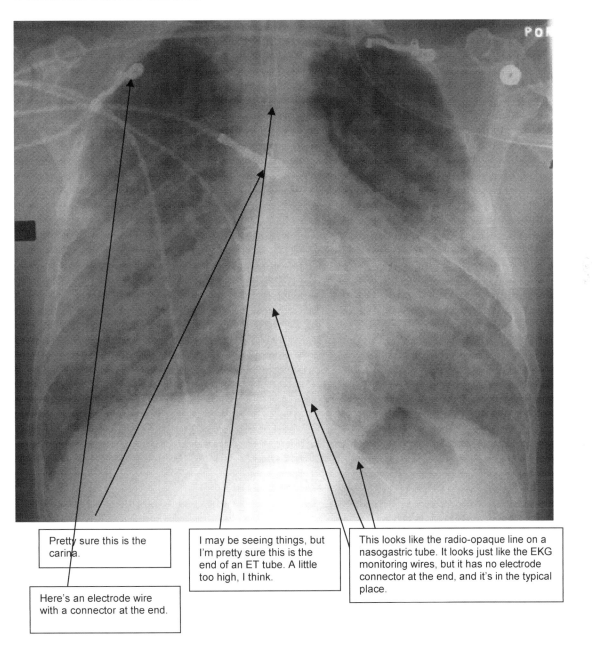

Pretty sure this is the carina.

Here's an electrode wire with a connector at the end.

I may be seeing things, but I'm pretty sure this is the end of an ET tube. A little too high, I think.

This looks like the radio-opaque line on a nasogastric tube. It looks just like the EKG monitoring wires, but it has no electrode connector at the end, and it's in the typical place.

d- Endotracheal tube in the right main stem.

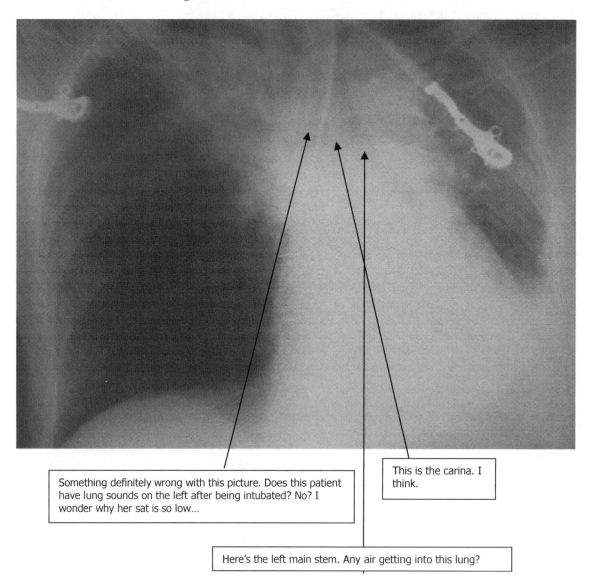

e- ET tube pulled back to the proper position.

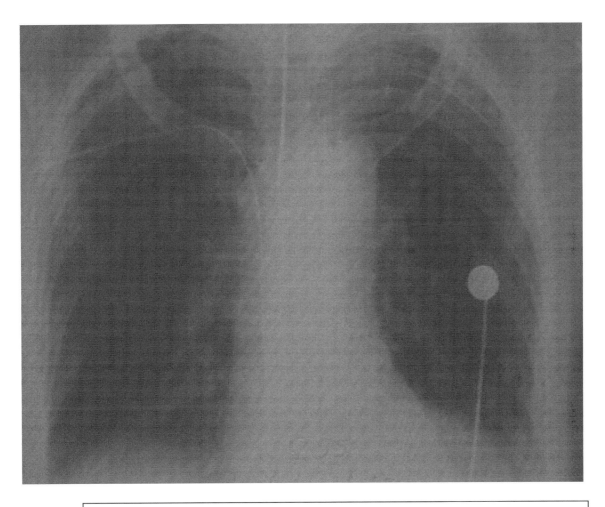

The web site said that this was the same patient, after the tube had been
repositioned (pulled back.) I'm not sure. But anyhow this person's ET tube isn't in
either main stem, and the left lung looks nicely aerated. (I can't see the carina
either.) What kind of central line does this patient have – meaning, is this in the
internal jugular, or the subclavian, or (hey, let's be creative) is it maybe a femoral
line? Is the tip where it ought to be?

f- Chest film with ETT, CVP line, and maybe an NG tube.

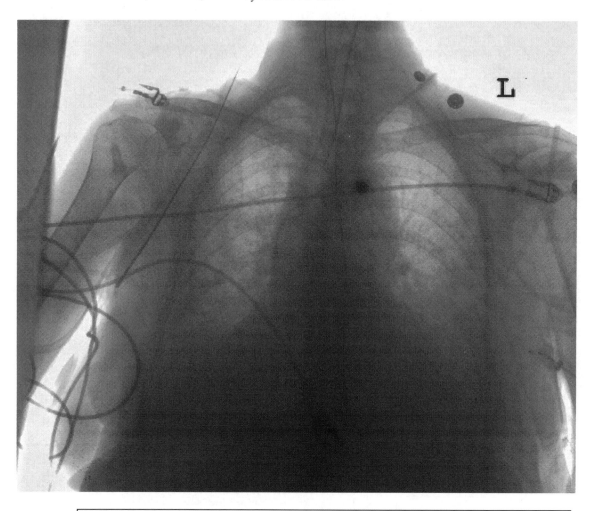

I have no idea why this image came out reversed, but there are a couple of things for you to try to find: ET tube look all right to you? What kind of central line does this patient have? Tip position okay? Is there an NG tube?

g- Chest film with a trach in place, and old sternotomy wire sutures.

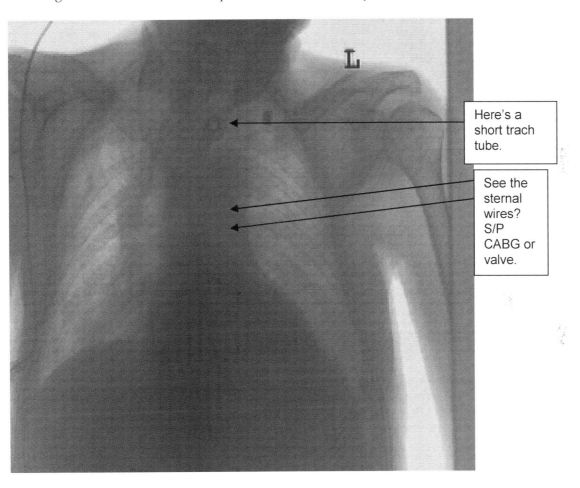

Here's a short trach tube.

See the sternal wires? S/P CABG or valve.

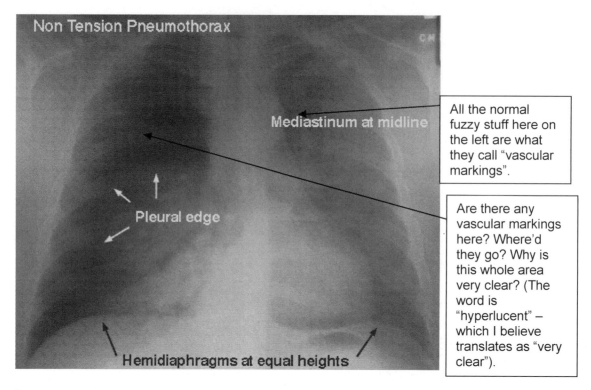

h- A non-tension pneumothorax.

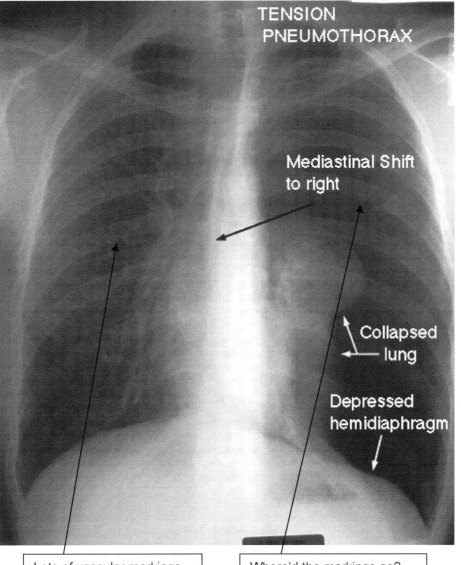

TENSION PNEUMOTHORAX

Mediastinal Shift to right

Collapsed lung

Depressed hemidiaphragm

i- Tension pneumothorax with a really neat mediastinal shift. (I guess the patient doesn't think it's so neat...)

Does everybody know the procedure for inserting an IV catheter into the chest to decompress a pneumothorax? Where does it go? Who puts it in? How far in should it go? What should you hear; and then maybe see the patient do? Fly around the room backwards?

Lots of vascular markings on this side.

Where'd the markings go?

This is definitely a much more dangerous situation than the one before it. This time, the pressure on the pneumo side has steadily increased, and now the heart is getting shoved forcibly over to the other side – definitely classed as a "big bad thing". Which service would you stat page to come see this patient?

Everybody knows how to set up a chest tube, right? And you all know what an air leak is? What maneuver could you make before the surgeons arrive?

If this patient had an arterial line, you might see a nice example of "pulsus paradoxus" – blood pressure that drops with inspiration, and rises with expiration – in fact, this might be your first clue that a tension pneumo might be developing. Take a look at the "Chest Tubes" FAQ for more on this ...

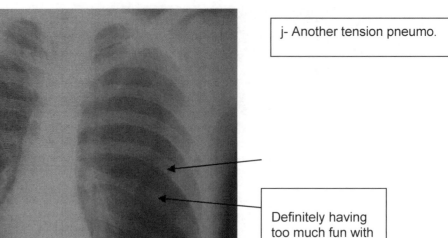

j- Another tension pneumo.

Definitely having too much fun with the arrows...

Why is this hemidiaphragm being pushed downwards?

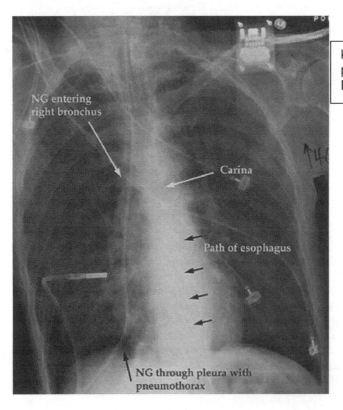

NG entering right bronchus

Carina

Path of esophagus

NG through pleura with pneumothorax

k- an NGT causing a pneumo. Looks like a Dobhoff.

Another really nice image from the Virtual Hospital.

Not a pretty picture, however. See the pneumothorax down there at the bottom? Actually, is there one on each side?

So, uh, did they never hear the phrase: "Stop when you feel resistance!"?

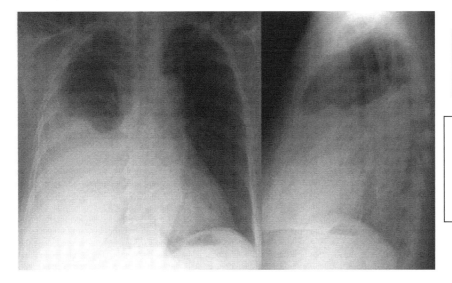

l.- A big pleural effusion.

Pretty big effusion over there on the patient's right. What should we do?

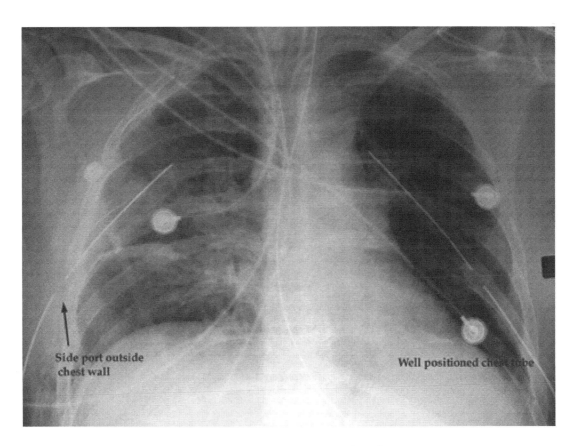

Side port outside chest wall

Well positioned chest tube

m.- A chest film with two chest tubes: one's in position, the other isn't.

Looking at the chest tube on the left – see the break in the line that travels along the side of the tube? That's where the drainage port is. Suppose that chest tube is hooked up to suction through a pleurevac box – what might you hear while standing close to the patient? What could you do about it as a temporary fix? What team would you call if you found this situation, and what would you have ready for them when they came?

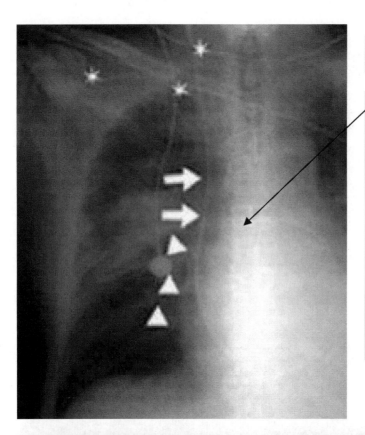

n- a PA line.

Awful picture, but you can see how the PA line curls around as it goes through the RA, the RV, and up around into the PA. My arrow is pointing to where I think the tip is - I think this line is probably not quite far enough in, and won't wedge. If the PA line were to slip back, say, to the RV – how might you know? What would you do about it?

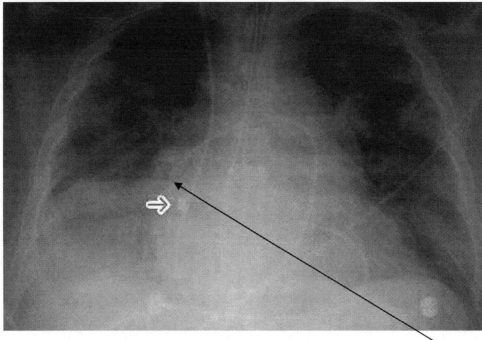

o.- A PA line
an interestin
object nearb

That's more like where a PA tip ought to be. I had to play with the contrast in this image to make the line a little clearer, so it's very dark. Any guesses as to what the white arrow is pointing at? What if I were to tell you that maybe the laryngoscope operator was a little hasty during intubation? Should we call the dentist if the patient codes?

p- An IABP tip. (Really?), and a PA line, probably not in far enough.

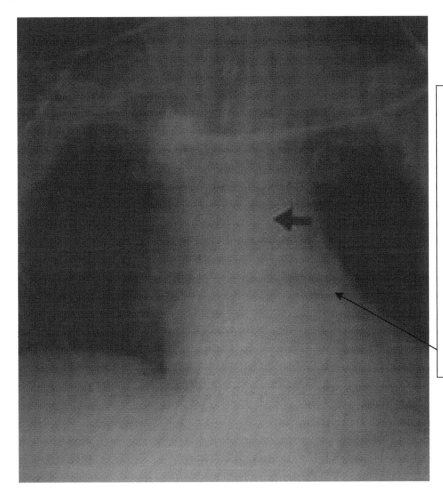

The story here was that the black arrow is pointing at the tip of an intra-aortic balloon pump. I think I see sternal wires, and my arrow I think maybe is pointing to the really misplaced end of a PA line, but I don't see any balloon tip. Which doesn't mean it isn't there...

q.- An abdominal film with dilated bowel loops.

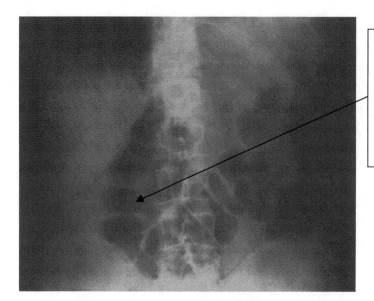

We don't spend all our time looking at the chest, you know. Has your patient been on a fentanyl drip? Gas collection can cause the bowel to distend for all kinds of reasons…time for Reglan? Or a surgeon?

r.- One patient, two films, before and after developing tamponade.

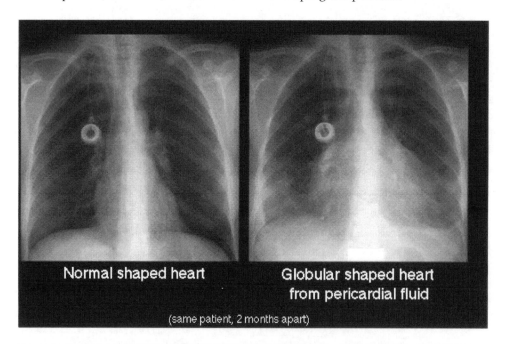

Normal shaped heart

Globular shaped heart from pericardial fluid

(same patient, 2 months apart)

What a difference two months makes! Bet this patient had some rub! That'll teach you not to forget your Indocin! There are three situations where you might see a clear pulsus paradoxus on your a-line wave, and this is one of them: pneumothorax, pericardial tamponade, and really severe dehydration/hypovolemia. Which one is this? The other clue is something you only might see now on the EKG monitor: "electrical alternans" – the QRS complexes are alternately big, then small, then big, then small. They may get a liter (!) out of this patient's pericardium…that's a portacath, right?

Here's a little sample of electrical alternans:

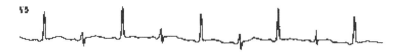

http://ecglibrary.com/elec_alt.html

And here's a sample of what pulsus paradoxus looks like on an a-line tracing:

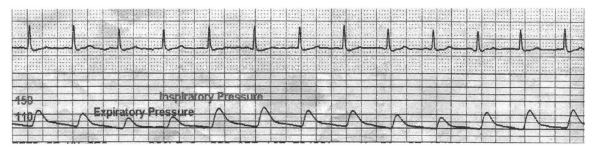

s.- Who is this, and what happened to him?

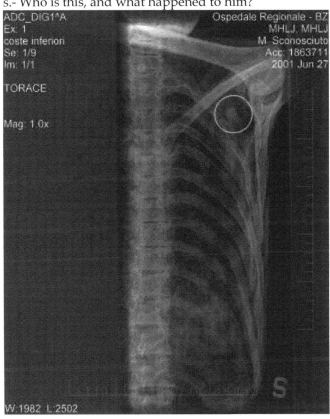

Any ideas? This turns out to be the "Iceman" – the poor guy that was found after being frozen for so long on that glacier in Switzerland. The pointed object in the yellow ring turns out to be the arrowhead that killed him. I thought the Swiss were neutral...

Thanks Iowa! ("Is this heaven?", "No, it's Virtual Iowa...").

One more…

t- The first-ever CVP line.

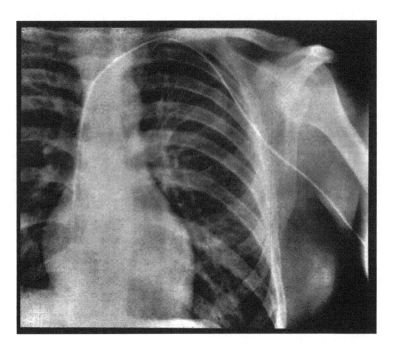

See it there, in white, coming up the left arm? This is apparently the original famous photograph taken by Werner Forssmann, back in 1929. Apparently in the grip of enthusiasm, he threaded a urologic catheter upwards into his own arm, then ran downstairs to the x-ray room where he got into a scuffle with a colleague who thought he was going nuts, kicked him in the shins to get by, and then shot this film. The rest, as they say, is – "Hey, would you just throw in a central line already? I can't keep this guy on peripheral neo forever, y'know!"

Sedation and Paralysis

Hi all – here's yet another FAQ file. Why did I get so sleepy writing this one? As usual, please get back to me if you find anything wrong, anything left out, or anything that shouldn't have gone in, and we'll fix it right away! Also as usual, please remember that this is not meant to be a final opinion on <u>anything</u>, but is supposed to reflect the information that a preceptor would pass on to a new orientee…

1- What is sedation?
2- Why do we sedate patients in the MICU?
3- What's the difference between 'regular' sedation and 'conscious' sedation, and why do we care?
4- What sedative drugs do we commonly us in the MICU?
  4-1-What is propofol?
    4-1-1- How much propofol do we use?
  4-2-What is fentanyl?
  4-3-How do we use morphine?
  4-4-What are the 'benzos' that we use in the MICU?
    4-4-1- How do we use Valium?
    4-4-2- How do we use Ativan?
    4-4-3- How do we use Versed?
    4-4-4- What do I do if my patient goes apneic with sedation?
  4-5 - How do we use Haldol?
  4-6- How do we use dilaudid?
5- How sedate does my patient need to be?
  5-1- Something to think about…
6- How do I document my patient's level of sedation?
  6-1- A sample nurse's note.
7- What should I do if my patient is oversedated, or undersedated?
8- How do we wean sedation?
  8-1- Weaning propofol
  8-2- Weaning 'benzos'
  8-3- Weaning fentanyl
9- What is paralysis?
10- Why do we paralyze patients in the MICU?
11- What drugs do we use for paralysis?
12- How paralyzed does my patient need to be?
13- What if my patient isn't paralyzed enough?
14- How do I assess my patient's level of paralysis?
  14-1- Problems with our paralysis system…
15- How do I assess my patient's level of sedation "under" the paralysis?
  15-1- What is BIS monitoring all about?
16- How do we wean paralysis?
17- How do I tell if my patient is ready for a wean?
18- What is a "paralysis holiday"?

19- How do I tell if my patient isn't tolerating the wean?
20- Steroids and paralysis.
21- What are some of the emotional issues around sedation?
      21-1- the patient
      21-2- the patient's family
      21-3- the nurse
22- What if I need sedation?
      22-1- Non-anesthetic techniques.
      22-2- Anesthetic techniques.
      22-3- What if I don't have kids, I hate cats, and I don't like horses either?

Sedation

1- What is sedation?

Sedation is actually used to mean two things in the ICU, because we have two goals: to either:

      - make the patient sleepy for one reason or another, or
      - give the patient pain relief, or
      - both,
      - safely!

To do this, we use a number of different meds in drips and pushes, depending on what we're trying to do. The meds may seem confusing at first, but mostly they all belong to only a couple of families: opiates, benzodiazepines, meds like haldol, and specialty meds like propofol. Sometimes we use meds like benadryl, but that hardly counts as ICU-type sedation…

2- Why do we sedate patients in the MICU?

Most often we sedate patients because they're fighting a ventilator, or because they're at risk for injuring themselves: an intubated patient with various invasive lines may become abruptly confused and start trying to climb out of the bed, either with or without those lines – this can lead to all sorts of dangerous situations, and it is your responsibility to keep your patient safe. There's a lot of debate about the legality and ethics of restraining patients, but there's not much disagreement that patient safety comes first.

Ventilation-dependent scenarios often require sedation, for a number of reasons. One of the simplest is that an agitated or confused patient may bite, hard and continuously, on his ET tube. Obviously a bad thing. I've seen patients code as a result of this – no oxygenation. (What's the common thing that patients will do, when they become abruptly hypoxic? How would you treat it?) Similarly, a patient in a serious respiratory situation – say, on 100% FiO2 for ARDS – can't be allowed to fight the ventilator, for the simple reason that she won't get oxygenated if she does.

A key concept in sedation: don't overdo it. You really want to keep the patient comfortable and free of distress or pain, but you don't want him anesthetized to the point where you can't assess his mentation. In fact, Jayne says that the Association of Critical Care Medicine's rule is that sedated patients need to be lightened every day – this really does make a lot of sense. Now that there are technical means of measuring sedation depth (BIS monitoring), it's apparently been shown that ICU patients are often oversedated, which keeps them in the unit longer, etc. - so by all means, if you need to, use the sedation that the situation requires, but remember to back off, and try to find the minimum amount required.

Another thing to keep in mind: <u>why</u> is your patient becoming confused? Obviously if your patient is at risk, your goal is keeping them safe, and that may mean quickly applying one form of sedation or other – but in the back of your mind you need to be thinking about what the causes might be. Just as a quick example, I remember a patient who became acutely confused: a relatively young man, maybe late 30's, who was otherwise stable, suddenly became agitated, frightened, very confused and combative – and we had no clue why. We did what we had to – as I recall we gave him some IV Haldol, and put him in soft restraints, but the medical team called the resident from the Acute Psych Service to look him over. To my amazement, they decided that his confusion was being caused by his cimetidine. This, I never heard of. Turned out they were exactly right. Remember that APS is always available to help sort things out if necessary.

Which brings up another critical point: what if the patient is adamantly refusing treatment? What if they're refusing and making sense? Or not making sense? Or intermittently making sense? (My wife says I usually fit in that last group…) Is the patient competent to refuse? Just make sure that you're not unlawfully attacking the patient – if there are questions of competency involved, Acute Psych gets a call.

3- What's the difference between "regular" sedation and "conscious" sedation, and why do we care?

I would call the main difference between regular sedation and "conscious" sedation scenarios the fact that the first group is usually intubated, and the second usually isn't, which can make things tricky. This second group is often going through a procedure like endoscopy, and there are a couple of key things to keep in mind:

Is the patient able to guard her airway during the procedure, or is she at risk for aspiration (how full is her stomach?), or airway obstruction?

Is she breathing at an adequate rate, or is she at risk for respiratory depression? Remember: an O2 saturation monitor <u>won't tell you</u> if your patient is breathing at a rate of 4, or even at a normal rate but much too shallowly, and becoming hypercarbic…<u>use your eyes</u>.

4-What sedative drugs do we commonly use in the MICU?

4-1- What is propofol?

Propofol is a very useful sedative drug. It's very powerful, and it both works very quickly, and wears off very quickly. This makes it very useful when you need to gain control of a situation in which, say, the patient is trying to extubate himself and climb out of the bed – it is also just as useful when you want to try, say a day later, to see if the patient has become more alert, and able to tolerate ventilator weaning.

A couple of important things to remember about propofol:

- It has no effect on pain at all. People get a little confused on this point at times. Propofol is not the drug to use alone when you have an agitated, intubated freshly postop patient.

- It is a very powerful respiratory depressant – **it will make your patient stop breathing**. This is not such a big deal when your patient is intubated, but you'd better be at the bedside and watching while it takes effect – if your patient is on some ventilator mode that lets him breathe for himself, he may suddenly need to be "put on a rate". Hospital policy: propofol patients must be on mechanical ventilation. There has been one exception in the past: we've gotten permission occasionally to run no more than 30mg/hour of propofol on patients who are getting face-mask ventilation. It's a situation I don't like from the get-go: here's a patient who's at risk of getting her stomach all inflated, and then you apply a sedative that may lower her ability to guard her airway – what if she then vomits into the mask?

4-1-1- How much propofol can we use?

Propofol is powerful medicine – it's easy to make a person lose blood pressure as well as respiratory drive. Depending on how large a patient is, I would start with 30-50mg per hour. Bolus doses can be given – we usually give 10-30mg boluses depending on what the patient needs, and we have an hourly limit of 300mg – this is a lot of propofol, and is usually enough to sedate anyone. (Not always! The trick to effectively sedating a patient often lies in finding out "What's their drug?" – some people never do well with Ativan or Versed, but respond excellently to Haldol. You have to try different things in different situations.)

A couple more things to remember about propofol:

- It's very easy to grow germs in propofol – like TPN. The tubing for syringe mixes needs to be changed (along with the syringe) every six hours, and the tubing for bottle mixes every 12.

- Run propofol alone.

- Let nutritional support know about the propofol – since it's mixed in a fat emulsion, they may need to decrease the amount of fat the patient gets.

4-2-What is fentanyl?

Fentanyl is a chemical cousin of morphine - an opiate. It's powerful – the doses are measured in micrograms - but like propofol, it's short-acting: works quickly, wears off quickly. We use fentanyl for patients who need long-term sedation, such as those with ARDS or BOOP – sometimes along with benzos prn.

The loading dose for fentanyl is 50-100mcg (at 50mcg/cc) by slow IV push – roughly 50mcg per minute. A drip can follow up to 200mcg per hour, or so says the policy, but I know that we've been authorized in the past to run higher doses when needed.

Things to remember about fentanyl:

- People develop tolerance to fentanyl pretty quickly – after a couple of days on a given dose, you may find that the patient needs more. Or not. Use your assessment skills. Does the patient have liver failure? Is the patient already drug-tolerant? Is the patient getting ready for extubation? Always try to fit the use of the drug to the situation at hand.

- Remember that opiate drips can always produce a paralytic ileus – this can ruin your plans for nutrition with tube feedings. (Save a port on every central line for TPN!) You'll see teams try giving narcan to try to get the gut to wake up while the rest of the patient stays asleep – there may be studies that show that this works, but I've never seen it do much. More recently they've tried erythromycin – anybody know if this works or not? Apparently neostigmine has been used this way with really impressive results.

Fentanyl will produce the small-pupil response that lets you know your patient is pretty well opiated. What if her pupils don't go small – what if she doesn't respond to the drug? What might be wrong?

4-3- How do we use morphine?

We don't use morphine drips much anymore – I seem to remember that one of the reasons that we changed to fentanyl is because morphine tends to provoke histamine release, which gets seriously in the way of asthma management. Still, morphine drips show up now and then, so a quick review of the policy:

- IV pushes can be 1-20mg over 4-5 minutes

- Drips can be 1-150mg/hour, titrated to response.

Remember that morphine can suppress respiration, that it can drop blood pressure, and that it can also create an opiate ileus, which may mean that your patient will starve for a week while you wait for the team to decide that it's time for TPN. It will also make patient's pupils shrink very small, like fentanyl. This isn't a bad thing in itself, but you can use it as a marker – if you shut the morphine drip off three days ago, and the patient's pupils are still tiny, then they may have a problem "cooking off" (metabolizing) the drug…

4-4- What are the "benzos" that we use in the MICU?

We use three "benzos" in the MICU: Valium, Ativan and Versed – although lately not much Valium, it seems to me. Just recently we've started using benzo drips: Ativan and occasionally Versed – I couldn't put my hands on policies for these drips right away, but they are cleared by pharmacy- check with them for any question, any time.

Update – lately we've shifted back to valium drips, specifically for etoh withdrawal. Got to be careful with this, if only for the fact that valium is really rough on the veins. Make sure you have a good blood return, that you're using a large vessel, that the site isn't starting to look unhappy… wow, these patients soak up a lot of drug!

Here's an interesting point: it turns out that ativan is renally cleared, while valium is cleared through the liver. When taking care of alcoholic patients, why would this be a useful thing to know?

4-4-1- Rules for using Valium:

- IV pushes are 2.5 -10mg, at 5mg per minute.

- For status epilepticus: 10-30mg at 5mg per minute.

- For delirium tremens – this gets a little hazy, and if this situation came up I would call pharmacy for guidelines. In my "too-many" years of ICU nursing, I've seen situations where people in acute DTs were given truly impressive amounts of IV Valium with no apparent effects on blood pressure or respiratory rate.

4-4-2- Rules for Ativan:

- For anxiety or agitation, we can push 1-4mg IVP

- For status epilepticus: 2-8mg IVP

- IV Ativan has to be diluted with NS to make a 1mg/cc concentration – it's very irritating to veins.

- Maximum dose in 24 hours: 30-40mg depending on response. Lately we've started using Ativan drips, and I am pretty sure I've seen them running at least at 3 or 4mg/hour, which would mean a daily total of what – 3 or 4 times 24 hours – more than the current policy limits. These drips are cleared by pharmacy – I'll follow up with them and get the latest info…

4-4-3- Rules for Versed:

- For anxiety or agitation: 0.5-2mg IVP.

- For maintenance: 1-2.5mg/hr. (I've seen patients arrive from other hospitals on versed drips, but I think we've only run them ourselves once or twice.)

- Maximum dose in 24 hours: 20-40mg depending on response.

- Policy says that these patients must be ventilated, or the med given in the presence of an MD trained in airway management. This is definitely for real – elderly patients seem to stop breathing very easily with versed.

4-4-4- What do I do if my patient goes apneic with sedation?

Let's stop and talk about this one for a second... what would you do if you gave your un-intubated patient a dose of versed, and they stopped breathing? First of all, you want to remember to be alert to this risk in the first place, right? Every time, right?

Okay, so there you are, and they're doing an upper endoscopy, and they've ordered you to push two mg of versed, and you do... and the patient stops breathing.

- First move? Tell the doctors doing the procedure that the patient has gone apneic. The scope needs to come right out. You are calling for assistance, right? You're watching the patient's heart rate and saturation up on the monitor, right?

- Second move – oral airway handy? They keep one in every room, and you know where it is? Put it in you know that little flipping maneuver, right? Know where the ambu-bag is? There's one of those in every room too... but of course you had them both at hand and ready, because you knew that this might happen – you are an ICU monster! (That was a compliment!)

- Third move – airway in place? How's the saturation? Are you bagging them yet? Good O2 flow through the bag? Nice control of the jaw, good chest movement with bagging? How long has it been – two minutes yet? Sat still okay? Heart rate still okay? What does the heart rate typically do if the patient's airway is obstructed? Three minutes – think the versed is wearing off yet? Should be...

Right. Deep breath – you, that is. Nice job. Sat okay? Heart rate, blood pressure, patient's physical skin color all okay? Nicely stabilized situation. Think you need to intubate this patient? Probably not – but is the versed still not wearing off? What drug do you want to have nearby? Do you want to give it or do you want to wait...? Why might you **not** want to give it? (Suppose you'd initially given fentanyl to the patient, or demerol – what drug would you want to have nearby if the patient had gone apneic in response to those...?)

4-5-How do we use Haldol?

We tend to use haldol when people are not intubated, and confused to the point where they may be trying to climb out of the bed, pull out their lines – situations like that, when all your explanations and reassurances aren't helping. It's a judgment call – sometimes benzos are a better choice; certainly if there's any question of ETOH withdrawal.

Here's a question. Why don't we treat impending DT's with alcohol? Seriously? I mean, if it would make the symptoms go away, and make gradual detox easier? Somebody shoot this idea down for me...

Haldol is a bit mysterious to me. Sometimes it works really well, other times it seems to do nothing. And yet apparently small doses, like 1mg bid have worked really well in controlling patients with panic attacks. Anybody know how this works?

The nice thing about Haldol though, is the fact that it doesn't seem to inhibit breathing very much, if at all. This may really be the way to go if you're trying to sedate a patient with respiratory problems that might be made worse with Ativan, or the like.

Rules for Haldol:

Initial Dose: 2 to 10mg IVP doses may be repeated every 20 minutes, up to 20 mg in one hour. 24 hour cumulative total dose is 240mg. (That's a lot of Haldol. Maybe that patient needs something else...)

Be careful of overdoing it – the drug can build up, and the patient may wind up knocked out for a long time.

Very important – and this turns out to be more important than we ever thought for a long time: be careful when using Haldol with cardiac patients, or even in non-cardiac patients. Haldol can prolong the QT interval, which is the bit with the line under it, below:

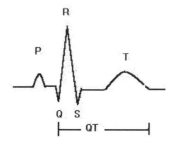

This increases the risk for something really unpleasant like "torsades de pointes" – also known as polymorphic VT, which sort of looks like a tornado on it's side on the monitor, in case you've never seen it. It has tornado-like effects on blood pressure too. We've actually seen haldol blamed for this several times over the years...

http://www.fbr.org/swksweb/ecg_long.JPG

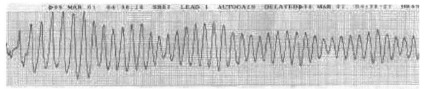

Nice strip!

http://www.ekgreading.com/AVB_torsades.jpg

So - what do you do for torsades?

4-6-How do we use dilaudid?

We've just started using dilaudid drips in the unit recently, as there seems to be a national shortage of fentanyl. (What, did the crop fail, out there in Idaho?) We run a drip of 1-20mg per hour – keep in mind that dilaudid is powerful stuff – according to a web reference I found, a milligram of dilaudid is roughly equivalent to 7 or 8 milligrams of morphine.

5- How sedate does my patient need to be?

Generally there are two goals for sedation: keep the patient safe, and/or keep the patient in "synchrony with the vent" – which is to say, to keep them from fighting the ventilator. We actually have a sedation scale on our flow sheets, which ranges from zero for "anxious and/or agitated", to 5 for "unarousable – does not respond to mild prodding or shaking."

Usually for ventilated patients, we shoot for somewhere around 3: "Drowsy/sedated, responds only after name is called loudly…" Of course, if we're trying to wean the patient, we'll lighten him up…

5-1- Something to think about…

Here's a question – we haven't gotten to discussing paralysis yet, but suppose you were caring for a chemically paralyzed patient, who was also on, say, a fentanyl drip. This patient is not going to "respond to mild prodding" in any way that you could see – or are they…? How could you tell if your patient was not sedated enough under their paralysis – say, awake and terrified at being unable to move? Or too sedated? Think this one over as we continue.

6-How do I document my patient's level of sedation?

Use the numbers on the assessment scale, but describe the patient's neuro status in your note. It doesn't have to be super detailed, but it should always cover the basics – first, are they in the same neurological state as they were when you started the shift? Pupils the same? Moving all extremities? No enormous, detailed assessment, but you sure want to know if a patient has blown a pupil on your time, and sedation will certainly hide symptoms – your assessment should be ongoing throughout your shift. Is the level of sedation meeting the patient's needs? Did you need to change it? How come?

6-1- A sample nurse's note.

Here's a sample of how I might write a note. Let's pick a scenario – say, an elderly patient who comes in, and who's been intubated in the ER for a COPD flare. She was given Ativan in the ER, because she'd been very combative and confused, and she'd needed sedation for a CT scan before she came up to the MICU.

Now she's been with me for six hours – it's 6 am, and I'm writing my note:

#2: Potential Alteration in Mental Status : Pt. arrived from CT scanner after ER admission, very agitated despite repeated attempts to re-orient, coughing and asynchronous with ventilation– per discussion with team, started on propofol at 50mg /hour with only fair effect, still trying to climb OOB despite explanations, reaching for ET tube – propofol titrated up to 120mg/hour with smooth effect, soft restraints x2 to wrists for safety. PERL, MAE with no apparent focal weakness…remains in phase with the ventilator, on PCV rate of 22/min, VT about 500…
In other words: she's not fighting the ventilator, she's safe and not in danger of extubating herself, and her tidal volume looks pretty good on pressure control ventilation (for more on what the ventilation terms mean, have a look at the "Vents and ABGs" FAQ). Make sure – right away - that the physicians are aware of the fact that you've applied restraints. You definitely have the legal authority and the right motivation in this case to apply them, but there must be an order written promptly, and the need for restraint must be carefully and continuously assessed. Remember – sedation is a form of restraint. What if the patient is completely competent, and is refusing all your treatment? While your first goal is to keep the patient safe when they may be confused, this is always something to keep in the back of your mind.

7- What should I do if my patient is oversedated, or undersedated?

This is why your assessment has to be ongoing. If your goal in the scenario above is to extubate the patient someday – well, you're going to have to lighten them up. So do it. But what if she doesn't tolerate it? Say her respiratory rate goes to 60, and her sat does the same? Yes indeed, you should re-sedate that patient, while informing the team that you are doing it, but – and this is an important "but" – document why you are doing it. No one from the team will stand there and argue with you if your patient is becoming hypoxic, diaphoretic, turning blue, and clearly not tolerating her sedative wean, but you must write down the essential information on your flow sheet while the events are occurring: the sat, the heart rate, the respiratory rate, the blood pressure... and send a blood gas while they look awful, to document their poor response to the wean. And another one afterwards to show how they benefited (or didn't) from re-sedation. This is the whole point of the exercise: to show what helps the patient, and what doesn't, and why.

Another critical point: in a situation like this, make sure the team is in close touch, that they understand every move you make, and why you made it. Don't be put off if they're deep in rounds discussion, or anything else – if your patient is in trouble, respond within the limits of your orders, get help from your teammates, drag those doctors physically into your patient's room, and keep them there until your patient is safe. Remember the essential point of survival in the ICU – always get help.

Let's do another example. Same patient, next day – lady with COPD, who was intubated, and needed sedation for agitation during a CT scan, right? Team makes rounds, says: okay, let's lighten her up and see if we can extubate her... you're not sure if this is actually going to be the way things go, but we do need to see how awake she is under her sedation... they have you turn the propofol off. Twenty minutes later, she's doing all those bad things we listed above – she's wild, blue, pulling at everything, tachycardic, she looks awful, maybe ischemic, she's sweating...

First move – get on the intercom, call to have the team come to your room immediately.

Quick second move- jot down the vital signs, whatever they are, somewhere – on a paper towel maybe. At the same time, keep your eyes on the patient and the monitor...

Third move – if you can, draw a quick blood gas, and get it sent off. Ask someone to send it for you – don't leave the bedside with your patient in trouble.

Fourth – got your propofol ready to restart? Team in the room? Everyone agrees? Start it back up, maybe with a little bolus first. Note the time – write it down.

Make sense? Sedation is a tool in your kit – and you have to use it! But do it by making the rules work for you, and for your patient.

8- How do we wean sedation?

Actually, you need to start thinking about weaning sedation as soon as the patient is started on it. This doesn't mean that you have to do it right away, but you do have to have some idea of where you're trying to go. Clearly, a patient who needs sedation to stay safely in synch with her vent, who is so sick that she clearly can't wean from that vent yet – that patient probably will do badly if her sedation is weaned.

In the event, you just have to do it. Turn the sedation down and see what happens. Document what does happen, and make sure the team knows – even better, pull them into the room and show them…

8-1- Weaning propofol.

The nice thing of course about propofol is how quickly it works, and how quickly it goes away. This makes it ideal for short-term intubation scenarios, say, a COPD flare that comes under control in a day or two. You can turn the propofol off, and the patient will be reasonably awake within minutes.

What would you do if she's not?

8-2- Weaning benzos.

I have to confess that we've been using benzo drips so infrequently that I really don't know much about how this is done- anyone from the group have anything to help out with this one?

8-3-Weaning fentanyl.

This one we do know about – we use a lot of fentanyl for long-term sedation cases, and if the patients have been on it for more than a week to ten days or so, weaning can become an issue. The general rule is to decrease the drip by 25% each day – this doesn't mean that the drip is off in four days; it means that if you start weaning at 1000mcg/hour, then your first move down is to 750. Next day – what's 25% of 750?: 187, subtracted from 750 – second day would run at 560mcg/hour. Next day, 25% less than that. So it actually probably takes something like 10 days… sometimes we'll wean the drip to a certain point and then apply a patch.

The symptoms of withdrawal are usually really obvious – the patients get tachycardic, hypertensive, maybe diaphoretic – clearly in distress, anyhow. Sometimes you just have to go back up on the drip for a while. Or give a small bolus and see if that helps things, at all.

Another anti-withdrawal maneuver that they make sometimes is to treat the patients with clonidine – usually a patch is applied, and the patient dosed po for a day or two until the patch starts to work. Micromedex says that clonidine has been used to control the symptoms of withdrawal to a bunch of things: opiates, benzos, nicotine, and alcohol, blocking the adrenergic release that's involved.

Paralysis

9- What is paralysis?

For some reason, people get confused about the difference between paralysis and sedation. Paralytic drugs do nothing to sedate your patient. Paralyzing drugs must be given with industrial -strength sedation: usually propofol or fentanyl, sometimes both. There are stories you can find in the literature about anesthetic failures in the OR, in which a patient was alert but chemically paralyzed throughout his surgery, and felt it all. Didn't the anesthetist notice all that tachycardia and hypertension? Give a lot of lopressor, did she? Yikes!

10- Why do we paralyze patients in the MICU?

The basic scenario in using chemical paralysis usually involves an effort to gain safe control when a patient is in severe respiratory trouble. Most of the time we can do this with effective sedation, but sometimes we just can't ventilate some patients effectively, and paralysis makes all the difference. I understand that it has to do with relaxing the muscles in the chest walls, and allowing better chest movement (if you want to be really cool, you call this "better excursion".) With better movement comes a larger tidal volume, and that allows for better clearance of CO_2. Remember that ventilation and oxygenation are different (you read the "Vents and ABGs" FAQ, right?) – ventilation specifically means "how well the patient is getting rid of CO_2".

Some scenarios for paralysis might be: severe asthma episodes (status asthmaticus), ARDS, sometimes big pneumonias - any condition that severely affects the volume of air that the patient can move in and out.

11- What drugs do we use for paralysis?

Over the years we've used a lot of different drugs to paralyze patients, including pavulon (pancuronium), and curare, which is the South American arrow poison. (Here's a question: if we are paralyzed by a plant, or sedated by a plant, does that mean that we're physically related to that plant?) Nowadays we paralyze our patients with Nimbex (cis-atracurium), or sometimes with vecuronium. Someone explained to me awhile back that we use the combination of Nimbex and fentanyl now, instead of the older curare and morphine, because they cause less of a histamine release. This can be really important in situations like asthma, which is "mediated" by the histamine-inflammatory thing. What do I know? I just hang the stuff and run it!

Up until just recently we dosed Nimbex by weight, using a range measured in mikes per kilogram, per minute. Lately we've been using a standardized scale of 1-10 mg per hour. It doesn't seem to have made much difference treatment-wise. Nimbex has to be loaded first, 10 or 15 mg, IVB. Usually what I do is give the load, and then start the patient in the middle of the drip range – that way you're not giving too much, but you know you're giving enough that they ought to have some response – then you titrate up or down by effect.

The only other paralyzing agent we see nowadays (rarely) is succinylcholine – anesthesia will use this when they're intubating. "Sux" has the very rare but really terrifying ability to produce super-rapid hyperkalemia… rare but deadly.

12- How paralyzed does my patient need to be?

Remember what your goal is: to keep the patient in synch with the vent, and to improve CO_2 clearance. If you meet those goals, there you are. If you can get there <u>without</u> paralyzing your patient, so much the better!

13- What if my patient isn't paralyzed enough?

Usually this is the way this goes: you give a loading dose – this is enough to initially paralyze the patient. Then you start a drip, which is supposed to keep them paralyzed. Each patient's metabolism is a little different – some patients will 'cook off' a loading dose faster than others, but they are also probably going to be the ones who also cook off the hourly amount they get at a faster-than-normal rate. Which means they may start to move around, drop tidal volume, and fight the vent. Usually we wind up repeating a loading dose, and then restarting the drip at a higher level. To me, it would only make sense in this situation to run the Nimbex at max: 10mg per hour, since your patient is in a life-threatening situation, or you wouldn't be doing all this in the first place, right? Your goal is to keep your patient safe. There's an old ICU nurse saying: "Sometimes your only goal is to be able to say that your patient is still alive at the end of your shift." Don't obsess about whether the next nurse will holler at you because the lines aren't dated – or even if the bed linen isn't clean. This is part of priority-setting – keep them alive. Cleanliness is next to godliness, but alive sometimes comes before clean!

14- How do I assess my patient's level of paralysis?

In the old days (I keep saying that…) there were only two positions on the "paralysis meter": "paralyzed enough", or "not paralyzed enough", and we'd increase or decrease the drip based on how well the patient was responding vent-wise.

Apparently the problem with this was that lots of patients took forever to become un-paralyzed, and they figured out that this was because the little muscle receptors were becoming too "saturated" with the paralyzing agent. In other words, we were giving too much drug, because we didn't have any precise way to measure the response to the doses we were giving, except for observing how flaccid the patients became, and what their response was on the vent. So we were taught to use the "Peripheral Nerve Stimulator".

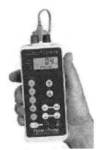

Cute! I love toys…

Here's the idea. The stimulator delivers a series of four electrical signals, (called a "train-of-four" – there's a button that says "TOF" on the box), to a specific site over the ulnar nerve. You hold the patient's hand as though shaking hands, with your thumb hooked in theirs. If the patient is not paralyzed at all, each of the four signals in the TOF will generate a "twitch" response in the patient's thumb – you'll feel it pull against yours: 1,2,3,4. If the patient is fully paralyzed, you won't feel any twitch response at all. Try the twitch with the output dial on the box at different settings – the knob can be set from 1-10. I try 5 at first, and I go to ten after that if necessary, then I try to find the lowest setting that gives a response. The whole procedure doesn't take more than a few minutes.

Here's how it's done. You find the ulnar pulse, and you put two sticky chest electrodes over the line that the pulse follows, moving upwards from the wrist. I put the electrodes right next to each other, with the gel part in the center over the points where I felt the pulse. Sometimes I use a doppler to find the pulse, mark the points with a pen, and benzoin the sites so the electrodes don't get sweated off.

Now you connect the wires of the PNS box, turn the box on with the dial, and try to assess the patient's response. The goal is a response of one or two twitches out of a train of four – meaning, you feel the patient's thumb twitch under yours once, or twice, in response to the first, or first two signals in the train. I guess they've done the studies: this level of paralysis means that your patient will be "paralyzed enough", but will not be so saturated with the drug that it takes too long to wear off.

14-1- Problems with our paralysis system …

There are a couple of problems with this system:

Some people don't seem to paralyze 'normally'. This is a weird but true thing – you can Nimbex load some of these people, and titrate the drip up to max, and they just won't paralyze. Doesn't happen often, but it happens enough that experienced RNs recognize it when it does. Just make sure that the patient is actually getting the drug – an infiltrated peripheral line will make the whole situation that much harder to figure out.

Some people paralyze properly, but they don't 'twitch' in response to the nerve stimulator. Clearly they are paralyzed: they're flaccid, and they respond the right way to the vent, but they won't twitch – maybe because they're very edematous. Some non-edematous people also just won't twitch. Any ideas about this one from the group? In this situation, you have to just assess the patient carefully, as we did in the old days, and try to titrate for the least amount of drug that keeps the patient safely in synch with the ventilator. Obviously, you want to be ready to re-bolus and re-titrate them if they need it. Also obviously, there are situations when the patient is so "tight" – moving so little air – that you wouldn't even want to think about letting them become un-paralyzed even briefly. Make sure that you and the team are clear about the paralysis plan for your patient.

15- How do I assess my patient's level of sedation "under" paralysis?

"I dunno – whadda you think? He looks sleepy enough to me…"

15-1- What is BIS monitoring all about?

This is a pretty neat thing, and provides us with yet another cool toy to play with... BIS stands for BiSpectral Index monitoring – it's a kind of EEG monitor. Apparently it works well enough that the anesthesia people believe in it – so I guess I do too.

The idea is to put a numerical value on the patients' level of sedation, in situations where they might not be able to show you – like when they're paralyzed...

Of course, there's always the old, "Wow, his heart rate is 140, and his blood pressure is 230 – ya think he's not sedate enough?"

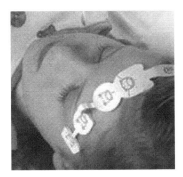

Here's the probe going on. Push hard, because the little wires in the pads have to contact the skin firmly. Not too hard!

http://www.aspectms.com/products/technology/default.mspx

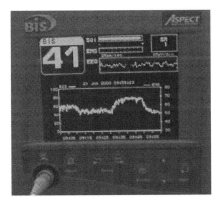

Here's the monitor box. The big number is the one to watch – 100 is fully awake, and zero would be – um... dead, maybe? Too sedate, anyhow - (grin!)

The usual goal for us is 40 – anesthesia tells us that if kept around 40, the patients won't remember much when we wake 'em up. Sounds good to me.

(The question remains: 40 what? I'll look into this and get back.)

http://www.vetmed.wsu.edu/depts-anesthesia/BIS/BIS_41~1.JPG

16- How do we wean paralysis?

Even though we try to titrate the dose and the effect very carefully, the net effect is that the patient is still either 'paralyzed enough', or 'not really paralyzed at all'. So when it comes time to 'wean' a paralytic drug, we usually just shut it off.

17- How do I know if my patient is ready for a wean?

Well, you're going to have to try it sometime. It can be a scary thing to do, if your patient was, say, critically acidotic going into paralysis, and only now is her pH above 7.2. (New RNs- remember why their pH would be so low?, and how paralysis would fix that?)

This is your basic medical judgment-call situation. Sometimes it's quite clear – you paralyze your patient for, say, status asthmaticus – your patient is moving a tidal volume of 75cc. Yikes! Afterwards, using a heliox mix (look at the Vents and ABGs FAQ for a little more on heliox and how cool it is), you get the tidal volume up around, oh, 300cc, running nebs continuously, but you still hear wheezing. Would you want to think about un-paralyzing this patient before their wheezes went away? Noooo, you would not! Judgment call. Suppose a physician came along and told you to do just that. Now what?

Take a look at the "Starting Out New in the MICU" FAQ for some ideas on "What should I do if I think the doctors are telling me to do the wrong thing."

18- What is a "paralysis holiday"?

This sounds like going off on Nimbex to the caribbean, right? Actually, the idea here is to do a 'trial run' off the paralytic, to see what happens. This is a better idea than just having someone give you an order to 'shut the drug off'.

Basic points apply here:

- Watch this patient very carefully if you think they might get right back into the trouble that they required the paralysis for in the first place. Watch them carefully anyway!

- Document what happens when the drug starts to wear off: heart rate, blood pressure, 02 saturation, respiratory rate, tidal volume - mark the times clearly, so that events make sense.

- Send off blood gases to document the patient's response.

- Have a plan ready in case your patient gets into trouble. This is precisely the kind of thing that house officers sometimes don't remember to do, often enough because they've been told by their higher-ups to 'do this', or 'do that' – 'shut off the nimbex – the patient will be fine.' Just make sure you are ready. What kind of plan could you have?

- Make sure the team is fully aware of everything the patient does, and of everything you do, want to do, plan to do, or think you could do. Physically pull them into the room if you think you need them there.

19- How do I tell if my patient isn't tolerating the wean?

This will usually be pretty clear – the patient will go right back into the same set of symptoms that got them paralyzed in the first place. As above, have a plan, and talk very seriously with the team if you think that weaning might be dangerous in the first place - such as that the patient's pH is still 7.10, and maybe that's why she needs so much Levophed? And maybe if she had another day or so to normalize acid-base-wise she could have more room to move on the vent? Sometimes we nurses have to be stubborn this way. Just make your case calmly and clearly, and lay out your reasoning – then document it in your notes, and describe what happened when you tried the wean.

20- Steroids and paralysis.

Apparently steroid myopathy can be made much worse by paralytic treatment, which in the MICU may mean that it will take an extremely long time for the patient to come out of paralysis. Weeks, maybe. We've heard about this for a while now in the MICU - as a result, we try to use deep sedation before paralysis if we can, especially in situations that are going to require a lot of steroid use – like severe COPD flares, or BOOP. In fact, we seem to be paralyzing less frequently lately. Something to remember, though.

21- What are some of the emotional issues surrounding sedation?

This is actually a pretty complicated question. First of all, there are a number of people involved:

- the patient (we knew that one)
- the patient's family
- the nurse caring for the patient
- the physicians caring for the patient

That gives us plenty to start with, so let's take them one at a time.

21- 1- The patient:

the goals here are relatively simple, although achieving them may not be:

- That the patient is given enough sedation so that he is comfortable, free of perceived pain and or distress, during the period that their condition demands it.

- That the patient is weaned from their sedation slowly enough that they can tolerate the process comfortably.

-That the patient is given emotional support and reassurance throughout the whole sedation period. And during a sedation wean. And afterwards.

There are various stories that come back from patients who've been sedated for long periods: most of them don't remember much, which is probably a very good thing! In fact, I'm pretty sure that's why we're seeing more Versed drips, for the "amnestic" effect. ("Huh?" - "It means: so they don't remember nothin…" "Oh - thanks!") But some of them do remember things – it's always been stressed, and I always do this – that you should talk to your sedated/paralyzed patients every time you do things to them, and even when you're not doing anything to them. Reassure them. Tell them that their loved ones called.

A word here about assessment. Your goal is to provide a smooth effect in the patient, right? You don't want to terrify them. Sometimes, passing along messages from loved ones will make a patient's heart rate shoot up. This tells you two useful things: first, they're alert to some degree under there. Second, you might not be sedating them enough. Remember, a patient can be quite terrified under paralysis if they're not receiving enough sedation.

21-2- The patient's family:

Strange to say, that part of a patient's sedation plan may include the family. Families will probably not benefit from seeing their loved one becoming very distressed while being weaned from sedation. Again, this should tell you two things: first, you may be weaning sedation too fast. Second, the family probably doesn't need to be in the room while most of this is going on. It's true that this is partly just my opinion, and this certainly varies from one family to the next. But I think that it doesn't really serve the families well to over-expose them to situations in which the patient may be going through periods of distress. Some distress is probably going to be unavoidable. Would you want to watch every minute of this, if it was your mom? I wouldn't.

I often tell families that they need to leave certain parts of this whole thing to the nurses. That is of course why The Great Supervisor made nurses. And that they, the family members, need to rest, and eat, and care for themselves, and let the nurses take the brunt of all this, because they, the families, need to be strong to get through all of this. And that they need to be strong in case decisions need to be made for their loved one: consents for procedures, getting bad news, even getting good news. It's often a long, tough roller-coaster ride for them.

21-3- The nurse:

Obviously very important, but too often ignored. Among the other twelve million things that nobody knows about nurses is the fact that we bear the emotional brunt of working with these patients, long-term, up and down, year in and year out, at an emotional distance of about eight inches. Maybe four inches.

Here it is in plain words: no one, no one gets as close to a patient, or stays as close to that patient, or is as involved with that patient, or for that matter suffers as much with that patient, as the ICU nurse. The family members go home, the respiratory therapists go from room to room, the physicians make their rounds, but a primary nurse will stay with his assigned patient for as long as it takes. Which may be months. Until the patient either gets better, or until they die. At a distance of four inches. Maybe eight inches. And they follow this career for what, maybe 30 years?

It's worth asking, at some point anyhow, what this does or doesn't do to the nurse as a person. And actually, this is not an unrelated digression here, because how the nurse is coping with all this may affect her perception of her patient's suffering. In other words, is the nurse interpreting her patient's need for sedation through her own colored lenses?

This brings up the question of relative distance. We spend weeks almost completely in bed with these patients, and we sometimes get angry when doctors stand back, and give what may seem like relatively cold, clinical opinions about this, or that point of patient management.

Here's my point: we need both perspectives to be at work at the same time – we nurses do, and the patients do. We need to have people almost in the bed with the patients, tuned into them at close range, and we also need people to stand back and be clinical, more "unemotional". I'll tell you – many of us are soft-hearted, very empathetic, and many, many is the time that we turn to each other and say something like: "Why in the world are they wailing so hard on this poor person? Why can't they just stop all this?". This is not inappropriate. This is patient advocacy.

But! How many times have I been amazed – to see some of these same patients, who with all my experience I honestly never thought would leave the MICU – go out? Go home? Enough times, I'll tell you, to know that the folks standing at a clinical distance are often right not to stop pushing. Not always. But enough to make me think about it, and to force my opinion to change sometimes. Their kind of work is also patient advocacy – exactly the same, except different. (Old joke…)

My point is that I don't think that either of these positions would serve the patient well without its opposite also being in place.
How does this bear on sedation issues? The nurse, depending on her level of experience, life conditions, age, whatever – the nurse may be at risk of being emotionally overwhelmed by her close proximity to genuine patient suffering.

And here comes a real problem. The nurse at the bedside may have trouble handling this daily emotional burden. So there may be difficulties when it comes to how much sedation she may think her patient needs.

The essential thing is: nurses, take care of yourselves. Remember, this is one of the very hardest jobs there is in the world: think about this – eight inches away from the near-dying for 30 years? You have to find a way to either deal with these stresses, or get out from under them. But keep an eye on your heart, and remember that there's no shame if it turns out that the MICU isn't for you – for 30 years, anyhow. And this of course brings us to our next question:

22- What if I need sedation?

I recommend several things, sometimes in order, sometimes all at once:

22-1- Non-anesthetic techniques: (some are mine, some are from my co-workers…)

- Keep a supply of "high-octane" ice cream handy in the unit for the nurses at all times, preferably any flavors containing certain key words: "fudge", "triple", "New York", "chunk"… there are some others. This is not sedation, actually. But when your heart is hurting, it's amazing what Waffle Cone can do…

- Own a cat. Probably two cats, so they can keep each other company. Name them after your co-workers. Don't like cats? Like horses? Go riding twice a week. I like dogs, myself, and I have two, and they understand everything I tell them. About the unit, anyway.

- Send lots of emails to lots of people, check them several times a day, and answer them with weird e-cards attached.

- Take a couple of vacation trips a year if you can, and spend a lot of time figuring out the details. I never get to do this – but I try to have fun at the grocery store. I need to get out more... (It was more fun in the grocery store when my kids were small...)

- Take karate lessons. Two women I work with have been doing this for years, (actually we have a kick-boxer, too), and one of them just got her black belt. Celebrate black belts at work with more ice cream.

22-2- Anesthetic techniques:

I prefer Heineken, myself, at home, with the spouse, and the kids, and the dogs, as a combination with HBO. Or if deep anesthesia is required, as a combination with congressional house tv coverage. Very effective. What were we talking about?

22-3- What if I don't have kids, I hate cats, and I don't like horses either?

Team up with your co-workers and friends. Eat out with friends every day. Eat at home with friends every day. The point is: ICU nursing is a group effort at every level. Don't carry the weight alone.

Blood Products and Transfusion:

Hello all. It's been a while between projects – here's a new FAQ article on blood: components, transfusion, bleeding situations, coag- and anti-coagulation – you get the idea. For this one we asked for audience participation, which came mostly from two sources (who also seem to enjoy this kind of self-torture) – SF and Becky. The material after their answers is mine, and I did the editing, so any errors in this article only come from me. They get a lot of thanks for going over the questions in detail, and taking the time to provide their own answers. They may not yak as much as I do, but they've both been there, done that, and wear the t-shirt. ("My mom transfuses blood in emergencies, and all I got was this lousy t-shirt.") Thanks, ladies.

As usual, please remember that these articles are not meant to be official references, but to represent what an experienced ICU preceptor passes on to a new RN orientee. (Plus some homework to fill in the gaps.) Let us know when you find errors or omissions, and we'll fix them right away. Thanks!

1- What do we use blood for in the MICU?

Blood Counts

2- What are some normal blood values?
3- What is a normal hematocrit?
4- What if the hematocrit is too high?
5- What if it's too low?
6- What is a "dilutional" crit drop?
7- What is a "delusional" crit drop?
8- What does iron have to do with it?
9- What is a normal white cell count?
10- What if the white count is too high?
11- What if it's too low?
12- What are the different kinds of white cells?

- Neutrophils
- Lymphocytes
- Eosinophils
- Monocytes
- Bands

13- What is "bandemia"?
14- What is "band-aid-emia?
15- What is "leukopenia"?
16- What is a normal platelet count?
17- What if the platelet count is too high?
18- What if it's too low?
19- What does "thrombocytopenia" mean?

47- When does GI get called in to look at the patient?

48- When does surgery get called in to look at the patient?

49- What is plasmapheresis?

50- What is dialysis?

51- What is "liver dialysis"?

52- What are some of the situations in the MICU when I would give blood products?

   - Cardiac
   - Pulmonary
   - GU
   - Bone Marrow Diseases
   - Postop Situations
   - Neuro
   - GI Bleeds

53- What do I need to know about GI bleeds?

54- How can you tell the difference between an "upper" GI bleed and a "lower" one?

55- What are "coffee grounds"?

56- What is melena?

57- What is the difference between testing gastric contents for blood, and stool for blood?

58- Why might be GI bleed patient need to be intubated?

Upper GI Bleeds

59- How are upper GI bleeds treated?

60- What is endoscopy all about?

61- Who does endoscopy?

62- What can endoscopy treat, or not treat?

63- What are "bands"?

64- What if the bands come off?

65- What do they use the epinephrine for?

66- Does the patient need to be intubated for upper endoscopy?

67- What kind of conscious sedation do we use for endoscopy if the patient isn't intubated?

68- What is a blakemore tube?

69- Who puts in the blakemore tube?

70- What are the different balloons and lumens for?

71- How long does a blakemore tube stay in?

72- Should patients with varices have NG tubes put in? Taken out?

73- How often should I monitor my patient's counts?

74- What is a TIPS procedure?

75- What is portal hypertension?

76- What is a porto-caval shunt?

77- Why do these patients become more encephalopathic?
78- What is a normal ammonia level?
79- Should I give lactulose to a patient with a GI bleed?
80- Should I give tube feedings to a patient with a GI bleed?
81- Can variceal bleeds be prevented?
82- What is helicobacter all about?
83- How can h.pylori infections be diagnosed?
84- What antibiotics are used to treat helicobacter?
85- What about carafate?
86- What about cimetidine, ranitidine, famotidine, James Dean?
87- What about Prilosec? If a person is taking Prilosec, and has bad breath, do I have to sit Nexium?
88- What about liquid antacids?

Lower GI Bleeds

89- How are lower GI bleeds treated?
90- Do they use endoscopy for this too?
91- How are GI bleeds treated in the angiography suite?
92- What are some clues to tell me that my GI-bleed patient may be heading for trouble?
93- Why does it matter if he's beta-blocked?

Cancer

94- What do I need to know about patients with low blood counts from chemotherapy?
95- What is a nadir?
96- How long does a nadir last?
97- What if the nadir doesn't go away?
98- What is aplastic anemia?
99- Who is Ralph Nadir?
100- What kinds of blood products should these patients get?
101- What shouldn't they get?
102- What is epogen?
103- What is neupogen?
104- Why isn't there something to stimulate platelet production, the way there is for red cells and white cells?

Kidneys

105- Why does it always seem like chronic renal-failure patients have low hematocrits?
106- Should my renal failure patient be transfused?
107- What about patients on CVVH?
108- Are we anticoagulating the machine, the patient, or both?
109- What about hematuria? What is a Murphy drip?

1- What do we use blood for in the MICU?

- Becky: "Postop, trauma, GI bleeds, hemorrhage, DIC."

- SF: "Everything!"

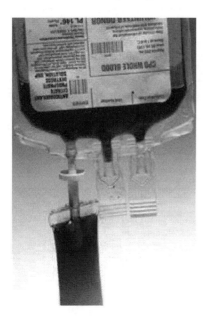

We give a lot of blood products in the unit, for lots of reasons. Some common situations that we see: upper or lower GI bleeds (I hate GI bleeds), and patients who've had some internal blood loss after a procedure. Patients in liver failure will often need frequent transfusion with fresh frozen plasma, since they can't make their own clotting factors any more – the transfused plasma gives some back. Patients in some acute cardiac situations seem to generally do better if their hematocrit is kept up around 30 – so do septic patients.

http://www.infusionpartners.com/images/blood_transfusion.jpg

There have been some changes in recent years in choosing who, or when to transfuse. The numbers that the physicians use as their goals have changed some – apparently there's been some mega-number-crunching on the studies that show what things hurt patients in hospitals, and blood transfusion is one of them. This can make it a little frustrating when a house officer doesn't want to treat a crit of 24, and for 17 years you've been transfusing for anything less than 30… just when you think you know something, they go and change it. All the time.

Blood Counts

2- What are some normal blood values?

Our patient's counts are usually far from normal, and we get very used to seeing numbers that would scare anyone else. So it's probably a good idea to go over the ranges that you'd like to at least hope for. (!)

A very nice lab website, although for non-professionals: http://www.labtestsonline.org/

3- What is a normal hematocrit?

Becky: Hmmmm. Don't often see that number.

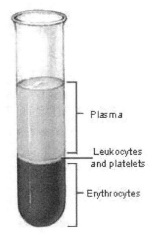

Plasma

Leukocytes
and platelets

Erythrocytes

It helps to remember exactly what a hematocrit is: draw some blood into a spec tube, spin it in a centrifuge for a bit, and then hold it up to the light. If the column in the tube is half full of red cells (with the plasma collected at the top), then the hematocrit is 50%. Make sense? What's the hematocrit if the liquid is only ¼ red cells?

What's the hematocrit here?

I'm usually surprised when we see a patient come in with a hematocrit over 40 – in our patients, this usually means that they're either very dry, or unusually young and/ or (otherwise) healthy. So many of our patients hang out at lower numbers that we begin to forget what the normal ones are. A normal hematocrit is something 41-53%, although if we see a number that high, it usually means the patient is dehydrated.

> Becky: Lots of places don't follow hematocrits – they follow hemoglobin levels instead. "Our docs tend to accept any HB>10, but <18. We tend to follow HB more than Hct. The ratio of hemoglobin to crit is 1:3."

So to me, that would mean a hematocrit range of 30 to 54. Sounds roughly right. A crit of 30% is often the transfusion point for our patients.

4- What if the crit is too high?

> SF: Dehydration.

> Becky: Depends. Is it secondary to dehydration? Then rehydrate. If they're dry enough, and you rehydrate them, you may find yourself transfusing them. We have done phlebotomies on folks with Hb>18.

Hematocrits can change for a number of reasons besides blood loss – for example, the number will change as a patient becomes more or less hydrated. If you take a patient with a fixed volume of blood circulating around, with a crit of 50%, and add, say, 4 liters of IV normal saline, which way will the hematocrit go? Draw another specimen now, spin it, and hold it up to the light. Are there more red cells? No. Is there more "water"? Yes. So the number of red cells hasn't changed, but there are "relatively" less of them – less red cells in every cc of water that they're floating around in. The blood has become "diluted" by the added IV fluid – the patient is "hemodilute".

5- What if it's too low?

SF: They need blood! Check for bleeding lungs, guaiac, etc.

Becky: What you do depends on the situation. Is the patient a Jehovah's Witness? Is the patient fluid overloaded? Is the patient symptomatic? Has the patient reached the doc's "magic number" for transfusion?

Clearly, if there aren't enough red cells around, all the nice things that we like - such as gas exchange and oxygen transport - won't happen, or at least won't happen enough. This leads to all the bad things we hate: tissue hypoxia, buildup of lactic acid (why?), not to mention blood pressure problems. (Don't forget to spend some time thinking about <u>why</u> your patient is doing what they're doing.)

6- What is a "dilutional" crit drop?

SF: If the patient is tanked with IVF.

Becky: Secondary to fluid resuscitation or fluid overload, the crit will drop. If it's because of fluid overload, the crit will be falsely low. A drop after successful rehydration may reflect a true state.

This is what we were talking about above. Say a person comes in with low blood pressure – little old person, hasn't been feeling well for a week, hasn't had much fluid intake, very "dry". Which way has his crit gone – up or down? What does their spun tube of blood look like? Up? – correct. Remember that crit is expressed as a percentage. Does this mean that the number of red cells has gone up? No - the same number is still there, but the fraction has increased because a lot of the water has gone away. The little old person's crit – assuming nothing else is going on – will go up: maybe to 50% – blood gets thick like sludge at really high crit levels. They say that Indian folks up in the Andes live all the time with crits like that. (Why?)

A similar situation: a person who's been developing DKA over a week or so may be "down" something like 8-10 liters, or more – which is called their "free water deficit". That's pretty dry. Which way has their crit gone? Now let's "water" the patient – sometimes treating a hypotensive situation will leave the patient "positive" - six, eight, even eleven liters positive in a day. Which way will this patient's crit go? Dilution. Less red cells per cc of circulating fluid. Should the patient be transfused?

7- What is a "delusional" crit drop?

Becky: *** please let me know!

This is when a nurse **thinks** his patients' crit has dropped.

An absolutely true "Peanuts" strip – Charlie Brown is looking very hot out on the pitcher's mound – sweaty, a little dizzy. Linus comes out from behind the plate and asks him what's wrong. "I feel dizzy, and I have a feeling of impending doom."

Linus: "Maybe you're hyponatremic, Charlie Brown."

Which way is his crit going?

8- What does iron have to do with it?

Becky: Better question – what does calcium have to do with it? If your calcium is too low your blood doesn't like to clot. You should watch the ionized calcium. A regular one doesn't reflect the whole picture if the albumin's low.

You have to have enough iron. Not enough – anemia. Too much: hemochromatosis. To tell the truth, that's all I know – somebody fill in the gaps here?

9- What is a normal white cell count?

Becky: Don't see too many of those either, LOL.

Lots of places use different ranges – in my mind, it's roughly 4 to 11 thousand. More important is to have some idea of why the count is what it is, and which way it's going.

10- What if the white count is too high?

SF: Infection/ steroids

Becky: Infection/ inflammatory response, steroids, leukemia (I think) The diff tells a lot more than the total count.

A white count that rises above the normal range immediately makes me think of infection – generally the higher the count, the worse the infection is, since the patient is cranking out more to fight it off – the range may be from, say, 14 to 40 thousand. Patients in the middle of a nasty septic episode can have the "bad white cell sign" – what we say when the white count is higher than the crit. ("That's your basic bad sign, right there." This is similar to the "more than six infusion pumps running at once" sign.)

Infectious white counts don't usually go much higher than that, but patients with bone marrow problems will crank out zillions of them, with counts up above a hundred thousand. Steroids will make a white cell count rise – this can be confusing if your patient is infected too. (Steroids and infection are usually a really bad combination…)

Update: Now we're starting to see septic patients get cort-stim tested, because apparently sepsis will shut off some patient's adrenals. If the cort-stim is negative, meaning the adrenals aren't working, they go on hydrocortisone q 6 hours. Apparently sometimes makes all the difference. Who knew?

11- What if it's too low?

SF: neutropenia (Ca? – chemotx recently?)

Becky: Really bad infection/sepsis, bone marrow suppression, ?leukemia

Something isn't right with the bone marrow. Maybe the patient has been getting cancer chemotherapy – this produces a hit to the bone marrow, and the counts drop – you just have to wait this out, and the patient may need component transfusion until it passes. The oncology people are pretty good at telling you when you should expect the counts to start rising again. The patient should definitely be on "reverse" precautions, and maybe in a "positive pressure" room - blows the incoming germs away from them.

12- What are the different kinds of white cells? What is a "differential"?

A differential is a breakdown of how much of each kind of white cell is present in a given spec.

There are lots of kinds of these, but we worry mostly about a few:

- Neutrophils: These are also called granulocytes, and they fight off bacterial infection – they're the ones, apparently along with the monocytes, that swallow up the bad guys. Your patients definitely want to have enough of these.

- Lymphocytes: Apparently a very complex system. There are several kinds: the B cells and the T cells. These what CD4 cells are.

- Eosinophils; ("Send a urine and blood for eos, okay?") These show up – among other things- in a patient's allergic or drug reactions. Sometimes we'll send specs for eos if the patient has been having fevers for no obvious reason, and the team suspects a drug reaction.

- Monocytes: apparently these respond to certain bacterial infections like TB, also to rickettsiae.

- "Bands" – here's the CNS (my wife) on bands: "They're immature white cells (neutrophils), and then when you have an overwhelming infection, the immune system releases anything it can to fight it off." (Then she checks in the book: "See, I was right. Can I have a kiss?") "You're not supposed to have any bands – they're supposed to wait until they're grown-up neutrophils before they go out into the world."

13- What is "bandemia"?

SF: sign of new infection?

Becky: Left shift? Inflammatory response – bone marrow churning out immature WBC's (bands).

Lots of bands. (Doh!) Bandemia tells you that you have a response to bacterial infection on your hands, rather than a viral one.

14- What is "band-aid-emia"?

SF: a clumsy nurse!

Becky: Too many venipunctures, LOL.

Wasn't that the concert with Willie Nelson, for all those farmers with cuts and scratches back in the '80s?

15- What is leukopenia?

Becky: Decreased white cell count.

Low white count: a post-chemo patient might have a total white count of, say, 2000. However, if the patient has enough neutrophils, they can still stay off isolation precautions, since they can still fight off infections – I know that there has to be some absolute number or percentage – does anyone know? Absolute neutrophil count?

16- What is a normal platelet count?

Becky: Something that makes surgeons very happy. LOL. (For non-nerds, LOL stands for "Laughing Out Loud") Unfortunately, you can have a "normal" platelet count and the platelets can still be dysfunctional due to situations like renal failure.

Again, the values vary, but the range is usually consistent from one institution to the next – you want to have roughly 150 thousand to 350 thousand platelets.

The dysfunctional platelet renal failure thing is actually quite real – sometimes if these patients are bleeding, the docs will order a dose of DDAVP, aka desmopressin, aka vasopressin, which apparently helps the platelets work more better.

17- What if the platelet count is too high?

Becky: CLOTS CLOTS CLOTS

I think this happens when the bone marrow gets confused, and I think I remember being told that these platelets don't work very well, being immature. (My wife said something like that about me just yesterday...)

18- What if it's too low?

SF: ?autoimmune reaction to transfused platelets, maybe plasmapheresis?

Becky: Spontaneous bleeding. A quick story: one of my coworkers once had a patient with thrombocytopenia (I forget why). This fellow had a scab on his upper lip from a shaving nick. She couldn't stand the look of the scab, so she – you got it- picked it off. And he bled, and bled, and bled. Lesson learned!

Couple of things: first of all, you have to worry that the patient may not have enough plates to clot with – in fact, if the count goes low enough, say below 10-15,000, they may bleed spontaneously. In scary places: lung… head… not a happy thing.

Second thing - and this points out that you need to think a bit about why the count is dropping – the patient may be developing DIC (more about DIC later).

Third thing: lately we've been seeing more and more patients who are turning up positive for HIT – the antibody that reacts badly with heparin to make the patient's platelet count drop. (You can actually watch it go down, spec by spec. Scary.) We've changed our policy from hep-saline to saline pressure bag lines for this one, because it seems like even saying the word "heparin" in such a patient's room can have a bad effect. Make sure the patient isn't getting sq heparin to prevent DVTs, and put on air boots instead. On the patient. ☺

Balloon pumps tend to destroy platelets – according to Gary the balloon tech, this is because the balloon "literally squishes them".

19- What does thrombocytopenia mean?

Becky: Low platelet count. Folks on platelet inhibitors act thrombocytopenic. Mention the word "Plavix" around a surgeon and listen to the screaming…

Low platelet count. Practice saying words like "thrombocytopenia" in front of the bathroom mirror, or in the car. It took my wife and me several weeks before we could say the words for ERCP.

Transfusion and Typing

20- What is transfusion?

Becky: Technically, it's the most common transplant. Quick rule of thumb: for each unit of PRBC's given, the HB should raise by 1.

So for me, that would translate into the crit going up by 3. Most everyone's seen transfusion, or done it by the time they get to the ICU. Like lots of things in the ICU, this can either be a lifesaver or a killer – and, like most things in the unit, it depends on you understanding what you're doing. Fortunately, we spend a lot of time remembering how to do it, and keeping strictly to the rules will keep you and your patient safe. Refer to the hospital's policies and procedures for the rules, and stick to them.

21- What blood components do we give in the MICU, and what do I need to worry about when giving each of them?

Becky: PRBC's, FFP, platelets, cryoprecipitates, salt poor albumin…

Red cells:

I can't remember if I've ever given red cells in any other form than "packed cells" – which is to say, red cells only, with the plasma and platelets removed. Once in a blue moon a patient will receive whole blood – I think maybe in the ER, but I don't think I've ever done it myself. We usually give one unit of red cells at a time, and usually over at least 2-3 hours. Obviously when a patient is really bleeding, we hang more than one red cell at a time – make sure you get an order for this, because normally you'd want to know which of the four PRBC's the patient got is the one responsible for the reaction he had…

When things are really hairy, we hang red cells, plasma, platelets – everything going at once. This is a pretty hazardous maneuver, but if the patient is in danger of dying, you do what you have to do.

Things to worry about with red cells:

- The big one comes first: transfusion reaction. You will definitely know if this is happening within a very short time. Minutes. More on this later.

- If you give red cells too fast, as with any kind of volume bolus, you may push your patient into CHF before you know it's happening. Try to stay aware of your patient's volume state.

- We use a new tubing set for each unit of red cells that goes up

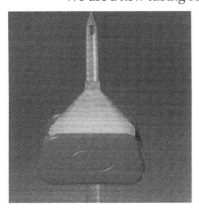

- If you're going to be transfusing your patient a lot, there are multi-unit filters available – these orange guys here on the left. These get hooked to regular, large-drop IV tubing (not more blood tubing), and you can run a total of ten units of red cells and/or FFP through them. I put a sticker on the tubing with numbers: 1 to 10, and cross them off as I go.

http://www.obex.co.nz/images/SQ40%20Filter.JPG

- White Cell Filters: These are big round filters that are rather a pain to use, but they filter out white cells from PRBCs being given to patients who can't defend against them. These will be patients who are immunocompromised, or pre-transplant. The filters are a little tricky to use, so get someone to show you how. Lately we've been getting packed cells up that are pre-filtered, irradiated, and CMV-reduced. I swear some of them glow in the dark…

Fresh Frozen Plasma:

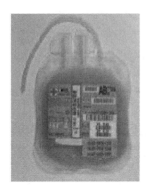

"FFP's" – this is the blood serum – the remainder after the red cells have been washed out. FFP replaces clotting factors when the patient can't manufacture their own, as well as volume. We run these in pretty fast if we need to – this is usually a coagulopathic situation where the patient can't make her own clotting factors. So, if we're going to insert a central line, chest tube, or even if the patient has only been having "slow leak" blood losses (usually GI), we try to correct the coagulopathy – temporarily - with FFP. These patients usually have elevations in both PT and PTT, and the problem is usually liver failure or DIC.

http://www.hokkaido.bc.jrc.or.jp/supply/img03/photo_ffp_.jpg

- What does albumin have to do with it? What is "oncotic pressure"?

Another nice thing about FFP is that it tends to stay in the blood vessels for a while after being infused. Lots of patients rapidly become "third-spaced" in the unit, because they don't get nutrition quickly enough, or because they're horribly catabolic, or both. These folks lose "water" from their vasculature into their tissues, and get that scary swollen look – the point is that the main thing holding water inside the vessels is the patient's albumin level. The "oncotic pressure" that does this isn't what we usually think of as a "pressure", in the sense of something squeezing something else – it's more like "stickiness". The lower the serum albumin, the lower oncotic pressure, therefore more water tends to leak out.

Now, remember the three parts of a blood pressure: pump, volume, and squeeze? (Maybe we could make a breakfast cereal…) Which part are we talking about here? Volume, right – a low-albumin patient losing lots of water from the blood into the tissue is only going to have worsened volume problems. Add to this the "capillary leak syndrome" that raises its ugly head along with dilated vessels in sepsis – this patient is going to have serious problems maintaining a blood pressure.

As usual, there's lots of argument as to how to treat this problem – most places including mine treat low-volume states with lots of "crystalloid" ("clear-as-crystal" IV fluids). This works for a while, and certainly if the patient is a corn-fed Iowa halfback at the age of 17, the serum albumin will stay nice and high for quite a while – he won't start third-spacing for days, and you can give him all the crystalloid you want (unless his hematocrit is 12…). But elderly Mr. Yakowitz in room 84 isn't very well nourished, and has a low albumin to start with – he'll start losing volume from his vessels by ten pm tonight. Maybe 9pm.

You could give "colloid", ("protein-based fluid suspension") – which is what we were talking about above – FFP will hang around longer in the vessels than D5W will. Or you could give albumin, it's true – but what this patient really needs is **nutrition**. Try to get something appropriate started right away – don't let the patient go 3 days without tube feeds, and if they need TPN – fight for it. I've seen both given at once.

Things to worry about with FFP:

I don't think I've ever seen a patient react to FFP, but you should remember to think about volume. It's not unusual for the team to order 6 units of FFP (usually adds up to more than a liter) in a coagulopathic patient if they're going to insert a central line.

You definitely want to recheck the patient's PT and PTT after giving FFP. After all, you're trying to figure out if it had the effect you wanted.

Platelets:

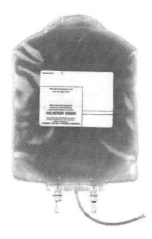

My experience is that if your patient is going to react, most commonly it'll be to platelets. At the same time, most reactions that I've seen to platelets are not the full-on, tidal-wave kind that red cells produce. Platelet reactions are usually more like a temperature spike, maybe rigors, maybe a drop in blood pressure, maybe all three. A lot of these reactions are avoidable by giving the platelets slowly, maybe a couple of hours for a single transfusion.

http://www.cobebct.com/Images/platelets.jpg
What are "cryos"?

Cryoprecipitates are a plasma product, which replace specific missing clotting factors – the cryo unit contains a number of them, including Factor VIII (that's "8" for the rest of us), which is what hemophiliacs don't have. There are a couple others – one at least is the factor needed in von Willebrand's disease. (Shelties apparently get von Willebrand's…any dog people out there?)

22- Can you please review the basics of blood typing?

Becky: Remember that you get one gene from your Mom, and one from your Dad. That's why an A mom and a B dad can have an O baby without causing divorce.

Ask an easy one, why don't you? As usual, I'll explain it as I understand it, and if I have it totally wrong, then hopefully lots of people will leap all over me and correct me, for which I will thank them. I suspect that I'm not too far off, because I've been hanging blood products for a long time, and I haven't hurt anyone yet.

Let's take it in short bites:

Red Cells

People are divided into groups that share a common blood type. There are only a few major ones: A, B, AB, and O. (Is this ethnic? Anybody know if all the people from Yakutsk are type AB, or something? Interesting question.)

The red cells in your body are <u>all</u> of one type – say, A. The cells in a B type person are all B's. Likewise O.

For the discussion, you could visualize the antigens as little raised patches on the surface of the red cells in the form of letters – zillions of little "A"s all over the cells of an A-type person, and B's all over the cells of a B person.

Now about antibodies. Antibodies are proteins floating about in the plasma, and people inherit them from their parents. Antibodies attack foreign invaders – in this case, transfused red cells with the wrong antigen on them. The result is the blood reaction – be careful!

O-type people have <u>neither A nor B antigens</u> on their red cells. (You could think of the O as a large "zero", meaning "zero" antigens, which isn't really true, but it works for the basic idea.)

What you <u>don't</u> want to do is to give a patient red cells that his body won't like. I'm an A person – if you put B cells into my bloodstream, my body will become <u>very</u> upset – producing all the bad things we think of in connection with a transfusion reaction.

Likewise B people – if you give them A type red cells, they'll attack them, and react.

AB people carry <u>both</u> antigens on their red cells – as a result, they can get either A, B, AB (duh) or O (no antigens) blood. Nice! AB's are called the "Universal Recipients" they can get just about anything. (Who just yelled: "What about Rh!"? – that's coming.)

Okay so far? All set with the A's and the B's? Onwards.

What about O people? O people, remember, have neither A nor B antigens on their cells. Can you <u>give</u> them A blood? Not! Their cells won't recognize the newcomers as friends, since it's the antigen on those cells that marks them as invaders to be attacked. Can't give them B blood either, or AB, for the same reason. O's only get O blood.

It does work the other way though – O people, having neither A nor B antigens (is there an O antigen?) can give blood to A's, B's, AB's, and other O's – this is why they're called "Universal D<u>on</u>ors" – they can give to anybody, practically speaking.

Making sense? Don't give people antigens that they don't want.

FFP:

FFPs have no red cells in them, or at least they're supposed to, and so they don't carry a significant risk of reaction. No red cells, no antigens, no reactions. (Uh huh, but they do carry antibodies, right? What does that have to do with it? Time to take the transfusion class again.)

Platelets:

Used to be, platelets were ABO-compatibility matched, but nowadays that's not the case.

23- What about Rh? What is RhoGam?

> Becky: An OB question! I think I remember. RhoGam is given to an Rh negative mom so that she doesn't make antibodies against an Rh positive baby.

Rh is another kind of antigen that lives on red cells, and it's a lot simpler than the ABO business – you either have it or you don't. If you do have it, you're Rh positive - if not, you're negative.

When giving red cells, can you give an Rh positive person some Rh positive blood? Sure, as long as it's the same ABO type.

Can you give them Rh negative blood? Also yes – there's no Rh antigen present if the red cells are Rh negative.

Can you give an Rh negative patient Rh positive blood? No. That would be giving them red cells with the antigen attached.

So ABO-typed blood also has to be checked for Rh, and any given unit of red cells will be clearly marked that way: A+, A-, AB+, AB-, O+, etc. (They leave out the "Rh", and just put "+" or "-".)

RhoGam: Wow – how long ago did I take the boards? (Quickly looking up RhoGam on the web).

Here's the situation. Pregnant mom is Rh negative. Dad is Rh positive. Junior is Rh positve – got it from Dad. Mom may attack Junior's Rh positive red cells, leading to bad things for Junior. To prevent this bad thing, Mom gets RhoGam shot. This prevents Mom from forming anti-Rh antibodies that will attack Junior. The shot's effects last for 12 weeks. There is, of course, lots more to it than that – I don't think I've ever even seen a vial of RhoGam. Or a bottle. Envelope? Shaker?

24- What does a transfusion reaction look like?

SF: rising temp, chills, rigors, change in mental status

Becky: A very long shift. There are a few types: febrile, with a temp increase greater than 2 degrees F; anaphylactic, allergic, hemolytic...

Transfusion reactions are scary, and at least part of the problem is that you can't be sure right away whether the patient is having a "minor" reaction – these are usually called the "febrile, non-hemolytic" reactions – or a major one: "hemolytic". Either kind of reaction will almost always occur during the first few minutes of the transfusion, which is why policy requires a set of vital signs recorded before, and a few minutes after the start of any transfusion.

Minor, febrile reactions: These are actually not so rare. The patient usually spikes a fever, probably has rigors, may break out in hives.

Major, hemolytic reactions: These are the bad ones. A partial list of the unpleasant things that can occur: hypotension, renal failure, bronchospasm, DIC...not a pleasant scenario.

25- What should I do if I think my patient is reacting?

SF: Stop the blood!

Becky: STOP THE TRANSFUSION!!!! Call the doc and the lab. We have a form which spells out exactly what needs to be done.

Stop the transfusion. Call for help right away. The plan is not to give the patient any more of the red cells that are causing the problem. Take the transfusion tubing down with the red cell bag – don't run anything through that tubing into the patient! I would aspirate the line that the patient was being transfused through, if I could, so that even the tiny amount of blood in the heplock or CVP lumen was removed.

26- How is a reaction treated?

SF: Benadryl, reaction documentation, urine and blood followup

Becky: Depends on what type of reaction. Febrile – usually just Tylenol and the docs usually say to continue, but running the blood slower. Hemolytic, allergic, anaphylactic – your patient may just code on you. That's why we check the vitals and the patient so frequently during the first 15 minutes. That's also why we have 2 licensed people check the blood before hanging it.

Treatment this depends on which kind of reaction is going on. For febrile, non-hemolytic reactions, antihistamines like benadryl will help, and tylenol will help with fever. Sometimes a small dose of IV demerol will help with acute rigors. These patients usually will get premedicated with tylenol and benadryl about half an hour before being transfused again.

Hemolytic reactions are obviously another thing altogether. These patients are really in trouble – they may need lots of volume and/or pressors for hypotension and to improve renal clearance, bronchodilators, FFP replacement during DIC, maybe platelets – these people are going to need central line access, maybe intubation, maybe dialysis. These reactions are really rare - I've never seen one happen. Remember that keeping strictly to the transfusion rules will prevent most of the possible problems.

27- What is involved in follow-up for a transfusion reaction?

Becky: The blood is tested: the patient's and the donor's, urine spec to the lab, supportive measures for the patient.

The blood bag and the tubing need to be sent back to the blood bank – there are some specs to be drawn from the patient as well. It's been years since I've had to do this, so check the lab book to see what's current.

28- Can a person have a reaction to fresh-frozen plasma?

Becky: Aren't drugs dissolved in protein? Can the patients react to that?

I haven't seen it happen.

29- What about platelets?

Becky: Yes, and it's ugly.

Platelets can be a problem- if they're run in too quickly, they can produce fever reactions, sometimes drops in blood pressure. I always try to run platelets in over at least an hour, two if possible, which really minimizes the problems.

30- What is a Coombs test?

Coombs testing has to do with the detection of antibodies attached to red cells, and helps with the diagnosis of hemolytic reactions.

Giving Blood Products

When to Get Ready

31- What kinds of procedures can make my patients lose blood?

Becky: Anything that punctures a vein or an artery. Harpoon one of those bad boys, add a little coagulopathy, and off you go running to the blood bank. Seriously: cath lab interventions, angio interventions, chest tube insertions sometimes, line placements…

Well, where should we start? Keep in mind: what were the patient's counts and coags before the procedure started? Many times the team will order a couple of different blood products for some coagulopathic patient before placing a central line. You probably ought to know if the numbers improve after you've given them…

For sure, any time anyone punctures your patient, there may be bleeding involved. This seems stupidly obvious until you realize that in lots of situations you may not know right away that a significant blood loss is happening. Cardiac cath patients are a good example. Lately the technique seems to have improved a lot, but I remember lots of patients who developed large hematomas into their femoral tissues, with impressive hematocrit drops – once in a while a vessel will develop an acute "pseudoaneurysm" – which may require a quick trip to the OR with vascular surgery.

Or retroperitoneal bleeding: any time you "hardware-ize" a patient's fem, the artery may be stuck – either on purpose or not, (and even with the best technique and the most experience these things do "just happen" sometimes, usually I hear because the patient's anatomy isn't straight out of the textbook). The artery can be pierced all the way through – and begins to leak pressurized blood into the patient's abdomen, retroperitoneally, settling towards their back. It may take a day or so for the hematomas to become visible, but you need to be thinking about possible "occult blood losses."

32- What about bleeding from a line insertion site?

Becky: If they're not coagulopathic, sometimes just a little pressure will stop it. Sometimes someone needs to add a stitch at the site.

This also sounds simple, but may not be. Suppose your patient inadvertently pulls out his IJ central line? Is he bleeding from the site, or has he pulled some air into his venous circulation and sent it merrily along to cause an air embolus in his lung? Was he anticoagulated? (Or pressor dependent, but that's a different FAQ – take a look at "Pressors and Vasoactives" for more on that topic.) Apply steady sterile pressure to the site – not too hard! Have you ever seen the maneuver technically referred to as "doing the neck thing"? – that's to say, the carotid body massage, used to try and break a tachycardic rhythm? (Nowadays they use adenosine instead of compressing the patient's carotid.) You're doing it now. Don't press on a neck site so hard that your patient becomes bradycardic!

33- Why does it matter where they put the lines?

Becky: Think "compressible vessel". How do you first try to stop bleeding? – hold pressure. How do you hold pressure on a subclavian artery? (I don't know how.)

What if it was a subclavian line that came out? Not a very compressible site, since the vein is mostly hiding under the clavicle. As always – do your best. Apply pressure to the site, call for help, get the team in the room – what labs would you probably want to send at this point? How would you know if your patient was having an air embolism, and what might you do? Would you want to get an x-ray? What does subcutaneous emphysema feel like, and what do you do if you find it? And, uh, what might you be doing while the patient is without pressors!?

34- What if my patient needs a line, and is anticoagulated?

SF: ? FFP before the procedure

This is why you need to know where your patient is lab-wise. The team may want to stop heparin treatment for a while, or not – follow up carefully.

35- Should my patient get FFP before line placement? Or platelets?

Becky: Maybe. Depends on where the doc is "going", how out of whack the numbers are, and the skill of the operator.

We looked at this before – I see this done a lot in coagulopathic situations. Platelets are also sometimes given before procedures, but giving platelets frequently makes for trouble, since the patient may stop responding to the transfusions for immune reasons.

36- What if I find a hematoma somewhere on my patient for no apparent reason?

SF: ?HIT

Tell the team. Mark the edges of the hematoma with a pen. Watch the patient's counts – crit going down? Where is the hematoma at? – on her back, two days after cardiac cath? Do you need to be measuring her abdominal girth every 4 hours? Or is it on her neck after a central line insertion, and if it's growing, is her airway being threatened? Or all over in patches – has the platelet count been falling – does the patient need an HIT spec sent? (Change the line flushes to saline (with an order) if this may be happening.) Heparin running – is the PTT too high? Or is it something really unpleasant like DIC? (More on DIC later on.)

37- What about embolus formation?

Be aware of the dangers: clots can form on the ends of central lines, which is why you're always supposed to aspirate them if they plug, not flush them. Be very aware of a patient in "paroxysmal atrial fibrillation" – clots may form in the atria and get shot out into the circulation whenever the patient switches to sinus rhythm.

(Why don't (insert religion here) people ever come out of a-fib? Because they don't convert!)

(Jayne, covering her eyes: "Tell me you did not put that in there…")

Try to be aware in general of what's going on in any part of the body that has a line of one kind or another inserted into it. Arterial lines of any kind can threaten the perfusion of whatever is downstream from them – intravascular devices are thrombogenic by nature. (My son loves to make fun of six-dollar words; he likes to know what they mean in regular English – in this case, "clots like to form on it". His current favorite is "epistaxis": "Dude, this kid had, like, wicked epistaxis at school today". But he's sixteen – I guess he's doing what he's supposed to.) Anyway, check the distal pulses!

38- What is an embolectomy?

Sometimes, no matter how careful you are, and no matter how perfect the numbers may be, bad things can happen. This can really be a source of guilt and frustration on the part of the caregivers, but it's important to remember: the best you can do is the best you can do. Some patients are going to bleed unexpectedly when anticoagulated. And some, despite your best care, are going to form clots – whether DVTs on the venous side, or embolic thrombi on the arterial side.

There are several situations that can lead to arterial clots getting thrown downstream – one is paroxysmal a-fib. Another is valve vegetation – as I understand it, usually this happens on the right side, because the venous circulation is where germs are going to get injected into the circulation, say during dentistry. (Where do hunks of vegetation from the right side of the heart go if they break loose? Which valve are they forming on?) Another might be recent vascular-repair surgery.

The one I always think of is the balloon pump. The balloon itself, the inflatable part, is very thrombogenic - which is why these patients are always anticoagulated. Even with the best practice, sometimes clots form, break loose, and float downstream to the nearest artery that's small enough to stop them – in the case of the IABP, this might be something minor like, say, the femoral artery. (I know, too detail-oriented. I mean really!) So every now and then a patient winds up in the OR because his leg went blue and cold from the knee downwards, below his balloon-insertion site. (If the patient is balloon-dependent, the balloon probably needs to be reinserted, usually in the other fem. Check the distal pulses!)

Tools

39- What kinds of blood transfusion tubing do we use?

> Becky: "Platelets have a special tubing which doesn't let them get caught up in the filter. We have 2 kinds of tubing for PRBC's and FFP. One is used for the pump and the other has chamber which when filled allows us to "hand-pump" a unit in 5-10 minutes, or use with a pressure bag."

The point to understand about transfusion tubing is that it has a filter built into it to catch clots. The size of the openings in the filter varies: one size for red cells, another for platelets. Regular blood tubing has to be changed with each transfused unit of blood component. Pressure bags are nice, but <u>don't use them on peripheral lines</u> if you can help it – the veins can't take the high pressure flow.

There are some nice images of transfusion tubing and pump bags in our article on Peripheral IVs for Beginners... www.icufaqs.org/PeripheralIVs.doc

40- What is a multi-unit transfusion filter?

SF: Used for blood and FFP, up to 10 units, I think.

See the picture back on question 21? This is a very helpful gadget – it goes between the blood bag and <u>regular</u>, maxi-drip tubing – no second filter. You can run ten units of blood components through it before changing – I flag the tubing with a sticker marked 1-10, and check off the numbers as I go.

41- What kind of IV access should my patient have for transfusion?

SF: At least two 18 gauge peripherals. Preferably a big cordis if they're really bleeding!

Becky: Minimally – two 18 gauges peripherally. My preference – an introducer/venous sheath, a triple lumen CVP line along with the two 18s.

Basic, basic rule of the MICU – access is everything. If your patient is really losing blood "briskly", then central access is a must. We have enormous Cordis introducers normally used for PA lines that run "like stink" – meaning, really well. Like a garden hose. Get the team to use the femoral vein site – you won't have to wait for an x-ray to use it. Make sure there's a blood return in the line!

42- Can I hang more than one unit of blood at a time?

SF: If they need it, yes!

Becky: In an emergency or if your patient is crashing, YES, and get 'em in quick. Routinely, no. They're supposed to run over 2-4 hours, and how would you tell which one caused a reaction?

If you need to, definitely – get the team to write an order for "concurrent blood products". Sometimes we have four or six running at a time. Under normal circumstances you want to know which unit provoked the reaction – if the patient has one. With six up and running the problem gets much more complicated.

43- Can I hang more than one kind of blood product at a time?

SF: Yes!

Yes again, but only if you need to. Get an order written.

44- What is a blood warmer?

Becky: We use Hot Line. It warms the blood to body temp for pts with cold agglutinins (cause the cold blood to clump), cold patients or folks you don't want to make cold (cold blood doesn't clot.)

We don't use these much for some reason – they seem to be more of a surgical-ICU device. What I have seen of them I don't like much – anything that gets more equipment between my bleeding patient and her blood bag is just something else in my way. I'm probably wrong about this though. Is that really true about the cold blood?

45- What is a rapid-infuser?

SF: Exactly what it says: it runs PRBC's through in five minues using a heated system.

This a neat device that I've never had the occasion to learn to use – I've seen them at times though, and I understand they work really well when your patient needs really large volume resuscitation. The surgical ICUs use them for traumas.

46- What if it looks like I'm losing the race?

SF: Sometimes there's no endpoint set…

Becky: According to the surgeons: "All bleeding eventually stops."

It can often feel like a race – your patient is having blood pressure problems, you're sending labs, writing down signs, spiking blood bags, changing tubing, constantly trying to stay a little ahead of the patient, wishing surgery would show up already…and you just can't seem to get your hands to move quickly enough. For twelve hours, maybe. Maybe less. Maybe for the second time in a day on the same patient.

The answer is very simple – get help. Your resource nurse should be standing right behind you, checking blood, helping keep track of what's up, what's in, how much has been lost, when the last counts and coags were sent, what they were, keeping the team in the room, helping you argue for central access with the team … if she's not right behind you, she should assign someone to back you up. Get help any way you can – lots of it – right away. Classic ICU crisis, with a classic answer – <u>don't face it alone</u>. And eat something – this is <u>not</u>

optional - I keep a couple of power bars in my bag for situations like this. Don't get so wrapped up in what you're doing that you pass out in a sweat with a blood sugar of 12…it doesn't help you to push that hard, and it certainly doesn't help the patient if you're not staying alert. Know your limits, stay within them.

But SF is raising another really important point – how long, and how hard are you going to push on this particular situation…?

Special Help

47- When does GI get called in to look at a patient?

Any time you have a patient who is seriously GI bleeding, GI are the first specialty team to get contacted. If your patient suddenly develops BRB pr, or per NGT – they need to get a call. The first maneuver will obviously be transfusion, but it's the GI team that's going to go in with a scope, and take a look around to see what can be done.

48- When does surgery get called in to look at a patient?

> SF: (A comment expressing frustration.)

> Becky: We usually call them in fairly early so that if/when the patient goes south, surg. has already evaluated them.

If you have a substantial bleeding situation, surgery should be paged early on in the process so that they're aware of the patient and any developing crises. The team should be making sure that surgery stays in the loop as things progress.

49- What is plasmapheresis?

Plasmapheresis is actually simpler than it looks – the technique is to remove blood from the patient, separate the red cells from the plasma, and then reinfuse the red cells with fresh donor plasma. The idea is to get rid of antibodies and the like that are creating problems. Plasmapheresis is done for several conditions: myasthenia gravis, Guillain-Barre, and TTP are the ones I remember.

Here's my plasmapheresis story. At her request, I took my mother to a specialty hospital when her standard chemo treatments had finally failed to stop the spread of her lung cancer. Among other things, she developed liver mets and got very encephalopathic, which really got to me – she had always been very smart, very verbal. I came back from several days away taking care of her household, and there she was: very yellow, very confused, incontinent. High ammonia, probably. It was awful. I'd been an RN for less than a year.

So anyway, after a week or so of this, watching her get worse, and for whatever reason that I can't remember 20 years later, her docs decided to do plasmapheresis. I got to the hospital that day after the procedure was done, and there was mom: alert, oriented, intact, happy to see me, wondering where I'd been, and wondering why I'd suddenly burst into tears. That night she got confused again – that was the last conversation I ever had with her, and it came as a surprise gift.

50- What is dialysis?

> Becky: Hemodialysis: think of it as a washing machine for the blood. We have regular HD nurses, and it takes 2-4 hours. They watch and monitor the patient. CVVH is what we do ourselves. It's done over several days (although a setup is only good for 72 hours.) It gently cleans and removes excess fluid. Nephrology determines the fluid removal/replacement rate. SCUF only removes excess fluid.

Dialysis uses osmosis to remove nitrogenous wastes from the blood. The blood flows along one side of a permeable membrane, and the dialysate flows along the other side – the membrane is designed to let certain molecules pass through, but not others, depending on how big they are. The membrane can be a synthetic filter, or it can be the membranes in the abdomen (peritoneal dialysis), but the principle is the same – water and waste substances travel across the membrane to the hypotonic side, and then get discarded.

We have an article on CVVH here: www.icufaqs.org/cvvh.doc

51- What is "liver dialysis"?

> Becky: We aren't doing this…

This is apparently the "latest and the greatest" – I understand that it involves using live liver cells in a filtration system to clear hepatic wastes. I don't know much more than that, and I've only ever seen it done once or twice, but supposedly it holds great promise. More info when it becomes available.

Giving Blood Products

52- What are some of the situations when I would give my patients blood components?

Let's try going through these system by system:

Cardiac:

> Becky: "CABG, valve replacement, AAA, vascular surgery, LVAD, blood loss from procedures, IABP, anticoagulation."

Lots of cardiac situations require transfusions, or sometimes anticoagulation, and there definitely hazards involved.

A common example is atrial fibrillation. I can remember the time when there was lots of argument about anticoagulating patients in a-fib; now it's almost routine. The danger is that the heart may pop in and out of a-fib: paroxysmal AF. The fibrillating atria sometimes allow clots to form inside them – a quick switch to sinus rhythm will shoot those clots into the circulation: to the lungs from the right side, causing PE, or into the arterial circulation from the left side, where they could go to all sorts of unpleasant places. These patients are heparinized short-term, and coumadinized long-term.

A question to think about – your patient comes in, in AF, let's say fairly rapid. Do you want to cardiovert him?

Pulmonary:

Becky: "Thoracic surgery, hemothorax, ruptured pulmonary artery…"

Hemoptysis is the big problem here, and of course the severity varies with the cause. We see lots of patients with this, some requiring intubation, some not. Recently we had a patient whose platelet count was super-low during a chemo nadir – he had a pretty big blood aspiration. Actually, anesthesia told us that if you have to aspirate something, blood is much better than stomach contents: no acid, for one thing. Blood is apparently broken down, absorbed, and cleared out much more easily than other aspirated liquids. The quick maneuver to make in the case of rapid hemoptysis is to call respiratory – they'll get the bronchoscopy cart down in case either the pulmonary fellow or thoracic surgery want to go in and take a look around.

The other scenario that comes to mind here is PA rupture. **This is why you want to know if your patients' PA line is stuck in wedge.** A PA line can poke a hole in the lung, right through the walls of the vessel that it's in – the results can be spectacular. I've seen vent-tubing suddenly collect a scary amount of BRB. Handling this takes some quick work by anesthesia and by the interventional radiology people – the first places a fogarty balloon into the bronchus where the bleeding is coming from, using a bronchoscope as a guide. The IR team will try to float a catheter into the PA circulation and inject gelfoam or something else to try to plug the leak from within the vessel. Cool, but scary.

GU:

We see a couple of these situations. Sometimes, despite the best care, some patients will get foley-catheter related trauma, producing hematuria. I tend to have a great deal of sympathy for this situation. Ow. The big question here: are there any clots in the urine? The danger is that the foley will plug up, the urine won't drain, the bladder will get over full, and problems may ensue that I really don't even want to think about. We treat these situations with saline bladder irrigant drips that run really fast by gravity through a 3-way Foley (www.icufaqs.org/FoleyCatheters.doc) – the idea is to flush the bladder continuously so that clots don't have time to form. Clearly, you want to know if what's coming out more than matches what's going in – otherwise, the catheter may need changing.

Bone marrow diseases:

We see these situations once in a while. Patients will frequently drop their counts after cancer chemotherapy, and depending on what they need and what problems they have, will receive component transfusion of one kind of another. I think this is the only situation in which I've seen white cell transfusion used.

Postop situations:

We get patients from the OR sometimes – sometimes as Surgical ICU overflow, and sometimes our own patients will go for one procedure or another. Our policy is clear: the nurse takes postop report from the anesthesia person involved – you should get a clear idea of what was done, what fluids were given, what the blood loss was, and how much urine was made by the patient during the case. (This last tells you a lot about how well perfused the patient was.) We routinely send off the basic "one of everything" labs when a patient is postop – routine lytes, CBC, coags, maybe a CK/iso/troponin. Get the numbers, assess for possible postop blood losses, and go from there.

Neuro:

This covers a pretty large area – which is why neurology has an ICU to itself. It's not saying too much to just point out that anything increasing the pressure inside the head – like bleeding - is your basic bad thing. Anticoagulated people, auto-anticoagulated people, thrombocytopenic people, very hypertensive people – are all at risk for bleeding into the head. So your liver-failure patient who suddenly seizes may be doing just that – just another unpleasant possibility that you need to keep in the back of your mind.

GI Bleeding

53- What do I need to know about GI bleeds?

> Becky: "Bleeds, postops, liver trauma, liver failure, ischemic/infarcted bowel, ulcerative dz…"

Just a personal thing – I hate GI bleeds. I'm not sure what my problem is – I get really happy if I know some real cardiogenic crash is coming my way: balloon pump, twelve drips, vent, paralysis, CVVH, all that – I love that stuff. But I hate GI bleeds.

54- How can you tell the difference between an "upper" GI bleed and a "lower" one?

Anatomically, I think the difference is whether the bleed is above or below the pylorus. You can't really tell until you go in there with a flashlight and look around, but there are two or three rough clues you can use to tell: as I understand it, the difference lies in relation to the pyloric valve at the end of the stomach. Blood exposed to gastric acid (above the pylorus) turns black, and gets passed through the gut as that tarry stool we all know so well. Blood lost below the pylorus doesn't get exposed to the acid in the stomach, so it stays red, or maroon – "melanotic".

Some other clues: is the patient vomiting blood? Probably upper GI bleed. BRBPR? (Bright Red Blood Per Rectum?) – probably lower GI bleed. Either way, endoscopy from one end or the other comes next.

55- What are "coffee-grounds"?

> Becky: Partially digested blood in emesis or NG aspirate looks like the coffee grounds in your coffee maker.

Slow bleeding (as opposed to "fire-hydrant" bleeding) in the upper GI tract will collect in the stomach – when you drain this through an NG tube, it has a characteristic look something like the stuff left in the filter long after the coffee is gone.

56- What is melena?

> Becky: Blood that's made it's way through the colon.

Melena is the reddish liquid or semi-liquid stool produced in lower GI bleeding. It can be dark or bright, large or small in volume, and you definitely want to keep track of how much is produced.

57- What is the difference between testing gastric contents for blood, and stool for blood?

You need to make sure that you use the right tester – guiac cards for stool are not the same as gastroccult cards for stomach specs.

58- Why might my GI bleed patient need to be intubated.?

> Becky: Which end?

An excellent question, which sometimes doesn't get raised quickly enough. It certainly seems to me a sort of basic idea that a patient who has an active upper GI bleed, who may be frequently vomiting, and who may need a prolonged endoscopy would probably benefit from having a cuffed ET tube in place. Aspiration is never a nice thing, although I have been told that if you have to aspirate something, blood is the way to go – it's more easily reabsorbed by the body than, say, milk. Or a cheeseburger… anyway, if the patient is bleeding actively, and there's any chance that he might become confused or agitated – think about pushing for intubation. Not only will the cuffed tube help guard against aspiration, but the ability to safely sedate your patient may make all the difference in getting him through the whole process. It's a classic example of the intubation rule – if you have a chance to electively tube your patient safely, you may want to take it, because you may find yourself in a real mess later, such as when your patient aspirates and codes later on…

Upper GI Bleeds

59- How are upper GI bleeds treated?

Becky: "H2 blockers, carafate, oversewing ulcers, resection."

The first thing you want to do – in any bleeding situation - is to stabilize the patient's blood pressure if you can. Make sure you have some way of frequently measuring this – whether automatic cuff, or arterial line. Obviously you're going to have your patient on a cardiac monitor too – watch the heart rate for quick changes upwards. If the patient is starting to "open up", (which you may not see right away if they're bleeding internally into the gut), the heart rate will abruptly rise to try to maintain blood pressure – the same as it would in any other hypovolemic shock state. Jayne: "Unless they're beta-blocked." Absolutely true. What happens to the blood pressure in that case?

Here's an interesting quote on this subject: "An inexperienced house officer was dealing with a patient with a GI bleed. The nursing staff were becomng rightly concerned that the patient had an ever increasing trachycardia. The house officer wanted to prescribe beta-blockers to control this. Fortunately, the nurses refused! The tachycardia is a crucial physical sign." (From the Student British Medical Journal website.)

What the " &*@#%" is that supposed to mean: "Fortunately"?!

Second critical thing: let's say it again - access is everything in these situations. If your patient is at all unstable blood-pressure-wise, insist on central IV access along with an arterial line for pressure monitoring. Not only can you get volume into the patient more rapidly this way, but you can monitor the CVP, give several infusions at once, give pressors if you need to - it's the most useful tool you can have in an unstable situation. The best rapid-infusion line that we use is a PA-line introducer - they're very large-bore, and you can really get volume into your patient rapidly. Don't forget: if the situation is critical, a femoral central line will usually go in more quickly than a neck or chest line, and won't need an x-ray to confirm placement. ("He's very repetitive.") (That's for a reason!)

Frequent hematocrit measurements are critical here – if your patient is actively bleeding, send count specs at regular intervals, so you'll know which way the trend is going. Keep an eye on the PT/PTT and the platelet count as well – problems tend to come in clusters, and you wouldn't want to miss anything. As you're transfusing, try to keep as accurate as you can your estimate of how much blood the patient is losing. For example, don't just write "Lg melena stool" on your output sheet – try to estimate. 300cc of melena? A liter? Definitely helpful.

60- What is endoscopy all about?

Becky: "We know it's in there, let's go look!"

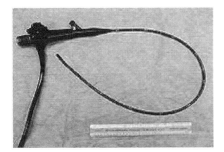

Hm – that a ruler, or a yardstick?

http://www.petvets.com/img/newsletter/endoscope.jpg

We see an endoscopy in the unit at least a couple of times a week. The idea is simple enough – they use a fiberoptic scope that looks about ten feet long, (but which probably isn't, but it sure looks that way) to look into one end of the patient or the other. The scope has suction attached, and some tools for treating what they find.

61- Who does endoscopy?

Becky: "GI, surgeons. The endo team brings equipment and monitors/assists after hours."

At night (the only shift where the <u>real</u> nursing goes on), the GI fellow on call will come in with a scope and a cart with lots of video equipment. It's standard now for the procedures to be videotaped, and images of whatever interesting things they find get printed out in full color to be put in the patient's chart.

62- What can endoscopy treat, or not treat?

Becky: "Treat – varices, diagnostic, biopsies. Not treat – hemorrhagic gastritis, erosion, ulcers, Mallory-Weiss tears."

Here's some information from a senior ICU person who wants to remain anonymous:

"Endoscopy can definitely diagnose gastritis, GI ulcers, diverticulosis, and polyps, and conditions such as Crohn's disease and irritable bowel. Endoscopy can be lifesaving in stopping an acute GI bleed with cautery or sclerosis. ERCP can relieve acute cholecystitis by removing gallstones. Percutaneous endoscopic gastrostomy allows for non-surgical placement of G-tubes. Transesophageal echo can detect thrombi in the atria when elective cardioversion is being considered and there is no time for anticoagulation…"

Upper endoscopy can often treat small acute bleeding sources, such as varices. I think I've seen them used to treat small arterial bleeds (which come from gastric erosion by too much acidity). Lower endoscopy can remove small polyps in the colon, which get sent off to pathology to check for malignancy. Both upper and lower scopes can take tissue biopsies. For situations that can't be managed by sclerosis or banding with a scope, the patient will have to go to the OR.

63- What are "bands"?

This is a pretty clever idea – the maneuver is to locate a swollen, bleeding esophageal varix, and to clamp it shut by fitting a tight rubber band around the leak. The image I have in mind is of a swollen vessel with a ballooned area sticking out from the side, leaking blood – the band gets fitted around the "neck" of the balloon. I know that varices show up in the stomach too, do they band those too?

64- What if the bands come off?

SF: they re-bleed!

They don't always. But it does seem to happen pretty often – the GI people will apply maybe five or six bands, and then maybe they lose a couple during the procedure – I know that I've found bands coming out the other end, which is always interesting. Little tiny blue rubber bands – I wash them off and put them in a sterile specimen cup to show the team. They never seem very happy to see them… I'm not sure how effective the bands are in the longer term anyway. Often enough, a patient will come in with a big bleed, and endoscopy will show lots of blood, but no source. Frustrating - even if the bands don't go on, sometimes a bleed will stop by itself. Maybe because of hypotension? Yow!

65- What do they use the epinephrine for?

The scope has a needle injector, and sometimes a bleeding source can be injected with epi, which scleroses the tissue at and around the bleeding site – another maneuver to stop bleeding at specific sites.

66- Does the patient need to be intubated for upper endoscopy?

SF: Not always.

Becky: Not unless the airway is compromised by something like aspiration.
We thought about this a little earlier. If the situation is an active upper GI bleed, you can't always depend on nasogastric tubes to keep the patient's stomach empty – they get plugged easily, and big clots in the stomach aren't going to come out through that tube anyway. I've seen some pretty impressive clots come up and out, certainly big enough to block an airway. Assess the patient. If they need airway protection, start pushing for it.

This reminds me of a situation we saw recently. An intubated patient was receiving a go-lytely prep overnight for a colonoscopy in the morning (a lower GIB situation). The prep liquid was being infused by a tube feed pump into an NG tube at 300cc/hour. How often would you check that patient's gastric aspirate?

67- What kind of conscious sedation do we use for endoscopy if the patient isn't intubated?

SF: "Versed/Ativan"

Becky: "Versed, Ativan, morphine, demerol. Personally I prefer it when the patient is intubated..."

The docs will tell you what they want given – I've seen small doses of IV demerol or fentanyl used, sometimes small doses of Versed. This is tricky of course, and gets into the area of "conscious sedation" – I'm never quite comfortable in this kind of situation, but that's probably just because I'm old, and I worry about things.

Intubating the patient, if only for endoscopy, makes my job about six times easier, not least because I can safely sedate the patient to the point where they can tolerate the procedure much more easily than they would the other way. Versed sometimes makes elderly people stop breathing – without an ETT tube in place, what would you do? What drug would you want to have next to you? What equipment?

68- What is a blakemore tube?

SF: Esophageal balloon for varices, gastric balloon, placed to traction.

Becky: "It's been many, many years since we used one."

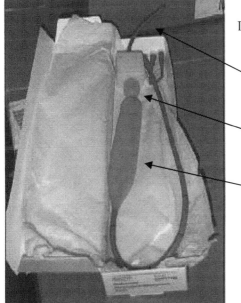

Looks like the squid from the deep...

This bit goes in to drain the stomach.

Here's the gastric balloon.

And the esophageal one.

The three red ports up top are a gastric drain, and inflation ports for the balloons.

http://www.ec.gc.ca/MERCURY/images/products/blackmore_tube.jpg

This is a neat idea. A blakemore tube is a soft nasogastric tube with two balloons built into it. The one at the end is about the size of a tennis ball, and the long one above that looks like an enormous hot dog spitted on a stick. The balloons are inflated to squeeze the bleeding vessels shut, and then left in place for a while.

It's rather a spectacle: the whole device is about four feet long, red along the central lumen, with the two tan balloons: one at the end and, and another along the lumen. The tube is usually inserted nasally and advanced into the stomach. Before any balloons get inflated, a KUB film needs to be shot to make sure of the tube's position.

The balloons are inflated to a pressure between 20 and 45mm of mercury – the physicians do the inflating, and the pressure is checked with a pocket manometer.

69- Who puts in the blakemore tube?

SF: Definitely not me!

I've only seen these inserted by GI.

70- What are the different lumens and balloons for?

The lower balloon is inflated and then pulled upwards to compress bleeding vessels in the upper stomach. The upper balloon inflates against the walls of the esophagus to compress bleeding varices there. There are a lot of lumens, but they make sense pretty quickly – there are two to inflate the balloons, and one to empty the stomach like an NG tube. I think there's another to drain the area between the balloons of any blood or gastric liquid that gets trapped there.

The strange-looking part is that the whole apparatus is put to traction, pulling away from the patient's face, which puts upward compression pressure on the gastric balloon. I've heard that some hospitals put the patient's head in a football helmet, and then attach the tube to the face guard after traction is applied – what we do is to actually use a traction bar apparatus attached to the bottom of the bed. A cord is attached to the end of the tube and run over a pulley on the bar to a weight – the GI physicians choose the weight, but I think it's never more than 5 pounds.

71- How long does a blakemore tube stay in?

SF: Pressure up for 24h?, or can cause erosion, perf, etc.

I think that I've never seen one left in place for more than two days – usually they stay in place for less than 24 hours.

72- Should patients with varices have NG tubes put in? Taken out?

SF: Out, especially if the patient has esophageal varices.

This is one of those situations that I let the docs worry about. I think that patients with bleeding varices are always at risk of vomiting, so I think that it only helps to have something in place to help keep their stomachs empty. At the same time, an NG tube won't evacuate large clots, and placing one may start more bleeding, or pop off some bands. A day or so after compression or sclerotherapy it may be safe to insert or remove an NG tube, but the GI docs make that call.

73- How often should I monitor my patient's blood counts?

SF: Q 2-4 hours.

In any situation involving significant bleeding, it's wise to monitor a CBC pretty often – either every couple of hours, or after every round of transfusions, or whenever you think you need to see one. If your patient is starting to have blood pressure or heart rate changes, send counts right away.

74- What is a TIPS procedure, and why is it included in the section about upper GI bleeds?

Becky: "Basically this procedure is a liver angioplasty with stent placement."

TIPS stands for Transjugular Intrahepatic Portosystemic Shunt. The process involves threading a "harpoon" tipped catheter down the jugular vein into the liver, where the tip is used to punch a tunnel from the hepatic vein into the hepatic artery. This lets a lot of the blood bypass the liver instead of going through it for filtration – and lowers the pressures in the portal venous system. A coil-spring stent is placed to keep the shunt lumen open.

75- What is portal hypertension?

The liver is normally a soft organ, and blood perfuses through it at low pressure. If the liver is stiffened up by cirrhosis, the blood doesn't flow through the liver tissue as easily. The pressure in the portal venous system backs up into the esophageal veins, making them bulge out, as varices. (One is called a "varix".) You've seen people with variceal veins in their legs? Same idea. Now imagine that these bulging veins are sitting there in the esophagus, and suddenly along comes a poorly-chewed piece of hard candy. Poof – a bleed. Or a bleed can happen just from the pressure in the bulging vessel.

76- What is a porto-caval shunt?

This is the same idea as a TIPS procedure, except that the shunt is created surgically – a connection is made directly between the hepatic vein and hepatic artery, lowering the pressure in the portal system. The idea is that the bulging varices then decompress, and shrink back into the walls of the esophagus, lowering the risk of re-bleeding.

77- Why do these patients become more encephalopathic?

Remember the blood that was supposed to be going through the liver, but which is now bypassing it through the shunt and going back into circulation? Didn't get detoxified, did it? Now the ammonia that normally gets removed by the liver starts to rise, and it produces the hepatic encephalopathy we all know and love so well. Time for lactulose.

78- What is a normal ammonia level?

Becky: It's important to remember that blood lying in the gut will raise this.

Where I work the number is less than 30, I think – I'll check on this. Above 100 usually means an unresponsive patient. Above 150 usually means an intubated patient. Lactulose works, but it's effectiveness depends on how rapidly the patient is making the ammonia in the first place… and Becky makes a useful point. Ammonia is a nitrogenous waste of protein digestion – and, so, what's blood? Right! So a gut full of blood can mean a big spike in serum ammonia…

79- Should I give lactulose to a patient with a GI bleed?

Becky: It brings down the ammonia released by digestion of blood lying in the gut.

I don't think so – the bleeding needs to be controlled first. Although they do give LGIB patients an oral golytely prep for colonoscopy…

80- Should I give tube feedings to a patient with a GI bleed?

Becky: "Some say yes – a slow trickle to coat the stomach and prevent bacterial translocation."

I'm not sure I would – I would ask GI what they wanted to do.

81- Can upper GI bleeds be prevented?

SF: Sometimes?

Becky: "Depends on what's bleeding and why. Mallory-Weiss tears? Varices? Ulcers? Maybe if detected early enough. Stress ulcers – we start prevention ASAP, like on admission."

Probably much of the time, although we'd have to stop people drinking alcohol. (Varices do happen for other reasons though…) Upper GI bleeding can come from Mallory-Weiss tears (tears at the g-e junction), and although I haven't seen too many of these, I don't think that the bleeding is anything like that of a variceal situation. The CNS who sits next to me points out that taking a lot of any of the NSAIDS (ibuprofen, etc.) can produce gastric bleeding, and that lower GI bleeding usually comes from intestinal polyps or tumors. (I'm getting close to 50. Do I get to look forward to the scope every year? If I get through enough of them, do I get frequent-flyer miles? Do they serve Versed in-flight?)

82- What is helicobacter all about?

Now see? - here I thought I understood something. But no – apparently the winds of wisdom are changing again… for a long time, no one ever thought that gastric hyperacidity and ulcers could be caused by an infection, because germs weren't supposed to be able to live in the gastric stomach acid. Then along came a bright doc down in Australia who did some cultures, and sure enough there they were: helicobacter pylori. I understand that the study results were very clear – infecting people's stomachs with h. pylori gave them ulcers when they hadn't had them before, and getting rid of the h. pylori with antibiotics got rid of the ulcers.

So for some years, it became this really neat revolutionary idea to treat chronic gastric ulcerative disease with anti-pylori antibiotics when the germs were cultured out. Now my turn with GERD has come along, and here I am, taking my prilosec, and now I'm getting tested for h. pylori, and it's negative. Twice! Great. This totally cool revolutionary discovery doesn't do anything for me at all – now I get to have an upper endoscopy. They better sedate the heck out of me.

83- How can h. pylori infections be diagnosed?

Originally, I understand that they used to use direct culture during upper endoscopy. Nowadays a blood test can tell if you've developed antibodies to h.pylori, meaning presumably that you've got the infection.

84- What antibiotics are used to treat helicobacter infections?

One source that we checked mentioned Flagyl, tetracycline, Biaxin, or Amoxicillin, along with H2 blockers and proton pump inhibitors. ("But Captain, that's only been done in theory!") Bismuth – probably in the form of Pepto-Bismol or the like, comes into it as well.

85- What about carafate?

Becky: We use 1 gram slurry q 6 hours.

Drugs go in and out of fashion. A couple of years back, we were crushing or dissolving these guys every day, sometimes four times a day, on what seemed like almost all of our patients. These days I hardly see it any more. Anybody know why not?

86- What about cimetidine, ranitidine, famotidine, James Dean?

Becky:" The first two can cause thrombocytopenia, which is why we've switched to famotidine – pharmacy tells us that it doesn't cause it (as much?) James Dean has been known to cause tachycardia in a susceptible population."

Cimetidine is really out of fashion now, ever since we noticed lots of patients dropping platelet counts when getting it. I think it's also a monster in the Ranitidine is still around, and my wife's hospital uses famotidine, but we don't.

As for James Dean – since my daughters became teenagers, just thinking about guys like James Dean gives me stomach pains. I mean, that hair! All that bear grease…

87- What about Prilosec? If a person is taking Prilosec and has bad breath, do I have to sit Nexium?

The proton-pump inhibitor group of meds is apparently the current version of the greatest thing since sliced bread. They work really well, don't screw up the body as a result, and seem to be safe to take for long periods of time. Nexium is apparently the even cooler cousin of prilosec – I've seen it used, but I have no idea if it's more effective than the original.
It can be difficult to get prilosec down an NG tube. The instructions say that you can't crush up the tiny pill-things inside the capsule, but I understand that it's okay to dissolve them in some bicarb solution, such as the stuff inside an injectable bicarb syringe.

88- What about liquid antacids?

Now I'm really starting to feel old. I remember giving 60cc of liquid antacid through an NG tube every four hours – when I think about it, this was nearly 20 years ago. Holy cow – where has the time gone? These days in the MICU we hardly use these any more, except for Amphogel, which we use to lower serum phosphate in renal-failure patients. Sometimes it's comes in handy – a patient with substernal chest pain may feel better after 30cc of Mylanta – tells you something. (Although you'd better do the EKG too.)

Lower GI Bleeds

89- How are lower GI bleeds treated?

Becky:" Order a bleeding scan (grin!). Vasopressin, angioembolization, surgical resection."

Some of them stop on their own. Frustrating when they do the whole deal, and the report says "no source of bleeding identified".

90- Do they use endoscopy for this too?

Becky: "Yes, and you have to prep them with go-lytely (ordered by the gallon).

Yes. I understand that the same cautery maneuvers can be made during colonoscopy. Also, I think that the scope has a "snare" that can be used to take out polyps, which sometimes are the bleeding source.

91- How are GI bleeds treated in the angiography suite?

Becky: "Embolization of the offending vessel. There's a critical-care-trained nurse there (most of the time...)".

This is interesting: instead of cauterizing the bleeding vessel from the outside, the angiographers use all sorts of special equipment, IV dyes, and radiology cameras to locate the source of bleeding from the blood-vessel side – they inject a plug of some solidifying material into the vessel that's leaking.

92- What are some clues to tell me that my GI-bleed patient may be heading for trouble?

SF: If he loses too much blood, he has nothing to pump!

Becky: "Tachycardia, drifting BP, thirst. How about just not looking right? Beta-blocked folks can't necessarily generate the tachycardia that they need."

I think I mentioned before that tachycardia is absolutely the giveaway in this situation – I always get a chill if I see this starting in a GIB patient.

93- Why does it matter if he's beta-blocked?

SF: If he's beta-blocked, his heart rate will be held down.

We thought about heart rates earlier. Remember the three parts of a blood pressure are pump, volume, and arterial squeeze – losing volume, the patient's heart rate will rise to try to keep blood pressure up. (What will happen to their SVR?) – remember the nurses who wouldn't let the doctor give a beta-blocker? If the patient were beta-blocked, then she wouldn't be able to raise a compensatory heart rate – big trouble, because now she has no effective compensation mechanism left – if her blood volume drops, her pressure will drop immediately.

Cancer

94- What do I need to know about patients with low blood counts from chemotherapy?

This is really specialist stuff – not my area at all. Generally the oncology people are closely involved, and they can be very good at predicting the effects of one kind of chemo or another on the bone marrow – and on the production of blood cells of one kind or another.

95- What is a nadir?

This is the "low point" that the patient's counts will reach after a round of chemotherapy treatment.

96- How long does a nadir last?

This apparently varies – I guess with the type and severity of the disease process, the type and duration of the chemo – as I say, I have no strong knowledge base here, but it makes sense to list the questions because they do bear thinking about. We find that the nurses up on the oncology floors love to answer these.

97- What if the nadir doesn't go away?

Sounds pretty bad to me. As I understand it (everyone please correct me where I'm wrong), the reason that chemotherapy can be lethal lies in it's effect on bone marrow. So the idea in breast cancer, say, would be to give a "lethal" dose of chemo, which hopefully knocks off the tumor process along with the marrow, (but not the rest of the patient), and then giving a bone marrow transplant to rescue them.

98- What is aplastic anemia?

This is what happens when your marrow fails. All the patient's counts drop, because the factory has closed.

99- Who is Ralph Nadir?

Wasn't he the doctor that gave chemotherapy during the presidential election and made the Democrats so mad?

100- What kinds of blood products should these patients get?

Again – not really my area. But from my limited experience I can say that they may need any kind of cell transfusion: RBCs, platelets, and recently I see that they've been doing white cell transfusions. I used to hear about these long ago when I worked the floors, but not since – have they gone out, and then come back into fashion?

101- What shouldn't they get?

Apparently along with ABO and Rh typing, these patients should only get filtered, irradiated, CMV negative blood products. The idea is to get rid of white cells in the blood to be transfused, to prevent febrile reactions. Obviously white cell transfusions aren't treated this way…

102- What is epogen?

Becky: Stimulates the bone marrow to produce RBCs. All our dialysis patients get this.

Stimulates red cell production. This is one of those modern miracles of science - epogen is the brand name for a recombinant form of erythropoietin – the hormone secreted by the kidneys that stimulates the production of red cells in the marrow. It is "… produced in the Chinese hamster ovary cells…". Oh really? I'm not sure I want it now…

103- What is neupogen?

Neupogen is the same as epogen, except different. It is also a miracle – a recombinant form of human granulocyte colony stimulating factor: G-CSF. Stimulates the production of white cells.

104- Why isn't there something to stimulate platelet production ("Plate-ogen"?), the way there is for red cells and white cells?

I understand that they've tried this, but that it hasn't worked so far.

<u>**Kidneys**</u>

105- Why does it seem like chronic renal-failure patients always have low crits?

They don't make enough erythropoietin.

106- Should my renal failure patient be transfused?

Transfusion is always a judgment call. Most of our dialysis patients are put on epogen shots. If the crit drops below whatever threshold has been deemed necessary, then transfusion may need to happen – cardiac patients for example are usually kept >30% nowadays.

107- What about patients on CVVH?

CVVH is a whole world unto itself. But the point to understand is that this enormous scary machine (Jayne calls it the "octopus from hell") needs to be anticoagulated one way or another or it will clot up. Heparin is used sometimes, or sometimes we use a citrate solution which actually works pretty well as long as the patient tolerates it – we've had systems stay up for 3, maybe 4 days before needing to be changed, which is pretty good for us. Transfusion-wise, if the system clots, the patient may lose the blood in the setup – about 150cc, and so might need a packed cell to replace it.

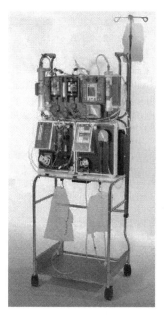

This is the interestingly named BM-25… nice machine, we used it for years.

http://www.hepanet.de/images/mars/BM25%20gr.jpg

108- Are we anticoagulating the machine, the patient, or both?

Probably both. When we use bicarb solution, the machine tends to be more, uh, thrombogenic (my son is grinning over there in the kitchen), and the systems have to be changed more often. If the patient can handle it we sometimes heparinize the system, and if the patient needs to be anticoagulated anyhow, then the whole thing can work out nicely.

109- What about hematuria? What is a Murphy drip?

Hematuria can happen for a couple of reasons – the main ones are catheter trauma and anticoagulation, or maybe a combination of both. This is not a trivial source of blood loss - we had a patient recently whose catheter got traumatized, and he had to be transfused for a couple of days until the bleeding resolved.

My main worry in this situation is clots – it's pretty obvious that if the catheter gets plugged with a clot, the bladder will get into trouble. What we call a Murphy drip is just a rapid infusion of normal saline into the bladder, flushing blood out before it forms clots in there. (Why does it seem like the Irish are making a lot of money here? And how about Kelly clamps – that guy is really selling a lot of those.)

One point about these rapid bladder flushes: we make a pretty big point of **not** putting these on pumps – you have to be <u>very</u> careful about measuring the true hourly urine. Make sure that more is coming out than went in – and you <u>don't</u> want to be using a pump to force fluid into a distended bladder! Here's our article of Foleys for Beginners:

www.icufaqs.org/FoleyCatheters.doc

<u>Coagulation and Anticoagulation</u>

Anticoagulation

110- What kinds of situations do we use heparin for in the MICU?

> Becky: Prophylaxis for DVT, patients with DVT, unstable angina awaiting cath lab, pts with MIs, PEs, IABP, new onset a-fib. We use a weight-based heparin protocol which tells us the bolus dose, pre-treatment labs, PTT timing, dose adjustments, and when to call the MD. It's pretty goof proof.

We use heparin a lot, for various situations: for example anyone suspected of ruling in for an MI goes on heparin. Most patients with PE's go on heparin. Anyone on a balloon pump, anyone with DVTs or other clot formations probably will go on heparin. Heparin is a <u>very</u> <u>powerful drug</u> – be very careful with it.

111- What are DVTs?

> SF: Clots!

> Becky: Deep vein thrombosis – blood clots in the big veins in the legs. The prime starting point for pulmonary emboli.

"Deep Vein Thromboses" – these are the clots that form in the leg veins of immobile patients. (Remember the "Hazards of Immobility"?) Some really high percentage of hospitalized patients will get DVTs if they're not prevented. Some numbers I've seen: 25% risk overall for patients after general surgery, roughly the same for MI and (elective) neurosurgery, 47% after stroke, 48% after hip fracture, and 51% after elective hip replacement.

112- What are "LENIs"?

"Lower Extremity Non-invasive studies" – sonograms that look for DVTs in the legs. You <u>definitely</u> want to know if your patient's LENIs were positive or negative.

113- What are "filters" all about?

Becky: IVC umbrella, Greenfield filters. Looks like a tropical drink umbrella on x-ray.

Venous clots can break loose and float downstream, towards the larger veins. If they keep moving, where do they wind up? (After the heart, I mean.) Patients can go to Interventional Radiology and have a filter placed in the inferior vena cava to block clots from traveling to the heart.

114- What are the air boots all about?

Becky: "Leg squeezers" cyclically inflate and promote venous return from the lower legs.

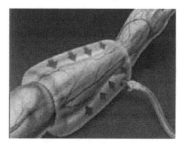

http://www.genasiabiotech.com/products/venodyne.jpg

It turns out that the air compression boots work really well for the prevention of DVTs. They look goofy, and they can be a pain to take on and off, but they really do the job. Do you want to apply air compression boots to a patient with a clot in his leg? Or an a-line in his foot?

115- Should the patient be getting air boots or heparin SQ to prevent DVTs? Does one work better than the other?

Becky: No, I don't really think it matters. The best thing is to be up and moving.

Apparently one is as effective as the other – they're used interchangeably. Some attendings like both.

116- What is so dangerous about a-fib? What about paroxsymal a-fib?

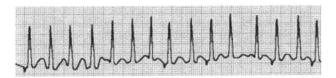

I clearly remember that back in the early 80's there were all sorts of arguments about whether a-fib patients should be anticoagulated or not. Apparently the anticoagulation group won out. It isn't the a-fib so much that's the danger – it's the possibility of suddenly popping back into, or in and out of sinus rhythm. Fibrillating atria tend to generate clots inside, which get shot very nicely out into the circulation if the rhythm changes to sinus, and the atria suddenly contract properly for the first time in a while.

117- What about PE's?

This is a big problem – this is what I was getting at when I asked: "where do venous clots go after they get to the heart?". PE's are a pretty common result of bedrest/immobility – they require anticoagulation for a certain period, initially with heparin, or maybe with a low-molecular-weight substitute for roughly 5 days, followed (normally) by oral coumadin treatment.

Hugeous PE's are sometimes treated with emergent lysis, but this is VERY hazardous, and needs very careful consideration, based on all sorts of criteria including: has the patient has recent surgery? CVA? Nosebleeds? I don't know them all, but it's a very dicey decision. Miraculous when it works though.

There's lots (lots!) more on the subject of DVTs and PEs here:

www.icufaqs.org/PulmonaryEmbolism.doc

118- What about cardiac stents?

We get our share of cardiac patients, and in recent years the technique of inserting coronary-artery stents has really gotten going, so it makes sense to think about them a bit. Stents are a nice alternative to having a full CABG procedure – the cardiologists send a catheter along the artery to the narrow spot, slide the stent into it, and click it open. Works quite well. What you don't want is to have it clot up closed afterwards! Preventing this calls for the use of anticoagulation and/or some of the newer platelet-aggregation inhibitors. (Sometimes also a balloon pump for a day or two after the stents are placed.) The cath people are very good about leaving very clear orders about what they want done – the IV stuff runs for a certain number of hours, and then the patient is started on oral meds for maintenance. Make sure you understand the plan, and if you have any questions about anything at all – ask!

119- What is the goal PTT range for patients on heparin?

The ranges have been changed around recently, and the goal range is lower now than it used to be for most of our patients: 50 to 70 seconds.

120- When should I check my patient's PTT?

Turning the drip up or down usually gets a recheck in five or six hours.

121- Are we checking PTT's frequently enough?

Interpreting PTT numbers can be tricky. If a patient had results coming back consistently too high, my feeling would be that we weren't checking often enough.

Or the problem may be spec contamination: an arterial line contaminated with heparinized saline flush, or even drawing the tubes in the wrong order can throw the results off. If you're getting weird results you may or may not want to believe them – in this situation I would let the team know, explain why I might think the result might be bogus, and try doing a peripheral stick for another stat test. Once you think your patient is in a stable relationship with his heparin, our rules call for checks q twelve hours.

122- What is an ACT?

Becky: Activated Clotting Time. We use this to guide heparinization for CVVH. One cardiologist uses this to determine when to pull cath sheaths.

Activated Clotting Time is a bedside test that can be used to assess anticoagulation on heparinized patients. I've only seen this used with patients on ECMO, where the ACT is checked every hour – maybe we should think about this for patients on heparin until we know where they are? Something to think about.

123- What does it mean if my patient is "HIT positive"?

This shows up now and again – an article I saw said it hits (ha!) about 5% of the population - but we see it often enough to remember it, and include in the (long) list of things we learn to think about over the years. "Heparin Induced Thrombocytopenia" is this nasty process wherein even <u>saying</u> the word "heparin" in your patients' room seems to make the platelet count drop. It's not common – one study I saw on the web found 9 cases out of some 350 patients studied, and another cited that figure of 5%, but as with so many things we see in the unit, "I don't know much about it, except that I definitely don't want it."

The test itself detects an antibody that your patient either has or doesn't – if they do, then even the small doses of heparin in an arterial-line flush will make their platelet counts drop drastically. If your patient turns up HIT positive and needs anticoagulation, she may need something else.

124- When do we use coumadin in the MICU?

Becky: Chronic a-fib, valve replacement, converting DVT folks from heparin.

We don't, actually. Not much, anyhow – most of our patients are pretty acute. It takes something like 3 days for a coumadin change to take effect – our patients definitely don't want to wait that long.

125- What is the goal PT range for patients on Coumadin?

Becky: Maybe this should read "therapeutic range", which is 1.5 times control.

We're mostly trying to get PT's to come down, rather than go up. It's not unusual to see liver-failure patients become "auto-anticoagulated" because they just don't make the normal clotting factors that they need – sometimes you'll see PT's of > 50. (That's, uh, pretty high.) Someone like that is in immediate danger of bleeding from everywhere: GI bleeding, spontaneous hematuria, bleeding into the head…

126- What is INR all about?

SF: International Normalized Ratio

Once again, showing my age (SF knew this one. I guess young people can be useful…grin!). INR - "International Normalized Ratio"- is another way of expressing prothrombin time – used in measuring the effect of coumadin. The normal number in an untreated patient is somewhere around 1.2 , and the usual goal for treatment is 2 to 3, and 2.5 to 3.5 for heart valve patients.

127- What are "low-molecular-weight" heparins? No PTT's?

They call these "LMW" heparins – apparently these are the latest and the greatest in the anticoagulation biz. There are several varieties (Lovenox/enoxaparin is one, Fragmin/dalteparin is another), and it turns out that they may have some real advantages over traditional heparin. (As usual, the debate rages on, but we're starting to see these drugs used fairly often in the unit, so the studies must be saying something good…)

First, they seem to give a steady-state drug delivery rate that gets rid of the need for checking PTT's. However, this varies from one drug to the other – make sure you know which is which! (I should've researched this better – any volunteers?)

Second – there seems to be less risk of HIT reactions threatening the platelet count.
The dose is weight-based, and given as a SQ injection once or twice a day.
Apparently not all the data are in yet, but LMW heparin works well for preventing and/or treating DVTs.

Sometimes the injections are combined with air-boot treatment, sometimes not. I think I'm going to ask for both... actually, I hear that there are surgical guidelines for choosing one, the other, or both, involving age, other conditions, and the procedure being done.

128- What are "platelet-aggregation inhibitors" all about?

These meds, such as Integrilin and Reopro, are used mostly in cardiac situations – you'll see patients get these after cardiac cath lab procedures like stent placement. The goal is to prevent platelets from sticking to the new stent and plugging it up. The basic concept here is different from that of anticoagulation, which interrupts the clotting cascade. Platelet aggregation inhibition seems to work really well – the patient may have to stay on an oral form of the med: Plavix is one, although apparently it works differently from the drips.

129- What if I'm too inhibited to ask about them?

I know exactly how you feel, but nursing is a profession that demands self-sacrifice, and we all have to make the effort. Stop complaining.

130- What if I have a beer first? Two beers? What were we talking about? Hey, do they have salsa here?

Quick, somebody anticoagulate this guy!

Coagulation

131- What should I know about Vitamin K?

Vitamin K is the reversing agent for the part of the clotting cascade affected by coumadin – namely, the PT-INR part. Patients with a little too much coumadin on board get 3 doses of Vitamin K SQ, qd for three days. (Update – now it turns out that it can be given po with good effect. Same dose, three days.) You'll occasionally see an order for IV Vitamin K – from what I understand this can be a truly dangerous maneuver, and I've never done it.

132- What about protamine sulfate?

Protamine is the med used to reverse the other part of the clotting cascade that we work with – the PTT part. I think I've seen it used once or twice in my whole nursing life.

133- When should I think about giving my anticoagulated patient FFP?

Patients who are in an auto-anticoagulated situation like liver failure are usually going to be the ones that you give FFP for any invasive maneuver.

134- What about lysis?

Lysis is much more of an ER procedure than something we do in the unit. We do get patients sometimes after the lysis is done – usually they arrive with heparin running as part of the treatment protocol. Just be aware that lysis drugs can really aggravate bleeding from other places – any other puncture sites, IV's, etc. There's a lot of discussion nowadays about lysing PE's and embolic strokes, but most of our patients are in no condition to stand up to lysis, which requires passing all sorts strict criteria. A quick example – you wouldn't want to give TPA for an MI if the patient had had a recent CVA. Or maybe CHF, complicated by PAF, who might be on PD, or even CVVH, or who knows maybe IABP!

(FBI, CIA, CBS, IDDM, PDQ, FUBAR…100% extra credit to any reader of this article who knows what FUBAR stands for. Hint: World War 2 word, taught to me by my stepfather, who didn't have any fun at all in the Pacific.)

135- What is DIC?

This is not a nice one. DIC is one of those complicated "syndromes" that sometimes occur when people are severely ill – often along with ARDS or sepsis. I've never read an explanation of DIC that didn't involve terrifying charts of clotting cascades, bradykinin waterfalls, interleukin mountains, and I'm sure that there's a cliff in there somewhere that I'd jump off if I had to learn all that stuff well enough to explain it.

Here's what I do know: DIC stands for Disseminated Intravascular Coagulation. If the patient's PT and PTT abruptly start to rise, and the platelet count begins to fall – rapidly – a little light goes on in my head that says "Uh oh. DIC?" Apparently these patients use up their own clotting proteins so rapidly that they don't have many left in circulation - factor deficiency then comes into the picture, and despite the zillions of mini-clots that they're making, they can start bleeding from all sorts of unpleasant places. Bladder. Nose. Rectum. Into the head. These patients may get everything and anything to help them clot: FFP, Vitamin K, cryoprecipitates, platelets, and red cells to replace the ones that they're losing in all directions. Relevant labs: along with the regular coags is fibrinogen (goes down), and d-dimer (goes up).

Treatment involves fixing the underlying condition – if and when the sepsis clears, hopefully the DIC should too. Scary.

136- An anticoagulation error, and a lesson learned…

Everyone makes errors. It's what we do. But sometimes there are errors that people learn <u>really</u> important lessons from, and it's to their credit when they do…

I was the charge nurse – they call it the "resource" nurse, nowadays, as though changing the name made the job any different… a pump goes off, alarms. I'm wandering around the unit, helping out, setting priorities, looking for hot spots… answering pumps. I go in – there's the pump, saying: "I'm done!" - it had been set to give 125cc over – probably – an hour. Antibiotic dose? I check the bag – I was going to tell the nurse that her dose was done. Holy smokes… argatroban!

Argatroban is one of the systemic anticoagulation drugs that's come into use to replace heparin, for people who can't tolerate it – HIT people and the like. It's given in very controlled doses – mikes per kg per minute… comes to something like 6cc per hour out of the bag. This person had just gotten half a bag in 30 minutes…

This is not good. As in, really, very seriously, not good. I call in the nurse. I tell her as gently as I can. She offers to go to pieces. I get out the duct tape, and we manage to hold her together.
It's interesting how some people are finally brought to realize the seriousness of what they're doing. Some of them, you think they never will – young people, busy with their agenda, looking to get married, looking for this, or that… sometimes they 'master" their profession along the way, as though it were just as series of tasks, instead of the deadly serious whole that it is.

This nurse was one of those. Busy girl. Lots to do, men to meet. Not a bad nurse at all, but… busy. I think this was the first really serious error she'd ever made – she'd been a nurse for – mm, a year or two?

She took it very hard, which was a reassuring thing. I mean – if she hadn't, what would that have said about her? It was definitely a professional growth experience for her, I'd say. She cried, and wanted to run out the door screaming… with some help, she held it together, and we worked the problem through with the team. We got her through the night. The patient, too – it turns out there's no specific antidote for an argatroban overdose – all you can do is to give ffp, vitamin k, and hope for the best. It turned out all right. Very scary.

The next time I saw her, she said, "Oh – I'm so paranoid now! I check everything six times, I check the names, I worry so much about EVERYTHING!"…

I looked at her, and I said, as gently as I could: "Susie… how did you think it was <u>supposed</u> to be?"

Two Interesting Situations:

1-   A patient with pulmonary hypertension.

1-1: Nice pair of lungs.
1-2: How about this one?
1-3: A PA line.
1-4: These lungs are <u>very</u> stiff.
1-5: Blood is having a hard time getting through these stiff lungs.
1-6: A really impressive diagram of the closed foramen ovale.
1-7: A diagram of a patent foramen ovale.
1-8: Floating a swan.
1-9: Wedging the swan.
1-10: Doing an inhaled nitric oxide trial.
1-11: Pulmonary Vascular Resistance.
1-12: A whole lot of numbers with a yow!
1-13: The situation in a nutshell. Nice arrows.
1-14: What are the numbers telling us?

- Baseline numbers.
- Numbers after 15 minutes on 100% O2.
- Back to baseline.
- After 15 minutes on 20ppm inhaled nitric oxide.
- Back to baseline.

2:   A patient with a right-ventricular MI.

2-1: A pretty cool 12-lead EKG.
2-2: What happens during an RV MI?
2-3: A whole lot more numbers. Different yow.
2-4: Following the stroke volume.
2-5: Two hours later.
2-6: Two hours after that.
2-7: Two more, plus the Starling curve, and setting goals for central pressures.
2-8: SVR comes down, and the pH does what?

Some nice hemodynamic numbers: These aren't really discussions for beginners, although I hope that I've been clear enough for anyone – I usually try new articles out on my kids ("Not again!"), and if they seem to get it, I think I'm doing the right stuff. It may take a while getting used to PA lines and "shooting numbers" before all this stuff makes sense.

A couple of scenarios that came up over the past week or so showed a really nice use of the PA line numbers that we "shoot": one was a pulmonary hypertension lady who was getting a nitric oxide trial, and the other was a gentleman who was unfortunately having a big RV MI.

1- A patient with pulmonary hypertension.

Let's take the pulmonary hypertension one first. This was a woman who came in short of breath – a street person who had any number of social and life difficulties, but who now showed up with dyspnea, which worried her enough to bring her into the ED. Turns out that as an alcoholic, her portal hypertension had backed up pressures into her lungs, creating pulmonary hypertension – anybody else ever heard of this? Not us – who knew? We wondered if a TIPS would help the woman…anyhow, she came into the MICU as part of a protocol workup to see if inhaled nitric oxide would help bring her pulmonary pressures down. She came to the MICU where the team placed a PA line.

The purpose of the exercise: I guess the data show that if a patient like this is given inhaled nitric oxide under controlled conditions, you can tell whether or not they'll respond to oral calcium channel blockers to help the PH or not – but you have to do the measurements first.

1-1: Nice pair of lungs:

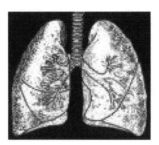

Look familiar? So here's the idea: lungs are like lots of other organs in the body – normally they're nice and soft, rather than stiff. The liver is like that: normally soft, but expose it to enough alcohol and it becomes stiff – cirrhotic. Lungs that are soft are said to be "compliant" – stiff lungs are: big surprise, "noncompliant". A patient with stiff lungs will be obviously hard to "bag" with the ambu…you'll see new nurses looking at the bag in surprise, trying to figure out what's wrong with it.

1-2: How about this one?

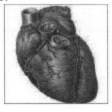

www.netdoctor.co.uk/focus/ heart/index.html

Who said "Liver!"?

So - there's the problem: stiff lungs. Any idea how to measure just exactly how stiff they are?

1-3: A PA line.

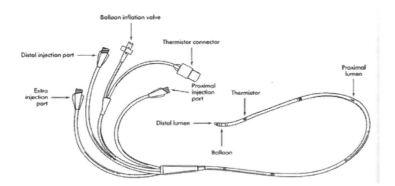

Yes – a PA line, because why? Because when the balloon is down, remember, the transducer "sees" what? The pressures all around it in the lung, very good. Also known as "ambient" pressures. As opposed to what it sees when the balloon is up – when it can only see what's ahead of it, over there into the left side of the heart, right through the pulmonary capillaries and all. How it does that I have no remote clue.

Anyhow. If you put a PA line in me, hopefully you'd see normal lung pressure numbers – that's what the PA numbers are, remember? They reflect the ambient pressures in the lung. Normal would be something like 30ish over 12ish, right? Something like that. This lady had pressures of about 105/60. In her <u>lungs</u>. Which means a couple of things:

1-4: These lungs are <u>very</u> stiff.

1-5: Blood is going to have a hard time getting through these stiff lungs – the pulmonary arterial system is tight, right? So the pressures are high. So is the resistance to flow. Now let's look at an incredibly sophisticated cardiological-type diagram:

1-6: Closed Foramen Ovale

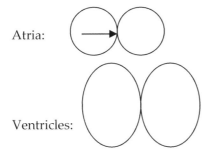

Wow – is that just some kind of really cool diagram or what? Now, anybody remember what it is that babies have that goes between the atria, where the arrow is pointing? Remember that stuff? The foramen ovale? (Not the same as the foramen O'Malley, which is where the beer goes…ow! Editing doesn't mean you have to <u>hit</u>, y' know!) Otherwise known as an atrial septal defect – an opening between the atria. Fetal blood flow.

It turns out that lots of people walk around with these, it's just that they stay closed most of the time. They have a "not-patent" foramen ovale.

Let's ponder this a second. What pumps blood to the lungs? The right side of the heart, very good. What if the lungs stiffen up over time? Well – you're going to get hypertrophy on the right side of the heart, that's for sure, because it's going to grow, just like any muscle will, if stressed.

Now – pumping against those stiff lungs, the pressure on the right side is going to go up. And up. Eventually the pressure becomes high enough on the right side that if you still have a foramen ovale that's just sitting there being closed – well, it's not going to stay closed if the RA pressure gets high enough. See that?

So. Now the pressure in the lungs is so high that the blood doesn't want to go through them any more, not if it can find an easier route. And there it is: it's going to go through that little opening, from the right side of the heart to the left, taking the easy way, instead of going through those stiff lungs.

But – does that blood pick up oxygen? No, it does not! Does it drop off carbon dioxide to get exhaled? No, it does not! What it does do is stay de-oxygenated, and just goes right back around into the arterial circulation. It gets shunted over there, from the right side to the left side, through the foramen, which has been forced open by the pressure. Patent foramen ovale.

1-7: The patent foramen ovale.

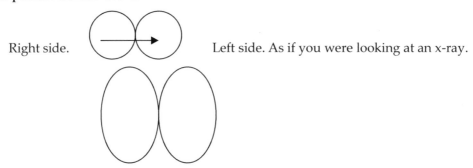

Right side.   Left side. As if you were looking at an x-ray.

Ha! Now you know what a right-to-left shunt is! Didn't see that one coming, did ya!? And you thought that was a big mystery…

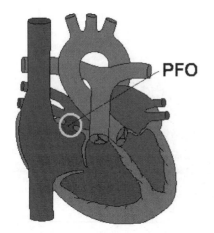

PFO

Here's a nice image – see the opening?

For the anatomists in the audience – this is a veterinary image – it's a canine heart… good diagram though.

Remember that if you're reading this article online, you can always grab a corner of the image and drag it, making it bigger, for a better look.

http://www.vmth.ucdavis.edu/Cardio/cases/case7/balloon.htm

Okay so far? So this person is going to be short of breath, probably even at rest, because some significant part of their blood isn't going through the lungs – instead, it's being shunted across the atria. That's the "shunt fraction" – I would imagine that you'd want it to be something like zero, normally.

1-8: Floating a swan.

So – what to do? Well – let's float in our swan:

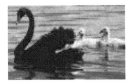

1-9: Wedging the swan.

Okay – now let's wedge the swan:

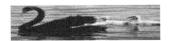

Right. Anyhow – okay, here comes the swan. Sure enough, PA pressures are really high: almost as high as the patient's systolic pressures. Scary.

1-10: Doing an inhaled nitric oxide trial.

Now the nitric trial, which involves shooting a lot of numbers:

1- a set of numbers at baseline:
2- a set of numbers after 15 minutes at 100% mask oxygen
3- another set after 15 minutes back on room air
4- a set after 15 minutes on 20ppm of inhaled nitric oxide
5- another set back at baseline.

Let's see if I can do a table without the kids:

1-11: Pulmonary Vascular Resistance

Just to be clear – everybody knows what these numbers are, right? Cardiac output, SVR, and so forth? **PVR** turns out to be "Pulmonary Vascular Resistance" – everybody remembers that Systemic Vascular Resistance is the number telling you how tight the arterial "bed" is – the arterial system as a whole. High is tight, low is loose, and the SVR is the "afterload" for the left ventricle – it's what the ventricle has to push against to perfuse the body. Right?

1-12: A whole lot of numbers, with a yow!

So the right ventricle has an afterload too. Be smart now – if the arterial system is the afterload for the LV, what's the afterload for the RV? Well, what are we talking about here? Lungs! Very good – yes, the RV pumps against the resistance created by the lungs. Tight pulmonary vasculature – you get a high PVR. See that? So if I tell you that normal is about 100, and you take a look over on the right there in the first row, what do you see? Yow! Eight and a half times normal. Pretty tight lungs there, man!

PA pressures	CO	SVR	CVP	PCW	PVR
- baseline	102/ 62	2.3	2400	26	13	855 (yow!)
- 100% O2	95/ 44	2.7	2050	22	16	745
- back to baseline	100/ 58	2.2	2480	26	12	875
- 20ppm NO	88/47	3.2	1900	16	18	655
- back to baseline	104/60	2.2	2450	25	14	845

1-13: The situation in a nutshell. Nice arrows.

Here's the situation in a nutshell:

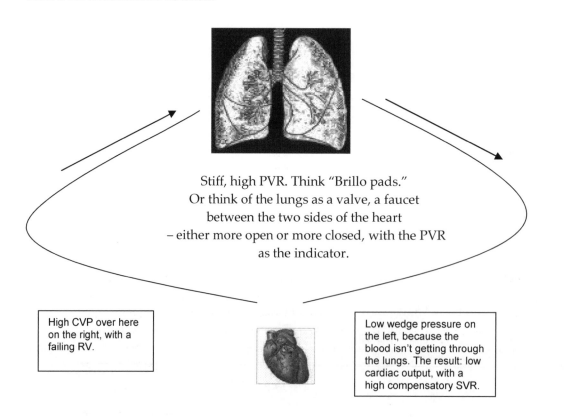

Stiff, high PVR. Think "Brillo pads."
Or think of the lungs as a valve, a faucet
between the two sides of the heart
– either more open or more closed, with the PVR
as the indicator.

High CVP over here on the right, with a failing RV.

Low wedge pressure on the left, because the blood isn't getting through the lungs. The result: low cardiac output, with a high compensatory SVR.

1-14: What are the numbers telling us?

So what we're trying to do is see if we can open the valve with inhaled nitric. The numbers tell the tale.

Baseline numbers:

Let's flip pages back and forth now a little, going back to the chart. Everybody see that first row, the baseline row? How's the cardiac output? Kind of stinky. The SVR is really high – how come? Because it's the same kind of thing as cardiogenic shock – if the output is stinky, then the only thing the body knows how to do is to squeeze the arterial bed to keep up the systemic blood pressure. See that? How about the CVP? Really high, ain't it? Why? It's 'cause that right side of the heart can't empty itself very well against those tight lungs, against that high PVR. Can't empty itself. Stays too full. CVP goes up.

How about the wedge pressure? Sort of low? Precisely the opposite volume problem, except on the other side of the heart: instead of too much, as on the right side, the blood is just not getting through to the left side, because it's being held back by the stiff, high-PVR lungs. Low wedge.

Numbers on 100% O2:

A little better! It's all about the PVR – see that? The PVR came down, so the resistance was less. CVP came down – less resistance for the RV to empty against, right? PCW came up – better flow through the lungs. Cardiac output – a little better.

Back to baseline:

Rats. Well, what did we expect? But do you see how the pattern works out? See how cool these numbers are?

After 15 minutes on 20 ppm of inhaled nitric:

Whoa! Looks better to me! CVP is down, wedge is up, output is up, SVR is better because the LV has a better supply and the CO is up. The PVR is much better. Bet she felt better too, and I bet you could feel her peripheral pulses now for the first time. (Why?)

Back to baseline:

Rats. But it was a useful test.

Unfortunately for the patient, it wasn't useful enough. I guess the data shows that the patient has to have something like a 20% improvement in the PA mean for the study to indicate that the patient can then go out and take calcium channel blockers on the outside and have them do any good. As a street person, the patient was not a candidate for flolan.

2- A patient with a right-ventricular MI.

The second patient with cool hemodynamic things going on was an unfortunate lady who was having an RV MI. By definition this means an extension of an inferior infarct (in Boston we say: "She took an infahction!") – Jayne says that something like 30% of people with IMIs infarct enough inferior territory (RCA infarct – leads II, III and AVF) to produce an RV MI.

2-1: A pretty cool 12-lead EKG.

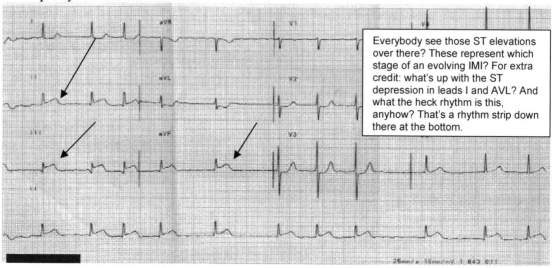

Everybody see those ST elevations over there? These represent which stage of an evolving IMI? For extra credit: what's up with the ST depression in leads I and AVL? And what the heck rhythm is this, anyhow? That's a rhythm strip down there at the bottom.

http://www.netmedicine.com/img_ekg/ekg12.jpg

2-2: What happens during an RV MI?

So in an RV MI – what happens? You need to think about what each side of the heart is doing, and what happens if it stops doing it.

Most of the time when we think of a patient taking an infahction we think of them having chest pain, maybe having trouble breathing – things like that. That's certainly true of almost all anginal episodes, or chest pain associated with an MI. But there are specific differences that start to make sense when you think of what each side is trying to do.

Left side of the heart: anterior and lateral territory, LAD and circumflex, respectively. The left atrium and ventricle drain the volume arriving from where? The lungs – okay. Suppose the LV takes a hit – and isn't pumping so well. Now it can't empty itself properly, and what happens to the wedge pressure? Goes up. What happens to the lungs if the LV doesn't empty? The pressure backs up into the lungs from that over-full LV, and water begins to leak across the capillaries around the alveoli: CHF.

So – left side ischemia or injury: CHF. Also hypotension maybe, from cardiogenic shock if the hit is big enough.

How about the right side – inferior territory, RCA? These folks have just as much chest pain as anybody else, but they probably aren't going to get into CHF problems. Instead, they develop bradycardias, maybe nausea and vomiting (apparently the innervation between the inferior part of the heart is shared with the stomach). If they take a big enough hit, a significant part of the RV is going to stop working and just sort of lie there, not moving much. "Inferior hypokinesis", which I believe translates as "just lying there, not moving much."

The hypokinesis is the problem – remember that each side of the heart has a preload, a source of incoming volume. Where does the LV get it's preload, its volume from? The lungs – right, we just said that. But what if the RV isn't pumping blood into those lungs? Will there be enough blood going through the lungs to get over there to the left side? No, there will not.

This can be a little hard to grasp, but important – bad push from the right side into the lungs, means poor blood flow coming from the lungs into the left side of the heart. Poor left sided preload. Low wedge pressure. Starting to sound familiar? Kind of like in pulmonary hypertension, sorta kinda? Not for the same reason, but producing a similar effect – low wedge, low blood pressure.

What to do? All other things being equal, it should be safe to give this person volume, right? They shouldn't go into ischemic CHF, or get easily pushed into CHF if the left side is working okay, right? These people get the opposite treatment of left-side disease people, who get diuresed all the time for failure – these RV folks get hydrated like mad. NS at 500cc/hour.

2-3: A whole lot more numbers; different yow.

So that's what we did: and interesting things happened. First of all, a look at the numbers:

	PA pressures	CO	SVR	CVP	PCW	SV
Start of the shift:	24/10	1.9	2800	10	7	18 (yow!)
Two hours later:	30/12	2.1	2550	12	9	21
Two more:	34/12	2.2	2400	13	9	23
Two more, even:	35/12	3.1	1700	17	14	42

2-4: Following the stroke volume.

This time instead of looking at the PVR at the end there, we're going to follow the stroke volume. SV remember, is how much blood gets pumped out of the LV with every beat: you get the number by dividing the CO in total cc's per minute, by the heart rate. Quick example: patient has a CO of 8 liters, which is 8000cc/minute. Heart rate is 100 bpm. So the stroke volume is 80cc. See that?

So let's look at the first set of numbers and try to interpret them. What's low, what's high? Cardiac output is awful low – should be 4-6 liters/ minute. SVR is real high – sound like anything? Sound like cardiogenic shock? Good try, especially since the patient's having an MI. But wait a sec – those central pressures are really kind of low, and what's with that stroke volume? Normal is something like 80-100cc/ beat. 18 sounds kind of low, like maybe super low. Yow!

Very good. This patient is dry. Or thinks he's dry – I mean, he may be up a couple of liters, but he's not filling his LV very well. Wait – RV MI, right? Aha – see? Time for dobutamine to get his output up? Nope – fluid. Why is his SVR so high?

2-5: Two hours later.

So we start NS at 500cc/hour after a liter bolus to get him going. Next set of numbers, a couple of hours later. A little better. CVP is coming up a little, wedge up a little, SV up a tiny bit, output too, and the SVR is coming down a little.

2-6: Two hours after that.

Two hours more: seems to be working. But slowly! Man, this patient is soaking up the volume! She was, too. By the end of the night shift she was up 4.5 liters since midnight, and she'd been up another 8 liters then! Hoo-wah!

2-7: Two more, plus the Starling curve, and setting goals for central pressures.

Two more: Now we're getting someplace. Took long enough! Something seems to have optimized here – suddenly things look a whole lot better: output and filling pressures are up, SV is up, SVR is really coming down. Probably that Starling curve thing, which is where you take a bunch of these little black birds, arrange them in a circle, and then do this sort of really cool nature dance with the kindergarten kids…(What? What do you mean "No, stupid!"? I've always done the dance with…what?)

Yeah, yeah. So: Starling says that at some point in filling up a ventricle, suddenly you hit a sweet spot and everything looks better. Not too full, or things get crappy again – so the thing to do is to make note of where you're at: "Hey Chuck, he seems to really like a CVP of about 14!" So that becomes your goal: "Titrate IV fluids to maintain a CVP of 14."

2-8: The SVR comes down, and the pH does what?

A last point: see how her SVR came down? As we filled her up, she opened up, loosened up. If the patient started the night with a pH of say 7.26 and a PCO2 of 40, what do you think might've happened to her pH as her SVR came down, and how come?

So - I'll tell you why: lactate. With a really high SVR like that, the distal perfusion can get really poor – you may not be able to feel the person's peripheral pulses as they clamp down so tightly. Since the perfusion to the periphery is bad, they do what any other shock-state patient does: their peripheral tissues switch from aerobic to anaerobic respiration, and instead of producing CO_2, they produce lactate. Metabolic acidosis. Loosen up that SVR, perfusion improves, everything switches back to the aerobic thing, the lactate gets washed out, the pH gets better.

Now: wasn't that just so cool?

Vents and ABGs

1- What are ventilators all about?

"All right. He's on pressure control at 25, on 100%, with a rate of 30, and 10 of PEEP, and look, his last gas was 65 – 72 - 7.15; I think you're in for a busy night. I've suctioned him twice with saline – he has no secretions at all, I guess that goes with the ARDS, but I don't see how he can go through all this without getting a pneumonia at some point…"

(Note to people who know about ABGs already: apparently I learned to write gases down backwards – unlike the rest of the known universe, we write pO2 – pCO2 – pH. Hey, just celebrating diversity, y'know.)

Here's a subject that could go on for ever, almost. Vents have been around for a while now – thirty years?, and they can do all sorts of things that they couldn't in years past. In the old days, vents did only two things – they'd push a given volume of air into a patient, at a given concentration of oxygen, and then let that volume come back out again. (Even that is a lot better than nothing: one of our RRTs came back from volunteering in post-earthquake Iran recently where, since they had no vent, they manually bagged a baby for 16-odd hours until he could be med-evacked out.)

Nowadays you can vary not only the size of the breath you give, but how hard that breath gets pushed in – this is called "pressure-limited" ventilation, and it's made all the difference in things like ARDS: everybody died of ARDS in the old days, and now most of them live. Ventilators can let the patient initiate her own breaths if she can, and support her more, or less, as desired, through the whole inspiration - expiration cycle. Or the vent can provide all the breaths for the patient. All these choices are tools in the kit, and have their own acronymic names: PSV, PCV, SIMV – you'll learn what these mean as you work with them, and which ones are used in different situations.

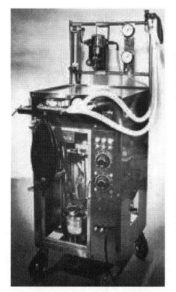

Oh my, how the time she does go by… I thought I'd find an image or two of the vents we used to use: this is a picture of an old Emerson vent, a "washing machine", which back in the Upper Cretaceous Period (middle 1980's) was all that we had. So off I go onto Google, looking around… well, look at the image link.

http://www.anesth.hama-med.ac.jp/Anedepartment/museum.asp

It's official – I'm a museum piece. They'll put me in a glass case next to one of these babies somewhere, with a little sign, something like "Nursus Criticalis, Earlious Ignoramus Extremius".

2- What is intubation?

Intubation is the placement of a clear silicone-plastic tube in a patient's trachea. "Call anesthesia and give them a heads-up – I think we're going to have to intubate Ralph's patient."

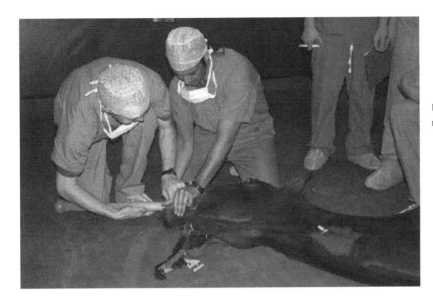

Uh, Ralph? You sure you got the right size tube, there?

http://www.ucd.ie/vetsurg/images/intubation.JPG

2-1- How is intubation done?

Intubation is done in our hospital by the anesthesia resident on call. Intubation has a whole FAQ to itself, and you can look there for lots more information.

2-2- How long can a person stay intubated?

We usually put a limit of about two to three weeks. We try to stretch the time limit a bit if we think that the patient will extubate soon, but after three weeks they usually wind up with a trach and a g-tube.

3- What is extubation?

Extubation is the removal of the tube, which ought to be a planned event: "That's the second time that Ralph's patient has made it to extubation. Except the first one was a self-extubation, right? I hope he flies this time."

3-1- How is a person extubated?

The patient's mouth and trachea are suctioned, the cuff is deflated, and the patient is briefly bagged to make sure there's a "leak" after the cuff is down. Then the tapes are removed, and the tube is taken out smoothly in one motion, on exhalation. We usually put patients on a 100%

corrugated face mask setup and then wean the oxygen, keeping saturations greater than 95-96%. Would you use that setup if your patient had severe COPD?

What if there was no leak when you deflated the cuff? Would you extubate that patient?

3-2- What are mechanics?

Mechanics are a set of numbers that tell you how ready your patient is to be extubated. We measure three things:

- Tidal volume – should be greater than ~ 500cc for a 75 kg patient.
- Vital capacity – the maximum exhaled volume after a maximal inspiratory effort – should be about 1500cc.
- Negative inspiratory force; "Ask respiratory, what's the patient's NIF?" - should be greater than - 50cm.

Acceptable numbers for all three of these means that your patient is strong enough to breathe on her own. What if "I've been suctioning her at least every hour for tons of secretions." Would you extubate her then?

3-3- How do I know if my patient can be extubated?

Basically because they'll look ready – comfortable on minimal vent settings, manageable amounts of secretions, good mechanics numbers, adequate oxygenation on near-room-air FiO2 – you'll know. One other important thing to keep in mind is the state of the trachea. A traumatic intubation, or other scenarios can provoke tracheal swelling, and once in a while it's severe enough that the ET tube is the only thing keeping the airway open.

The trick to assessing this is the presence of an air leak when the ET tube cuff is deflated. Dropping the cuff and bagging the patient should produce enough of an airflow back up through the patients' mouth that they could actually speak – this is a useful trick for communicating with intubated folks who are desperately trying to tell you something, but who can't write it out. Be sure to preoxygenate them, and suction them first, and watch for any signs of desaturation or distress when you try this.

4- What is an endotracheal tube?

This refers to the tube itself. "What size tube do you think they want? They've been putting in a lot of eights lately, because they're having to do so many bronchoscopies. "

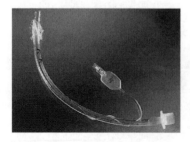

Not usually green…see the inflatable cuff at the end near the top of the picture? The thing floating on a string in the middle of the image is the "pilot balloon", which is inflated with air, and then passes that air along to the cuff.

http://www.pahsco.com.tw/imges2/10.jpg

5- What is FiO2?

"Fraction of Inspired Oxygen" – how much oxygen this patient is on. "What's his Fi02? 80%? But he's oxygenating really poorly – you think he's having a PE?"

6- What is O2 saturation?

The saturation number tells you how much of the hemoglobin in your patient's blood is saturated with oxygen, and is read by a probe that the patient wears on a finger. The probe actually looks at the pulsatile flow in the finger, and measures changes in the blood color as the saturation changes – better is brighter red. "You'd better call the team, this patient's sat is going down."

One problem comes from the fact that other things besides oxygen can saturate a hemoglobin molecule: carbon monoxide is the big one. Binds tightly, too – very hard to get off without a trip to the hyperbaric chamber. A patient with CO poisoning will have a lovely sat by finger probe, nice and high, around 100 – except that it's not oxygen his blood is carrying!

7- What is the oxygen-hemoglobin saturation curve, and why do I have to care about it?

(Uh –oh, a graph! This is getting scary… mommm!…Okay. Deep breath. Re-saturate yourself, there.

Y'okay? It's gonna be okay – really, it is!   Just stick with me here a minute.)

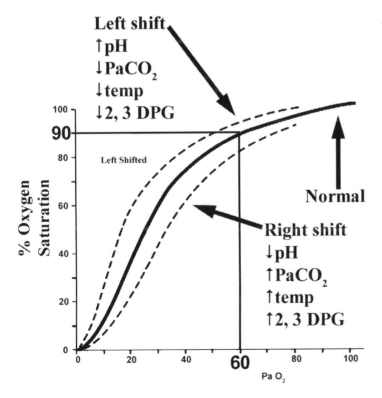

The left shift and right shift stuff has to do with the fact that changes in the patient's physiology will change the way the hemoglobin binds up the O's. Holy O's, Batman - can I remember this?

Or let's do it the smart way and figure it out from the chart. If your patient becomes, uh, **alkalotic, pH up**, and the curve moves to the left, then what happens? A sat of 90, instead of representing a pO2 of 60, represents what? Draw a line down to the pO2 scale: about 50. Oooh – a left shift is not a good thing.! **Harder** for the hemoglobin to saturate?

How about a right shift, say, for a patient with a **temp spike**?

This time the sat reads lower than it ought to – a sat of about 70 means a pO2 of 60. **Easier** to saturate? So a right shift isn't such a bad thing?

Now. See that dark curved line up there? See how it goes up rapidly, going from the left to the right? That means something very important. Here it comes: what it means is that even with a saturation that seems fairly high, like 90%, your patient's pO2 may be pretty stinky, like 60. See that? – that's what those straight lines are telling you.

That's pretty important. That steep curve means that your hemoglobin saturates quickly as you go upwards, and desaturates just as quickly on the way down. If you draw your own intersecting lines across the graph, you'll see that a sat of 80 actually means that your patient has a pO2 of something like – what? Stinky.

There are always exceptions, and stinkiness is no exception: some people walk around with a pO2 of about 50 – group, who are they? Y'all heard of the 50-50 club? Who are those people? What? Oh, sorry! I mean, "What subset of the general population admitted to the critical-care pulmonary facility comprises the sub-moiety which fits this physiologic demographic?" (Arrgh!)

8- What is tidal volume?

Tidal volume is a number that describes how much air a patient moves in and out of his lungs, both lungs together at the same time, with each breath, either in, or out, measured in cc of air. Bigger (within the normal range of roughly 300-450cc) is generally better. For example, an asthmatic may only "move" about 100 cc or less with each breath until they "break" – so if they start moving larger tidal volumes, that would represent improvement. But too big could be bad – pushing too much air into stiffened lungs could cause a barotrauma ("pressure injury"). This subject is complex , and the goals are often different in different situations– be patient, and spend lots of time observing at the bedside.

9- What is rate?

This one is easy: rate means the number of breaths delivered in a minute. Sometimes you want to control the patient, and control the rate – sometimes you want to let the patient initiate their own breaths. It depends on whether they're getting better, or worse, and what was wrong in the first place.

10- What is "minute ventilation"?

Minute ventilation is another number. Multiplying the rate, times the tidal volume, gives you the total air "moved" – that went in and out of the patient – measured in liters, in a minute. If you measured mine – say I was breathing 16 times per minute, with a tidal volume of about 400cc – my minute ventilation would be, 6400cc, or 6.4 liters. This goes up and down in different conditions – for example, an asthmatic in a flare might initially be able to keep her minute ventilation up near normal by breathing with a tidal volume of about 100cc at a rate of 60 breaths per minute, but she'd get tired pretty fast. Time for nebs, and heliox.

10-1- A very cool thing...

Just as an aside – this is so cool. Helium is lighter than air, right? Meaning that it's thinner, less dense than normal air, which is mostly nitrogen anyway, and rather thick and heavy by comparison. So, in asthma, when the bronchi are tightened up, the problem is that the thick, heavy normal air doesn't get in and out of those tight tubes very well – what to do?

Try this: mix your normal amount of oxygen, say 21%, with helium instead of nitrogen: "heliox". This thinner mix actually slips in and out of those tight tubes more easily than that nasty heavy nitrogen-type air we usually breathe, and can often help asthmatics avoid being intubated. So cool. Anybody know – do the patients talk funny on heliox? Divers do, I know, although they use heliox for different reasons.

11- What is "oxygenation"?

Oxygenation is how well oxygen is getting into the blood from the lungs, measured by P02. Clearly, if the alveoli are full of water, then the oxygen is going to have a hard time getting into the little exchange capillaries in the alveolar walls- which is why people oxygenate poorly in CHF. A normal PO2 is roughly 80-100. Suppose you had a patient who was on 100% oxygen, and they had a PO2 of about 85. An inexperienced person might look at that PO2 and say: "Well, they're oxygenating okay." – Nuh-uh!

Think about this for a second. What FiO2 are you breathing right now, at room air: 21%, right? And your P02 by blood gas is roughly 80 to 100, right? Okay, so, just by the numbers alone, the ratio of "21" to "80 to 100" is what, roughly... 1 to 4, or 1 to 5? In other words, your P02 should be roughly 4 or 5 times your Fi02, given normal lungs. So, if you intubated me, and put me on 100%, what should my P02 be? – roughly 400-500! So our friend in the paragraph above, who is on 100% oxygen, with a P02 of 85 – is he oxygenating well? No, he is not. He is oxygenating very poorly indeed. "Wow, this oxygenation is really awful."; "Yeah, I know – you think we should diurese him?"; "Probably, this is mostly CHF – he had a really wet looking chest x-ray."

12- What is "ventilation"?

<u>Ventilation</u>: how well CO2 is being removed from the blood, measured by pC02: a higher pC02 means that less C02 is being cleared – that ventilation is worse. With better ventilation, (with a higher "minute ventilation" number), the pC02 goes down. (It always helped me to think of C02 as 'exhaust gas'- it's the byproduct of aerobic respiration, like 'engine emissions' coming out of a tailpipe, it's what you want to get rid of.) The asthmatic who moves a small tidal volume will not clear pC02 very well – she will "retain" it. "Oooh, look at her pC02, it's up to 90." – "Yeah, she's retaining C02." "What should we do?" "Well, we need to ventilate her better. We probably need to turn the rate up on the vent."

Remember, <u>oxygenation and ventilation are different</u>, and mean specific things.

13- What is "PEEP"?

PEEP: this stands for Positive End-Expiratory Pressure. This means that at the end of an expiration, the vent doesn't let the lungs empty completely – instead, it uses a fixed amount of pressure, measured in cm of water (as though it were water in a column, exerting weight downwards), to hold the lungs open at the end of the breath. This does two things – it keeps the alveoli from collapsing ("atelectasis"), and it pushes the air forcibly, if gently, forwards into the lungs. This forward pressure helps oxygen diffuse into the alveolar capillaries, and raises the P02 – so if your patient is on high levels of oxygen, this can let you reduce the FiO2.

Did that make sense? You don't want to keep a patient on really high levels of oxygen – anything greater than 60% is considered "toxic FiO2", so if you can do things to reduce that level, you try to do them. (Too much oxygen for too long produces fibrotic lung damage.) PEEP is one of the maneuvers you can make – they call this "trading PEEP for FiO2" – the idea being that as you apply more PEEP, you can reduce the amount of oxygen you have to give through the vent. So PEEP is applied in increments of 2.5 cm, up to about 15 or 17.5. That's a lot of PEEP. Another way to think of PEEP is as "forward pressure" – the pressure the vent is using to push air into the patient's lungs. There are other forms of "forward pressure" that are used in different "modes" of ventilation, that we'll look at below.

13-1- What is a recruitment maneuver?

A creative application of the PEEP concept. Simple idea: you apply a really high level of PEEP in a long steady forward push – 20 seconds maybe, at a level of 30cm. (That's a whole lot of PEEP.) This hopefully blows open, or pops open all the little collapsed bunches of alveolar grapes that are closed on themselves. Often very helpful, sometimes not.

14- What is 'pressure-limited' ventilation?

We looked at this briefly up on page 2. In the olden days, at least back when I started in the units in the early 1980's, there was only one kind of ventilation – "volume ventilation" – the thought was that you wanted the machine to push a given volume of air into the patient for a tidal volume – say, 500cc. You would dial in a volume of 500cc, and turn on the vent, the old Emerson vents, and the machine would push that volume into that patient, no matter how hard it had to push to do it. So the volume was fixed, and the pressure varied with how stiff or flexible the patient's lungs were: if they had nice soft normal lungs, only a nice low pressure was needed to push the air volume in. Stiff lungs, and the machine had to push lots harder, and would! The problem was, you can only push so hard through the airways, until – blam!, a pneumothorax. We used to measure the 'PIP' – the Peak Inspiratory Pressure – the point at which the machine pushed the hardest, always measuring in cm of water pressure. 40 cm was a lot – 50 was scary, and at 60 you'd get out your chest tube insertion kit and pleurevac and set up, because you knew what was coming – you'd see ARDS patients with six chest tubes. And they almost all died.

Nowadays ARDS patients live – and one big reason is pressure-limited ventilation. Instead of the volume being fixed and the pressure varying as the lungs stiffened or loosened, now the pressure is fixed, and the volume varies. So instead of dialling in a volume of 500cc, we dial in a pressure level of "X", still measured in cm, and we watch what the tidal volume does. "Hey Chuck – how much are they moving now?" "Only about 200cc – his last PC02 was in the 80's, right? We might have to paralyze him." "Uh-oh, the team is going to hate hearing that."

There are two modes of pressure-limited ventilation that we use: Pressure Control, and Pressure Support. In pressure control – we control the rate. In pressure support, the patient controls their own rate, and we support it, with more or less forward pressure. So when you get report, the nurse will tell you that the vent settings are something like: "Pressure control, set at 18cm, rate of 22, PEEP of 10, and he's doing pretty good – he's moving about 400cc" – which means that the patient is getting pressure-limited ventilation, at a rate of 22 breaths per minute, with 18cm of forward pressure with each breath. The patient's lung compliance determines the tidal volume, - tighter lungs: smaller volume, right? In this case, he's doing pretty good – moving a normal tidal volume, and the machine is doing all the breathing for the patient. (Actually not "breathing" – right? The vent doesn't actually do gas exchange – that would be ECMO.) If the patient improved to the point where, say, you could lighten the sedation that they might've needed during their acute asthmatic episode, you could change the vent to let the patient initiate their own rate – which would mean changing from "pressure control" to "pressure support".

15- What is volume ventilation used for nowadays?

Just to keep it confusing – we do still use volume ventilation, but usually in situations where a patient only needs intubation to protect her airway – say, a drug OD. In this case there's no primary lung problem – she just isn't breathing. So we'll use a vent mode called "MV" for "mandatory ventilation". The settings might be: "35% Fi02, rate of 14, tidal volume of 500, PEEP of 5."

There is lots and lots more to this subject, and I probably have at least some of it wrong – which is why respiratory therapists go to school for years. The same principles always apply – keep your ears open, try to learn all the time, stay humble, and <u>always</u> ask if there's something you don't know.

A word about asking when you don't know: once, years ago, I changed jobs, and moved from a surgical ICU to a medical CCU in another hospital. Coming from the surgical setting, I thought I was doing pretty good when I asked a co-worker if I shouldn't probably hold my patient's diltiazem when his heart rate was a little low (no parameters had been ordered). I mean, I hadn't even held a dilt pill in my hands for years…the response was interesting. The interpretation was that I didn't know my stuff – and the leadership were very concerned at my apparent lack of critical-care-type knowledge. This was pretty much the universal attitude taken by the senior staff. The effect was predictable- new nurses would get one taste of that, and then fake it – putting on a show of never asking questions, but of appearing confident, of not needing help.

It's hard even now, after many years, for me to say how wrong I felt this was. Angry, I guess I mean. To say the least, this endangered the patients. It was professionally neglectful, and unconscionable. Don't do it. (Have you noticed that ignorance and arrogance so often go together? If you stay in the units, you'll see your share…)

16- How do I interpret my patients' ABGs?

"I think this must be a mixed acidosis, because look: his pH is 7.10, but his PC02 is only 50 – the pH goes down .08 for each 10 that the PC02 goes up, right? So that would make him 7.32, but he's a lot lower than that – I'll ask the team if they want me to send a lactate…"

This is another subject that takes a while to master. Try to remember that ABG numbers should be within certain close ranges, and that they ought to be near certain ideal fixed points:

17- What are the ideal ABG values, and why do we use them?

• P02 should be 80-100.

• PC02 should be (ideally) 40. (These are all plus/minus, but picking an ideal point helps you interpret what's going on.)

• Serum C02 (bicarb) should be 26-30.

• PH should be 7.40

Okay. Some simple concepts, very condensed, and with <u>lots</u> of lies thrown in. The body stays in acid-base balance through the operation of two systems: respiratory and metabolic. The blood chemical relative to acid-base balance that is regulated by the respiratory system is called the "pC02", or "partial pressure of carbon dioxide".

The chemical regulated by the metabolic side of things is actually bicarbonate – there are lots of others, but to keep things simple, we'll focus on bicarb alone. The problem is that bicarb is sometimes referred to as "serum CO2", because of the way the carbonic acid reaction runs. Do I remember all that chemistry stuff? No – but what <u>you</u> need to remember is that the "serum CO2" that comes back on a "chem-7", and the "bicarb" that comes back on a blood gas are essentially the same thing.

17-1- Respiratory effects on blood gases:

Changes in your patient's respiratory pattern are obviously going to affect both oxygenation and ventilation, but it's the acid-base stuff that's so confusing, so let's stick with that.

Carbon dioxide, as 'engine exhaust gas', is measured by the PC02 in a blood gas. If your patient breathes too slowly (too much morphine?), or loses the ability to exchange gas (lots of secretions in the airways?), then more CO2 is collects in the blood. Not <u>serum</u> CO2 (bicarb), but actually CO2 dissolved in the blood. Having more CO2 dissolved in the blood drives the carbonic acid reaction in the wrong direction – more acid gets made. The patient hasn't lost any bicarb – that would be a metabolic change. But now there's more acid around than there's supposed to be, so the pH goes down. Respiratory acidosis. Give some narcan. Suction out the airway.

How about the other way? What if your patient breathes too rapidly? Higher minute ventilation? Less CO2 in the blood makes the reaction go the other way: carbonic acid molecules break apart, the level of acid decreases. Has the serum level of bicarb changed? No – but there's relatively more of it now than there should be, so the pH changes – which way this time? Too much bicarb? Alkalotic? Yup – pH goes up.

17-2- Metabolic effects on blood gases:

So bicarb, the metabolic-side stuff, is measured by the level of serum C02 - not the pC02 . Confusing, right? If it helps to think of C02 as bicarb, do that. The bicarb number in the "chem-7" panel of basic electrolytes is reported as the "serum CO2" – not as bicarb. It is reported as bicarb on a blood gas. Please do not ask me why this is – I just work here.

Either way, the higher this number is, the more bicarb you have. If you have more bicarb, then you have a larger alkaline component, right? And your pH will go up or down? Which way is alkaline? – up, correct. So if for example your patient drank four bottles of Maalox, they would have a bicarb excess or deficit? Excess, correct. So their pH would go up, maybe 7.60, maybe higher. Dangerous. A metabolic alkalosis.

A patient can also develop a metabolic alkalosis by losing acid – gastric suction can do this, because he loses his gastric HCL. Or aggressive diuresis, because lasix will make your patient pee out not just the K^+ that you learned about, but also H^+, leaving him with an acid deficit. (Remember that acids are made of those H+'s, connected to other things. If you lose the H+'s, you lose acid.) This time the serum C02 - the bicarb - stays in the normal range. (This is called a "contraction alkalosis" – because when you diurese somebody, their circulating volume contracts – and they become, on balance, alkalotic from losing all that H^+ in their urine.)

The really common metabolic acidosis that we see in the unit is the lactic one that comes from one kind of shock or another. "Ralph, lactate is grey top tube on ice, right? Holy cow – his lactate was 12 last time!" In a hypotensive patient, lactate is produced by poorly perfused tissue out there in the distal areas – hypoxic, it switches from aerobic respiration to anaerobic, from producing CO2 as "exhaust gas" to producing lactic acid. Unless the perfusion improves, the lactic acid level just builds up, producing an acidosis. Metabolic. pH goes down.

18- An ABG scenario…

Okay - here's a scenario. Gentleman comes into the ER – oh, say, with a heroin overdose. Respiratory rate is 4 per minute. Is he going to clear his C02? No, he is not! Let us remember, the idealized pC02 is 40. (Forget the ranges for the moment - I mean, I know it's actually 35-45, but forget that for just now.) Okay, so, this guy's blood gas on room air is: p02 of 45, pC02 of 75, pH of 7.14. . Is that pC02 high or low? High, right. So his pH went which way? Down, right, because the extra carbon dioxide in the blood will drive the carbonic acid reaction, making more, well, carbonic acid! Making him acidotic. Has he lost or gained bicarb? No. Is his acidosis present simply for respiratory reasons? Yes. So – a pure respiratory acidosis. By the way – is his oxygenation normal? No? How come?

19- Another, related scenario...

Okay? Getting dizzy yet? No? Okay, one more. Another gentleman comes in, he's been bitten by a non-poisonous snake, but what does he know, it could've been a cobra, and he is so scared that he's breathing at a rate of 60. Blood gas shows P02 of 120, pC02 of 20, pH of 7.56. Okay – is the PC02 normal? No– high or low? – low, correct. So pH goes up or down? – this time we're driving the carbonic acid reaction the other way – actually using some up as the patient blows off pC02. Less PC02 – less carbonic acid – now, the patient hasn't gained or lost any bicarb on the metabolic side, but he has a <u>relative</u> bicarb excess – in relation that is, to the amount of carbonic acid he has, which is less than there ought to be. Result: alkalosis. Reason? Respiratory.

Give it time. After you get used to seeing the blood gases in relation to the scenarios yourself, you'll begin to say : "Hey, I remember this, I've seen this before – this is a metabolic acidosis with partial respiratory compensation in the presence of renal failure – probably a type 1 renal tubular acidosis – I mean, hey, look, he's got an old fistula here in his arm, and don't I know him from my part-time job in dialysis, and also a heroin overdose, and would you just intubate this guy already?!" No problem!

20- How should I suction my patient?

We use in-line suction catheters nearly all the time nowadays, for our vented patients. These save an incredible amount of time and trouble if you are trying to run into the room and suction your patient in a hurry. Some rules apply:

• Never forget to preoxygenate the patients. The vent has a setting that puts the patients on 100% O2 for five minutes.

• Never forget to warn the patient that you're about to cause him distress – a little reassurance goes a long way.

• Take the time needed to clear the airway of secretions as you bring the catheter out.

20-1- Should I use saline?

For reasons that I don't understand, there's a lot of argument about this. Some people say that saline instillation forces secretions downwards into the bronchi – I don't know about that, but all my experience tells me that saline is very effective in loosening thick secretions so they can be cleared by suctioning.

20-2- How high should I set the suction?

This is a matter of hospital policy. Obviously you need to use higher levels of suction if the patient has very thick secretions, occasionally as high as "line" pressure. This can also produce a tissue biopsy (grin!) – so be careful. Reset the suction to lower levels as soon as possible.

20-3- How often should I suction my patient?

The goal is to keep the airway clear, so this is a matter of assessment as well as treatment. There are clearly times when you want to avoid too much suctioning – anticoagulated patients are easily injured to the point of tracheal bleeding for example. Use your assessment skills.

21- What is non-invasive ventilation?

The idea here is that you're trying to provide some kind of vent support without actually intubating the patient. There are a couple of things that you're trying to do, which are actually pretty much the same as what you do with an intubated-ventilation setup:

- You're trying to oxygenate the patient better. Once you've gone up to 100% on a face mask there are only a couple of things you can do to try and stave off intubation, but you should be getting ready to tube the patient if they don't work:

    o You can put the patient on "high flow". This uses a regular face mask that's been attached, basically, to an oxygen typhoon – it delivers upwards of a hundred liters of oxygen per minute.

    o You can put the provide some steady forward pressure into the patient's airways to increase oxygenation. This is also known as "blowing" - but you can't say "blowing" in the MICU, on account of that ain't scientific, know what I'm sayin', yo?

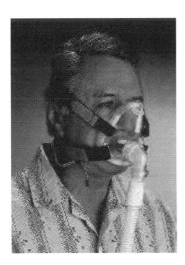

To do this, you're going to have to use a different kind of mask setup – this time the mask is going to have to seal up against the patient's skin, so that the air goes into her airways with a set pressure behind it, rather than leaking out the edges of the mask.

This is the basic idea. The broad edge of the mask is actually a sort of low-pressure balloon filled with air, which makes a nice seal against the face when you tighten up those nice velcro straps.

- You're trying to ventilate the patient better. This is where "Bi-pap" comes in.

http://www.cpap.ru/files/76_18.jpg

22- What is mask CPAP?

Once the mask makes a seal, you can apply a little constant forward pressure – like PEEP, except in this setting it's called CPAP, for "Continuous Positive Airway Pressure". 5cm of water forward pressure is the usual. This can really help in some situations – CHF comes to mind.

23- What is bi-pap?

Bipap is exactly the same as CPAP, except different. It uses two pressure settings, one each for inspiration and expiration, coming from a special ventilator.

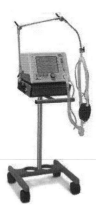

Here it is – this is called the "Vision" system. Smaller than a regular vent. Where's the silence button?

http://www.fuji-rc.co.jp/hospital/pickup/img/bipap_vision.jpg

24- What are "I-pap" and "E-pap"?

The idea is that you're providing positive airway pressure – that's the "PAP" part, but instead of using the same pressure continously, you're giving inspirations at one setting, and expirations at another. The I-pap pressure is usually the higher one – which makes sense, right?, as you're pushing air into the patient on inspiration? Positive pressure.

On expiration there's still positive pressure applied to the patient, but less. Also makes sense, since you're trying to let the air come out, correct?

25- How well does non-invasive ventilation work?

I don't like it much. If the patient has pneumonia – how are you going to help her clear her secretions? Even if they tolerate being taken off the mask, the forward pressure is pushing the secretions further on down, isn't it? What if they cough an enormous loogie up into the mask and can't breathe around it, and you're not in there? What it they vomit into the mask and can't get it off?

Another point – these jobbies don't provide much in the way of airway humidity. Regualar vents send nice moist air down into the patient's lungs – not these guys. The patients tend to develop very large, dry mucus plugs as a result, which means that you're going to have to take the mask off sometimes to do pulmonary toilet – what if they desaturate drastically every time you do that? Well – are they going to die of hypoxia, or die because you couldn't clean out their plugs? Both, seems like…I guess I'd agree that noninvasive ventilation works in a setting like CHF, where you're basically trying to send water back into the alveolar capillaries using air pressure. But not in pneumonia – you're just blowing the sputum back down, it seems to me. (Now there's an ugly mental image…!)

The Index!!!

This was a bear. Three weeks of manual entries, eyes red, everyone in the house saying, "Ok, <u>now</u> what is he doing with that book?" Then, with everyone called in to watch, we hit the indexer button, and in all of about three seconds – whoosh! Sixteen pages! And from – of all people - our skeptical son, came: "Whoa. Dad. Coooooool….."

646

I

Myoglobin, 289, 304

N

N95 masks, 364
nadir, 574, 597, 610
nadolol, 339, 355
Napoleonic Wars, 212
Narcan, 85, 93, 115, 307, 339, 349, 350, 392
Nardil, 339, 346
Nasal airway, 116
nasal cannula, 118, 256
nasal trumpet, 117, 125, 128, 129
nasogastric tube, 368, 369, 375, 383, 528, 604
negative inspiratory force, 178
negative pressure, 129, 130, 161, 173, 175, 178,
    184, 364, 374, 378, 388
Neisseria meningiditis, 364
neisseria meningitidis, 518
neostigmine, 361, 555
Neosynephine, 111
neosynephrine, 29, 105, 106, 108, 111, 345, 367
neosynephrine (phenylephrine), 459
Neosynephrine/phenylephrine, 340
nephrostomy, 32
Nepro, 381, 391
neupogen, 363, 574, 611
neurogenic bladder, 203, 213
neuroleptic malignant syndrome, 35, 345, 367
newbie, 85, 88, 98, 280, 294, 429, 432, 446, 448
nexium, 361
NG drainage, 120
NG tube, 33, 87, 101, 119, 120, 127, 130, 318, 361,
    373, 374, 378, 383, 384, 386, 392, 393, 527, 534,
    540, 599, 603, 604, 605, 608
NG tubes, 202, 369, 380, 573, 605
nicotine, 350, 356, 561
nifedipine, 339, 346, 355, 357, 366
nimbex, 17, 22, 566
Nimbex/cisatracurium, 339
nipride, 28, 34, 76, 83, 230, 231, 262, 274, 306, 340,
    347, 357, 466, 470
Nipride/nitroprusside, 340
nitrates, 30, 340, 357, 360
Nitrates, 47, 102, 104, 228, 357, 360, 498
nitric oxide, 12, 317, 621, 622, 625
nitroglycerine, 102, 104, 340, 357, 359, 361, 498,
    523
Nitroglycerine, 465, 523
Nobel Prize, 261, 328
Nodal beats, 41, 71
non-invasive ventilation, 631
nurse becomes confused, 224, 247

nurse manager, 5, 9, 402
Nurse Ruth, RN, 518
Nursus Criticalis, Earlious Ignoramus Extremius,
    632
Nutrition, 13, 381

O

O2 saturation, 12, 16, 553, 631, 635
obturator, 138, 397, 419, 485
octreotide, 137, 341, 359, 361, 466
oncotic pressure, 304, 381, 388, 584
open lung biopsies, 160
Opiate overdoses, 276
opiates, 22, 93, 274, 339, 348, 349, 350, 351, 392,
    393, 552, 561
Opiates, 289, 307, 339, 348
Opportunistic Infections, 292, 329
OR, 6, 8, 10, 20, 21, 105, 106, 130, 149, 181, 207,
    236, 249, 254, 263, 266, 303, 353, 367, 378, 382,
    393, 414, 439, 448, 562, 590, 592, 598, 602
oral airway, 28, 30, 63, 95, 98, 116, 285, 557
orogastric tube, 368, 370
osmolality, 34, 273
Osmolality, 289, 303
Osmolyte, 381
Osmosis, 272
output cable, 429, 430
Overdoses, 7, 35
oversedated, 448, 551, 553, 560
overwedged, 396, 410
oxycodone, 308, 349
Oxygen, 24, 47, 102, 104, 228, 357, 498, 635
oxygen typhoon, 643
oxygenation, 76, 117, 130, 229, 231, 257, 314, 552,
    562, 631, 634, 637, 640, 641, 643

P

P1, P2, and P3, 269
PA line placement, 137
PA lines, 11, 16, 19, 133, 136, 140, 142, 364, 395,
    397, 398, 399, 401, 404, 418, 455, 456, 457, 526,
    593, 621
pacemaker, 49, 52, 56, 58, 59, 67, 96, 194, 221, 241,
    247, 420, 421, 422, 424, 426, 427, 428, 431
pacemakers, 49, 56, 67, 98, 191, 197, 215, 221, 420,
    421, 422, 423, 426, 428, 531
pacing generators, 422
pacing wires, 347, 421, 431
paddle view, 197, 200
pain in the urethra, 202, 211
papillary muscles, 228, 497

W

X

Y

Z

Made in the USA
Monee, IL
16 May 2020